Bioactive Phytochemicals

Perspectives for Modern Medicine

— Volume 3 —

The Editor

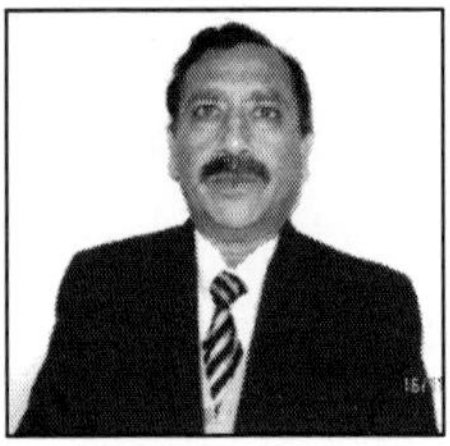

Dr. Vijay Kumar Gupta, Ph.D., FLS, London (born 1953-) Ex. Chief Scientist, CSIR- Indian Institute of Integrative Medicine, Jammu, India. He did his M.Sc. (1975) and Ph.D. (1979) in Zoology both from University of Jammu, Jammu-India. His research capabilities are substantiated by his excellent work on histopathology, ecology and reproductive biology of fishes, turtles, birds and mammals, which has already got recognition in India and abroad.

Dr. Gupta has to his credit more than 150 scientific publications and review articles which have appeared in internationally recognized Indian and foreign journals. Founder fellow, life member and office bearer of many national societies, academies and associations. He has successfully completed a number of research/consultancy projects funded by government, private and multinational agencies. His current areas of interest are histopathology, toxicology, pre-clinical safety pharmacology, reproductive efficacy studies of laboratory animals and biodiversity.

He is the Series Editor of the recently published multi-volume set of books, **"Comprehensive Bioactive Natural Products (Vols. 1-8)"**, published by M/S Studium Press, LLC, USA. He is also Editor-in-Chief of the books, " **Utilisation and Management of Medicinal Plants (Vols. 1-3)"**, "**Medicinal Plants: Phytochemistry, Pharmacology and Therapeutics (Vols. 1-4)"**, **"Traditional and Folk Herbal Medicine (Vols. 1-3)"**, **"Natural Products: Research Reviews (Vols. 1-4)"**, **"Bioactive Phytochemicals: Perspectives for Modern Medicine (Vols. 1-3)"**, **"Perspectives in Animal Ecology and Reproduction (Vols. 1-10**)" and **"Animal Diversity, Natural History & Conservation (Vols. 1-5)"**. The Editor-in-chief of the American Biographical Institute, USA, has appointed him as *Consulting Editor* of *The Contemporary Who's Who*. Dr. Gupta also appointed as Nominee for the *Committee for the Purpose of Control and Supervision of Experiments on Animals* (CPCSEA, Govt. of India). The *Linnaean Society of London, U.K.* has awarded fellowship to him in November 2009 in recognition of his contribution towards the cultivation of knowledge in Science of Natural History. Recently, Modern Scientific Press, USA has nominated Dr. Gupta as the Editor of the *International Journal of Traditional and Natural Medicine*.

Bioactive Phytochemicals

Perspectives for Modern Medicine

— *Volume 3* —

Editor
V.K. Gupta
Chief Scientist (Ex)
CSIR-Indian Institute of Integrative Medicine
Canal Road, Jammu – 180 001,
India

2015
Daya Publishing House®
A Division of
Astral International Pvt. Ltd.
New Delhi – 110 002

Cataloging in Publication Data—DK
Courtesy: D.K. Agencies (P) Ltd. <docinfo@dkagencies.com>

Bioactive phytochemicals : perspectives for modern medicine / editor, V.K. Gupta.
volume 3 cm
Includes bibliographical references (pages) and index.
ISBN 978-81-7035-778-0 (Series)
ISBN 978-93-5124-674-9 (Volume 3)
ISBN 978-93-5130-091-5 (Series- International Edition)
ISBN 978-93-5130-706-8 (Volume 3- International Edition)

1. Pharmacognosy. 2. Phytochemicals. 3. Antineoplastic agents. I. Gupta, V. K. (Vijay Kumar), 1953-, editor.
DDC 615.32 23

Published by : **Daya Publishing House®**
A Division of
Astral International Pvt. Ltd.
– ISO 9001:2008 Certified Company –
4760-61/23, Ansari Road, Darya Ganj
New Delhi-110 002
Ph. 011-43549197, 23278134
E-mail: info@astralint.com
Website: www.astralint.com

Laser Typesetting : **Classic Computer Services**, Delhi - 110 035

Printed at : **Thomson Press India Limited**

PRINTED IN INDIA

Editorial Board

Prof. Ian Fraser Pryme

Department of Biomedicine,
University of Bergen,
Jonas Lies vei 91, N-5009 Bergen, NORWAY
Tel: +47-55-586438
Fax: +47-55-586360
E-mail: ian.pryme@biomed.uib.no

Dr. George Qian Li

Herbal Medicines Research and Education Centre,
Faculty of Pharmacy, The University of Sydney,
NSW 2006, AUSTRALIA
Tel: 612 9351
Fax: 9351 8638
E-mail: george.li@sydney.edu.au

Dr. Julia Serkedjieva

Institute of Microbiology,
Bulgarian Academy of Sciences,
26, Academician Georgy Bonchev St.,
1113 Sofia, BULGARIA
Tel: +359 2 979 31 85
Fax: +359 2 870 01 09
E-mail: jserkedjieva@microbio.bas.bg

departamento de química
universidade de aveiro dqua

Artur M. S. Silva
E-mail: artur.silva@ua.pt
Telefone: +351234370714
Fax: +351234370084

Foreword

It is a great honour to have been asked to write the foreword to this book in which several distinguished experts in the field have, with enormous care and attention, detail important aspects that related secondary metabolites with promising new medicinal approaches.

During the last few decades natural products' research has advanced tremendously through the fields of chemistry and they are ubiquitous in our everyday life. Their presence as constituents of many medicines is certainly one of the most significant ones.

In the last years the search of more natural treatments is also being implemented in the so called developed countries and traditional medicine gained new supporters being the scope and completeness of this volume a gift to academic readers but also to the industrial chemists and pharmacologists.

The major aim of this volume is to provide an easy to read overview of natural bioactive products highlight their structure and source, but mainly their biological activity and health applications. It is rare to find a combination of so much interesting topics in a single book. There is something in this volume for everyone and, personally, I will read it from time to time, as well as using it as a reference resource.

This volume includes twenty one chapters covering most of the aspects of bioactive phytochemicals. There are chapters devoted to a single natural compound that showed important biological activities, such as lupeol and naringin, and also to important families, such as rotenoids and lignans. The majority are devoted to relate the natural source (usually the genus) with its bioactive phytochemicals, and doing that a relationship between secondary metabolites biological activities (mainly anticancer) and the plant traditional use can be inferred. Interesting aspects of secondary metabolites as source of inspiration to develop new drugs are also covered.

In summary, a wide variety of conceptually distinct approaches are presented in an attempt to cover the most recent development in the area.

We are deeply indebted to Professor V.K.Gupta for a magnificent compilation of issues that will contribute to enrich the literature with comprehensive information on many aspects of natural bioactive products.

Artur Silva

Dr. Artur M. S. Silva

(Full Professor of Organic Chemistry)
(Director of the Organic Chemistry Research Group)
(Director of the Master and PhD programmes in Chemistry)

Preface

Nature is a unique source of structures of high phytochemical diversity, many of them possessing interesting biological activities and medicinal properties. Primitive people in all ages have had some knowledge of natural medicines. The knowledge of the primitive man has been so modified with the advancement of civilization that know-a-days almost every type of medicine be that of Ayurvedic, Unani or even a number of allopathic medicines are obtained from plant sources. The medicinal value of drug plants is due to the presence of some chemical compounds in the plant tissue that produce a definite physiological action on human body. Early societies learned through trial and error that many plants contained substances with significant curative properties and over the years the phytochemicals became used in more refined ways leading ultimately to the use of pure single component "active ingredient" as drugs.

In the context of the worldwide spread of different diseases such as AIDS, chronic diseases and a variety of cancers, an intensive search for new lead compounds for the development of novel pharmacological therapeutics is extremely important. Medicinal plants would be the best source to obtain a variety of drugs and, therefore, such plants should be investigated to understand better about their properties. It has been proved that although the effects of natural remedies may seem slower, the results are sometimes better on the long run especially in chronic diseases.

Bioactive phytochemicals have served as an important source of drugs since ancient times and about half of the useful drugs today are derived from natural sources. Recently, a renewed interest in obtaining bioactive secondary metabolites from plants and microorganisms including fungal endophytes has been observed, notwithstanding the impressive progress competing methodologies such as combinatorial chemistry and high-throughput screening or genetic engineering. This world-wide attention on bioactive phytochemicals is based on their low or absent toxicity, their complete biodegradability, their availability from renewable sources, and their low cost compared with that of corresponding synthetic drugs. It is well known that the accumulated data in bioactive phytochemicals did bring not only a large amount of lead compound for drugs, but also the discovery and development of drugs.

It is owing to a world wide and sustained effort of scientist's that enormous information is being generated and there has been a series of publications on bioactive phytochemicals. Based on this rational, the present volume ***"Bioactive Phytochemicals: Perspectives for Modern Medicine- Vol. 3"*** of the book series presents edited information on 21 research and review communications received from eminent scientists and researchers from Bangladesh, China, Ethopia, India, Italy, Mexico, Nigeria and Portugal, providing recent and present state of the art data on therapeutic properties, action and uses of bioactive phytochemicals in combating a number of diseases and conditions for which there is lesser satisfactory treatment in modern medicine.

The aim of this publication is to enthuse the reader with this active and exciting area of research and to lay a solid foundation on which further study of its various facts may be based and the editor will consider himself to be amply rewarded if this humble piece of work proves to be useful for those it is meant. Finally, I would always remain debtor to all our well-wishers for their blessings, without which the present volume of the book series would not have come into existence.

V.K. Gupta

Contents

Bioactive Phytochemicals: Perspectives for Modern Medicine Vol. 3 (2015) *Pages* **1–16**
Editor: **V.K. Gupta**
Published by: **DAYA PUBLISHING HOUSE, NEW DELHI**

1

Lupeol as Anticancer Drug: A Review of its Anticancer Activities and Potential as an Anticancer Therapeutic

Md. Ezazul Haque[1], Abdullah-Al-Nahain[1], Rownak Jahan[2] and Mohammed Rahmatullah[1*]

ABSTRACT

Triterpenes (member of phytosterol family) are diversely found in plant, fungi and animal kingdom. Daily foods consumed by human are rich in triterpenes that are largely derived from edible oils, cereals, fruits and vegetables. Among several pentacyclictriterpenes, lupeol also known as fagarsterol, belongs to the lupane-type triterpenes, and exhibits an array of biological activities, which is currently of great interest for its ability to slow down, arrest or reverse the process of carcinogenesis. Experimental studies have shown promising inhibitory effects of lupeol in pancreatic cancer cells, human prostate cancer cells, and human metastatic melanoma cells. This chapter explores the various plant sources of lupeol and lupeol-derivatives along with their possible mechanisms of anticancer and chemopreventive actions and discusses the therapeutic potential of these compounds.

Keywords: Lupeol, Anticancer drug, Chemopreventive actions, Therapeutic potential.

Introduction

At present cancer is one of the most common causes of morbidity. Cancer can be described as not just a disease but a collection of many diseases in which abnormal

1 Department of Pharmacy, University of Development Alternative, Dhanmondi, Dhaka – 1209, Bangladesh

2 Department of Biotechnology and Genetic Engineering, University of Development Alternative, Dhaka – 1209, Bangladesh

* *Corresponding author*: E-mail: rahamatm@hotmail.com

cells start to divide without control and can invade other tissues or other parts of the body through the blood and lymph systems. There are more than 100 different types of cancer (NCI). According to World Health Organization cancer is referred as the second leading cause of death in the most developing countries. In 2012, World Health Organization (WHO) estimated that there were 8.2 million deaths worldwide due to different types of cancer (WHO, 2012). Among the main types of cancers and related deaths are – lung cancers caused 1.59 million deaths, liver cancers caused 745,000 deaths, stomach cancers caused 723,000 deaths, colorectal cancer caused 694,000 deaths, breast caused 521,000 deaths, oesophageal cancer caused 400,000 deaths. WHO also reported in 2012 that worldwide every year there are 14.1 million new cancer cases, 8.2 million cancer deaths and 32.6 million people living with cancer (within 5 years of diagnosis) (WHO, 2012). According to WHO, there will be 84 million deaths within 2005 to 2015 (WHO, 2009).

Various chemotherapeutics agents are widely applied to control or suppress this disease. But, the serious adverse effects to normal healthy cells are major drawbacks of present therapeutic regimes. Therefore finding out new agents having potential anticancer effect with lowest side effects compared to existing drugs is greatly needed (Dupuy *et al.*, 2013). Various phytochemical constituents have been reported to possess anticancer effects following different mechanisms. Lupeol is such a phytochemical that has been claimed to be a potential anticancer agent. Among all potential phytochemicals, lupeol has been playing a pivotal role against different diseases. Both *in vivo* and *in vitro* studies reported lupeol to have beneficial activities against inflammation, cancer, arthritis, diabetes, heart diseases, renal toxicity and hepatic toxicity (Basuroy and Gerner, 2006; Fernández *et al.*, 2001; Nagumo *et al.*, 1991; Novotny *et al.*, 2001; Saleem, 2009; Sudhahar *et al.*, 2008; Sudharsan *et al.*, 2006a, 2006b, 2006c).

The goal of this chapter is to highlight the therapeutic potentials of lupeol as a potent anticancer drug as well as the mechanisms through which it exerts its anticancer and chemopreventive activities.

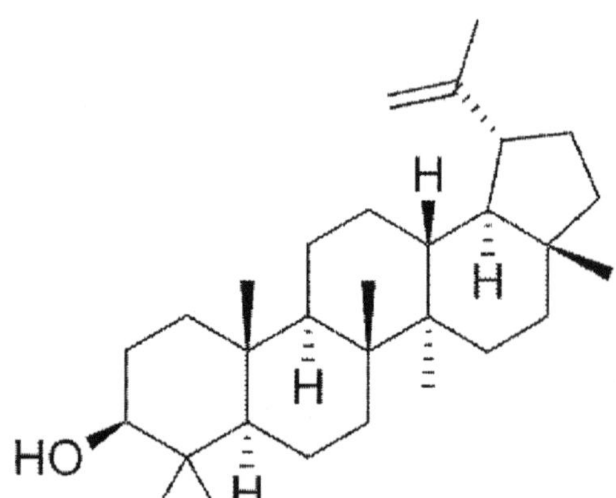

Lupeol

Figure 1.1: Chemical Structure of Lupeol.

Sources of Lupeol and Derivatives

A large number of plants have been reported to have lupeol. Table 1.1 represents the name of some plants and the parts of the plants that are reported to contain this phytochemical. Additionally, Figure 1.1 shows the chemical structure of lupeol.

Table 1.1: Table Shows Sources of Lupeol from different Plants and Plant Parts

Plant Name	*(Family)*	*Used Part(s)*	*Reference(s)*
Withania somnifera	Solanaceae	Branch point	Dhar *et al.*, 2014
Glycyrrhiza glabra	Fabaceae	Whole plant	Nasrollahi *et al.*, 2014
Millettia richardiana	Fabaceae	Stem bark	Rajemiarimiraho *et al.*, 2014
Wrightia tinctoria	*Apocynaceae*	Fresh Leaves	Srivastava, 2014
Scaphium macropodum	Malvaceae	Stem Bark	Al Muqarrabun *et al.*, 2014
Tephrosia purpurea	Fabaceae	whole plant	Palbag *et al.*, 2014
Juglans regia	Juglandaceae	Leaves	Salimi *et al.*, 2014
Euphorbia hirta	Euphorbiaceae	Stems, roots	Ragasa and Cornelio, 2013
Akschindlium godefroyanum	Fabaceae	Bark	Chaipukdee *et al.*, 2014
Ricinus communis	Euphorbiaceae	Root	Srivastava *et al.*, 2014
Ficus microcarpa	Moraceae	Bark	Kalaskar *et al.*, 2012
Lychnophora pinaster	Asteraceae	Aerial parts	Abreu *et al.*, 2013
Millettia richardiana	Fabaceae	Stem bark	Rajemiarimiraho *et al.*, 2013
Bauhinia purpurea	Fabaceae	Leaves	Negi *et al.*, 2012
Solanum schimperianum	Solanaceae	Aerial parts	Al-Oqail *et al.*, 2012
Garcinia livingstonei	Clusiaceae	Stem bark	Mulholland *et al.*, 2013
Cenostigma macrophyllum	Sapotaceae	Stem bark	Piaulino *et al.*, 2013
Manilkara zapota	Sapotaceae	Fruit	Fayek *et al.*, 2013, 2014
Illicium difengpi	Schisandraceae	Stem bark	Li *et al.*, 2013
Euonymus japonicas	Celastraceae	Stem bark	Tantry *et al.*, 2013
Oroxylum indicum	Celastraceae	Seeds	Wei *et al.*, 2013
Manilkara bidentata	Sapotaceae	Resin	Rhourri-Frih *et al.*, 2013
Bauhinia racemosa	Fabaceae	Root bark	Jain *et al.*, 2013
Artocarpus fulvicortex	Moraceae	Leaves	Jamil *et al.*, 2012
Chloranthus multistachys	Chloranthaceae	Root	Liu *et al.*, 2012
Centella asiatica	Apiaceae	Different parts	Alqahtani *et al.*, 2013
Camellia sinensis	Theaceae	Different parts	Alqahtani *et al.*, 2013
Oleae uropaea	Oleaceae	Different parts	Alqahtani *et al.*, 2013
Vaccinium myrtillus	Ericaceae	Berries and leaves	Szakiel *et al.*, 2012
Calluna vulgaris	Ericaceae	Flower and leaf cuticular wax	Szakiel *et al.*, 2013
Machaerium hirtum	Fabaceae	Leaves and branches	Ignoato *et al.*, 2012
Glochidion zeylanicum	Euphorbiaceae	Stem bark	Tanaka *et al.*, 2004
Alstonia scholaris	Apocynaceae	Flowers	Sultana *et al.*, 2013
Diospyro scuneata	Ebenaceae	Stem bark	Quintal-Novelo *et al.*, 2013

Contd...

Table 1.1–*Contd...*

Plant Name	(Family)	Used Part(s)	Reference(s)
Ficus racemosa	Moraceae	Leaves	Das *et al.*, 2013
Pentadesma butyracea	Clusiaceae	Fruit pericarp	Lenta *et al.*, 2011
Plicosepalus curviflorus	Loranthaceae	Leaves	Al-Taweel *et al.*, 2012
Pyrus communis	Rosaceae	Whole plant	Tomosaka *et al.*, 2012
Pyrus serotina	Rosaceae	Twig bark	Tomosaka *et al.*, 2012
Pseuderanthemum carruthersii	Acanthaceae	Root	Vo *et al.*, 2012
Catharanthus roseus	Apocynaceae	Leaf cuticular wax layer	Huang *et al.*, 2012
Lepidaploa cotoneaster	Asteraceae	Aerial parts	dos Santos *et al.*, 2012
Albiziaadi anthifolia	Mimosoideae	Stem bark	TamokouJde *et al.*, 2012
Klainedoxa gabonensis	Irvingiaceae	Stem bark	Wansi *et al.*, 2010
Clerodendrum chinense	Lamiaceae	Leaves	Wahba *et al.*, 2011
Clerodendrum indicum	Lamiaceae	Leaves	Wahba *et al.*, 2011
Clerodendrum glabrum	Lamiaceae	Leaves	Wahba *et al.*, 2011

Reported Anticancer Effects of Lupeol and Derivatives

Saleem's group has done extensive work to find out efficacy of lupeol as anticancer agent against different types of cancer. As a corollary, anticancer effect of lupeol was investigated against human prostate cancer cells alone and in combination with anti-Fas monoclonal antibody in athymic nude mice implanted with CWR22 Rnu1 cells (Saleem *et al.*, 2005a). Result showed significant inhibition of cell viability in a dose-dependent manner where lupeol exhibited higher cell death in comparison with the additive effect of the compounds alone. Anticancer effect of lupeol on human pancreatic adenocarcinoma cells AsPC-1 was investigated on cell growth and its effects on the modulation of multiple Ras-induced signaling pathways by the same group (Saleem *et al.*, 2005b). Lupeol showed a significant dose-dependent inhibition of pancreatic cancer cells. Saleem and co-workers also investigated the anticancer efficacy of lupeol against normal human melanocytes, and human metastatic (451Lu) and nonmetastatic (WM35) cells (Saleem *et al.*, 2008). Lupeol was administered thrice a week on athymic nude mice bearing 451Lu and WM35 melanoma cells and its effects on growth, proliferation, and apoptosis were evaluated. The results demonstrated that lupeol significantly decreased the viability of 451Lu and WM35 cells but had only a marginal effect on normal human melanocyte cells at similar doses. The significant growth reduction resulted from its effects on modulation of the expression of proliferation markers, apoptotic markers, and cell cycle regulatory molecules in tumor xenografts. Saleem (2009) also reported the chemopreventive effect of lupeol through inhibition of proliferation of human prostate cancer (CaP).

Cardioprotective effect of lupeol and its ester was observed against cyclophosphamide induced cardiac membrane damage in *in vitro* studies (Sudharsan *et al.*, 2006a). Significant cardioprotective effect was found with lupeol and lupeollinoleate (50 mg/kg body weight) respectively, dissolved in olive oil for 10 days and administered by oral gavage in male albino rats of Wistar Strain treated with a single dose of cyclophosphamide (200 mg/kg body weight) dissolved in saline. Prasad and co-workers found hepatoprotective effects of lupeol and mango pulp extract against 7, 12-dimethylbenz (a) anthracene (DMBA) induced alteration in liver of *Swiss albino* mice (Prasad *et al.*, 2007). Animals were administered with lupeol (25 mg/kg body weight) or 1 mL of 20 per cent w/v aqueous MPE/mouse and the cell population in the hypodiploid region was observed in both lupeol and MPE supplemented animals. Strong inhibition of apoptosis was obtained due to its effect on decreasing reactive oxygen species (ROS) level and restoration of mitochondrial transmembrane potential followed by decreased DNA fragmentation in DMBA treated animals. Following year, Prasad's group reported significant anticancer effect of lupeol against prostate cancer (Prasad *et al.*, 2008a). Testosterone was subcutaneously administered in male Swiss albino mice to induce prostate cancer which was exhibited by increasing enlargement of prostate. Administration of lupeol significantly arrested the enlargement of prostate in experimental mice. Another study by the group evaluated anti-proliferative and apoptotic activity of lupeol against pancreatic cancer (PCa), using human PCa cells (Prasad *et al.*, 2008b). Significant inhibition of the cell proliferation (12-71 per cent) at doses of 50-800 microM was observed in time dependent manner. Analysis of cell-cycle revealed that an anti-proliferative effect of lupeol (400-600 microM) was associated with an increase in G(2)/M-phase arrest(34-58 per cent). Further increase of dose resulted in caspase-induced apoptosis due to increase in reactive oxygen species, loss of mitochondrial membrane potential followed by DNA fragmentation. Apoptosis inducing effects of lupeol were studied in human epidermoid carcinoma A431 cells by Prasad and co-workers. The study revealed that apoptosis (14-37 per cent) was mediated by activation of mitochondrial cell death pathway and Akt/PKB, and inactivation of NFκB signaling pathways in a dose dependent manner (Prasad *et al.*, 2009). Investigation of antitumor activity and underlying mechanism of lupeol-3β-O-succinyl-lupeol (LD9-4), a derivative of lupeol has recently been carried out in human non-small cell lung cancer A549 cell line (Hao *et al.*, 2011). The study exhibited significant inhibition of cell proliferation by LD9-4. The anticancer effect was exhibited through apoptosis where accumulation of reactive oxygen species, up-regulation of Beclin 1 and inhibition of mTOR signaling pathway played the major role.

Wu and co-workers demonstrated that in appropriate concentrations lupeol inhibits the proliferation of gastric cancer cell lines BGC823, N87 and HGC27, and increase the killing effect of NK cells by promoting the proliferation of NK cells on gastric cancer cells (Wu *et al.*, 2013).

He and co-workers investigated lupeol's growth inhibitory and apoptotic effect on hepatocellular carcinoma (HCC) cell lines SMMC7721 and HepG2 (He *et al.*, 2011). *In vitro* studies showed that lupeol decreased the cell viability of two cell lines of HCC in a dose dependent manner; in *in vivo* studies, nude mice implanted with SMMC7721 cells and treated with lupeol subcutaneously for three times a week showed significant inhibition of tumor growth. Further investigation with combination of anti-tumor effect of lupeol and tumor necrosis factor-related apoptosis-inducing ligand (TRAIL) in HCC was also conducted. The result demonstrated that TRAIL alone could not achieve high level of anti-tumor effect, but lupeol in combination with TRAIL exerted chemo sensitization of HCC.

Cytotoxicity of lupeol, isolated from the different extract of the leaves of *Luehea candicans* Mart. et Zucc. (Tiliaceae) was evaluated against K-562 (leukemia), NCI-ADR (breast expressing the multidrug resistance phenotype), OVCAR (ovarian), MCF-7 (breast), NCI-460 and 786-O (human kidney) carcinoma cell lines. Lupeol, betulin, a mixture of steroids, (-)-epicatechin, vitexin and liriodendrin, present in the chloroform and methanol fractions extracted from the branches of the plant showed highest cytotoxic activity against these cells with GI(50) values between 27 and 40 μg mL(-1) (da Silva *et al.*, 2011).

Study by Siddique and co-workers revealed that lupeol possessed anticancer effect by inhibiting androgen-dependent phenotype (ADPC) and castration-resistant phenotype (CRPC) of prostate cancer (CaP) (Siddique *et al.*, 2011).

Liu *et al.* (2013) conducted *in vivo* evaluation of lupeol on hepatocellular carcinoma (HCC) cells model and reported that this phytochemical strongly inhibited the growth of HCC model without any side effect on body weight.

Using human colorectal cancer (CRC) cells that exhibit differential expression of Wnt/β-catenin signaling, Tarapore and co-workers demonstrated the effect of lupeol on CRC in mouse model and the results were dose-dependent decrease by lupeol in cell viability due to decreases in colonogenic potential, β-catenin transcriptional activity, expression of Wnt target genes and induction of apoptosis (Tarapore *et al.*, 2013).

Nitta and co-workers investigated tumor-suppressive effects of lupeol in melanoma bearing mice model following locally and systemic administration of lupeol (Nitta *et al.*, 2013). After seven days, tumor growth rates were determined. Immuno-histochemical staining for Ki-67 and proliferating cell nuclear antigen (PCNA) were also evaluated. They found that lupeol significantly inhibited tumor growth as well as arrested cell cycle. Lupeol also significantly decreased the areas positively stained for Ki-67 and PCNA in the tumor tissues compared to those in the NT and solvent control.

Anti-proliferative and apoptotic potential of lupeol was proposed by Nigam and co-workers (Nigam *et al.*, 2009). Significant preventive effects were observed with marked inhibition at 48, 72, and 96 h against DMBA-mediated neoplastic events in the skin of Swiss albino mice. Chemopreventive effect of lupeol was also reported by Nigam and co-workers on 7, 12-dimethylbenz[a]anthracene (DMBA) induced DNA alkylation damage in Swiss albino mouse skin. Both pre- and post-treatment with lupeol showed significant prevention of DMBA-induced DNA strand breaks in dose- and time-dependent manner. Increasing doses of lupeol (50-200 microg/mouse) were given topically at times of 24, 48, 72 and 96 h, respectively, prior or after the single topical application of DMBA (100 microg/mouse). The pre-treatment showed 56.05 per cent (200 microg lupeol/mouse) prevention, and post-treatment showed 43.26 per cent (at the same dose) prevention, at 96 h time interval, against DMBA-induced DNA strand breakage. The results suggested strong chemopreventive effects of lupeol on DMBA-induced DNA alkylation damage in Swiss albino mice (Nigam *et al.*, 2007).

Activity of lupeol was investigated in depth by Murtaza and co-workers (Murtaza *et al.*, 2009). Sensitization effect by lupeol on chemo resistant human pancreatic cancer cells to tumor necrosis factor-related apoptosis-inducing ligand (TRAIL) due to over expression of the cellular FLICE-like inhibitory protein (cFLIP) was investigated. Lupeol (40 mg/kg) thrice a week increased the TRAIL protein level and decreased the viability of AsPC-1 cells in both cFLIP-suppressed cells and in cFLIP-over expressing cells in athymic nude mice.

Wang reported the anti-tumor activity of lupeol derivative; where lupeolpalmitate showed strong activity against human cervical squamous carcinoma (Hela) cells (Wang, 2007).

Prevention of free radical mediated macromolecular damage and alleviation of benzoyl peroxide induced biochemical alterations in murine skin were investigated by Sultana and co-workers (Sultana *et al.*, 2013). *In vitro* study revealed significant reduction of the free radical mediated DNA-sugar damage and microsomal lipid peroxidation in an iron/ascorbate free radical generating system by lupeol and *in vivo* study showed inhibition of benzoyl peroxide (a known free radical generating tumor promoter, which causes oxidation of proteins) induced modulation in the activities of quinine reductase (Sultana *et al.*, 2013).

Zhang and co-workers investigated anti-tumor effect and associated mechanism SMMC7721 cells of lupeol in hepatocellular carcinoma (Zhang *et al.*, 2009). Significant inhibition of cell viability resulted depending on doses.

Anticancer activity of lupeol was investigated by Lee *et al.* (2011). They carried out their study in two types of cancer cells namely hepatocellular carcinoma (HCC) cell lines and clinical HCC samples. Lupeol significantly inhibited self-renewal activity of liver tumor-initiating cells (T-ICs) in these two types of cells. Besides, lupeol potentially inhibited tumorigenicity in nude mice.

Significant cytotoxic effect was also observed from the crude ethanol extract from the leaves of *Dendropanax* cf. *querceti* (Araliaceae) from Monteverde, Costa Rica, against Hep-G2, A-431, and H-4IIE tumor cell lines where lupeol was the main active phytochemical to show this effect (Moriarity *et al.*, 2005).

Reported Anticancer and Chemoprotective Mechanism of Lupeol and Derivatives

Saleem *et al.* (2005a) experimented to find out the underlying mechanism of lupeol against prostate cancer. They proposed that lupeol exhibited cell apoptosis through death-receptor dependent and Fas-associated apoptotic pathway through initiator caspase-8 and caspase-9 and by effector caspase-6. Besides, up-regulation of Fas expression by lupeol may play a role in enhanced cytotoxicity. In their next study they revealed that lupeol induced apoptosis of pancreatic cancer through activation of caspase-3, -8 and -9 (2005b). Lupeol also inhibited the promotion of pancreatic cancer by inhibiting PI3K/Akt signaling pathway; decreased the expression of phospho-p38 MAPK. Lupeol also inhibited IκBα phosphorylation, which suggested that the effect of lupeol on NFκB/p65 was through inhibition of phosphorylation of IκBα which in turn was regulated by Ras and PI3K/Akt pathways. Another study by

Saleem's group found a different mechanism towards apoptosis by lupeol in metastatic melanoma cells (Saleem *et al.*, 2008). They reported that apoptosis was caused by increasing the expression of Bax protein. The study demonstrated that lupeol inhibited metastatic melanoma by arresting cell cycle at G1 – S phase. Along with these mechanisms, lupeol also enhanced cell apoptosis by decreasing the levels of cyclin D1. Lupeol significantly increased the expression levels of p21 protein and decreased the cdk2 expression level. Mechanism of lupeol against melanoma bearing tumor mice was also studied by Nitta *et al.* (2013). Their study concluded that lupeol significantly reduced the Ki – 67 and PCNA (cell proliferative markers) thereby arrested cell cycle progression by inducing B 16 2F2 cell differentiation.

Molecular mechanisms of lupeol were elaborately evaluated by Prasad's group (Prasad *et al.*, 2009). In 2009, they showed that lupeol induced apoptosis following caspase dependent mitochondrial cell death pathway through activation of Bax, caspases, Apaf1, decrease in Bcl-2 expression and subsequent cleavage of PARP. Lupeol treatment also inhibited Akt/PKB signaling pathway by inhibition of Bad (Ser136) phosphorylation. Additionally, lupeol inactivated NFκB via upregulation of its inhibitor IκBα.

He *et al.* (2011) reported that lupeol induced apoptosis by increasing caspase-3 expression. Lupeol arrested G2/M-phase by inhibiting the cyclin B-regulated signaling pathway involving p53, p21/WAF1, cdc25C, cdc2, and cycling-B gene expression.

Lee group's found inhibition of proliferation of head and neck cancer where this phytochemical inhibited the phosphorylation of IκB and subsequently activity of NFκB (Lee *et al.*, 2007).

Study by Moriarity and others found that lupeol exhibited cytotoxicity through inhibition of topoisomerase II (Moriarity *et al.*, 2005). Another study reported that lupeol inhibited binary formation between topoisomerase II and DNA (Wada *et al.*, 2001). Investigation by Chaturvedula and co-workers also supported this mechanism (Chaturvedula *et al.*, 2004).

Zhang *et al.* (2009) investigated the effect of lupeol as an anticancer agent against hepatocellular carcinoma SMMC7721 cells. They found that lupeol exerted its effect through down-regulation of death receptor 3 (DR3) expressions along with activation of caspase 3 expression.

Cardioprotective effect of lupeol during cancer chemotherapy was due to the membrane preservation of membrane permeability of myocardial tissue (Sudharsan *et al.*, 2006a). In another study, Sudharsan and co-workers reported that lupeol and lupeollinoleate exhibited cardioprotective role against cyclophosphamide-induced cardiac mitochondrial toxicity through the restoration of mitochondrial structure and function which was damaged due to cyclophosphamide (Sudharsan *et al.*, 2006b). This group also showed that lupeol and its ester exhibited cardioprotective effects by preserving lysosomal integrity as well as increasing thiol levels (Sudharsan *et al.*, 2006c).

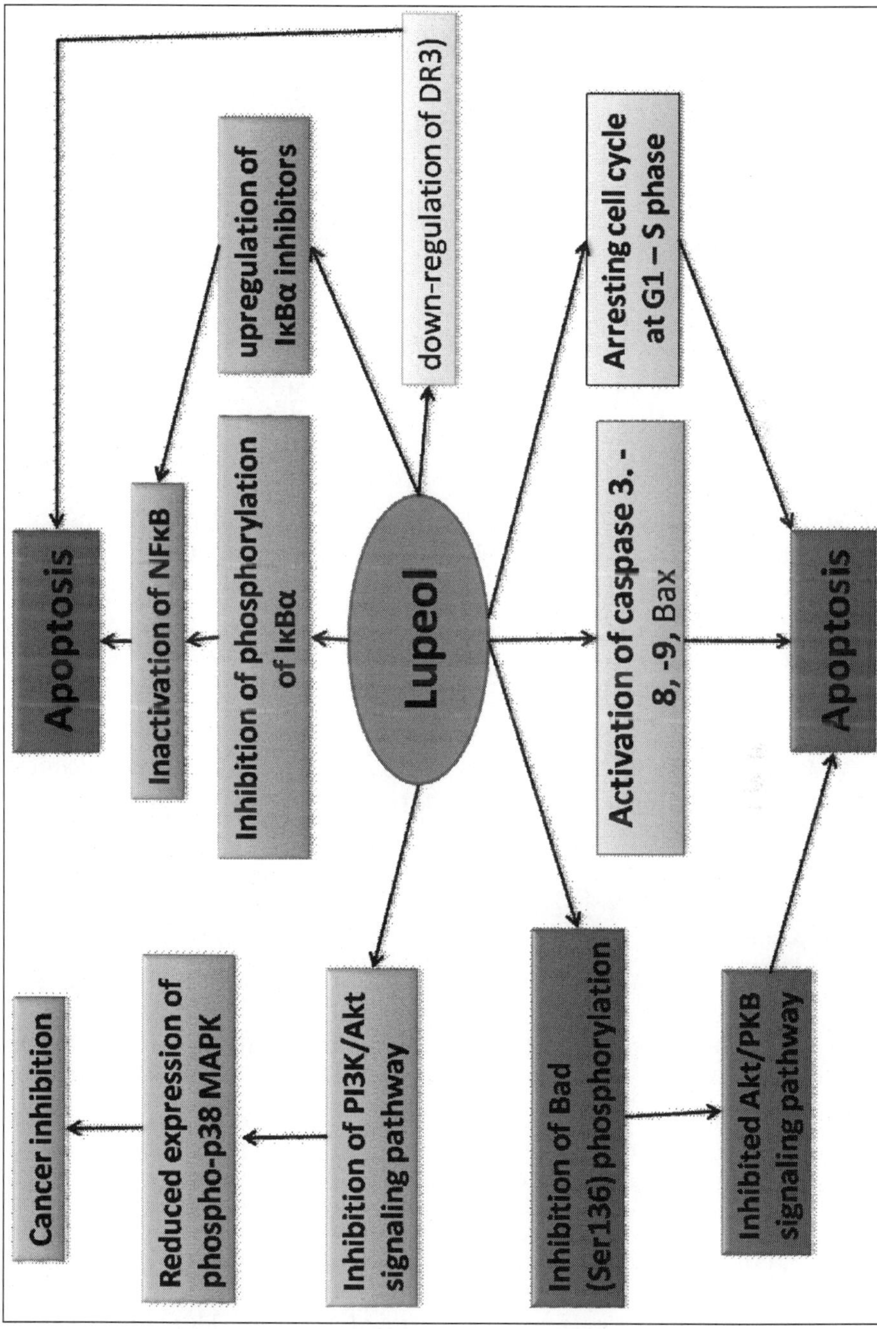

Figure 1.2: Possible Anticancer Pathways Induced by Lupeol.

Anticancer effect of lupeol by inhibiting angiogenesis has also been reported (Kässmeyer *et al.*, 2009). A summarized mechanism of lupeol is presented in Figure 1.2.

Conclusion

Present chemotherapeutic drugs suffer from the problem that they also affect normal cells and so cause various adverse reactions for the patient. A new generation of anticancer drugs is therefore necessary, which selectively kills cancer cells without affecting normal cells and causing adverse reactions in the body. Lupeol shows promise as one of the new generation of anticancer compounds. However, more studies are necessary to completely elucidate the anticancer mechanisms of lupeol as well as any associated adverse effects.

References

Abreu, V.G., Correa, G.M., Silva, T.M., Fontoura, H.S., Cara, D.C., Piló-Veloso, D., and Alcântara, A.F. (2013). Anti-inflammatory effects in muscle injury by transdermal application of gel with *Lychnophora pinaster* aerial parts using phonophoresis in rats. *BMC Complementary and Alternative Medicine*, **13**: 270.

Al, M.L.M., Ahmat, N., Aris, S.R., Norizan, N., Shamsulrijal, N., Yusof, F.Z., Suratman, M.N., Yusof, M.I., and Salim, F. (2014). A new triterpenoid from *Sapium baccatum* (Euphorbiaceae). *Naural Product Research.* **DOI**: 10.1080/14786419.2014.903396.

Al, M.L.M., Ahmat, N., Aris, S.R., Shamsulrijal, N., Baharum, S.N., Ahmad, R., Rosandy, A.R., Suratman, M.N., and Takayama, H. (2014). A new sesquiterpenoid from *Scaphium macropodum* (Miq.) Beumee. *Natural Product Research*, **28**: 597-605.

Al-Oqail, M., Hassan, W.H., Ahmad, M.S., and Al-Rehaily, A.J. (2012). Phytochemical and biological studies of *Solanum schimperianum* Hochst. *Saudi Pharmaceutical Journal*, **20**: 371-379.

Al-Taweel, A.M., Perveen, S., Fawzy, G.A., Alqasoumi, S.I., and Tahir, K.E. (2012). New flavane gallates isolated from the leaves of *Plicosepalus curviflorus* and their hypoglycemic activity. *Fitoterapia*, **83**: 1610-1615.

Alqahtani, A., Hamid, K., Kam, A., Wong, K.H., Abdelhak, Z., Razmovski-Naumovski, V., Chan, K., Li, K.M., Groundwater, P.W, and Li, G.Q. (2013). The pentacyclic triterpenoids in herbal medicines and their pharmacological activities in diabetes and diabetic complications. *Current Medicinal Chemistry*, **20**: 908-931.

Al, M.N.M., Mothana, R.A., Gamal, A.A., Al-Massarani, S.M., and Maes, L. (2013). In vitro antiprotozoal activity of triterpenoid constituents of *Kleinia odora* growing in Saudi Arabia. *Molecules*, **18**: 9207-9218.

Aristimuño, F.M.E., Vattuone, M.A., Audenaert, K., Catalán, C.A., and Sampietro, D.A. (2014). Antifungal and antimycotoxigenic metabolites in *Anacardiaceae species* from northwest Argentina: isolation, identification and potential for control of *Fusarium species*. *Journal of Applied Microbiology*, **116**: 1262-1273.

Basuroy, U.K., and Gerner, E.W. (2006). Emerging concepts in targeting the polyamine metabolic pathway in epithelial cancer chemoprevention and chemotherapy. *Journal of Biochemistry*, **139**: 27–33.

Chaturvedula, V.S., Zhou, B.N., Gao, Z., Thomas, S.J., Hecht, S.M., and Kingston, D.G. (2004). New lupane triterpenoids from *Solidago canadensis* that inhibit the lyase activity of DNA polymerase β. *Bioorganic and Medicinal Chemistry*, 12: 6271-6275.

Chaipukdee, N., Kanokmedhakul, S., Lekphrom, R., and Kanokmedhakul, K. (2014). Two new flavanonols from the bark of *Akschindlium godefroyanum*. *Natural Product Research*, **28**: 191-195.

Das, A.K., Mandal, V., and Mandal, S.C. (2013). Design of experiment approach for the process optimisation of microwave assisted extraction of lupeol from Ficus racemosa leaves using response surface methodology. *Phytochemical Analysis*, **24**: 230-47.

da Silva, D.A., Alves, V.G., Franco, D.M., Ribeiro, L.C., de Souza, M.C., Kato, L., de Carvalho, J.E., Kohn, L.K., de Oliveira, C.M., and da Silva, C.C. (2011). Antiproliferative activity of *Luehea candicans* Mart. Et Zucc. (Tiliaceae). *Natural Product Research*, **26**: 364-369.

Dhar, N., Rana, S., Razdan, S., Bhat, W.W., Hussain, A., Dhar, R.S., Vaishnavi, S., Hamid, A., Vishwakarma, R., and Lattoo, S.K. (2014). Cloning and functional characterization of three branch point oxidosqualene cyclases from *Withania somnifera* (L.) Dunal. *Journal of Biological Chemistry*, doi: 10.1074/jbc.M114.571919.

dos Santos, E.O., Meira, M., do Vale, A.E., David, J.M., de Queiróz, L.P.l., and David, J.P. (2012). Isolation and characterization of new ceramides from aerial parts of *Lepidaploa cotoneaster*. *Natural Product Communications*, **7**: 781-3.

Dupuy, L.O.A., Bonilla, V.J.A., Murillo, R., Taylor, P., Abad, M.J., González, L., and Juliao, A.J. (2013). *In vitro* effect of lupeol and casearin G on peripheral blood mononuclear and tumor cells. *Revista Medica de Chile*, **141**: 1150-7.

Fayek, N.M., Monem, A.R., Mossa, M.Y., Meselhy, M.R., and Shazly, A.H. (2012). Chemical and biological study of *Manilkara zapota* (L.) Van Royen leaves (Sapotaceae) cultivated in Egypt. *Pharmacognosy Research*, **4**: 85-91.

Fayek, N.M., Monem, A.R., Mossa, M.Y., and Meselhy, M.R. (2013). New triterpenoid acyl derivatives and biological study of *Manilkara zapota* (L.) Van Royen fruits. *Pharmacognosy Research*, **5**: 55-59.

Fernández, M.A., de las Heras, B., García, M.D., Sáenz, M.T., and Villar, A. (2001). New insights into the mechanism of action of the anti-inflammatory triterpene lupeol. The *Journal of Pharmacy and Pharmacology*, **53**: 1533–1539.

Hao, J., Pei, Y., Ji, G., Li, W., Feng, S., and Qiu, S. (2011). Autophagy is induced by 3 β-O-succinyl-lupeol (LD9-4) in A549 cells via up-regulation of Beclin 1 and down-regulation of mTOR pathway. *European Journal of Pharmacology*, **670**: 29-38.

He, Y., Liu, F., Zhang, L., Wu, Y., Hu, B., Zhang, Y., Li, Y., and Liu, H. (2011). Growth inhibition and apoptosis induced by lupeol, a dietary triterpene, in human hepatocellular carcinoma cells. *Biological and Pharmaceutical Bulletin*, **34**: 517-22.

Huang, L., Li, J., Ye, H., Li, C., Wang, H., Liu, B., and Zhang Y. (2012). Molecular characterization of the pentacyclic triterpenoid biosynthetic pathway in *Catharanthus roseus*. *Planta*, **236**: 1571-1581.

Ignoato, M.C., Fabrão, R.M., Schuquel, I.T., Botelho, M.F., Bannwart, G., Pomini, A.M., Arruda, L.L., Bersani-Amado, C.A., and Santin, S.M. (2012). Chemical constituents of *Machaerium hirtum* Vell. (Fabaceae) leaves and branches and its anti-inflammatory activity evaluation. *Natural Product Research*, **27**: 1556-1561.

Jain, R., Yadav, N., Bhagchandani, T., and Jain, S.C. (2013). A new pentacyclic phenol and other constituents from the root bark of *Bauhinia racemosa* Lamk. *Natural Product Research*, **27**: 1870-6.

Jamil, S., Taherb, M., Sirat, H.M., and Othman, N.A. (2012). Flavonoids and triterpenes from the leaves of Artocarpus fulvicortex. *Natural Product Communications*, **7**: 1587-8.

Kässmeyer, S., Plendl, J., Custodis, P., and Bahramsoltani, M. (2009). New insights in vascular development: vasculogenesis and endothelial progenitor cells. *Anatomia, Histologia and Embryologia*, **38**: 1-11.

The Wealth of India Raw Materials. Vol. 9. New Delhi: Publications and Information Directorate, Council of Scientific and Industrial Research; 1948–1976.

Kalaskar, M.G., and Surana, S.J. (2014). Pharmacognostic and phytochemical studies on *Ficus microcarpa* L. fil. *Ancient Science of Life*, **32**: 107-1.

Laszczyk, M.N. (2009). Pentacyclictriterpenes of the lupane, oleanane and ursane group as tools in cancer therapy. *Planta Medica*, **75**: 1549-1160.

Li, C., Xi, F., Mi, J., Wu, Z., and Chen, W. (2013). Two New 3,4;9,10-seco-Cycloartane Type Triterpenoids from Illicium difengpi and Their Anti-Inflammatory Activities. *Evidence Based Complementary and Alternative Medicine*, **2013**: 942541.

Li, X.J., Xie, Z., Wang, Y.H., Yan, Y.M., Pei, G., and Zhou, X.J. (2012). Study on the chemical constituents from the leaf of *Hydnocarpus hainanensis*. *Zhong Yao Cai*. **35**: 1782-4.

Liu, X., Liu, Y.L., Niu, X.F., and Qi, L. (2012). Study on the chemical constituents of *Chloranthus multistachys*. *Zhong Yao Cai*. **35**: 1254-6.

Liu, F., He, Y., Liang, Y., Wen, L., Zhu, Y., Wu, Y, Zhao, L., Li, Y., Mao, X., and Liu, H. (2013). PI3-kinase inhibition synergistically promoted the anti-tumor effect of lupeol in hepatocellular carcinoma. *Cancer Cell International*, **13**: 108 [doi: 10.1186/1475-2867-13-108].

Lee, T. K., Poon, R.T.P., Wo, J.Y., Ma, S., Guan. X-Y., Myers, J. N., Altevogt, P., and Yuen, A P.W. (2007). Lupeol suppresses cisplatin-induced nuclear factor-KB activation in head and neck squamous cell carcinoma and inhibits local invasion and nodal metastasis in an orthotopic nude mouse model. *Cancer Research*, **67**: 8800-8809.

Lee, T.K., Castilho, A., Cheung, V.C., Tang, K.H., Ma, S., and Ng, I.O. (2011). Lupeol targets liver tumor-initiating cells through phosphatase and tensin homolog modulation. *Hepatology*, **53**: 160-170.

Lenta, B.N., Kamdem, L.M., Ngouela, S., Tantangmo, F., Devkota, K.P., Boyom, F.F., Rosenthal, P.J., and Tsamo, E. (2011). Antiplasmodial constituents from the fruit pericarp of *Pentadesma butyracea*. *Planta Medica*, **77**: 377-9.

Murtaza, I., Saleem, M., Adhami, V.M., Hafeez, B.B., and Mukhtar, H. (2009). Suppression of cFLIP by lupeol, a dietary triterpene, is sufficient to overcome resistance to TRAIL-mediated apoptosis in chemoresistant human pancreatic cancer cells. *Cancer Research*, **69**: 1156-1165.

Nagumo, A., Takanashi, K., Hojo, H., and Suzuki, Y. (1991). Cytotoxicity of Betulinic acidcteriohopane-32-ol against mouse leukemia L1210 and P388 cells *in vitro*. *Toxicology Letters*, **58**: 309–313.

Nasrollahi, V., Mirzaie-Asl, A., Piri, K., Nazeri, S., and Mehrabi, R. (2014) The effect of drought stress on the expression of key genes involved in the biosynthesis of triterpenoid saponins in liquorice (*Glycyrrhiza glabra*). *Phytochemistry*, **103**: 32-37.

Negi, B.S., Dave, B.P., and Agarwal, Y.K. Evaluation of antimicrobial activity of *Bauhinia purpurea* leaves under *in vitro* conditions. *Indian Journal of Microbiology*, **52**: 360-365.

Nigam, N., Prasad, S., George, J., and Shukla, Y. (2009). Lupeol induces p53 and cyclin-B-mediated G2/M arrest and targets apoptosis through activation of caspase in mouse skin. *Biochemical and Biophysical Research Communication*, **381**: 253-258.

Nigam, N., Prasad, S., and Shukla, Y. (2007). Preventive effects of lupeol on DMBA induced DNA alkylation damage in mouse skin. *Food and Chemical Toxicology*, **45**: 2331-2335.

Nitta, M., Azuma, K., Hata, K., Takahashi, S., Ogiwara, K., Tsuka, T., Imagawa, T., Yokoe, I., Osaki, T., Minami, S., and Okamoto, Y. (2013). Systemic and local injections of lupeol inhibit tumor growth in a melanoma-bearing mouse model. *Biomedical Reports*, **1**: 641-645.

Novotny, L., Vachalkova, A., and Biggs, D. (2001). Ursolic acid: an antitumorigenic and chemopreventive activity. *Neoplasma*, **48**: 241–246.

Palbag, S., Dey, B.K., and Singh, N.K. (2014). Ethnopharmacology, phytochemistry and pharmacology of *Tephrosia purpurea*. *Chinese Journal of Natural Medicine*, **12**: 1-7.

Piaulino, C.A., Carvalho, F.C., Almeida, B.C., Chaves, M.H., Almeida, F.R., and Brito, S.M. (2013). The stem bark extracts of *Cenostigma macrophyllum* attenuates tactile allodynia in streptozotocin-induced diabetic rats. *Pharmaceutical Biology*, **51**: 1243-1248.

Prasad, S., Kalra, N., and Shukla, Y. (2007). Hepatoprotective effects of lupeol and mango pulp extract of carcinogen induced alteration in Swiss albino mice. *Molecular Nutrition and Food Research*, **51**: 352-359.

Prasad, S., Kalra, N., and Shukla, Y. (2008a). Induction of apoptosis by lupeol and mango extract in mouse prostate and LNCaP cells. *Nutrition and Cancer*, **60**: 120-130.

Prasad, S., Nigam, N., Kalra, N., and Shukla, Y. (2008b). Regulation of signaling pathways involved in lupeol induced inhibition of proliferation and induction of apoptosis in human prostate cancer cells. *Molecular Carcinogenesis*, **47**: 916-24.

Prasad, S., Nigam, N., Kalra, N., and Shukla, Y. (2008c). Protective effects of lupeol and mango extract against androgen induced oxidative stress in Swiss albino mice. *Asian Journal of Andrology*, **10**: 313-318.

Prasad, S., Madan, E., Nigam, N., Roy, P., George, J., and Shukla, Y. (2009). Induction of apoptosis by lupeol in human epidermoid carcinoma A431 cells through regulation of mitochondrial, Akt/PKB and NFκB signaling pathways. *Cancer Biology and Therapy*, **8**: 1632-1639.

Quintal-Novelo, C., Moo-Puc, R.E., Chale-Dzul, J., Cáceres-Farfán, M., Mendez-Gonzalez, M., and Borges-Argáez, R. (2013). Cytotoxic constituents from the stem bark of *Diospyros cuneata* Standl. *Natural Product Research*, **27**: 1594-1597.

Rajemiarimiraho, M., Banzouzi, J.T., Nicolau-Travers, M.L., Ramos, S., Cheikh-Ali, Z., Bories, C., Rakotonandrasana, O.L., Rakotonandrasana, S., Andrianary, P.A., and Benoit-Vical, F. (2014). Antiprotozoal activities of *Millettia richardiana* (Fabaceae) from Madagascar. *Molecules*, **19**: 4200-4211.

Rajemiarimiraho, M., Banzouzi, J.T., Rakotonandrasana, S.R., Chalard, P., Benoit-Vical, F., Rasoanaivo, L.H., Raharisololalao, A., and Randrianjah, R. (2013). Pyranocoumarin and triterpene from *Millettia richardiana*. *Natural Product Communication*, **8**: 1099-1100.

Ragasa, C.Y., and Cornelio, K.B. (2013). Triterpenes from *Euphorbia hirta* and their cytotoxicity. *Chinese Journal of Natural Medicine*, **11**: 528-33.

Rhourri-Frih, B., Renimel, I., Chaimbault, P., André P., Herbette, G., and Lafosse, M. (2013). Pentacyclic triterpenes from *Manilkara bidentata* resin. Isolation, identification and biological properties. *Fitoterapia*, **88C**: 101-108.

Saleem, M., Kweon, M.H., Yun. J.M., Adhami, V.M., Khan, N., Syed, D.N., and Mukhtar, H. (2005a). A novel dietary triterpene Lupeol induces fas-mediated apoptotic death of androgen-sensitive prostate cancer cells and inhibits tumor growth in a xenograft model. *Cancer Research*, **6**: 11203-11213.

Saleem, M., Kaur, S., Kweon, M.H., Adhami, V.M., Afaq, F., and Mukhtar, H. (2005b) Nov. Lupeol, a fruit and vegetable based triterpene, induces apoptotic death of human pancreatic adenocarcinoma cells via inhibition of Ras signaling pathway. *Carcinogenesis*, **26**: 1956-1964.

Saleem, M., Maddodi, N., Abu, Z.M., Khan, N., bin Hafeez, B., Asim, M., Suh, Y., Yun, J.M., Setaluri, V., and Mukhtar, H. (2008). Lupeol inhibits growth of highly aggressive human metastatic melanoma cells in vitro and in vivo by inducing apoptosis. *Clinical Cancer Research,* **14**: 2119-27.

Saleem, M. (2009). Lupeol, a novel anti-inflammatory and anti-cancer dietary triterpine. *Cancer Letter,* **285**: 109-115.

Salimi, M., Ardestaniyan, M.H., Mostafapour, K.H., Saeidnia, S., Gohari, A.R., Amanzadeh, A., Sanati, H., Sepahdar, Z., Ghorbani, S., and Salimi, M. (2014). Anti-proliferative and apoptotic activities of constituents of chloroform extract of *Juglans regia* leaves. *Cell Proliferation,* **47**: 172-9.

Siddique, H.R., Mishra, S.K., Karnes, R.J., and Saleem, M. (2011). Lupeol, a novel androgereceptor inhibitor: implications in prostate cancer therapy. *Clinical Cancer Research,* **17**: 5379-91.

Srivastava, R. (2014a). A review on phytochemical, pharmacological, and pharmacognostical profile of *Wrightia tinctoria*: Adulterant of kurchi. *Pharmacognosy Reviews,* **8**: 36-44.

Srivastava, P., Jyotshna, Gupta, N., Maurya, A.K., and Shanker, K. (2014b). New anti-inflammatory triterpene from the root of *Ricinus communis*. *Natural Product Research,* **28**: 306-11.

Setzer, W.N., and Setzer, M.C. (2003). Plant-derived triterpenoids as potential antineoplastic agents. *Mini Reviews in Medicinal Chemistry,* **3**: 540–556.

Sudhahar, V., Ashok, K.S., Varalakshmi, P., and Sujatha, V. (2008). Protective effect of lupeol and lupeol linoleate in hypercholesterolemia associated renal damage. *Molecular and Cellular Biochemistry,* **317**: 11–20.

Sudharsan, P.T., Mythili, Y., Selvakumar, E., and Varalakshmi, P. (2006a). Lupeol and its ester exhibit protective role against cyclophosphamide-induced cardiac mitochondrial toxicity. *Journal of Cardiovascular Pharmacology,* **47**: 205–210.

Sudharsan, P.T., Mythili, Y., Selvakumar, E., and Varalakshmi, P. (2006b). Lupeol and its ester inhibit alteration of myocardial permeability in cyclophosphamide administered rats. *Molecular and Cellular Biochemistry,* **292**: 39-44.

Sudharsan, P.T., Mythili, Y., Selvakumar, E., and Varalakshmi, P. (2006c). Lupeol and its ester ameliorate the cyclophosphamide provoked cardiac lysosomal damage studied in rat. *Molecular and Cellular Biochemistry,* **282**: 23-29.

Sultana, N, Saify, Z.S., Saleem, M., and Kamal, M. (2013). Two new triterpenes from *Alstonia scholaris* flowers. *Natural Product Research,* **27**: 1277-1286.

Szakiel, A., Nizyñski, B., and Paczkowski, C. (2013). Triterpenoid profile of flower and leaf cuticular waxes of heather *Calluna vulgaris*. *Natural Product Research,* **27**: 1404-1407.

Szakiel, A., Paczkowski, C., and Huttunen. S. (2012). Triterpenoid content of berries and leaves of bilberry *Vaccinium myrtillus* from Finland and Poland. *Journal of Agricultural and Food Chemistry,* **60**: 11839-11849.

Tamokou, J. D., Mpetga, D.J.S., Lunga, P.K., Tene, M., Tane, P., and Kuiate, J.R. (2012). Antioxidant and antimicrobial activities of ethyl acetate extract, fractions and compounds from stem bark of *Albizia adianthifolia* (Mimosoideae). *BMC Complementary and Alternative Medicine*, **12**: 99.

Tantry, M.A., Idris, A., and Khan, I.A. (2013). Glycosylsphingo lipids from *Euonymus japonicas* Thunb. *Fitoterapia*, **89**: 58-67

Tanaka, R., Kinouchi, Y., Wada, S., and Tokuda, H. (2004). Potential anti-tumor promoting activity of lupane-type triterpenoids from the stem bark of *Glochidion zeylanicum* and *Phyllanthus flexuosus*. *Planta Medica*, **70**: 1234-6.

Tarapore, R.S., Siddiqui, I.A., Adhami, V.M., Spiegelman, V.S., and Mukhtar, H. (2013). The dietary terpenelupeol targets colorectal cancer cells with constitutively active Wnt/β-catenin signaling. *Molecular Nutrition and Food Research*, **57**: 1950-8.

Tomosaka, H., Tamimoto, H., Tsukagoshi, Y., Suzuki, Y., Ooka, H., and Ota, M. (2012). Constituents of twig bark of pear cultivars (*Pyrus* species). *Natural Product Communication*, **7**: 987-8.

Vo, T.N., Nguyen, P.L., Tuong, L.T., Pratt, L.M., Vo, P.N., Nguyen, K.P., and Nguyen, N.S. (2012). Lignans and triterpenes from the root of *Pseuderanthemum carruthersii* var. *atropurpureum*. *Chemical and Pharmaceutical Bulletin (Tokyo)*, **60**: 1125-33.

Wada, S., Iida, A., and Tanaka, R. (2001). Screening of triterpenoids isolated from *Phyllanthus flexuosus* for DNA topoisomerase inhibitory activity. *Journal of Natural Products*, **64**: 1545-1547.

Wang, K.W (2007). A new fatty acid ester of triterpenoid from *Celastrus rosthornianus* with anti-tumor activities. *Natural Product Research*, **21**: 669-674.

Wansi, J.D., Chiozem, D.D., Tcho, A.T., Toze, F.A., Devkota, K.P., Ndjakou, B.L., Wandji, J., and Sewald, N. (2010). Antimicrobial and antioxidant effects of phenolic constituents from *Klainedoxa gabonensis*. *Pharmaceutical Biology*, **48**: 1124-1129.

Wahba, H.M., AbouZid, S.F., Sleem, A.A., Apers, S., Pieters, L., and Shahat, A.A. (2011). Chemical and biological investigation of some *Clerodendrum* species cultivated in Egypt. *Pharmaceutical Biology*, **49**: 66-72.

Wei, X.N., Lin, B.B., Xie, G.Y., Li, J.W., and Qin, M.J. (2013). Chemical constitunents of seeds of *Oroxylum indicum*. *Zhongguo Zhong Yao Za Zhi*, **38**: 204-207.

Wu, X.T., Liu, J.Q., Lu, X.T., Chen, F.X., Zhou, Z.H., Wang, T., Zhu, S.P., and Fei, S.J. (2013). The enhanced effect of lupeol on the destruction of gastric cancer cells by NK cells. *International Immunopharmacology*, **16**: 332-340.

Zhang, L., Zhang, Y., Zhang, L., Yang, X., and Ly, Z. (2009). Lupeol, a dietary triterpene, inhibited growth, and induced apoptosis through down-regulation of DR3 in SMMC7721 cells. *Cancer Investigation*, **27**: 163-170.

Bioactive Phytochemicals: Perspectives for Modern Medicine Vol. 3 (2015)
Editor: **V.K. Gupta**
Published by: **DAYA PUBLISHING HOUSE, NEW DELHI**

Pages **17–92**

2

Capparis Genus (Capers): A Critical Review on Bio-active Phytochemicals as Phytomedicine and its Pharmacology

P. Rajesh[1*], S. Chandru[1] and V. Rajesh Kannan[1]

ABSTRACT

Capparis genus is belongs to Capparidaceae (Capparaceae) family in the order of Brassicales consisting about 46 genera and 900 species; in particularly Capparis genus constitutes about 250 species. The Capparis is widely distributed around Asia, America and Africa in tropical and subtropical spaces. The present review summarizes various species of Capparis genus produced and derived phytochemical compounds, structures and its phytomedicine properties. The bioactive phytochemicals were derived and established from the normal flora of medicinal plant as Capparis. The bioactive phytochemicals are pioneering ailments to various pharmacological and therapeutical applications from various medicinal plants which are primary and secondary metabolites. The phytochemicals were classified from various researches such as glycosides, glucosinolytes, flavonoids, terpenoids, tannins and steroids. The above secondary metabolic compounds were reported about 400 compounds from Capparis genus which includes capparispine, glucocapparin, rutin, quercetin, quercetin-3-O-glucoside, kaempferol, kaempferol-3-rutinoside, kaempferol-7-rhamnoside, rhamnetin, glucosinolytes, (6S)-hydroxy-3-oxo-α-ionol-glucoside, proline betaine, polyprenols from 15 different Capparis genus were reviewed here. The phytochemicals were reported as treatment for various infectious diseases such as anti-inflammatory, anti-cancer, anti-bacterial, anti-ulcer, anti-diabetic etc., The critical review of phytomedicine and its chemical structures will be useful for further biological and pharmacological, medical approaches etc.,

Keywords: Capparidaceae, Capers, Cappariloside, Capperspine.

1 Department of Microbiology, Bharathidasan University, Tiruchirappalli - 620 024, Tamil Nadu, India

* *Corresponding author*: E-mail: raju19marc@gmail.com

Introduction

Herbal medicines are being used about 80 per cent of the world population primarily in the developing countries for primary health care. An increasing number of people are adopting alternative medicine or system owing to the irreversible effects of modern drugs and therapies. Also the medicinal plant products are widely less side effects and treatment for various acute and chronic diseases is gaining increased importance around the globe with the short term course. In perpetually herbal remedies are suitable for the quick response to inflammation is reported, *i.e.*, alfalfa is a good resource of minerals and chlorophyll; bilberry contains flavonoids; further cat's claw, ginger, goldenseal, paudarco, strawberries, red clove, yucca and turmeric were reduces inflammation and arthritis. They have stood through the test for safety, efficacy, cultural acceptability, lesser side effects and unfavourable reactions. Ancient literature also mentioned that herbal medicine cure for various diseases.

Herbalism is a traditional medicine or folk medicine practice based on the use of plants and their extracts. The scope of herbal medicine is sometimes extended to include bacterial, fungal and bee products, as well as minerals, shells and even certain animal parts (Acharya *et al.*, 2008). Many plants are synthesizing substances called as secondary metabolites that are useful to the maintenance of health in humans and other animals. These include alkaloids, flavonoids, glycosides, saponins, steroids, tannins etc. Many of them at least 12,000 compounds have been isolated and also estimated through identification of the compounds (Huxtable, 1992). In many cases, these substances (particularly the alkaloids) serve as plant defense mechanisms against predation by microorganisms, insects and herbivores. Many of the herbs and spices used by humans to season food yield useful medicinal compounds (Lai *et al.*, 2004; Tapsell *et al.*, 2006). People from all continents have used hundreds to thousands of indigenous plants for treatment of ailments since prehistoric times. About Capparidaceae family as Caper plants having different range of phytochemicals used as traditionally as Ayurveda, Siddha, Unani. The particular plant *Capparis* genus constituting medicinal purposes and its corresponding bioactive phytochemicals were reviewed here.

Bioactive Phytochemicals and Its Pharmacology of *Capparis* genus

Capparis aphylla

The results were reported that whole plant ethanolic extract of *Capparis aphylla* manifested an antifertility effect on male reproductive system in adult Wistar Albino rat model. The administration of ethanolic extract at varied doses led to alteration in both the histoarchitecture of testis, mainly caput epididymis and erratic spermatogenesis have been documented and reported. The data reported that functional sterility could be induced in male rats by whole plant ethanolic extract treatment, which promises to be a potential male contraceptive (Revathi *et al.*, 2010).

The active fractions methanol extract of stem part in *Capparis aphylla* on pancreatic cells and antioxidant enzymes in experimental streptozotocin induced diabetes in rats was reported to be significantly reduced blood glucose levels in diabetic rats. The above report was possessed remarkable reduction in glutathione, superoxide dismutase, catalase and glutathione peroxidase activity in the liver, heart and kidney of diabetic rats by scavenging of free radicals thereby reducing the risk of diabetic complications. The results were reported that *C. aphylla* stem extract treatment might effectively normalize the impaired pancreatic cells and antioxidant status in streptozotocin induced diabetes (Dangi and Mishra, 2011).

Capparis cartilaginea, C. deserti and *C. spinosa*

The *Capparis cartilaginea* and *C. deserti* growing in Egypt were investigated and reported for their glucosiolates and rutin content. From *C. cartilaginea* four isothiocynates were reported using GC and EI/MS chromatographic and spectroscopical techniques. The reported compounds were butyl isothiocyanate **(1)**, 6-methylsulphonylhexyl isothiocyanate **(2)**, 7-methylsulphonylheptyl isothiocyanate **(3)** and 5-benzylsulphonyl-4-pentenyl isothiocyanate **(4)**. In addition to compounds butyl isothiocyanate **(1)**, 6-methylsulphonyl hexylisothiocyanate **(2)**, 3-methylthiopropyl isothiocyanate **(5)** and 11-(2-butenylthio)-6-undecenyl isothiocyanate **(6)**, compounds were isolated and reported from *C. deserti* for the first time. Also, quantitative evaluation of main flavonoids compound as rutin **(7)** in the above two species were reported by TLC-densitometry analysis. The antioxidant activity was reported on using diphenylpicrylhydrazyl (DPPH) radical scavenging method in butanol fraction from *C. cartilaginea* and *C. deserti* with possession of significant antioxidant properties (Ahmed *et al.*, 2007).

The chemical composition of essential oils and antibacterial activity of crude extract fractions and their phytochemical screening from the aerial parts of *Capparis cartilaginea* and *C. spinosa* were examined and reported. GC-MS analysis of the essential oils revealed and reported a complex mixture of compounds including nitrogen and sulfur containing compounds, oxygenated sesquiterpens and monoterpene hydrocarbons. About 59 components were identified and reported in the oil of the *C. cartilaginea*. The essential oil of *C. cartilaginea* was dominated by methyl isothiocyanate **(8)**, isopropyl isothiocyanate **(9)**, isobutyl isothiocyanate **(10)**, 3-p-menthene **(11)**, occidol **(12)**, carissone **(13)** and ethyl isothiocyanate **(14)**. A total of 40 constituents were identified in the oil of the *C. spinosa*. *C. spinosa* was dominated and reported by butyl isothiocyanate **(1)**, methyl isothiocyanate **(8)**, isopropyl isothiocyanate **(9)**, 3-p-menthene **(11)**, 2-butenyl isothiocyanate **(15)** and 3-methylthio-1-hexanol **(16)** as major constituents. The antibacterial activity of petroleum ether, water, butanol, methanol and hexane crude extracts from the aerial parts of *C. spinosa* and *C. cartilaginea* and the fractions were most active against *Staphylococcus epidermidis* and *Streptococcus faecalis*. Water fraction of *C.cartilaginea* and *C. spinosa* contained and reported as presence of alkaloids, flavonoids and tannins. However, no secondary metabolites were detected and reported in petroleum ether, butanol, methanol and hexane fractions of *C. cartilaginea* and *C. spinosa*. While, alkaloids and tannins were reported in methanolic fraction of *C. spinosa* and butanol fraction of *C. spinosa* reported tannins (Ahmad Sultan, 2006).

Capparis decidua

Phytochemical investigation of aerial parts of *Capparis decidua* reported in the isolation of a new compound germacr-3β-ol-7,9-dien-6,14-olide-15-oic acid **(17)** along with several known compounds through ethyl acetate fraction of column chromatography (Mona *et al.*, 2012).

The ascorbic acid **(18)** contents of roots, shoots and fruits of three selected medicinal plants like *Capparis decidua*, *Cleome gynandra* and *Cleome viscosa* of family Capparidaceae have been analyzed and reported. Maximum ascorbic acid **(18)** contents were reported in the fruits of *C. decidua* while, minimum in the roots of *C. viscosa* (Kapoor and Raksha, 2013).

In the traditional system of medicine, the bark of *Capparis decidua* has been shown to be useful in the treatment of coughs, asthma and inflammation; roots used in fever and buds in the treatment of boils, anthelmintic and purgative. In Unani, leaves act as appetizer, helps in cardiac troubles, fruits used in bilious nessal veolaris and pyorrhea. The plant is reported to contain phytochemicals including alkaloids, terpenoids, glycosides and some fatty acids. The plant *C. decidua* have reported and possessed significant pharmacological activities such as antihypercholesterolemic, antiinflammatory, analgesic, antidiabetic, antimicrobial, antiplaque, antihypertensive, antihelmintic and purgative activities. The review analyses and reported on phytochemical and pharmacological potential of medicinal plant *C. decidua* as rutin **(7)**, methyl isothiocyanate **(8)**, ascorbic acid **(18)**, spermidine alkaloid **(19)**, codonocarpine **(20)**, isocodonocarpine **(21)**, capparisine **(22)**, capparisinine **(23)**, capparidisine **(24)**, decidua terpenolide A **(25)**, 14-N- acetylcodonocarpine **(26)**, 15-N-acetyl capparisine **(27)**, cadabicine **(28)**, stachydrine **(29)**, n-triancontanol **(30)**, β-sitosterol **(31)**, β-carotene **(32)**, phthalic acid **(33)** and glucocapparin **(34)** (Sushila *et al.*, 2010).

The plant *Capparis decidua* is traditionally used for curing a variety of ailments such as toothache, cough, asthma, intermittent fever and rheumatism in India was reported. There are no reports of quantification of β-sitosterol **(31)** from this plant. Hence, a TLC densitometric method has been reported for quantification of this marker compound using the solvent system of toluene: methanol (Sushila *et al.*, 2010a).

The chemicals rutin **(7)**, codonocarpine **(20)**, isocodonocarpine **(21)**, capparisine **(22)**, capparisinine **(23)**, capparidisine **(24)**, 15-N-acetylcapparisine **(27)**, β-sitosterol **(31)**, 14-N-acetylisocodonocarpine **(35)** were reported in root bark of *Capparis decidua* (Verma *et al.*, 2011).

Two sterols, one diterpine alcohol **(36)**, two aliphatic constituents and one diterpenic ester **(37)** were reported from root bark of *Capparis decidua*. β-sitosterol **(31)** was reported from the roots by extracting with ethanol and chromatography the alcoholic extract on neutral alumina with the eluents benzene, ether, chloroform and methanol successively. The structures of the sterols were established as 24-β-methylcholest-7-ene-22-one-3-β-ol **(38)** and 24-β-methylcholest-9-(11)-ene-22-one -3β-ol **(39)**. The structure of diterpene alcohol was reported as 3-methyl-7-hydroxymethylene-10-(12,16,16-trimethylcyclohex-11-enyl)-dec-9-ene-5-one-8-ol, butyl-3-oxoeicosanoate **(40)** and 25-oxooctosan-1,20-diol were the aliphatic constituents. The diterpenic ester **(37)** was reported as 9-(11,15,15-trimethylcyclohex-11-ene-13-one-yl)-one-6-hydroxymethylene-7-one-yl, 4-me heptanoate (Rai, 1987). From the root bark of *C. decidua*, spermidine alkaloid **(19)** like isocodonocarpine **(21)** were reported (Ahmed *et al.*, 1989), capparisinine **(23)** (Dahot, 1993; Ahmad *et al.*, 1985, 1987a), capparidisine **(24)** (Ahmad *et al.*, 1992) were reported. Six oxygenated heterocyclic constituents capparisesterpenolide (3-carboxy-6,17-dihydroxy-7,11,15,19-tetramethyleicos-13-ene-d-lactone) and deciduaterpenolides (d-lactone derivatives of 1,3,3-trimethyl-1,4-cyclohexadien-6-one) A **(25)**, B, C, D and E from alcoholic extract of root bark of *C. decidua* have been reported (Gupta and Ali, 1997). The root bark also reported as alkaloids such as15-N-acetylcapparisine **(27)**, cadabicine **(28)** and 14-N-acetyl isocodonocarpine **(35)** (Ahamad *et al.*, 1987b); further rutin **(7)**, codonocarpine **(20)**, capparisine **(22)** and stachydrine **(29)** were reported (Gaind and Juneja, 1970).

The phytochemicals such as codonocarpine **(20)**, capparisine **(22)**, capparisinine **(23)**, capparidisine **(24)**, 15-N-acetyl capparisine **(27)**, β-sitosterol **(31)**, glucocapparin **(34)**, diacetyl capparisine **(41)**, capparisininediacetate **(42)**, O-N-diacetyl capparisine **(43)**, L-stachydrine **(44)**, 3-hydroxy stachydrine **(45)** were reviewed and reported in the plant *Capparis decidua* (Pradeep *et al.*, 2011).

The study was reported in the toothache reliever activity on aqueous extract of *Capparis decidua* and oral acute toxicity study. However, the rats reported in signs of depression and inappetence. Using the intraperitoneal route, the rats were reported that dose dependent signs of toxicity ranging from inappetence, depression, unsteady gait, tremors and respiratory distress to death. No gross changes were observed and reported in the lungs of rats following extract administration. This result suggested and reported that the aqueous extract of a *C. decidua* to be used for toothache reliever by oral route administration (Pokharkar *et al.*, 2007).

The seeds of *Capparis decidua* are found and reported to contain non-edible oil in a wide range. The study has been demonstrated and reported the cost effective new source of energy by single step reaction *i.e.* production of oil by combining extraction and reaction of extract with the mixture of alcohols. The effect of catalyst concentration, time, water content and temperature on in-situ transesterification is reported to obtain optimum yield and fatty acid methyl ester (Biodiesel). The fuel characterization tests also reported the striking similarity of various physical and chemical properties and capers to ASTM standards (Raghunath*et al.*, 2008).

The plant *Capparis decidua* extract produced a significant dose-dependent decrease in the levels of total cholesterol (TC), triacylglycerol (TG), low density lipoprotein cholesterol (LDL), with a significant increase in the level high density lipoprotein-cholesterol (HDL) and reported to possessed a hypolipidemic potential (Neelkamal, 2009).

The pharmacological activities such as antidiabetic, antiatherocslerotic, antihypertensive, antihelmintic, purgative, anti-inflammatory, analgesic, antimicrobial, antiplaque, depressant, hypercholesterolemic, hepatoprotective and hypolipidaemic activity were reported in root bark of *Capparis decidua* (Baby Joseph, 2011).

The study has been reported on various solvents *i.e.,* acetone, chloroform, petroleum ether, methanol, hexane and aqueous extracts of stem, root and flower of *Capparis decidua* were evaluated for insecticidal activity against the *Rhizopertha dominica* (Upadhyay, 2012).

Moisture, phosphorus, magnesium, iron, zinc, copper, sodium, calcium, crude protein, proline, total carbohydrate, soluble carbohydrate, starch, crude fiber, NDF, hemicelluloses, cellulose, lignin, crude fat, total ash were identified and reported in the chemical analysis of *Capparis decidua* (Sushil Kumar *et al.,* 2013).

The reported study has been evaluated the effect on *Lymnea acuminata* and their cercarial larvae while treating with alcoholic extracts of *Capparis decidua* flowers due to its wide presence of phytochemicals (Jyotsna Shekhawat and Naresh Vyas, 2013).

Antimicrobial screening of ethyl ether and alcoholic extracts of leaves of four selected such as *Capparis decidua, Eclipta alba, Pedalium murex* and *Pulicaria crispa* showed and reported reactions against bacterial pathogens *viz., Staphylococcus aureus, Escherichia coli* and a fungal pathogen *Candida albicans* (Kapoor and Mishra, 2013).

Capparis grandiflora

The study was reported to screen the antimicrobial activity of dried root powder of *Capparis grandiflora. In vitro* antimicrobial activity of various extracts from the roots of *C. grandiflora,* by using *Staphylococcus aureus, Bacillus subtilis, Bacillus pumillus, Escherichia coli, Klebsiella pneumonia, Proteus vulgaris, Candida albicans* and *Aspergillus niger*. The *C. grandiflora* extracts that reported and possessed significant antimicrobial activity and none of any antifungal activity (Karanayil *et al.,* 2011).

Capparis humilis

The *Capparis humilis* has been reported to possess many active constituents such as proline betaine **(46)**, N-methyl proline **(47)**, 3-carbomethyoxy-N-methoxypyridinium (trigonelline) **(48)**, quaternary ammonium compounds **(49)**, glucosinolates **(50)**, alkaloids **(51)**, polyprenals **(52)**, saccharose **(53)** and kaempferol-3,7-dirrhamnoside **(54)** were reported using NMR techniques (Rajesh *et al.,* 2009).

Capparis masakai

Detailed chemical, degradative and spectroscopic studies have been reported to possess 2-hydroxyethyl glucosinolate **(55)** from the seed of *Capparis masakai*. This study is the first report of glucosinolate, which is the group of glucosinolates which spontaneously cychze upon treatment with thioglucoside glucohydrolase (myrosmase), thereby yielding oxazohdme-2-throne **(56)** (Zhong *et al.*, 1989).

Capparis ovata

The phytochemicals such as palmitic acid **(57)**, stearic acid **(58)**, oleic acid **(59)**, linoleic acid **(60)**, linolenic acid **(61)** were reported from the *Capparis ovata* and *C. spinosa* (Haydar *et al.,* 2011).

Capparis orientalis, C. sicula and *C. spinosa*

The flavonol content of commercial capers (pickled flower buds of *Capparis spinosa C. sicula* and *C. orientalis*) has been reported and they were quercetin-3-rutinoside

(62), kaempferol 3-rutinoside **(63)** and kaempferol-3-rhamnosyl-rutinoside **(64)** as well as the aglycones (quercetin **(65)** and kaempferol **(66)**) were reported by HPLC technique coupled with a diode-array detector (Cristina *et al.*, 2000).

Capparis sepiaria

The phytochemicals such as oleic acid **(59)**, N-methylhomopiperazine **(67)**, 3-pyridinecarboxylic acid-1,2,5,6-tetrahydro-1-methyl-methyl ester **(68)**, 8-azabicyclo(3,2,1)-ocatan-3-ol-2-bromo-8-methyl-(exo, exo)- **(69)**, pyrrolidine-1-(1-oxobutyl) **(70)**, benzofuran-2,3-dihydro **(71)**, 2-methoxy-4-vinylphenol **(72)**, 2-furanmethanol-5-ethenyltetrahydro-α,α,5-trimethyl-,cis- **(73)**, 2H-indeno(1,2-b)furan-2-one,3,3a,4,5,6,7,8,8b-octahydro-8,8-dimethyl **(74)**, 1,2,3,4-cyclohexanetetrol **(75)**, 3-tert-Butyl-4-hydroxyanisole **(76)**, ethyl-α-d-glucopyranoside **(77)**, aspidospermidine-3-carboxylic acid-2,3-didehydro-methyl ester, (5α, 12β, 19α)- (Synonym: Vincadifformine) **(78)**, 3,7-cycloundecadien-1-ol, 1,5,5,8-tetramethyl- **(79)**, pentadecanoic acid-14-methyl-methyl ester **(80)**, n-hexadecanoic acid **(81)**, hexadecanoic acid, ethyl ester **(82)**, 9,12-octadecadienoic acid-(Z,Z)-methyl ester **(83)**, 9-octadecenoic acid-(Z)-methyl ester **(84)**, phytol **(85)**, 9,12-octadecadienoic acid-ethyl ester **(86)**, ethyl oleate **(87)**, octadecanoic acid ethyl ester **(88)**, 1,2-benzenedicarboxylic acid diisooctyl ester **(89)**, squalene **(90)** and τ-tocopherol **(91)** were reported in GC-MS analysis in ethanolic extract of aerial parts of *Capparis sepiaria*(Rajesh *et al.*, 2010).

The plant *Capparis sepiaria* reported on preliminary phytochemical evaluation of the ethanolic extract of revealed that the presence of reducing sugar, flavonoids, steroids, tannins, glycosides **(92)**, alkaloids, gums, resins, amino acids, proteins and anthraquinones **(93)**. The results of the various phytochemical tests indicated that the plant to be rich in various biologically active compounds which could serve as potential source of the crude drugs and in addition the plant is not toxic to the experimental model was reported (Rajesh *et al.*, 2010a).

Capparis sikkimensis

The plant *Capparis sikkimensis* has reported a active constituent as 3(4H)-one-6-methoxy-2-methyl-4-carbaldehyde **(94)** (Rajesh *et al.*, 2009).

Capparis spinosa

A plant, namely *Capparis spinosa* was studied from chemical standardization and nutraceutical point of view (hexane and chloroform extract). Along with HPTLC, GC-MS profiles, chemical standards such as organoleptic standards, test for purity, extractive values were measured and reported. The XRF and FPM data also reported that the plant is rich in minerals like K, Ca, Mg and P. Such standardization and validation studies report will help in developing standard and quality herbal dietary supplements (Manikandaselvi and Brindha, 2014).

The phytochemicals like, n-hexadecanoic acid **(81)**, hexadecanoic acid, ethyl ester **(82)**, phytol **(85)**, 9,12-octadecadienoic acid, ethyl ester **(86)**, octane **(95)**, hexanal **(96)**, 2-heptenal-(z)- **(97)**, nonanal **(98)**, octanoic acid **(99)**, 2-decenal-(z)- **(100)**, nonanoic acid **(101)**, 8-nonynoic acid **(102)**, 2,4-decadienal **(103)**, 2-dodecenal **(104)**, n-decanoic acid **(105)**, 13-tetradece-11-yn-1-ol **(106)**, 2(4H)-benzofuranone, 5,6,7,7a-tetrahydro-

4,4,7a-trimethyl **(107)**, dodecanoic acid **(108)**, tetrahydrofuran-2-one,5-(1-hydroxyhexyl)-**(109)**, tetradecanal **(110)**, tetradecanoic acid **(111)**, 2-hexadecen,3,7,11,15-tetramethyl-(R-(R*,R*-(E))) **(112)**, 3,7,11,15-tetramethyl-2-hexadecen-1-ol **(113)**, 2-pentadecanone-6,10,14-trimethyl **(114)**, hexadecanoic acid, methyl ester **(115)**, octadecanamide **(116)**, penta triacontane **(117)**, hexatriacontane **(118)** and tetratriacontane **(119)** were identified through GC-MS on chloroform extract of *C. spinosa*. The chemicals such as hexadecanoic acid, ethyl ester **(82)**, 9,12-octadecadienoic acid, ethyl ester **(86)**, octane **(95)**, hexanal **(96)**, 13-tetradece-11-yn-1-ol **(106)**, 1-Propane, 1-(2-propenyloxy) **(120)**, (E)-2-Hexanone **(121)**, 1-undecyne **(122)**, heptanes,5-ethyl-2,2,3-trimethyl **(123)**, undecane, 2,8-dimethyl **(124)**, decane, 3,7-dimethyl **(125)**, sulfurous acid, di(2-ethylhexyl) ester **(126)**, decane,2,3,7-trimethyl **(127)**, dodecane **(128)**, 3-octadecene,(E)- **(129)**, undecane, 2,3-dimethyl **(130)**, dodecane, 2,7,10-trimethyl **(131)**, Benzene, 1-methoxy-4-(1-propenyl)-**(132)**, tridecane, 4-methyl **(133)**, tridecane, 2-methyl **(134)**, heptadecane, 2,6,10,15-tetramethyl-**(135)**, n-decanoic acid **(136)**, pentadecane **(137)**, benzene, (1-butylhexyl) **(138)**, benzene, (1-propylheptyl) **(139)**, benzene,(1-ethyloctyl) **(140)**, Benzene, (1-methylnonyl)- **(141)**, benzene,(1-butylheptyl) **(142)**, benzene, (1-propyloctyl) **(143)**, benzene, (1-ethylnonyl)- **(144)**, benzene, (1-methyldecyl) **(145)**, benzene, (1-butyloctyl) **(146)**, benzene, (1-propylnonyl) **(147)**, benzene, (1-ethyldecyl) **(148)**, tetradecanoic acid, ethyl ester **(149)**, benzene, (1-methylundecyl) **(150)**, benzene,(1-propyldecyl) **(151)**, (E)-9-octadecenoic acid ethyl ester **(152)**, benzene, (1-ethylundecyl)- **(153)**, pentadecanoic acid, ethylester **(154)**, benzene, (1-methyldodecyl) **(155)**, ethyl 9-hexadecenoate **(156)**, heptadecanoic acid, ethyl ester **(157)**, octadecanoic acid, ethyl ester- **(158)**, 9,12-Octadecadien-1-ol, (Z,Z)- **(159)**, nonadecanoic acid, ethyl ester **(160)**, androstan-7-one, 3-(acetyloxy)-(3a,5a) **(161)**, 1,2-benzenedicarboxylic acid, mono-(2-ethylhexyl) ester **(162)** and eicosanoic acid, ethyl ester **(163)** were identified and reported through GC-MS on hexane extract of *C. spinosa* (Rajesh *et al.*, 2009;.Manikandaselvi and Brindha, 2014).

The adjuvant arthritic rat model was developed and reported to evaluate the antiarthritic effects of different fractions of ethanol extraction from *Capparis spinosa*. The ethanol water fraction was reported to possess most significant antiarthritic activity. The chemical constituents of this fraction were reported as seven known compounds such as stachydrine **(29)**, p-hydroxy benzoic acid **(164)**, 5-(hydroxymethyl) furfural **(165)**, bis-(5-for-mylfurfurly)-ether **(166)**, daucosterol **(167)**, α-D-fructo furanosides methyl **(168)** and uracil **(169)** (Xiaolu Feng *et al.*, 2011).

The caper bush as *Capparis spinosa* has been reported to possess different flavonoids such as quercetin-3-rutinoside **(62)**, quercetin-7-rutinoside **(170)**, quercetin-3-O-glucoside-7-O-rhamnoside **(171)**, kaempferol-3-rutinoside **(172)**, kaempferol-3-glucoside **(173)** (Sharrif *et al.*, 2012).

The plant *Capparis spinosa* leaf oil was composed and reported to possess phytochemicals likely isothiocyanates **(174)**, n-alkanes **(175)**, terpenoids **(176)**, a phenyl propanoid **(177)**, aldehyde **(178)** and fatty acid **(179)**. The main components of this oil were butyl isothiocyanate **(1)**, isopropyl isothiocyanate **(9)**, thymol **(180)** and 2-hexenol **(181)** reported. The volatile oils of the ripe fruit and the root were composed mainly of the methyl isothiocyanate **(8)**, isopropyl isothiocyanate **(9)** and sec-butyl isothiocyanates **(182)** was reported (Ahmed *et al.*, 1972).

Table 2.1: Phytochemical Compounds of *Capparis* genus (Chemical structures drawn through ISIS Chemdraw).

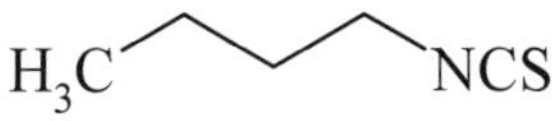 **Butyl isothiocyanate (1)**	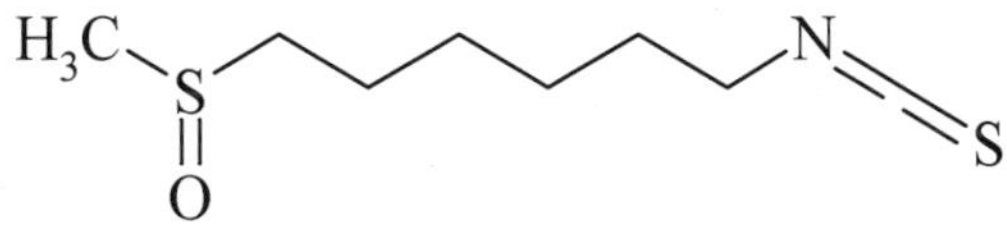 **6-Methylsulphonylhexylisothiocyanate (2)**
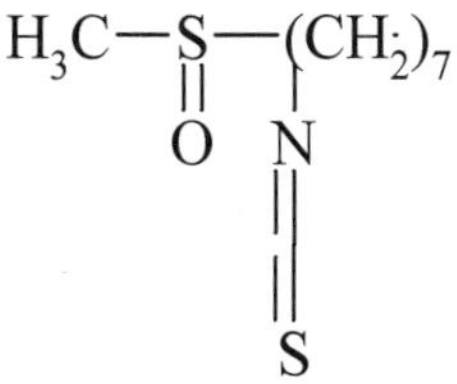 **7-Methylsulphonylheptyl isothiocyanate (3)**	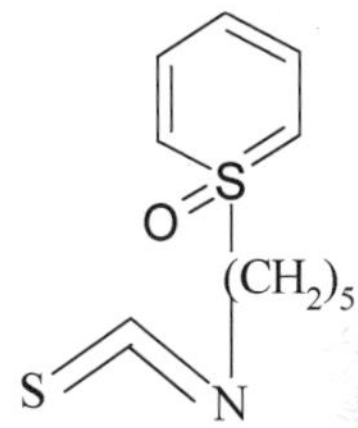 **5-Benzylsulphonyl-4-pentenylisothiocyanate (4)**
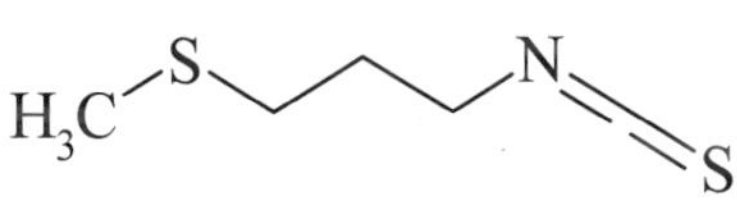 **3-Methylthiopropyl isothiocyanate (5)**	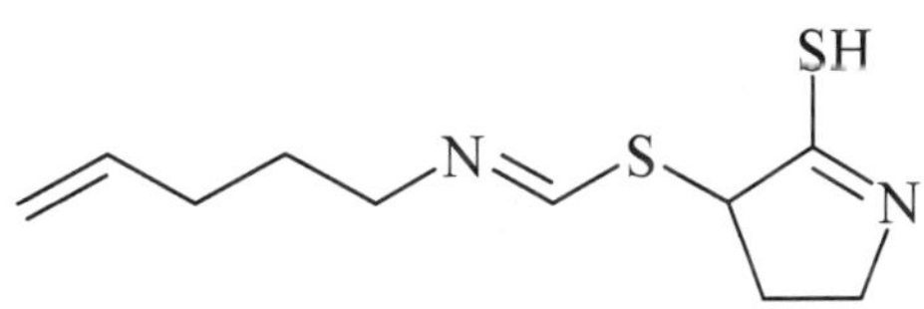 **11-(2-Butenylthio)-6-undecenyl isothiocyanate (6)**
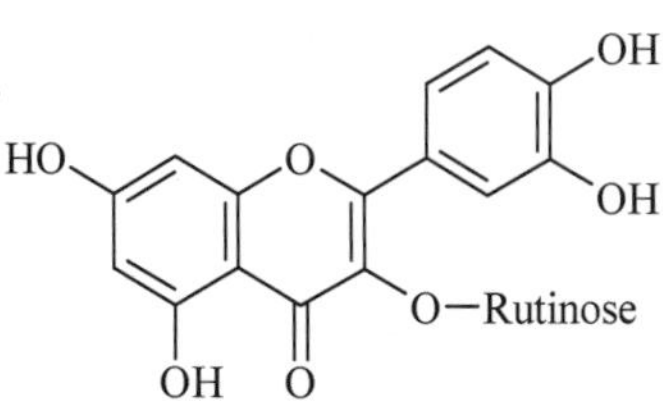 **Rutin (7)**	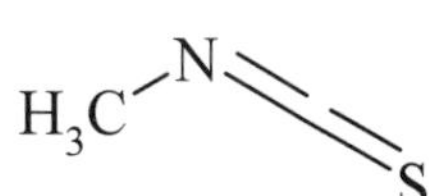 **Methyl isothiocyanate (8)**
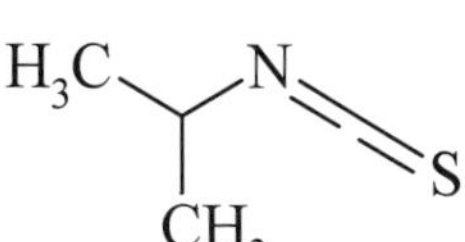 **Isopropyl isothiocyanate (9)**	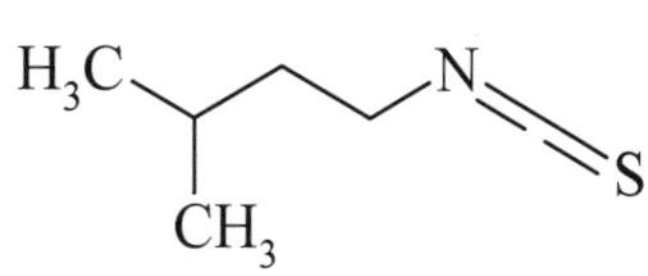 **Isobutyl isothiocyanate (10)**

Contd...

Table 2.1–*Contd...*

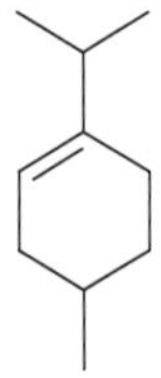

3-p-Menthene (11)

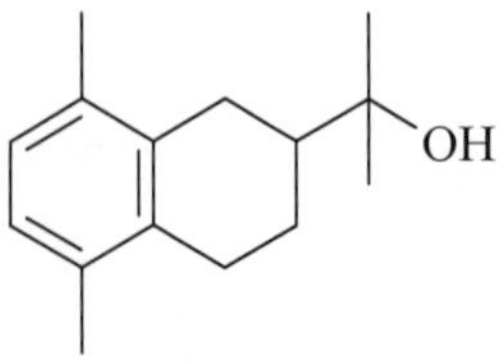

Occidol (12)

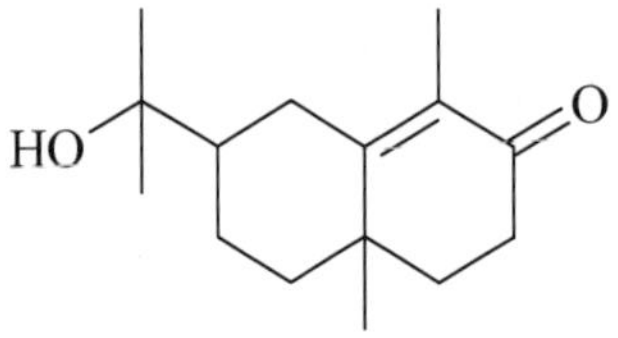

Carissone (13)

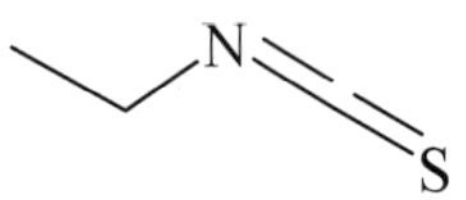

Ethyl isothiocyanate (14)

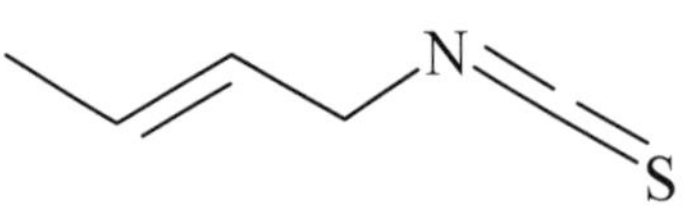

2-Butenyl isothiocyanate (15)

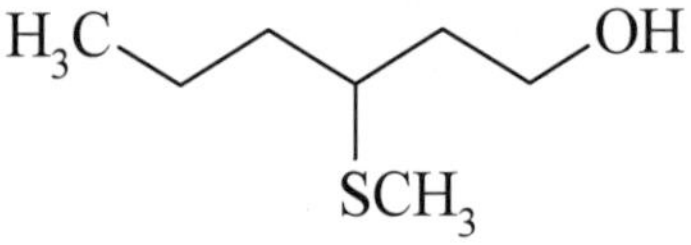

3-Methylthio-1-hexanol (16)

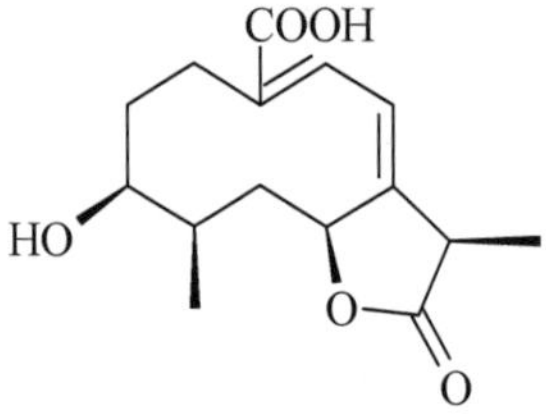

Germacr-3β-ol-7,9-dien-6, 14-olide-15-oicacid (17)

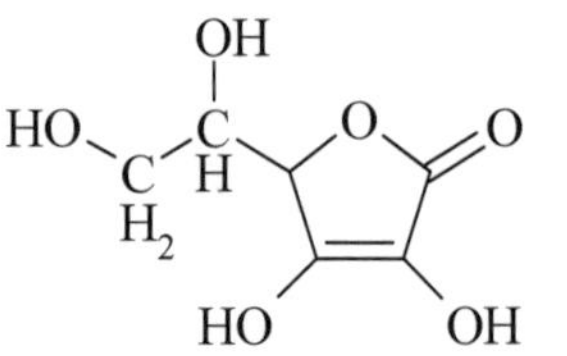

Ascorbic acid (18)

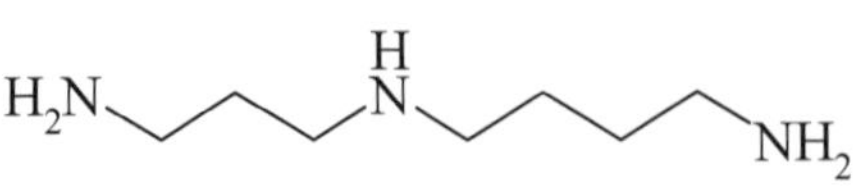

Spermidine alkaloid (19)

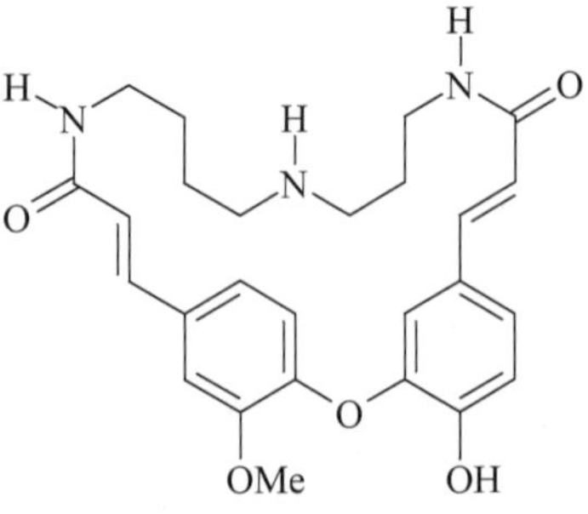

Codonocarpine (20)

Contd...

Table 2.1–*Contd...*

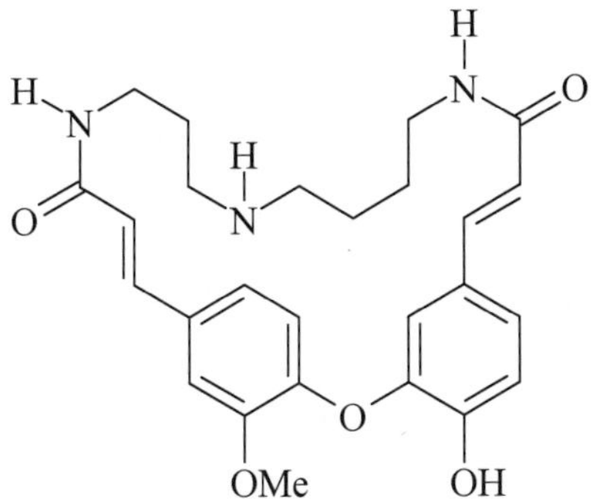

Isocodonocarpine (21)

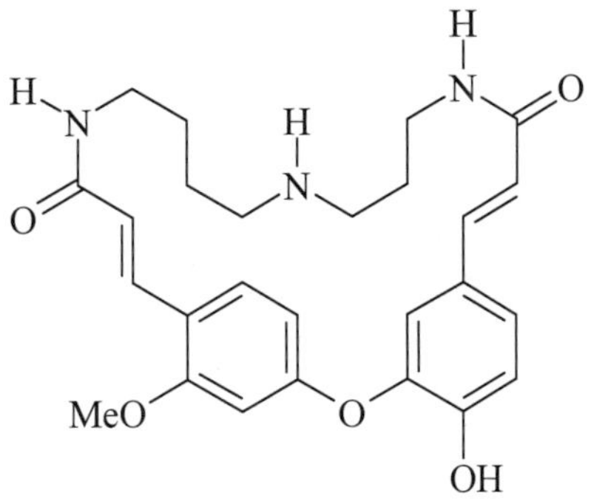

Capparisine (22)

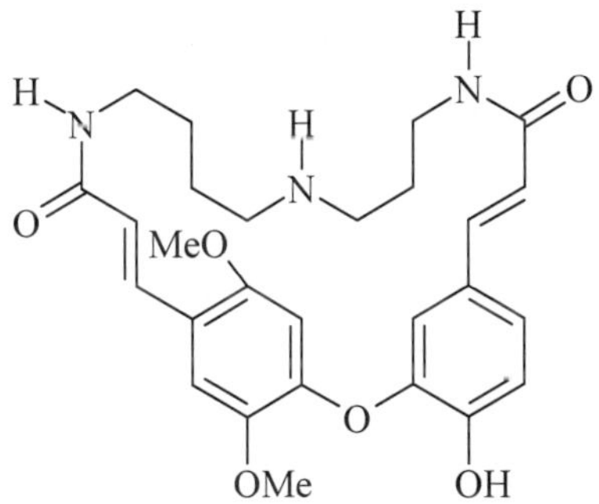

Capparisinine (23)

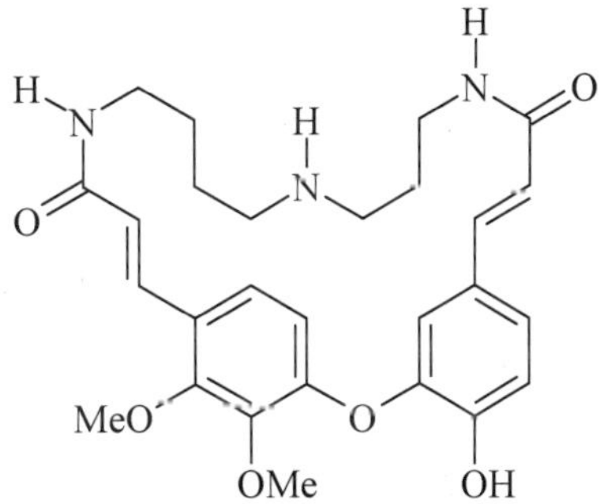

Capparidisine (24)

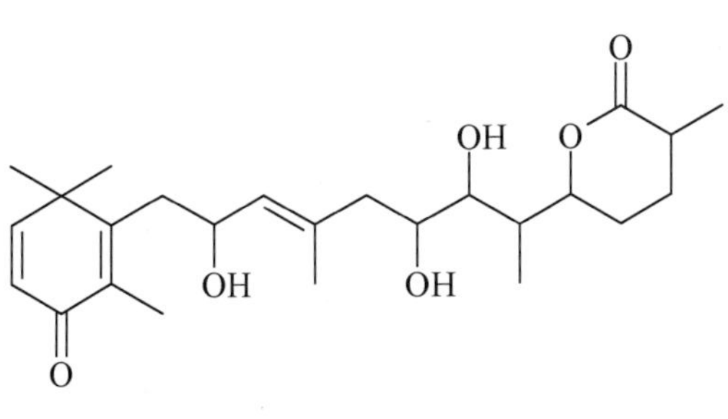

Decidua terpenolide A (25)

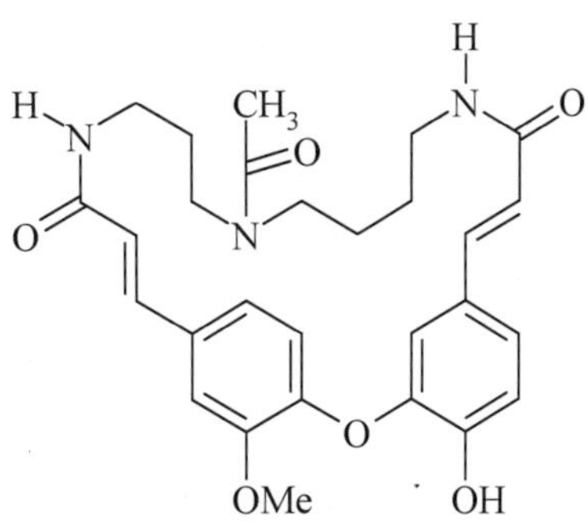

14-N-Acetylisocodonocarpine (26)

Contd...

Table 2.1–*Contd...*

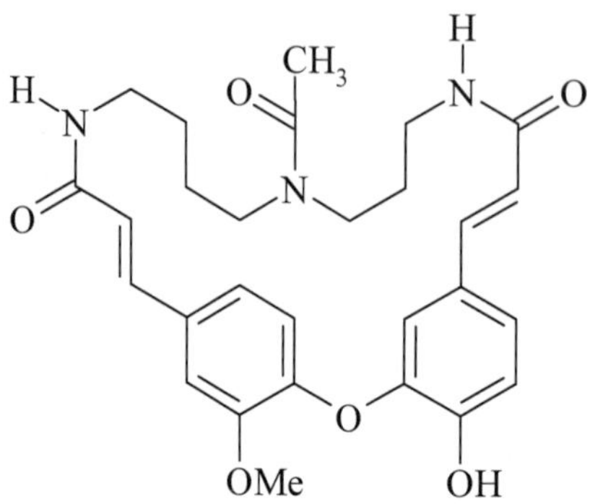

15-N-Acetyl capparisine (27)

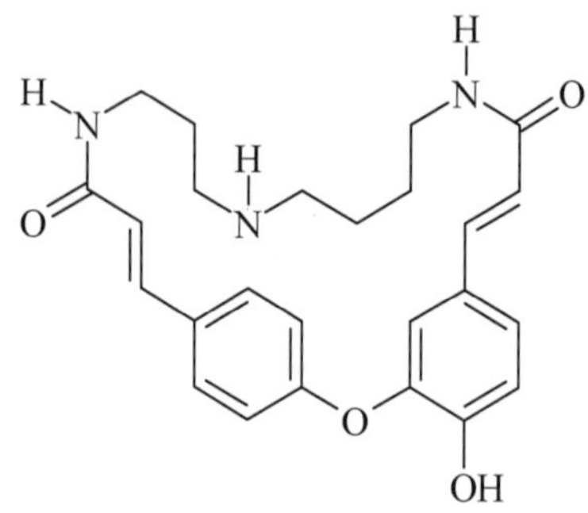

Cadabicine (28)

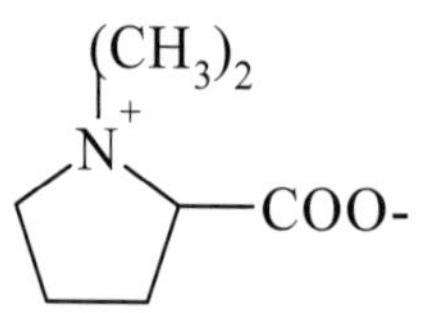

Stachydrine (29)

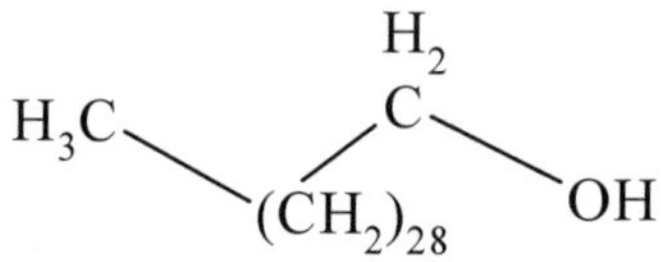

n-Triancontanol (30)

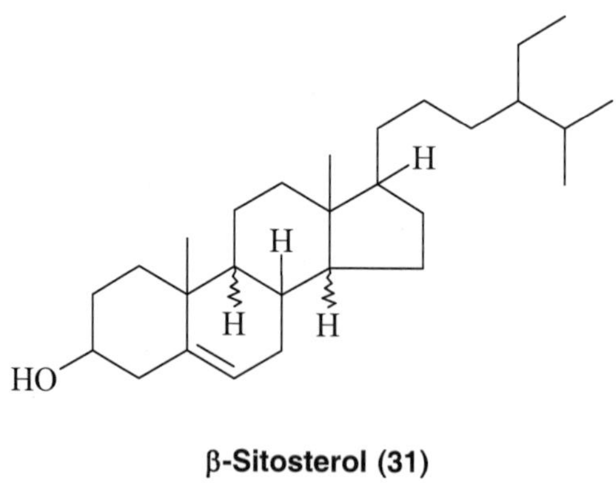

β-Sitosterol (31)

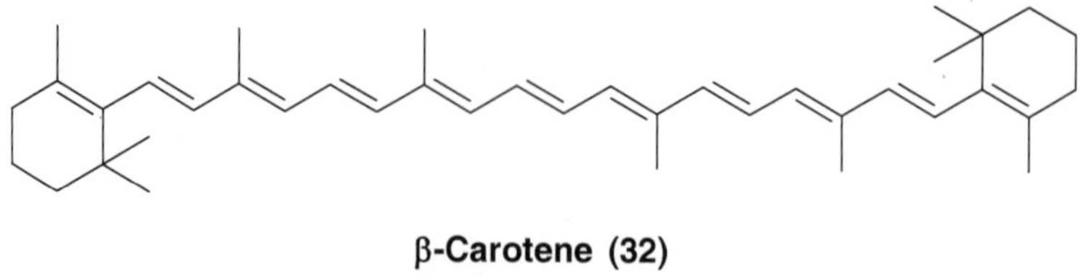

β-Carotene (32)

Contd...

Table 2.1–*Contd...*

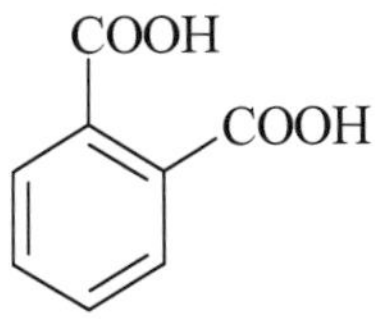

Phthalic acid (33)

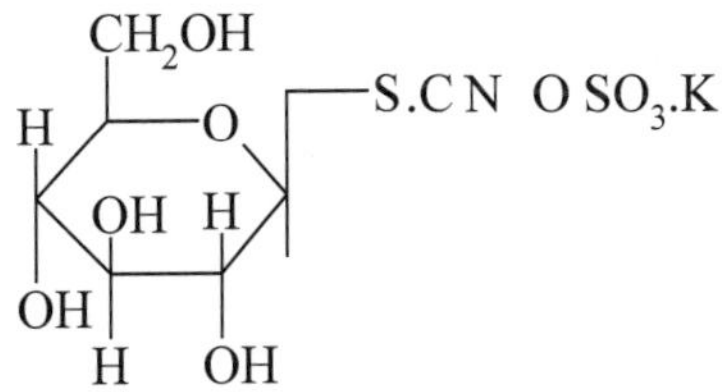

Glucocapparin (34)

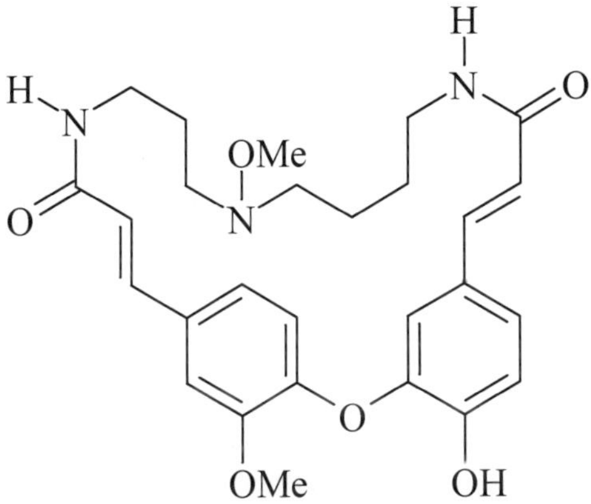

14-N-acetyl isocodonocarpine (35)

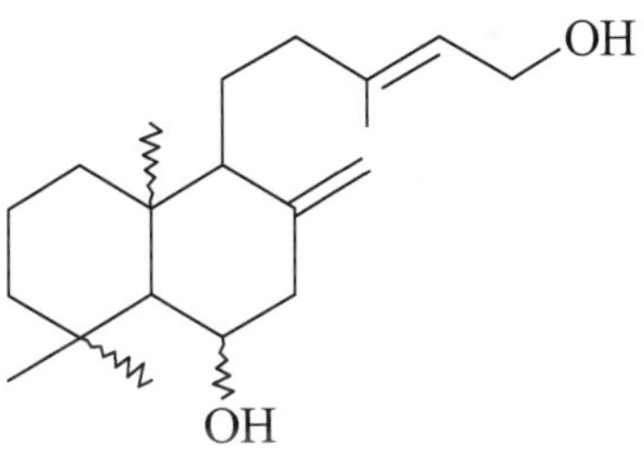

Diterpine alcohol (36)

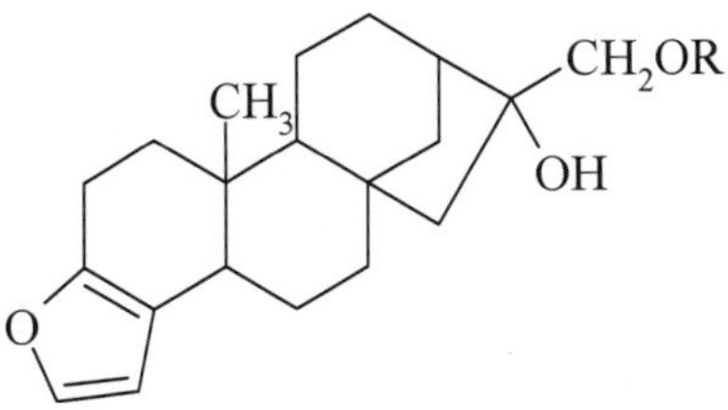

Diterpenic ester (37)

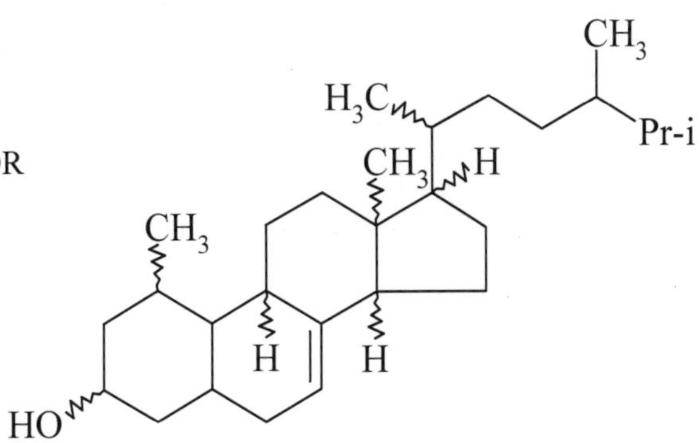

24-β-Methylcholest-7-ene-22-one-3-β-ol (38)

Contd...

Table 2.1–*Contd...*

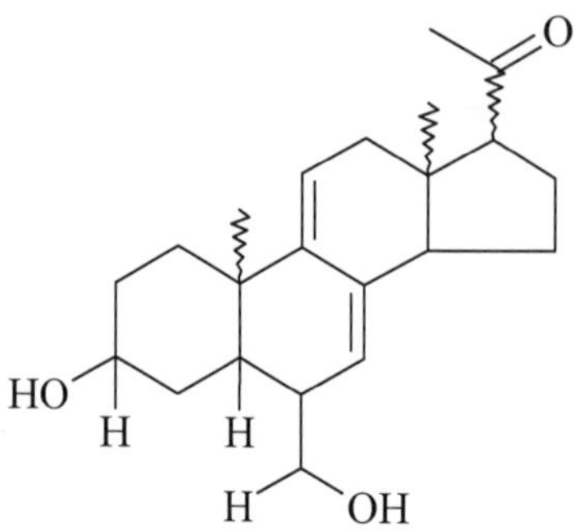

24-β-Methylcholest-9-(11)-ene-22-one-3β-ol (39)

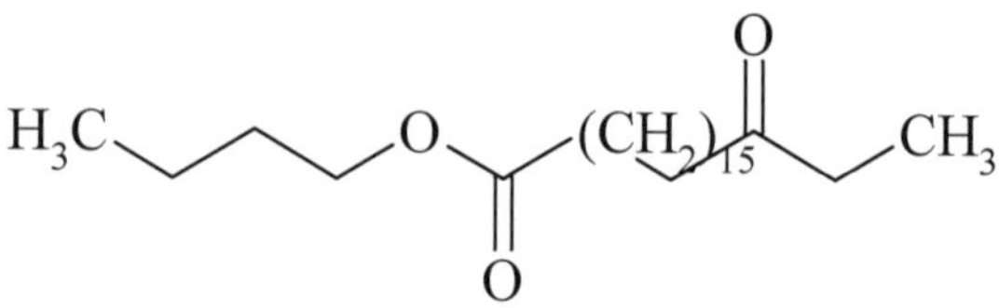

Butyl-3-oxoeicosanoate (40)

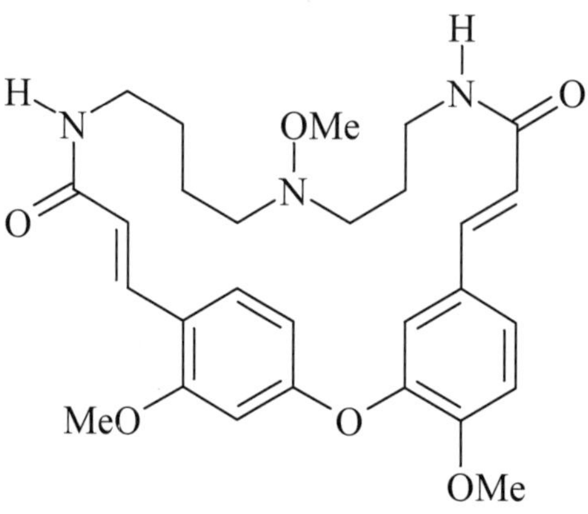

Diacetylcapparisine (41)

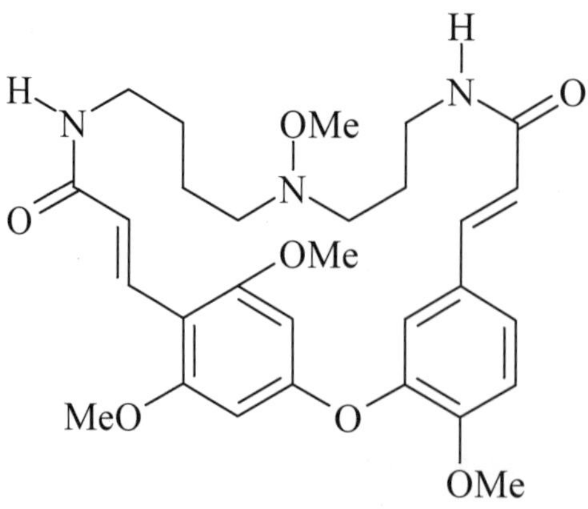

Capparisinine diacetate (42)

Contd...

Table 2.1–*Contd...*

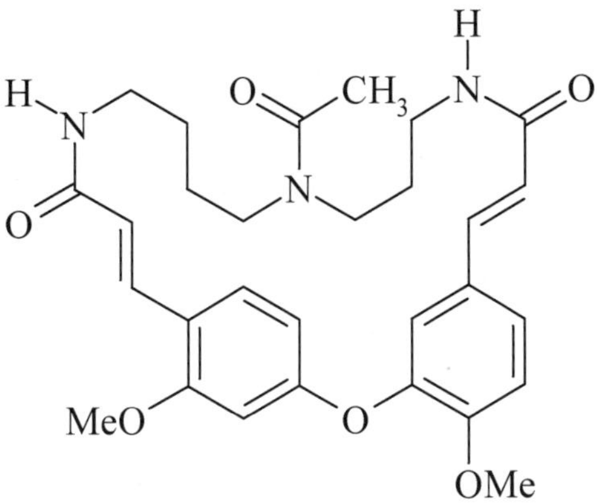

O-N-diacetylcapparisine (43)

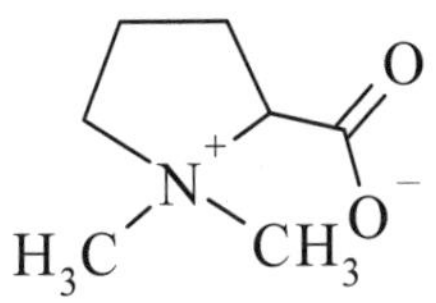

L-Stachydrine (44)

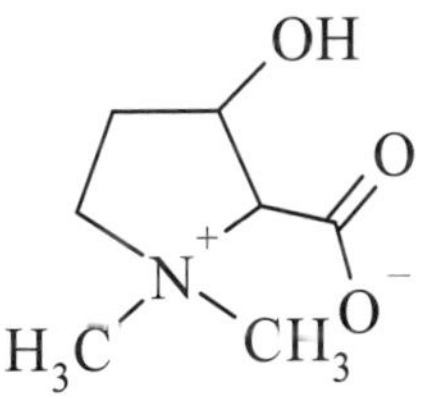

3-Hydroxy stachydrine (45)

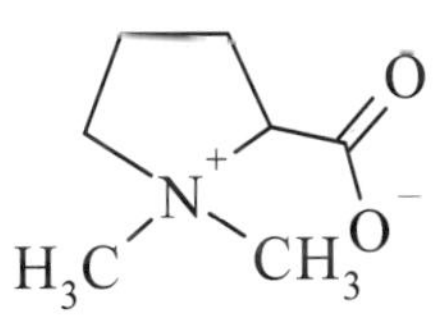

Prolinebetaine (46)

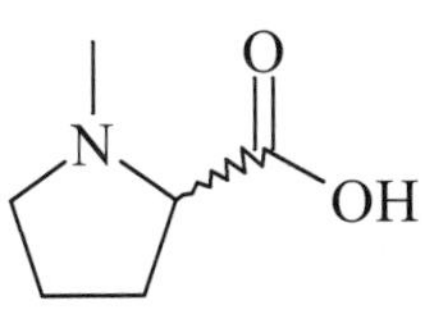

N-Methyl proline (47)

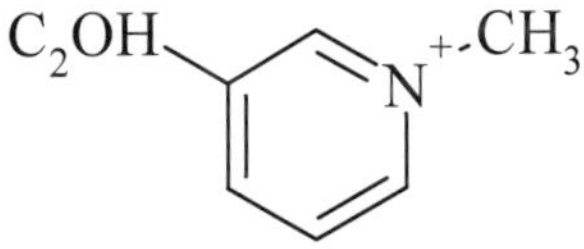

3-Carbomethyoxy-N-methoxypyridinium (trigonelline) (48)

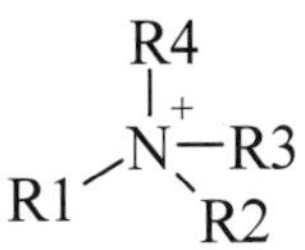

Quaternary ammonium compounds (49)

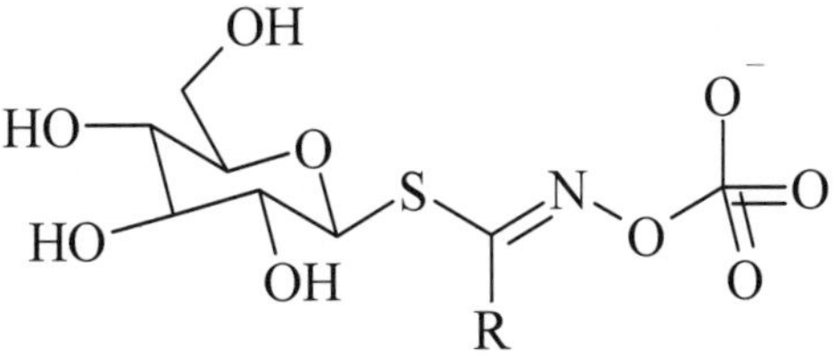

Glucosinolates (50)

Contd...

Table 2.1–*Contd...*

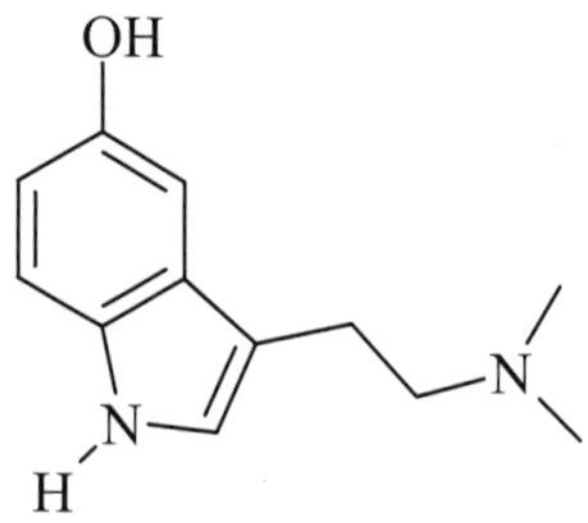

Alkaloids (51)

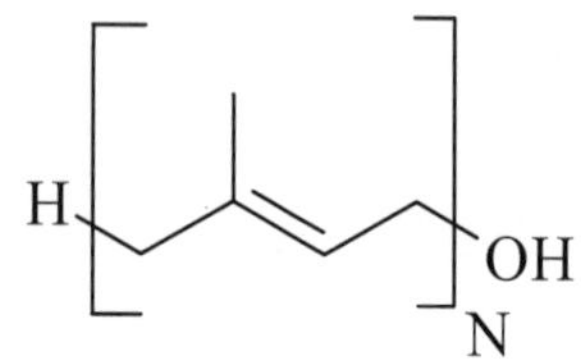

Polyprenals (52)

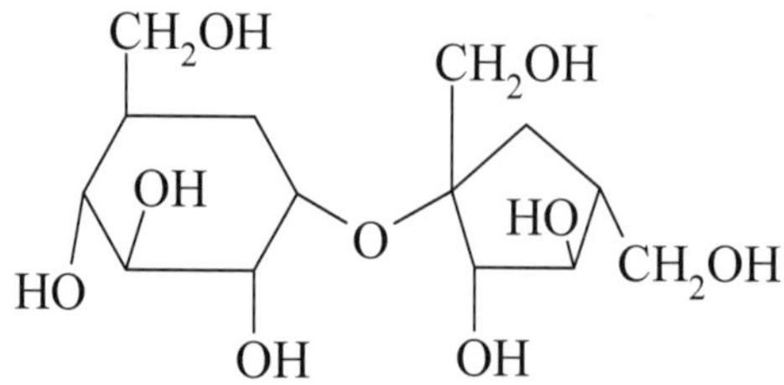

Saccharose (53)

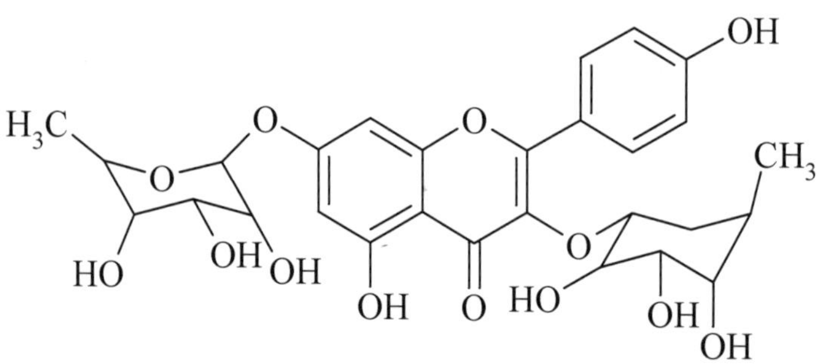

Kaempferol-3,7-dirrhamnoside (54)

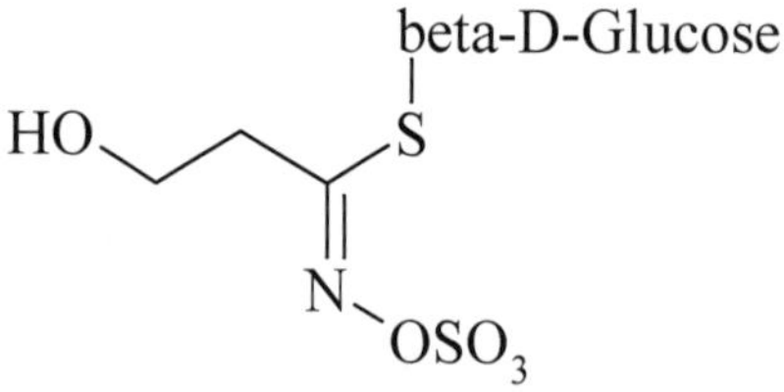

2-Hydroxyethyl glucosinolate (55)

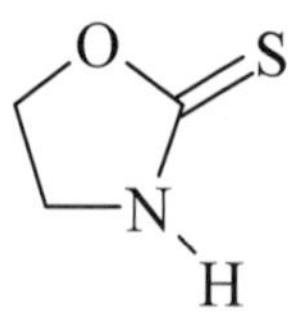

Oxazolidine-2-thione (56)

Contd...

Table 2.1–*Contd...*

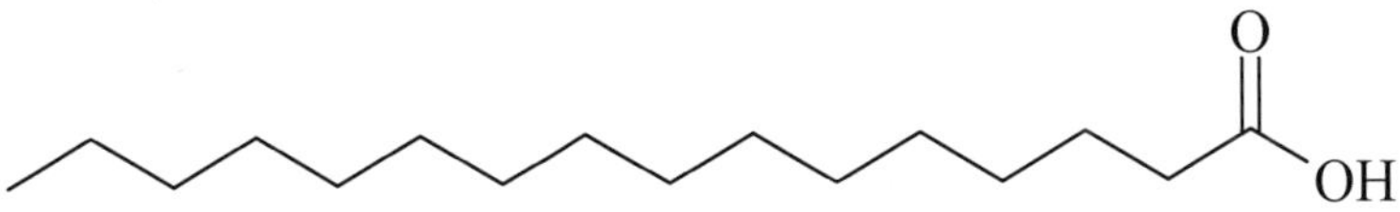

Palmitic acid (57)

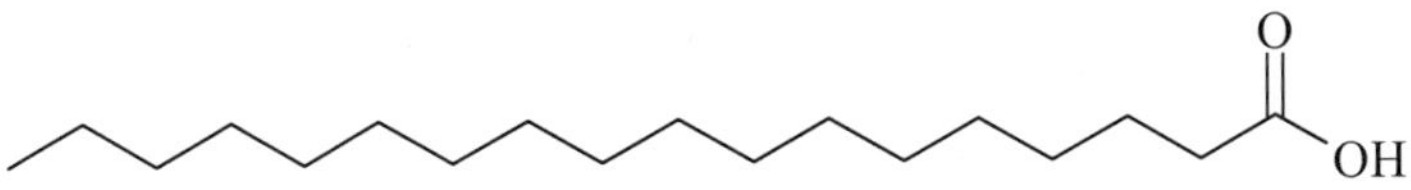

Stearic acid (58)

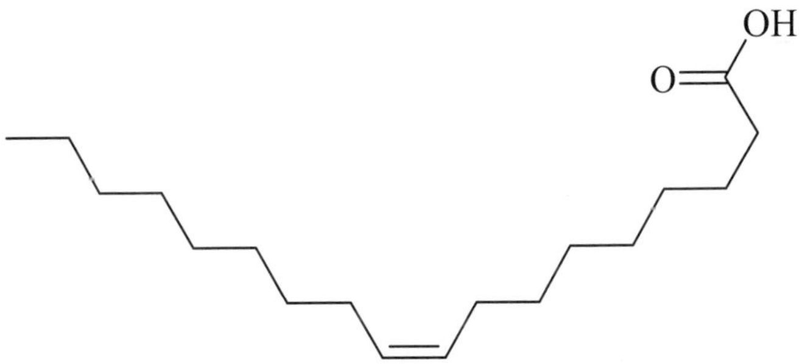

Oleic acid (59)

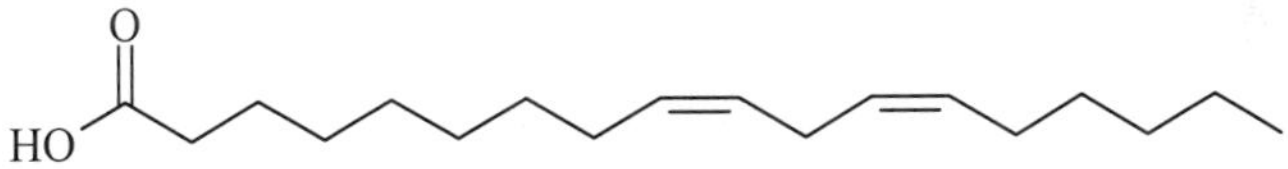

Linoleic acid (60)

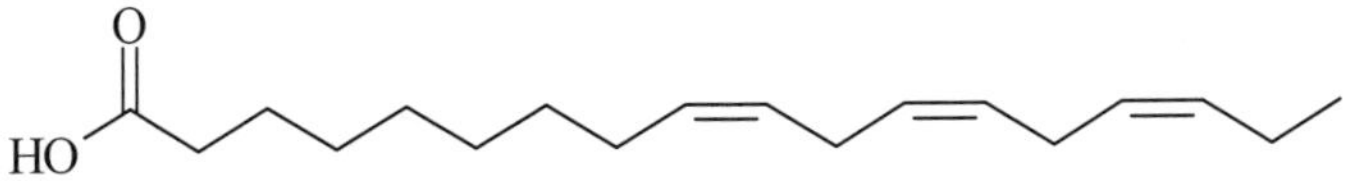

Linolenic acid (61)

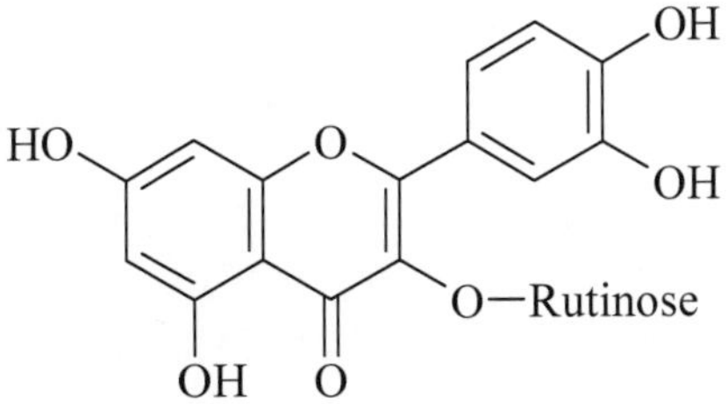

Quercetin-3-rutinoside (62)

Contd...

Table 2.1–*Contd...*

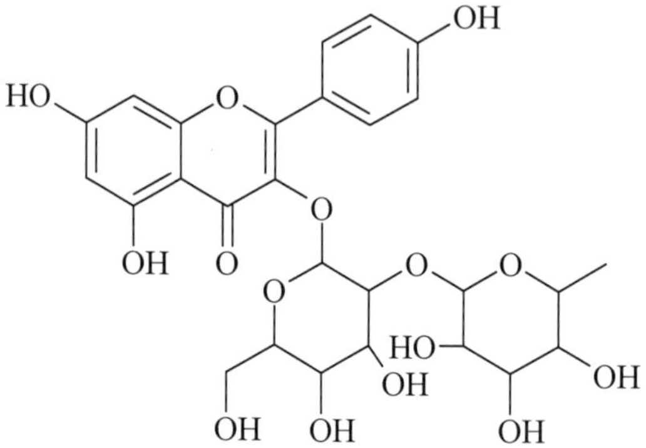

Kaempferol-3-rutinoside (63)

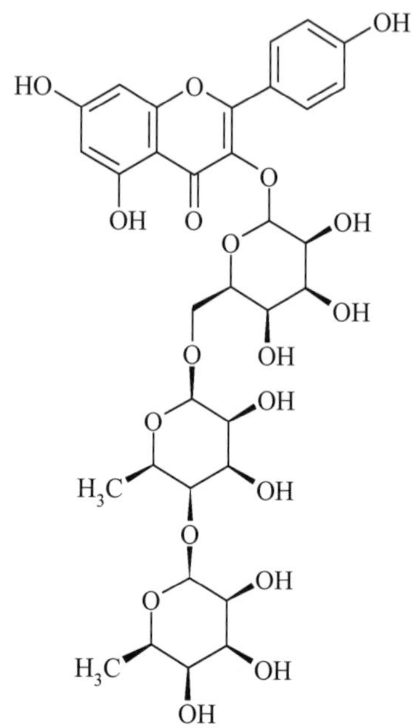

Kaempferol-3-rhamnosyl-rutinoside (64)

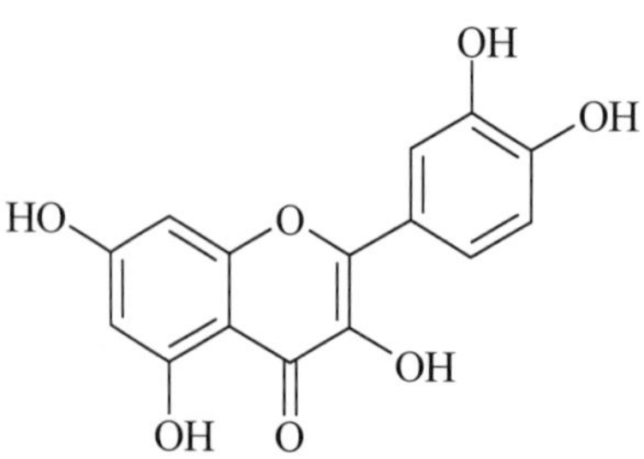

Quercetin (65)

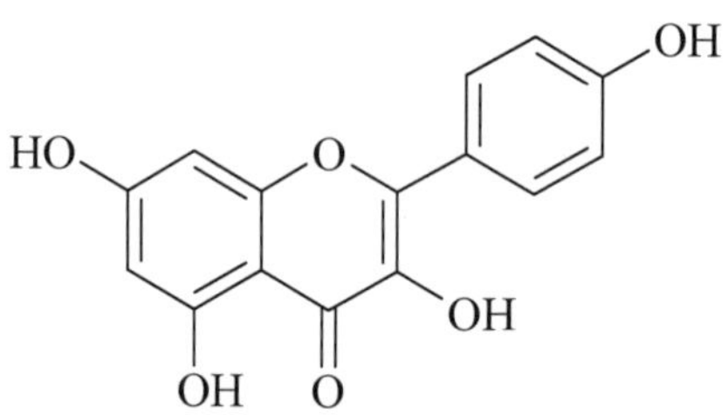

Kaempferol (66)

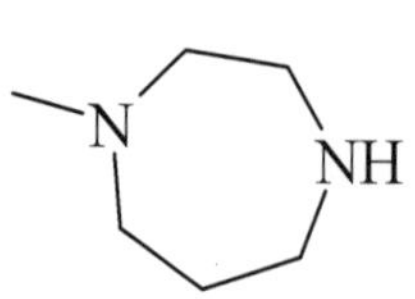

N-Methylhomopiperazine (67)

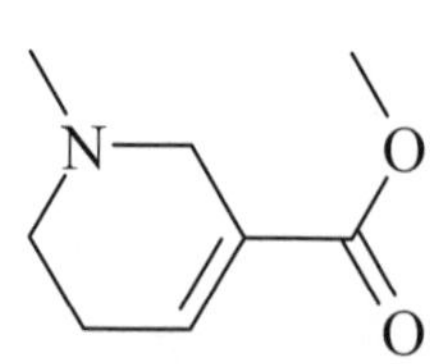

3-Pyridinecarboxylic acid-1,2, 5,6-tetrahydro-1-methyl-methyl ester (68)

Contd...

Table 2.1–*Contd...*

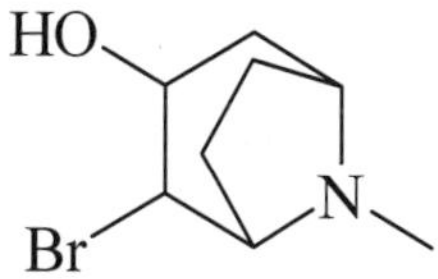

8-Azabicyclo(3,2,1)-ocatan-3-ol-2-bromo-8-methyl-(exo, exo) (69)

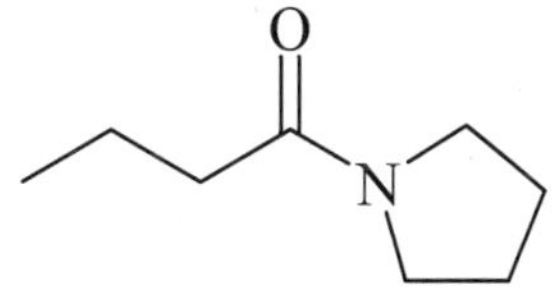

Pyrrolidine-1-(1-oxobutyl) (70)

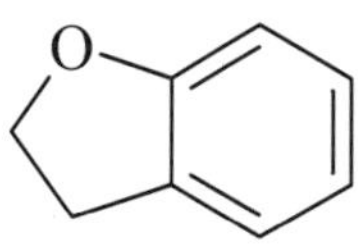

Benzofuran-2,3-dihydro (71)

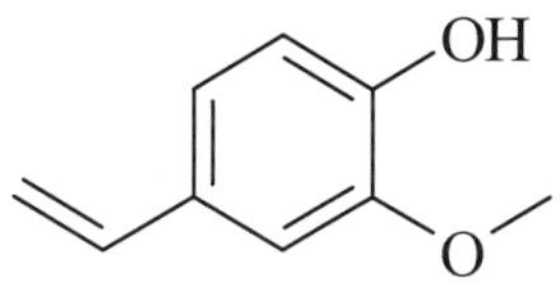

2-Methoxy-4-vinylphenol (72)

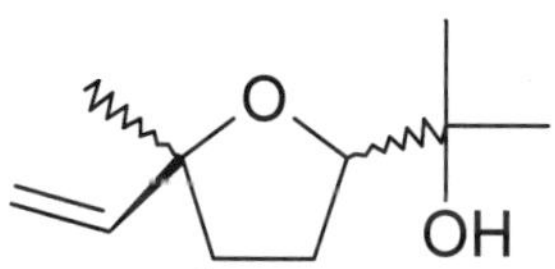

2-Furanmethanol-5-ethenyltetrahydro-α,α,5-trimethyl-,cis- (73)

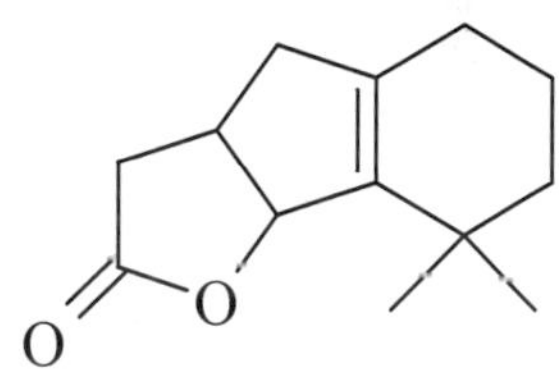

2H-Indeno(1,2-b)furan-2-one,3,3a,4,5,6,7,8,8b-octahydro-8,8-dimethyl (74)

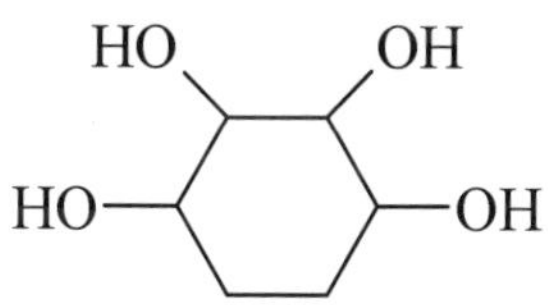

1,2,3,4-Cyclohexanetetrol (75)

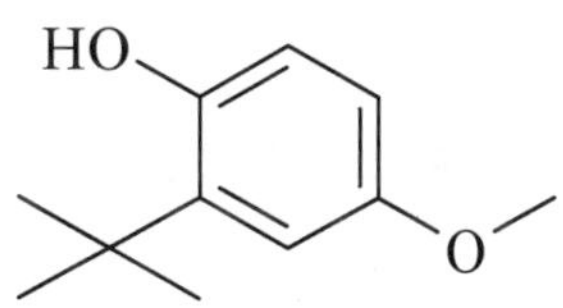

3-Tert-Butyl-4-hydroxyanisole (76)

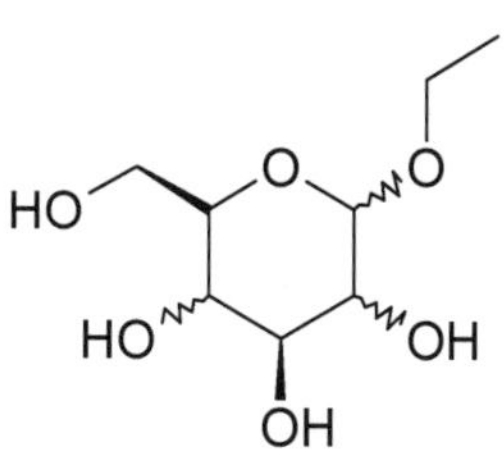

Ethyl-α-d-glucopyranoside (77)

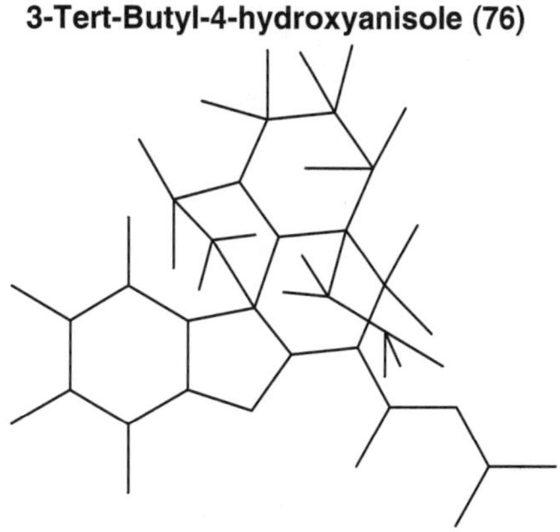

Aspidospermidine-3-carboxylic acid-2,3-didehydro-methyl ester, (5α, 12β, 19α)-(Synonym: Vincadifformine) (78)

Contd...

Table 2.1–*Contd...*

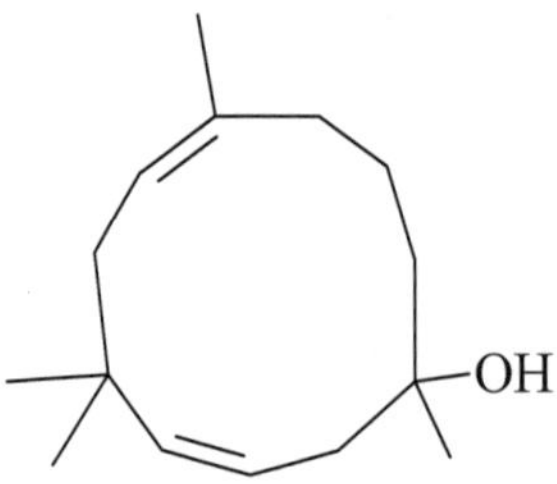

3,7-3,7-Cycloundecadien-1-ol, 1,5,5,8-tetramethyl- (79)

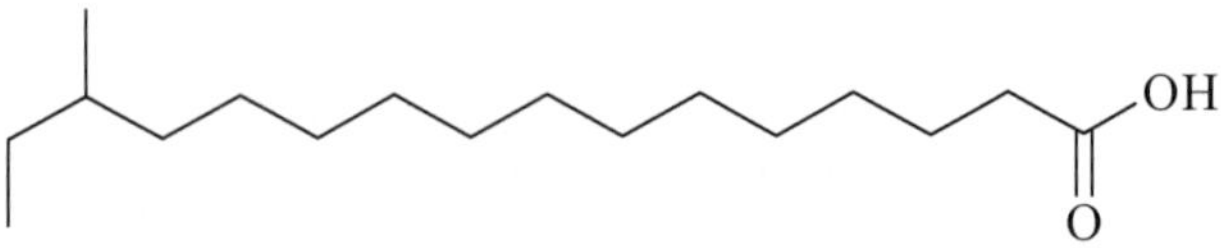

Pentadecanoic acid-14-methyl-methyl ester (80)

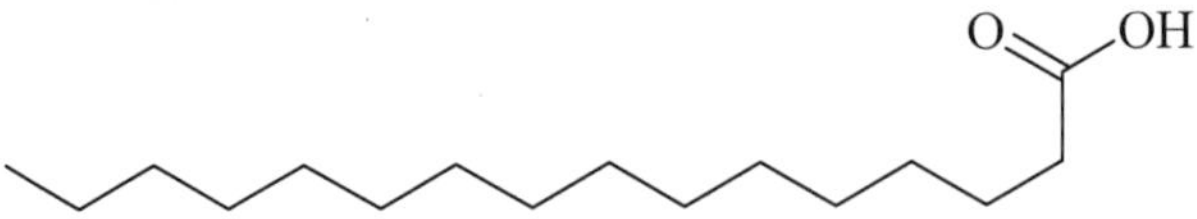

n-Hexadecanoic acid (81)

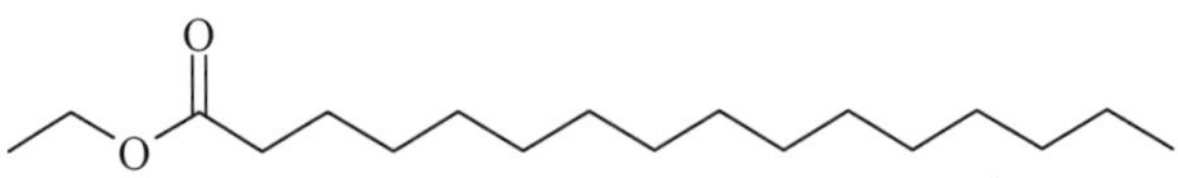

Hexadecanoic acid, ethyl ester (82)

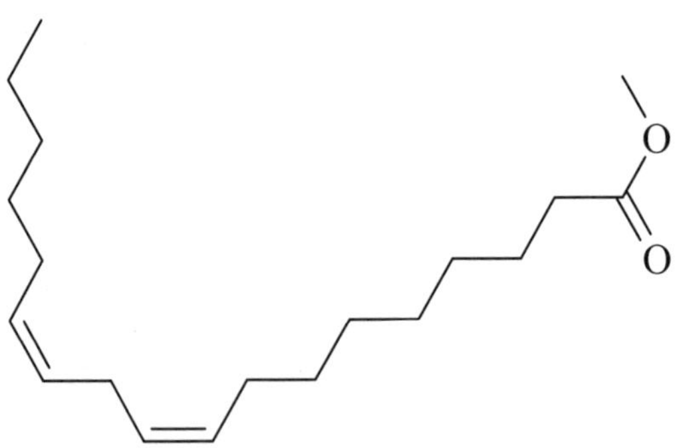

9,12-Octadecadienoic acid-(Z,Z)-methyl ester (83)

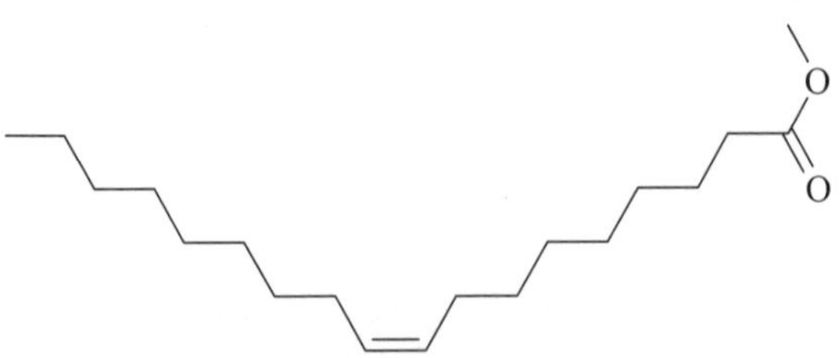

9-Octadecenoic acid-(Z)-methyl ester (84)

Contd...

Table 2.1–*Contd...*

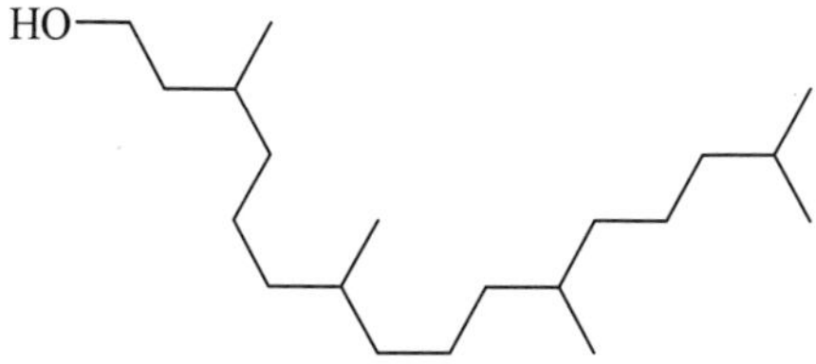

Phytol (85)

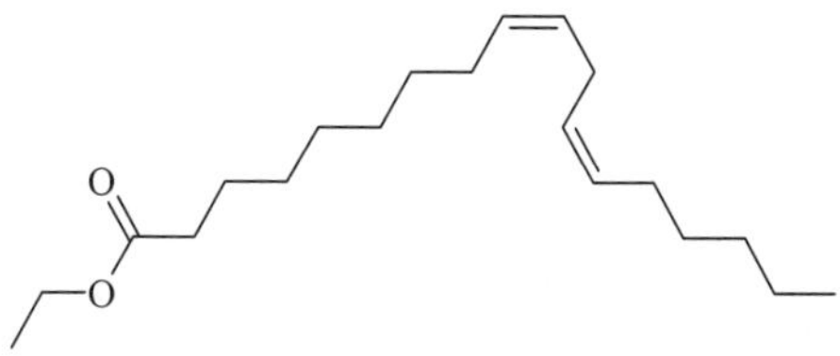

9,12-Octadecadienoic acid, ethyl ester (86)

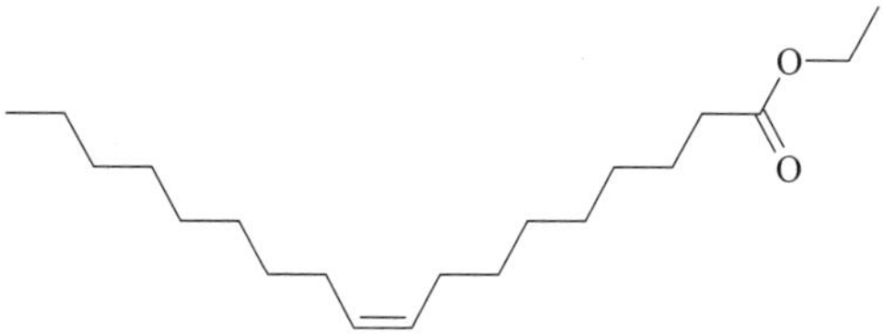

Ethyl oleate (87)

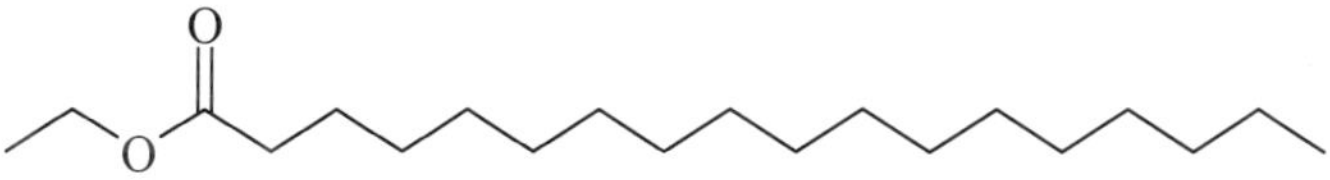

Octadecanoic acid, ethyl ester (88)

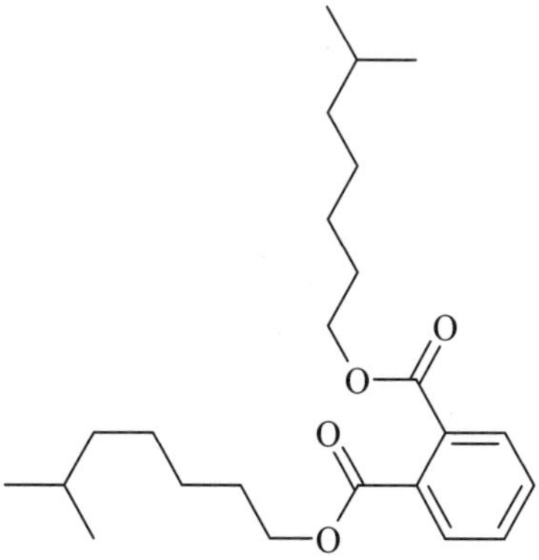

1,2-Benzenedicarboxylic acid, diisooctyl ester (89)

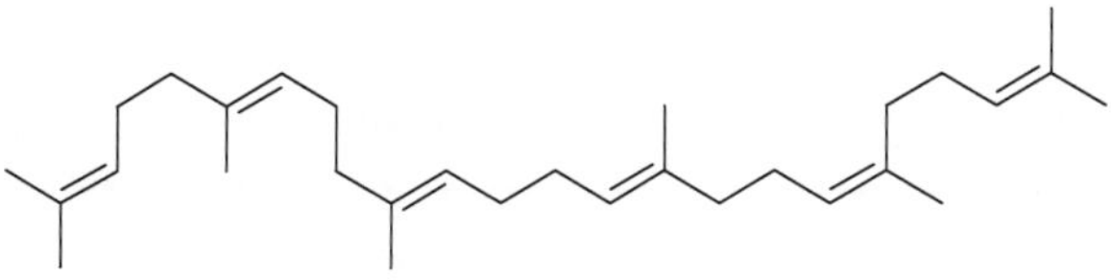

Squalene (90)

Contd...

Table 2.1–*Contd...*

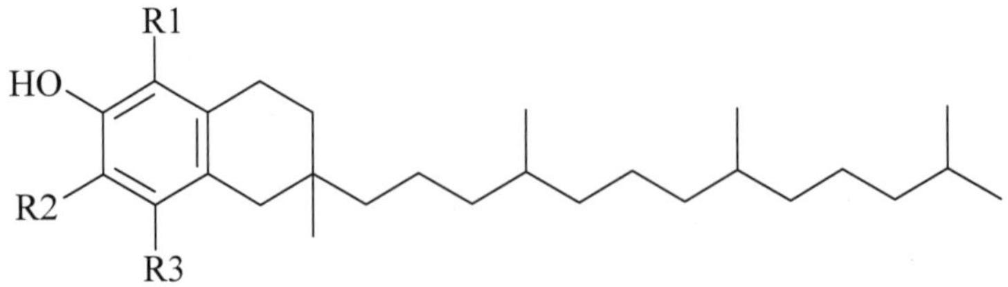

τ-Tocopherol (91)

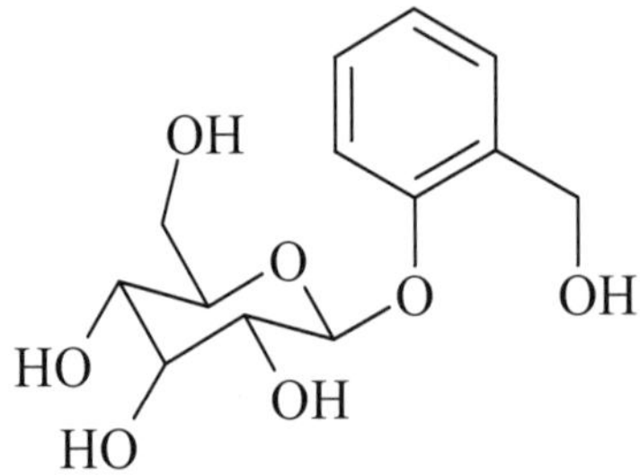

Glycosides (92)

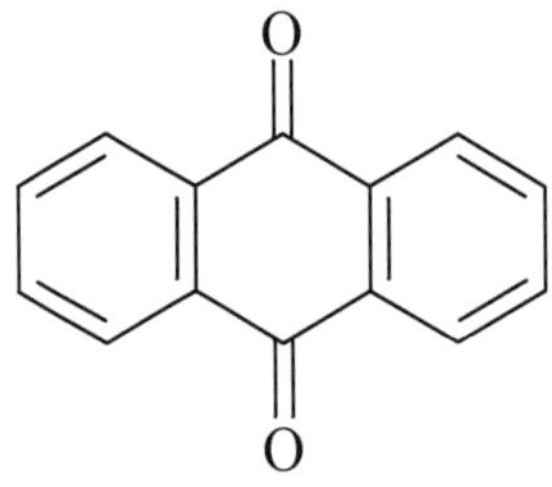

Anthraquinones (93)

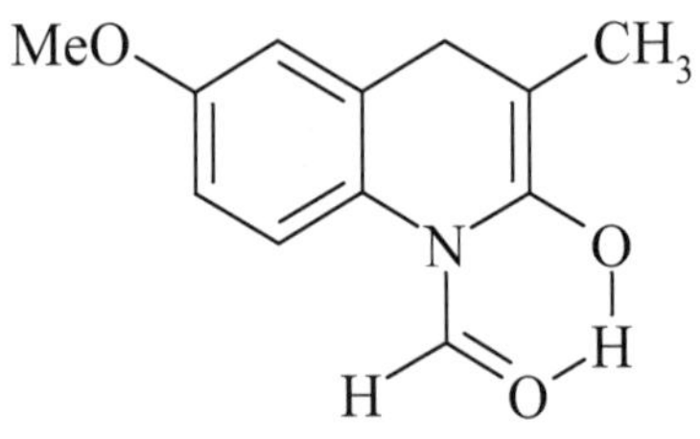

3(4H)-One-6-methoxy-2-methyl-4-carbaldehyde (94)

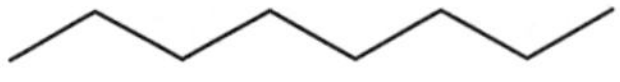

Octane (95)

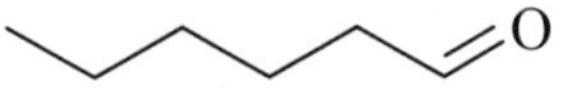

Hexanal (96)

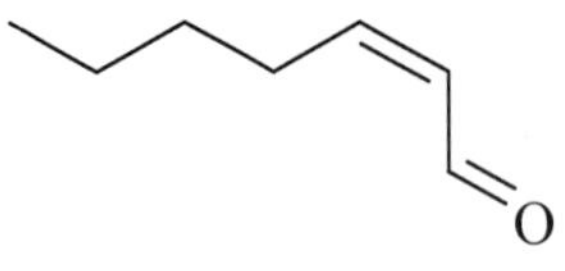

2-Heptenal,(z)- (97)

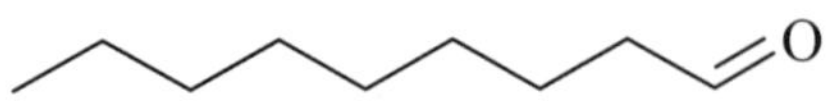

Nonanal (98)

Contd...

Table 2.1–*Contd...*

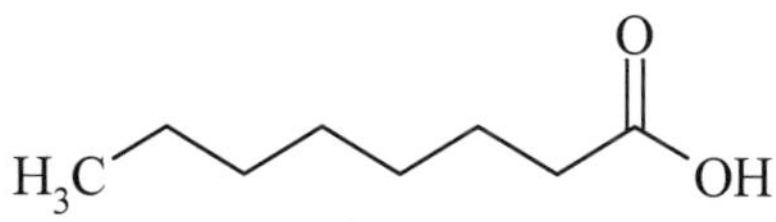

Octanoic acid (99)

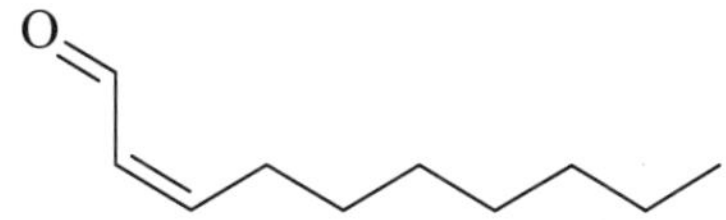

2-Decenal-(z) (100)

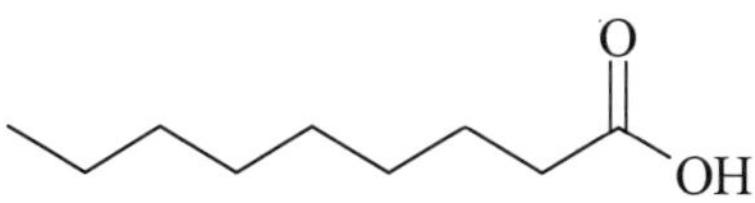

Nonanoic acid (101)

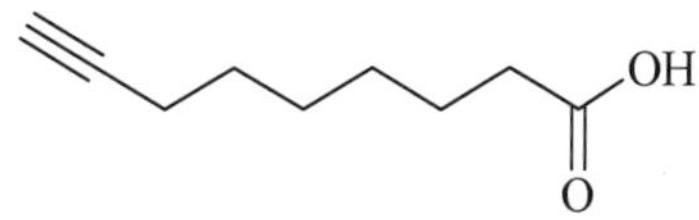

8-Nonynoic acid (102)

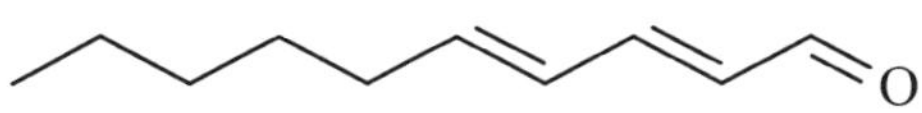

2,4-Decadienal (103)

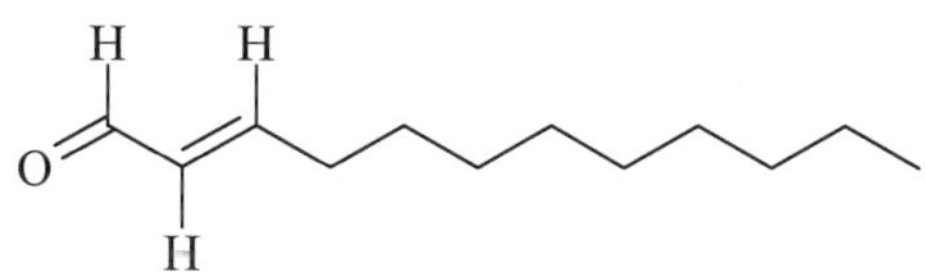

2-Dodecenal (104)

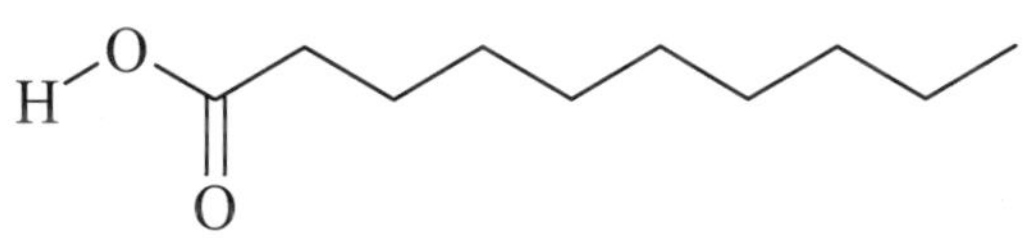

n-Decanoic acid (105)

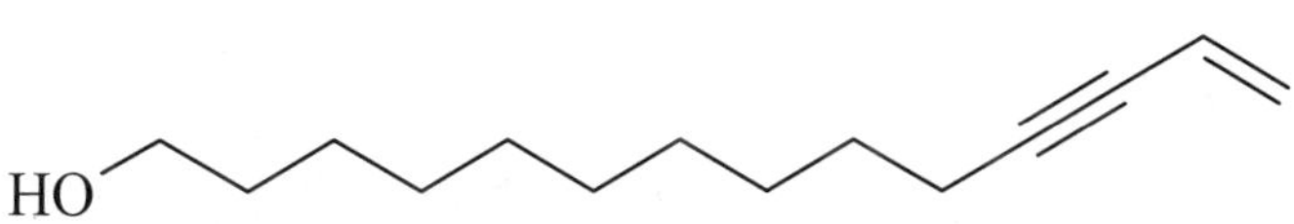

13-Tetradece-11-yn-1-ol (106)

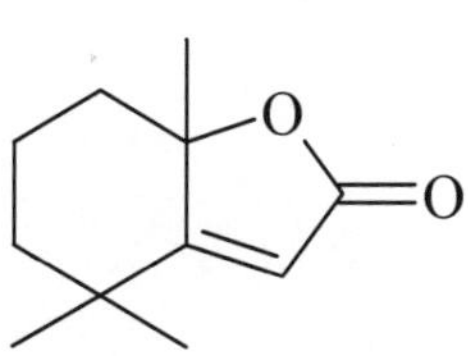

2(4H)-Benzofuranone, 5,6,7,7a-tetrahydro-4,4, 7a-trimethyl (107)

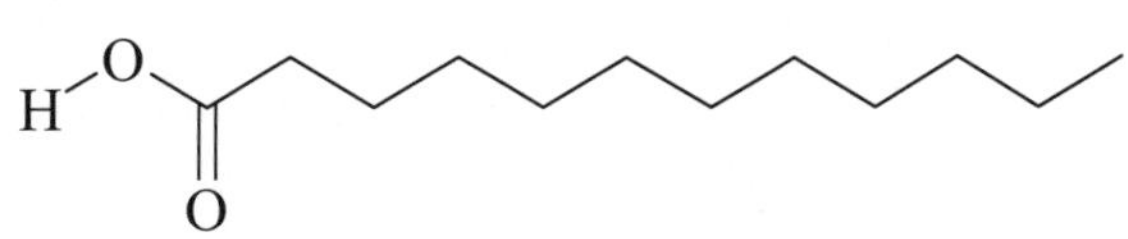

Dodecanoic acid (108)

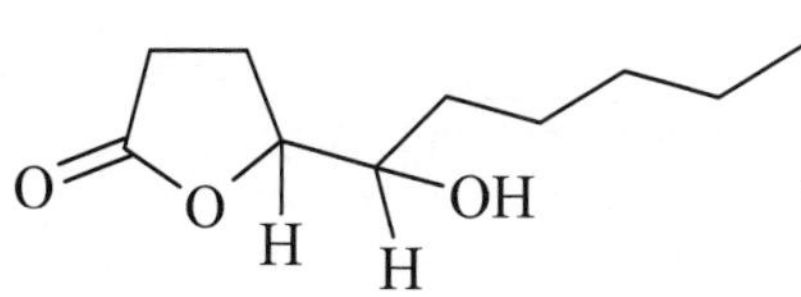

Tetrahydrofuran-2-one,5-(1-hydroxyhexyl)- (109)

Contd...

Table 2.1–*Contd...*

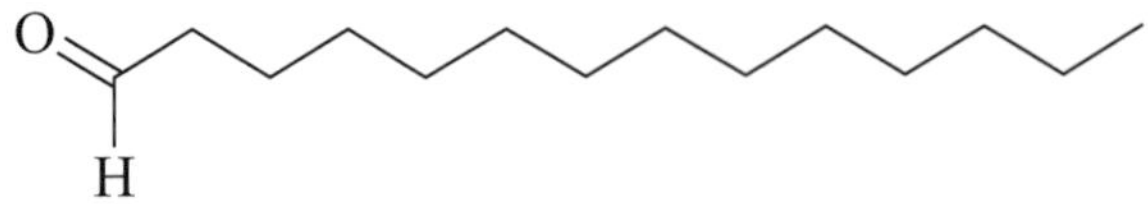

Tetradecanal (110)

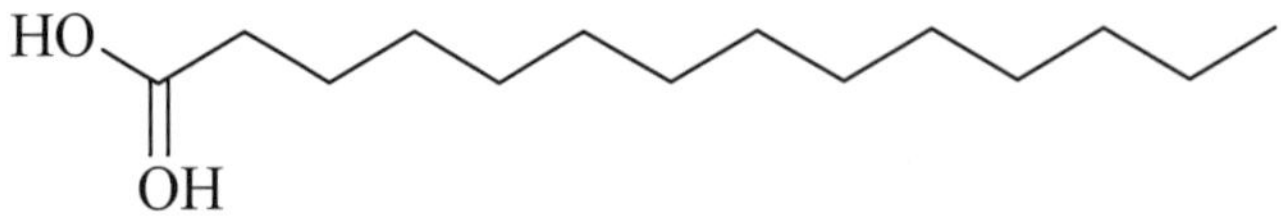

Tetradecanoic acid (111)

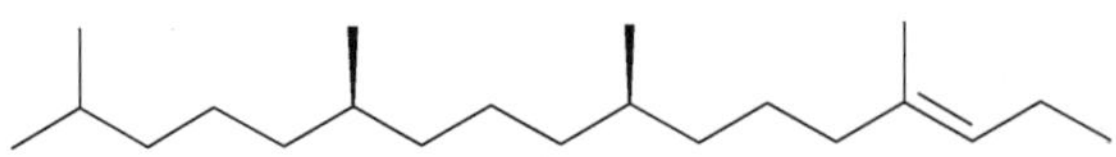

2-Hexadecen,3,7,11,15-tetramethyl-(R-(R*,R*-(E))) (112)

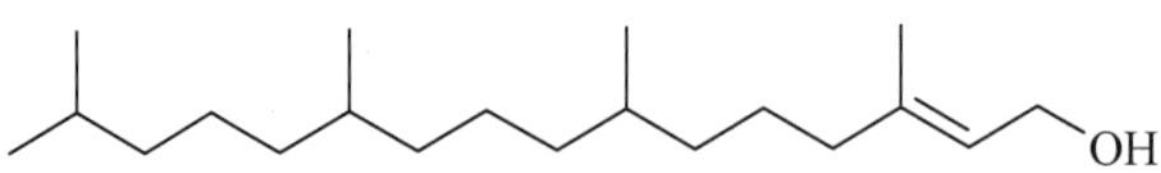

3,7,11,15-Tetramethyl-2-hexadecen-1-ol (113)

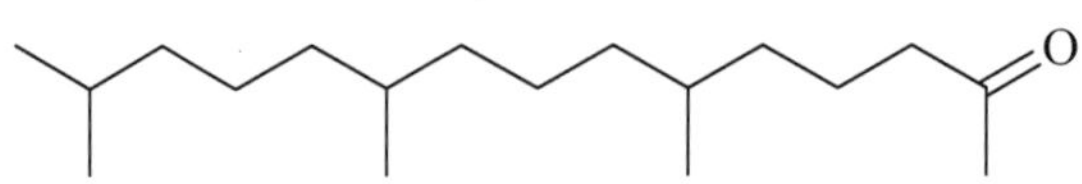

2-Pentadecanone-6,10,14-trimethyl (114)

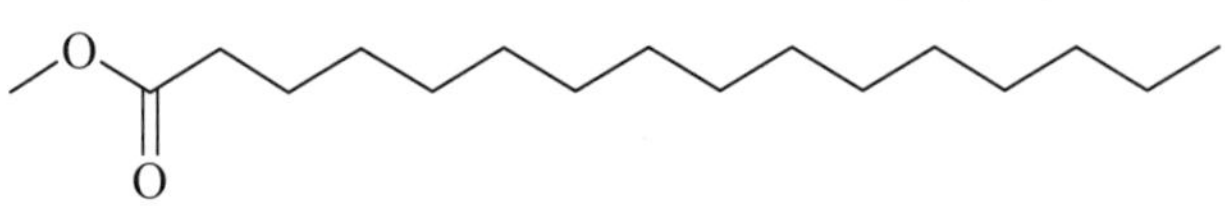

Hexadecanoic acid, methyl ester (115)

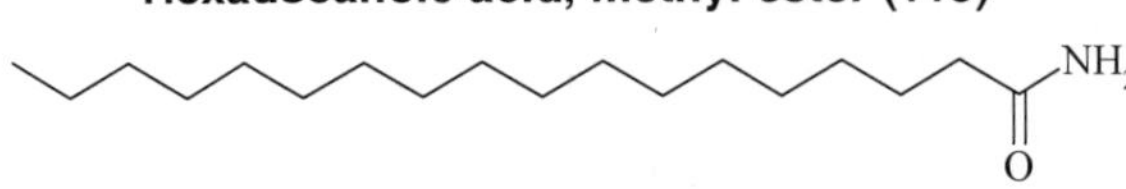

Octadecanamide (116)

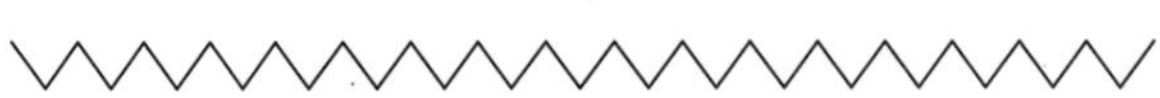

Pentatriacontane (117)

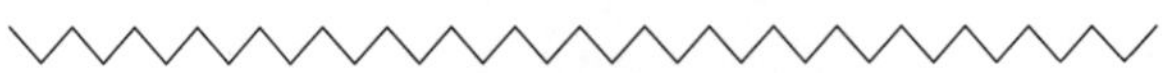

Hexatriacontane (118)

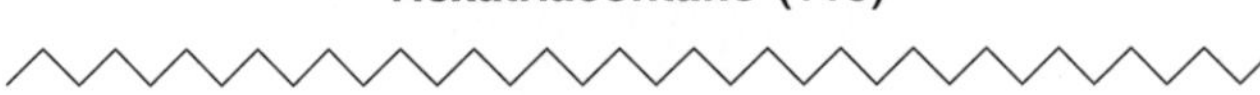

Tetratriacontane (119)

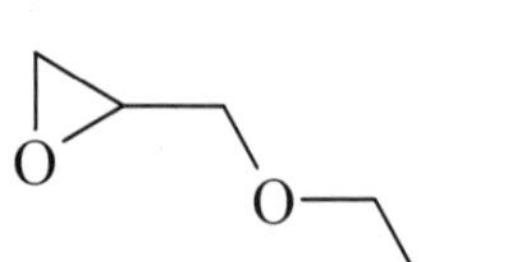

1-Propane, 1-(2-propenyloxy) (120)

Contd...

Table 2.1–*Contd...*

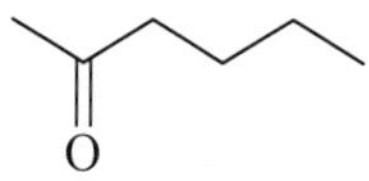

(E)-2-Hexanone (121)

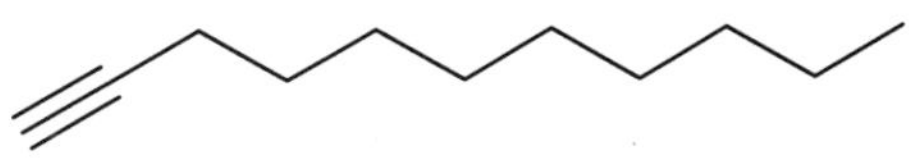

1-Undecyne (122)

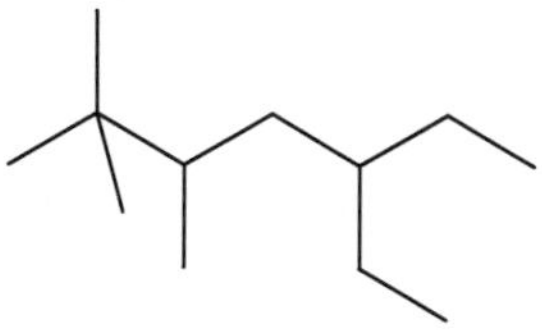

Heptanes,5-ethyl-2,2,3-trimethyl- (123)

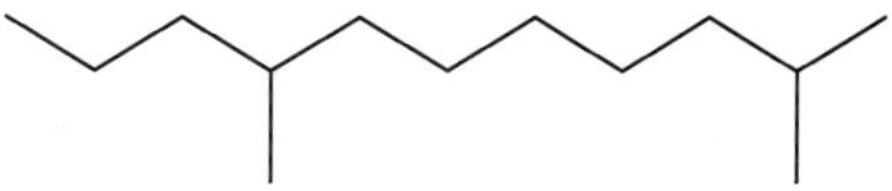

Undecane, 2,8-dimethyl- (124)

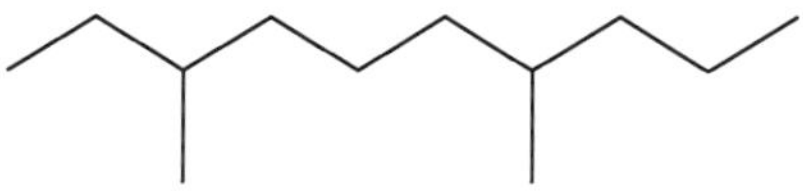

Decane, 3,7-dimethyl- (125)

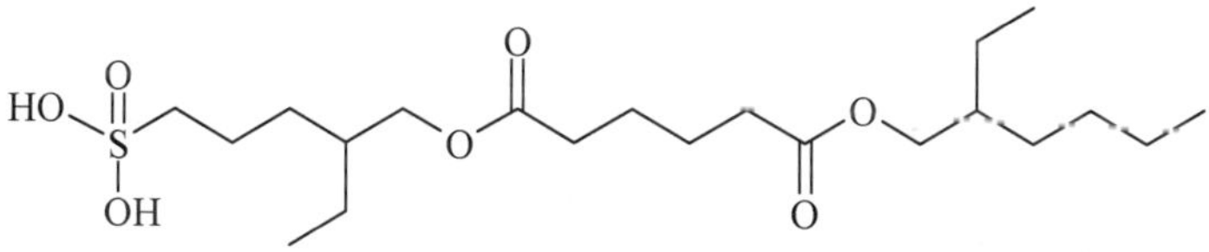

Sulfurous acid, di(2-ethylhexyl) ester (126)

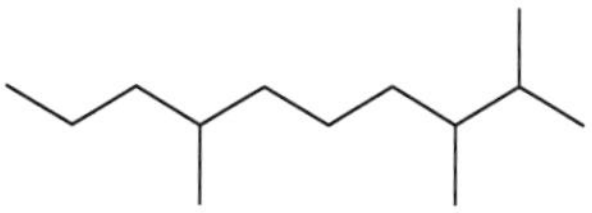

Decane,2,3,7-trimethyl- (127)

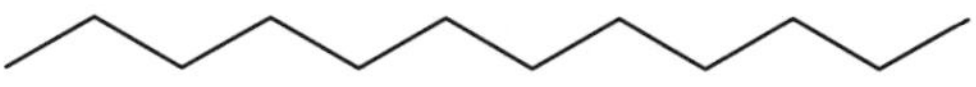

Dodecane (128)

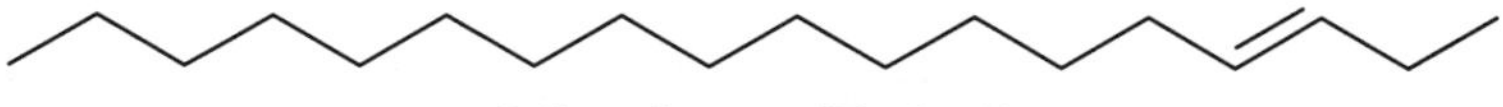

3-Octadecene,(E)- (129)

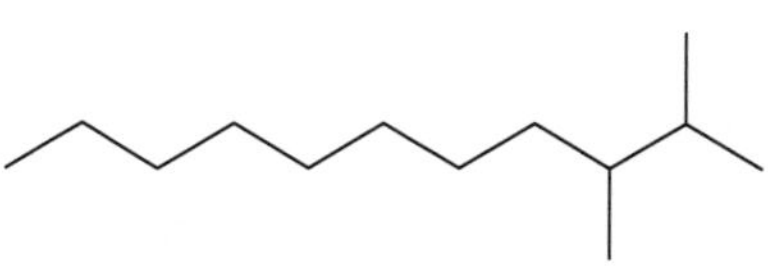

Undecane, 2,3-dimethyl- (130)

Contd...

Table 2.1–*Contd...*

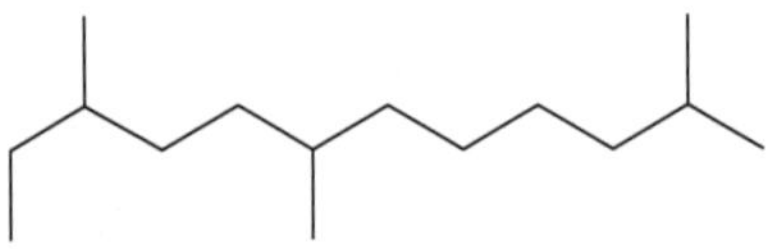

Dodecane, 2,7,10-trimethyl- (131)

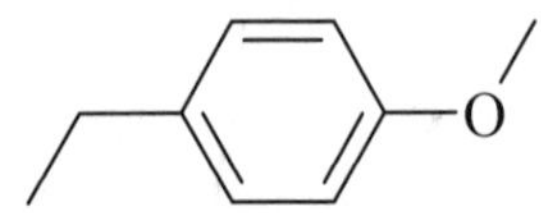

Benzene, 1-methoxy-4-(1-propenyl)- (132)

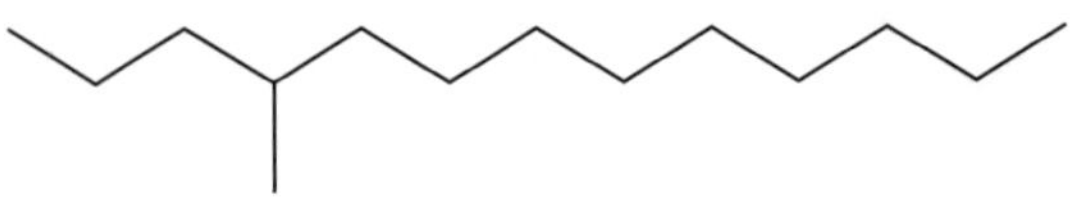

Tridecane, 4-methyl- (133)

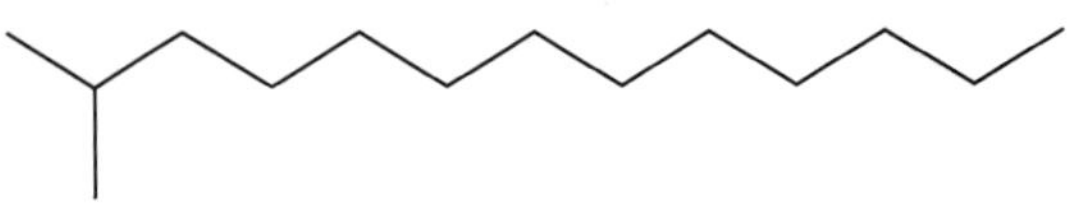

Tridecane, 2-methyl- (134)

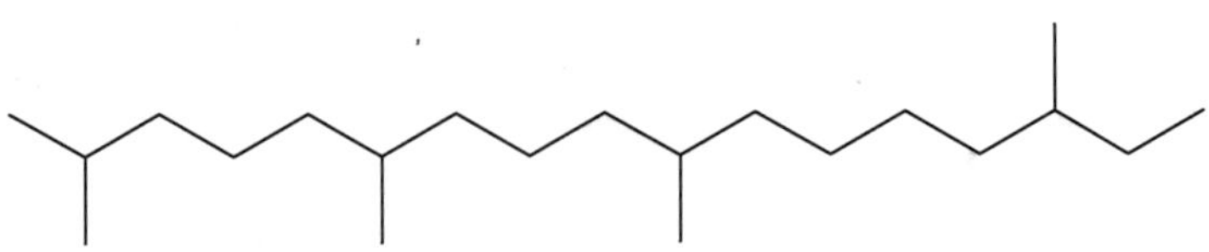

Heptadecane, 2,6,10,15-tetramethyl- (135)

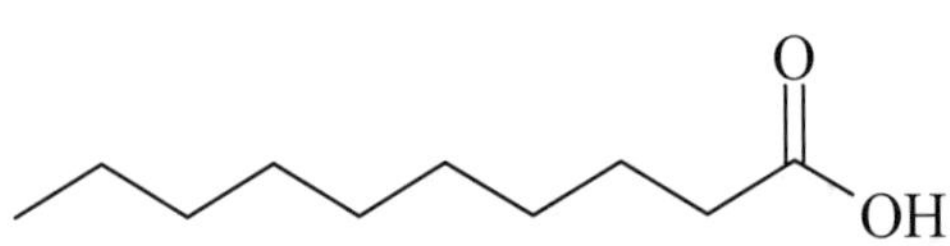

n-Decanoic acid (136)

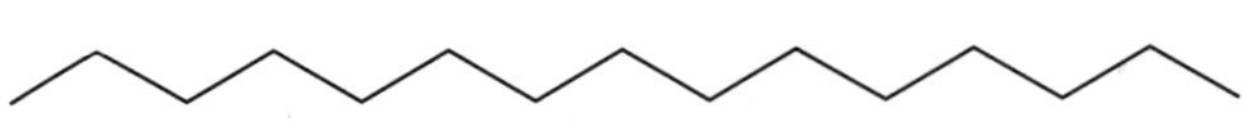

Pentadecane (137)

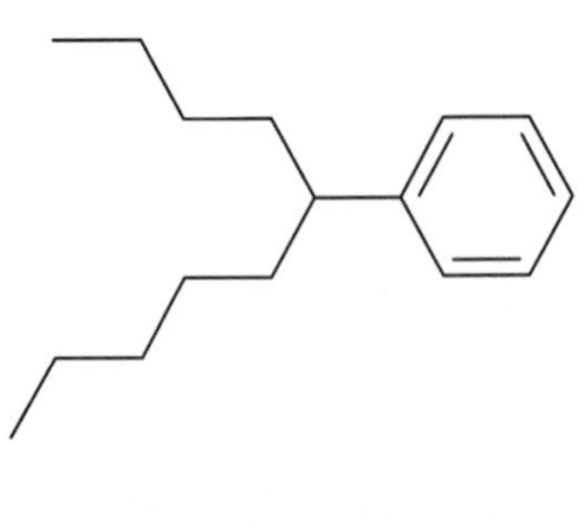

Benzene, (1-butylhexyl)- (138)

Contd...

Table 2.1–*Contd...*

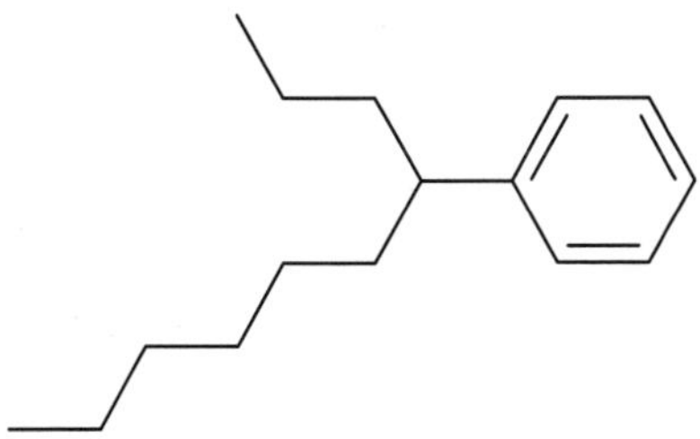

Benzene, (1-propylheptyl)- (139)

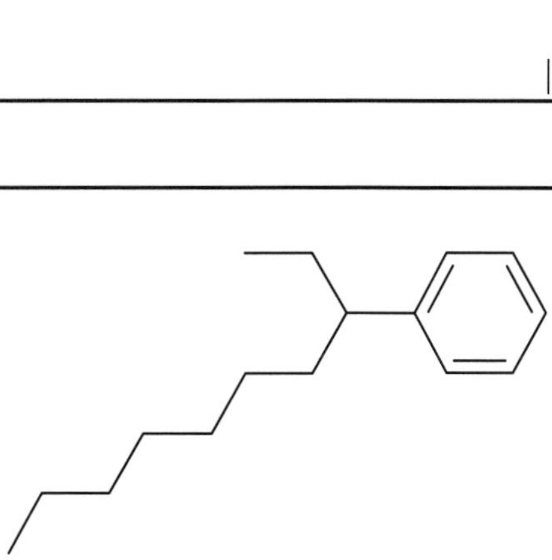

Benzene, (1-ethyloctyl)- (140)

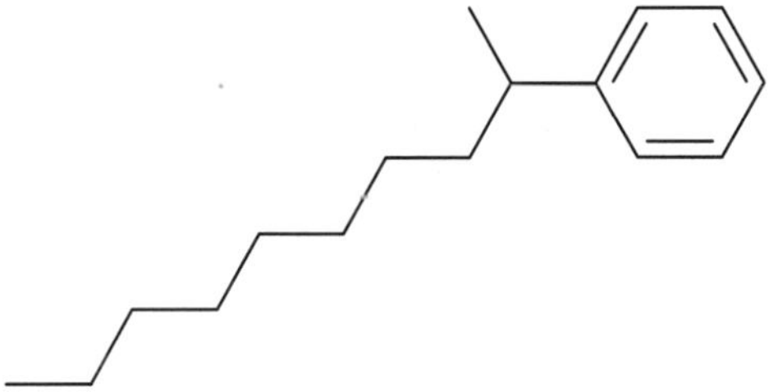

Benzene, (1-methylnonyl)- (141)

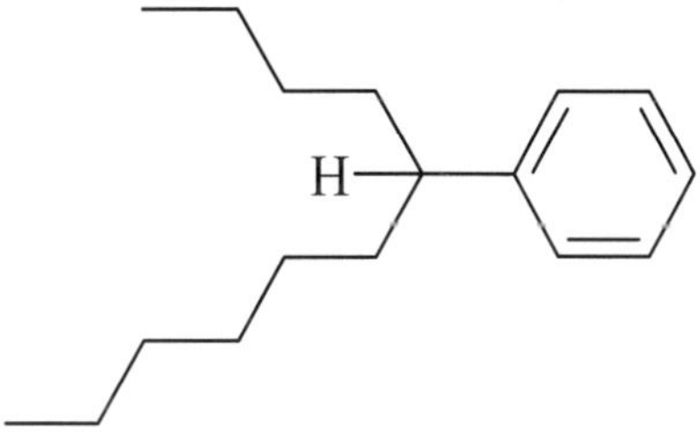

Benzene, (1-butylheptyl)- (142)

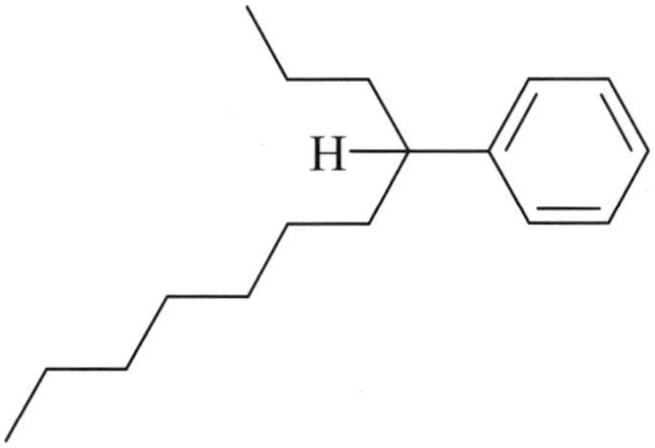

Benzene, (1-propyloctyl)- (143)

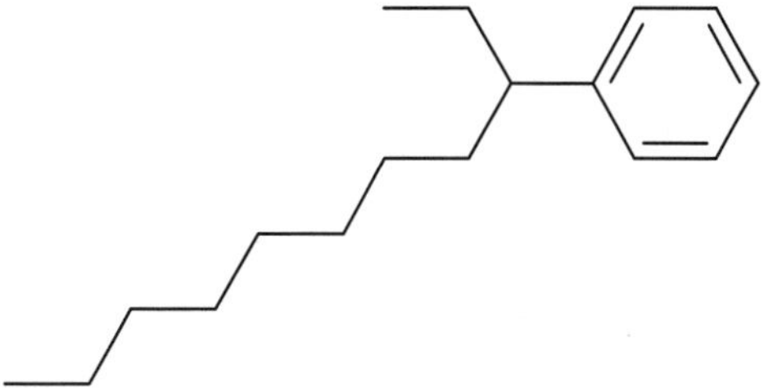

Benzene, (1-ethylnonyl)- (144)

Contd...

Table 2.1–*Contd...*

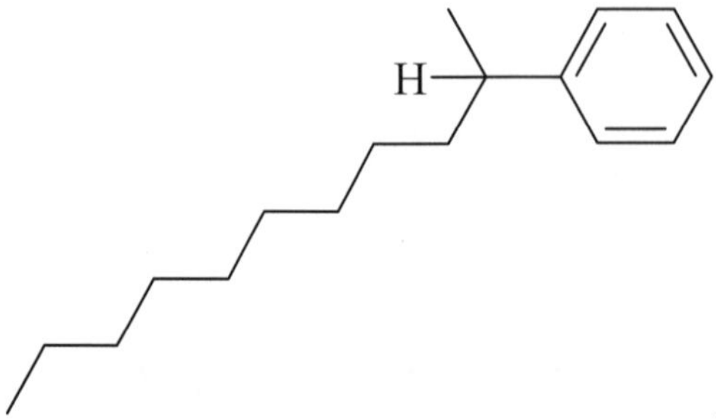

Benzene, (1-methyldecyl)- (145)

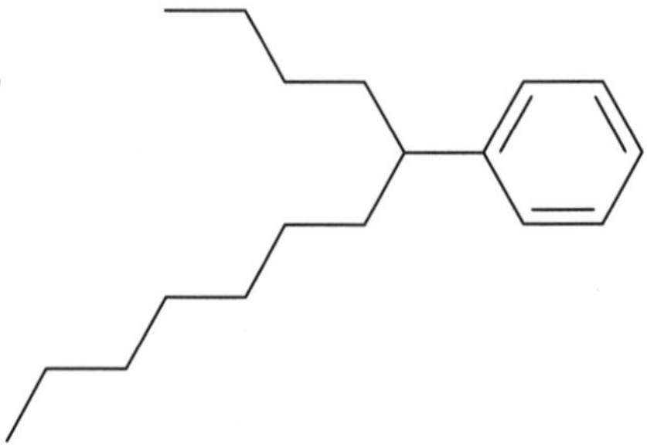

Benzene, (1-butyloctyl)- (146)

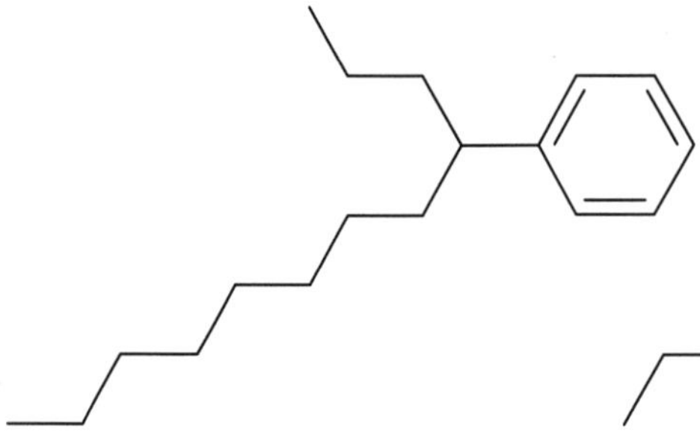

Benzene, (1-propylnonyl)- (147)

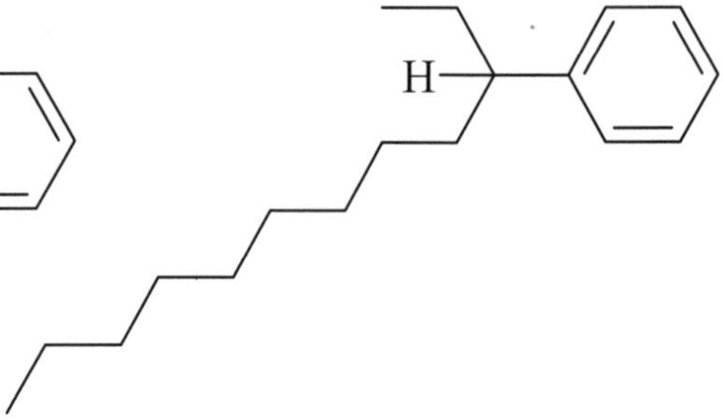

Benzene, (1-ethyldecyl)- (148)

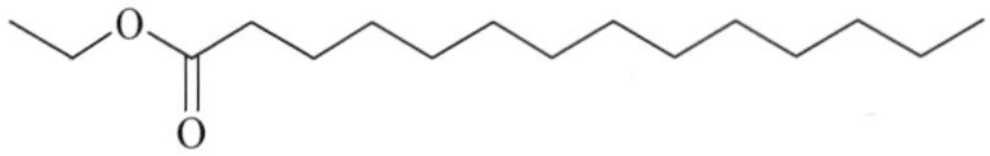

Tetradecanoic acid, ethyl ester (149)

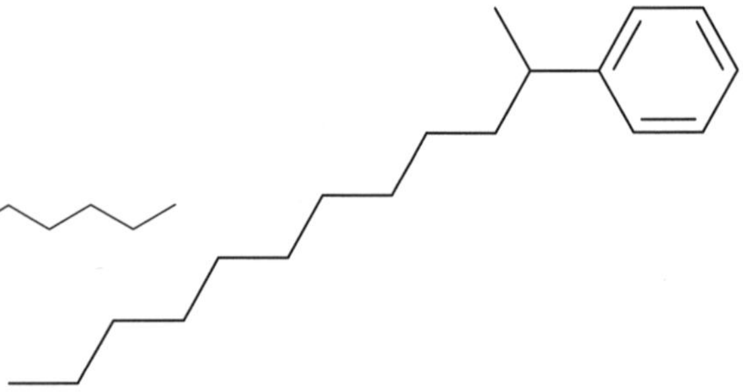

Benzene, (1-methylundecyl)- (150)

Contd...

Table 2.1–*Contd...*

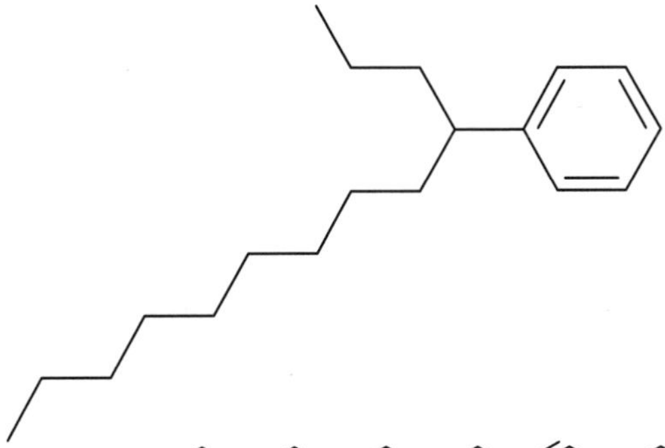

Benzene, (1-propyldecyl)- (151)

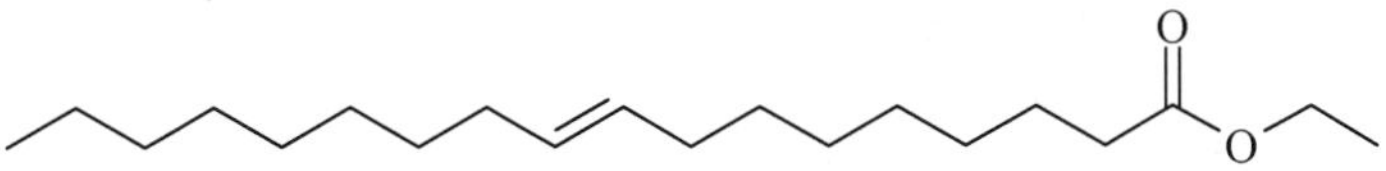

(E)-9-Octadecenoic acid ethyl ester (152)

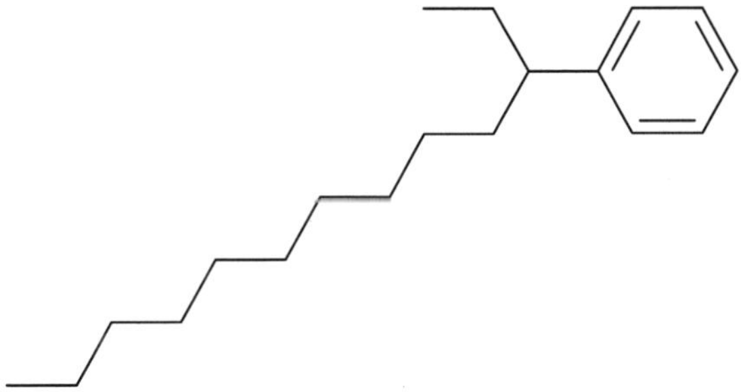

Benzene, (1-ethylundecyl)- (153)

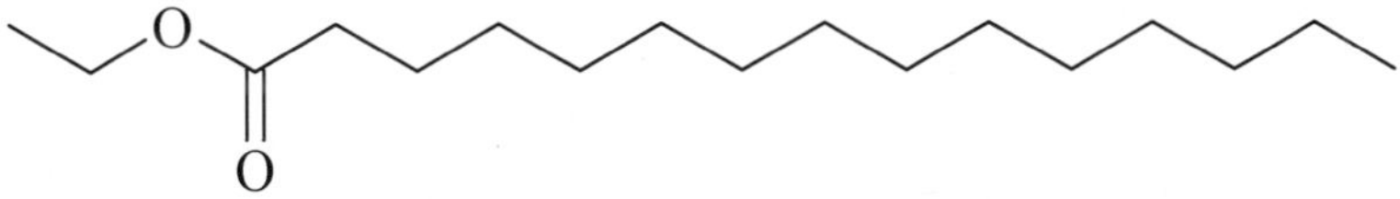

Pentadecanoic acid, ethylester (154)

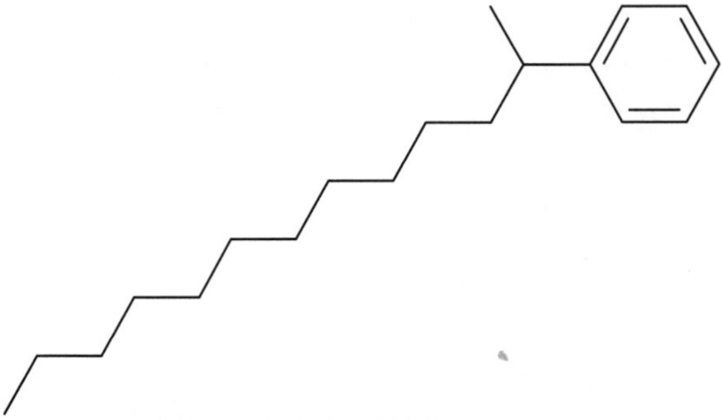

Benzene, (1-methyldodecyl)- (155)

Contd...

Table 2.1–*Contd...*

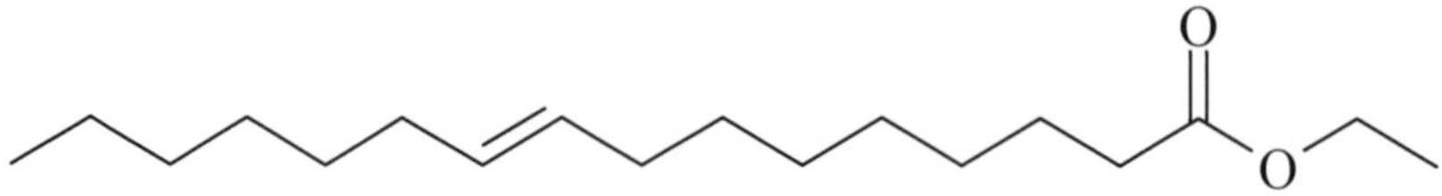

Ethyl 9-hexadecenoate (156)

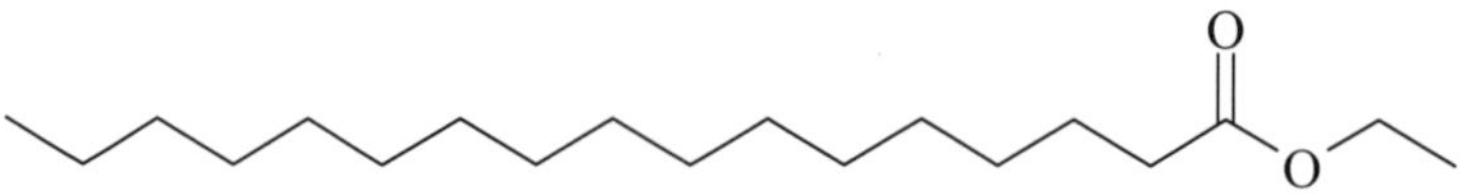

Heptadecanoic acid, ethyl ester (157)

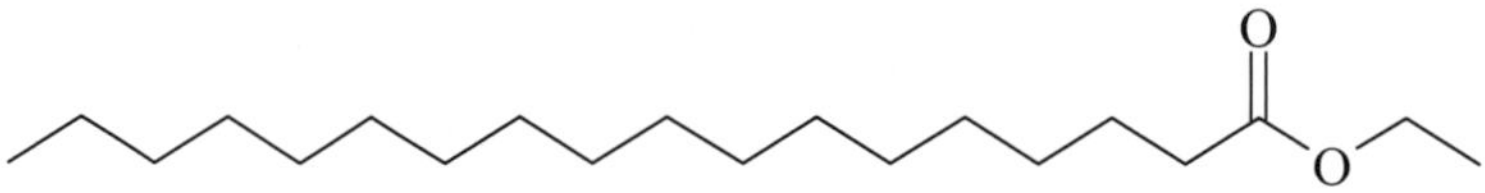

Octadecanoic acid, ethyl ester- (158)

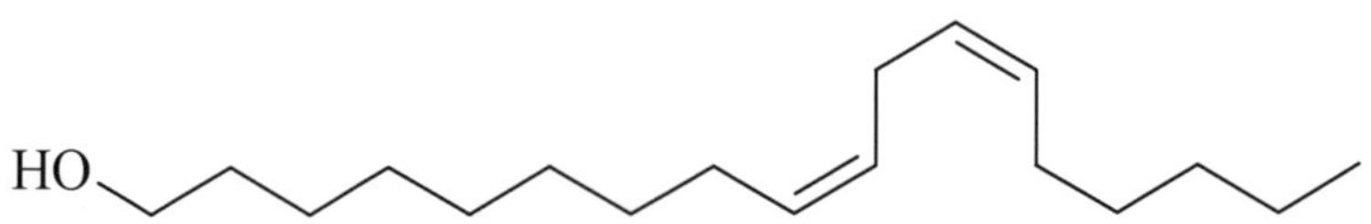

9,12-Octadecadien-1-ol, (Z,Z)- (159)

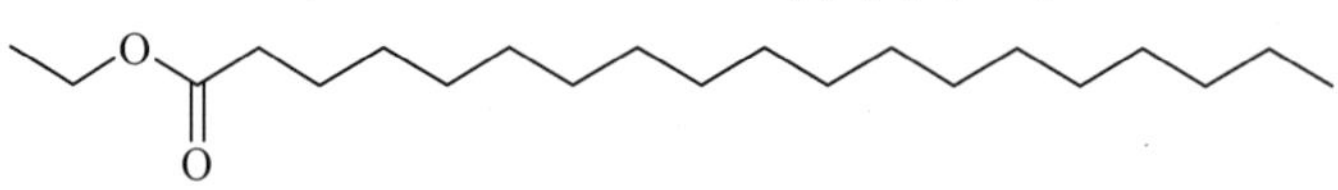

Nonadecanoic acid, ethyl ester (160)

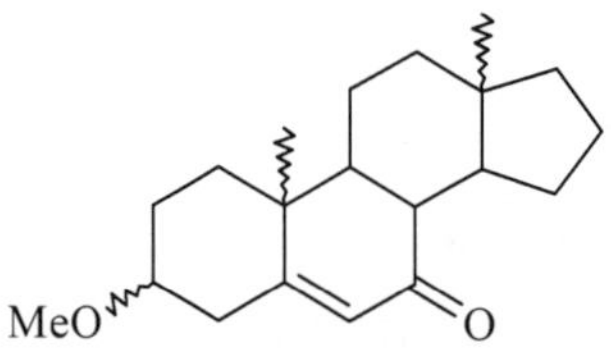

Androstan-7-one, (161) 3-(acetyloxy)-(3a,5a)

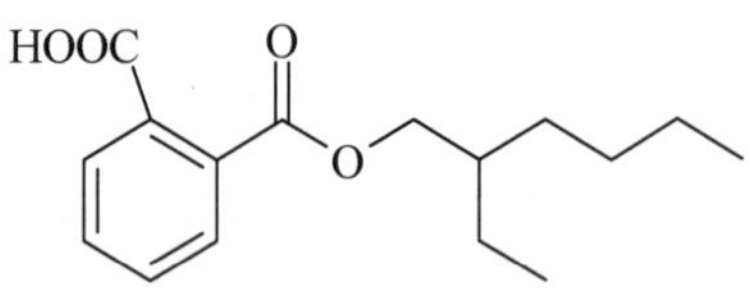

1,2-Benzenedicarboxylic acid, mono-(2-ethylhexyl) ester (162)

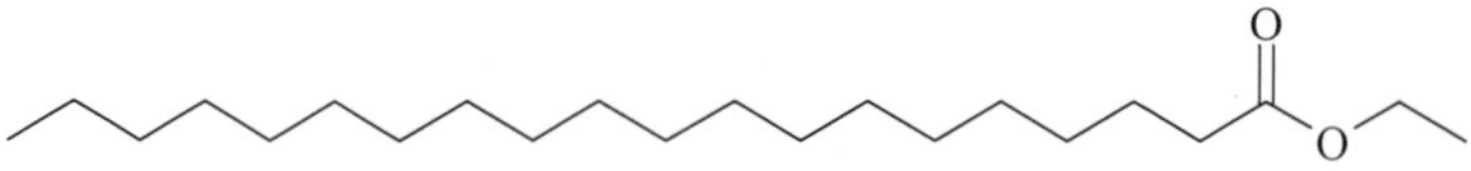

Eicosanoic acid, ethyl ester- (163)

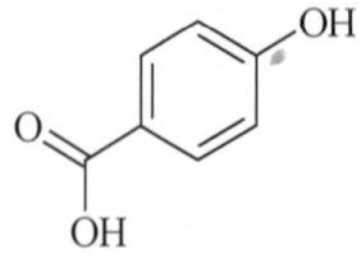

p-Hydroxy benzoic acid (164)

Contd...

Table 2.1–*Contd...*

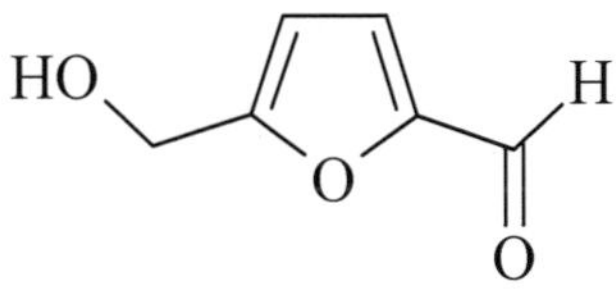

5-(Hydroxymethyl) furfural (165)

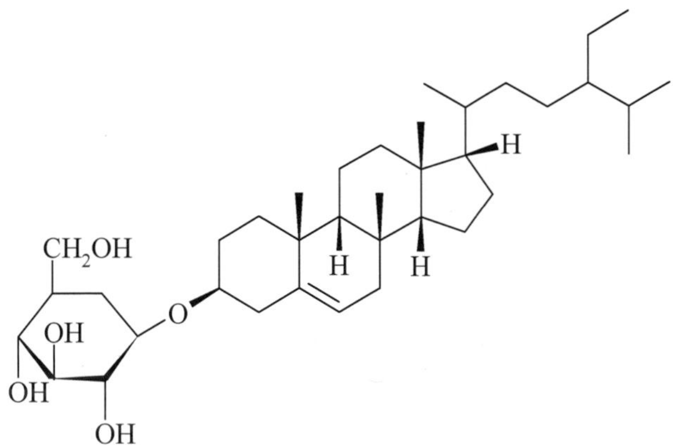

Bis-(5-formylfurfuryl)-ether (166)

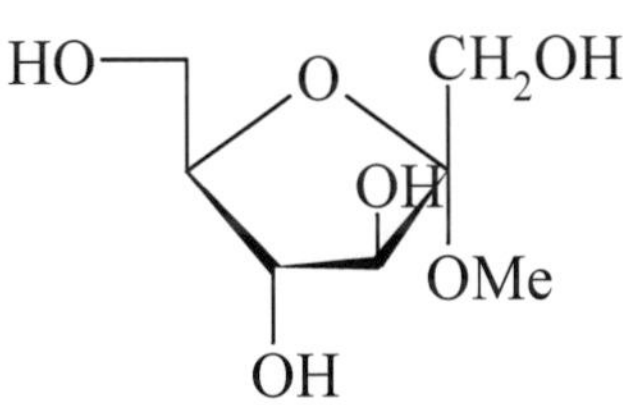

Daucosterol (167)

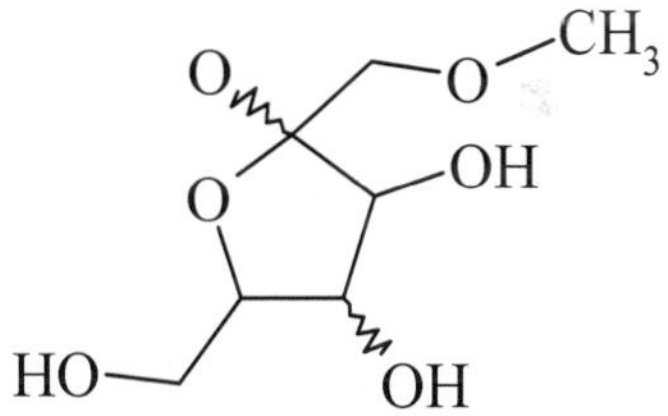

α-D-Fructofuranosides methyl (168)

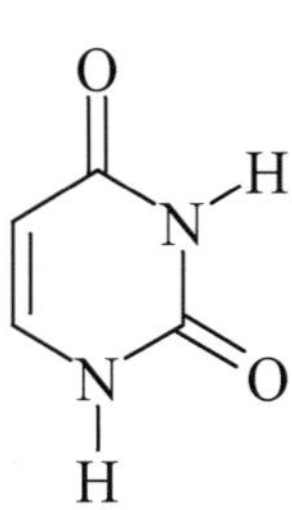

Uracil (169)

Contd...

Table 2.1–*Contd...*

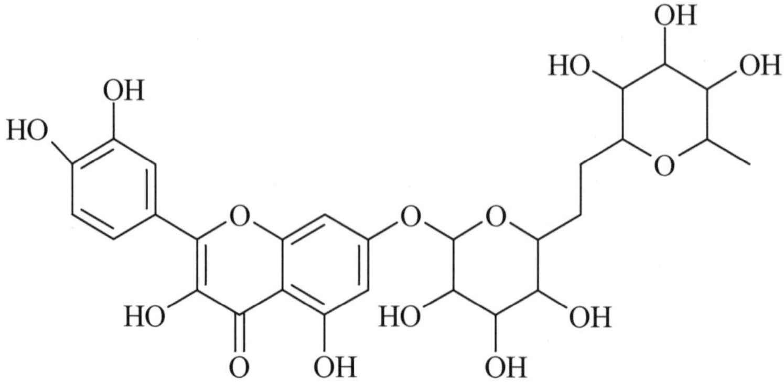

Quercetin-7-rutinoside (170)

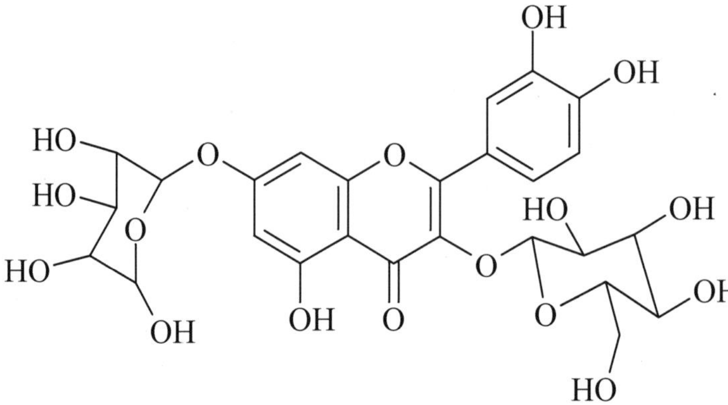

Quercetin-3-O-glucoside-7-O-rhamnoside (171)

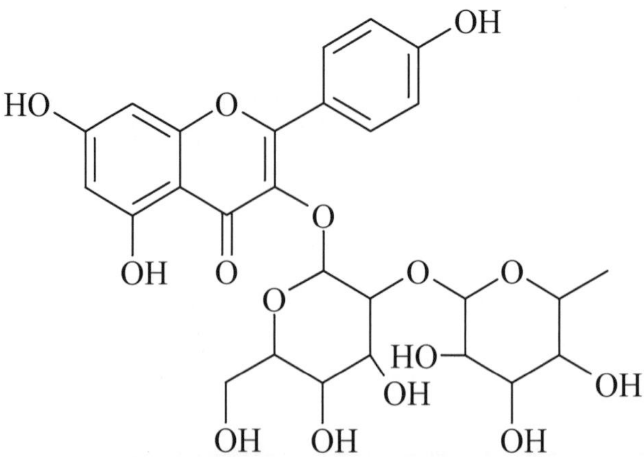

Kaempferol-3-rutinoside (172)

Contd...

Table 2.1–*Contd...*

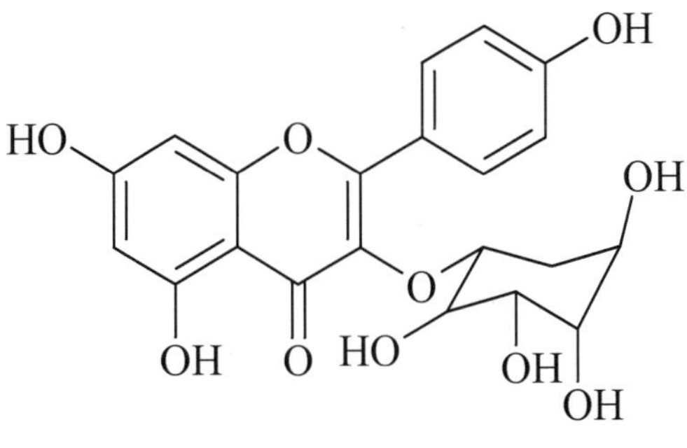

Kaempferol-3-glucoside (173)

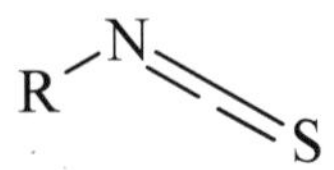

Isothiocyanates (174)

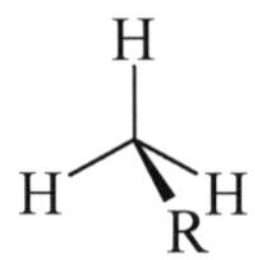

n-Alkanes (175)

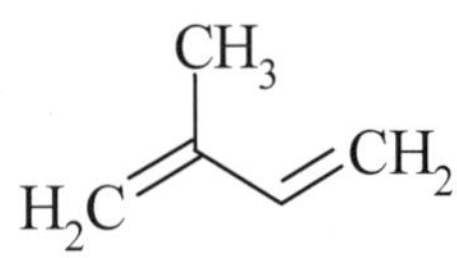

Terpenoids (176)

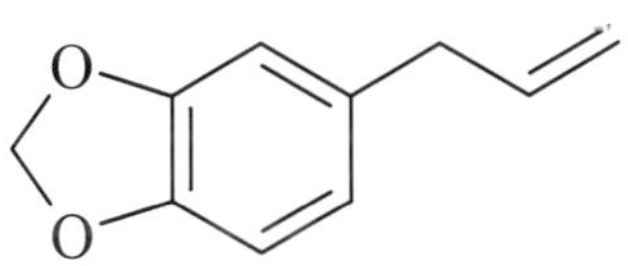

Phenyl propanoid (177)

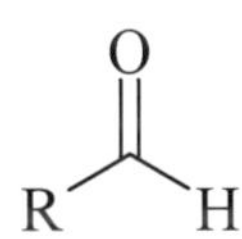

Aldehyde (178)

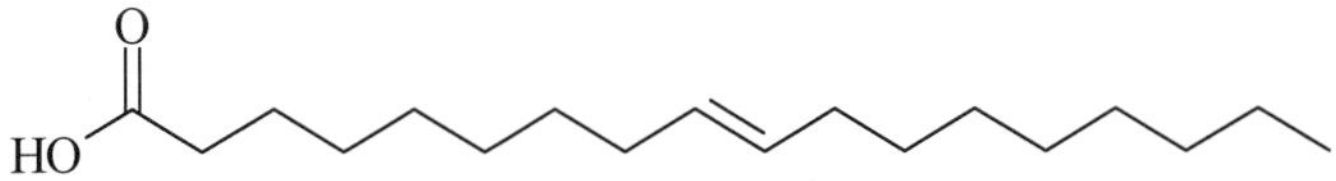

Fatty acid (179)

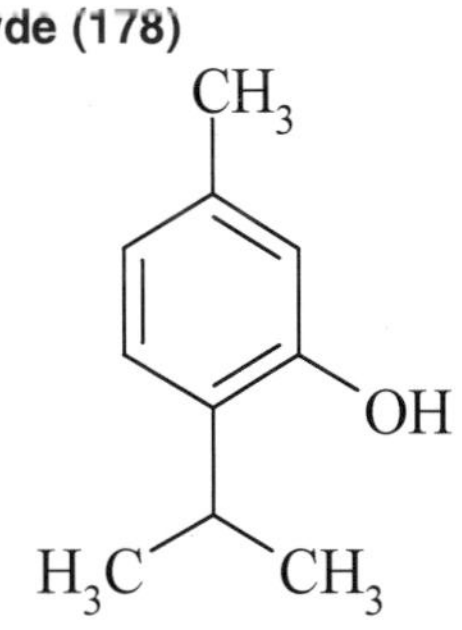

Thymol (180)

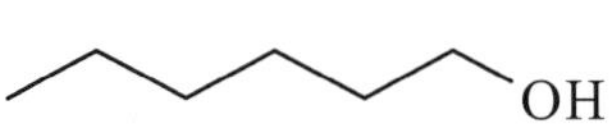

2-Hexenol (181)

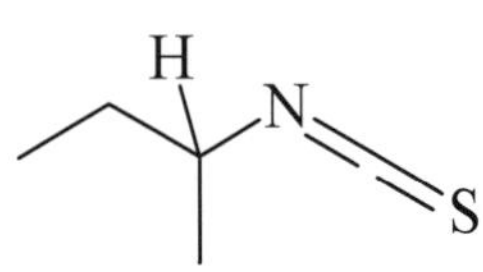

Sec-butyl isothiocyanates (182)

Contd...

Table 2.1–*Contd...*

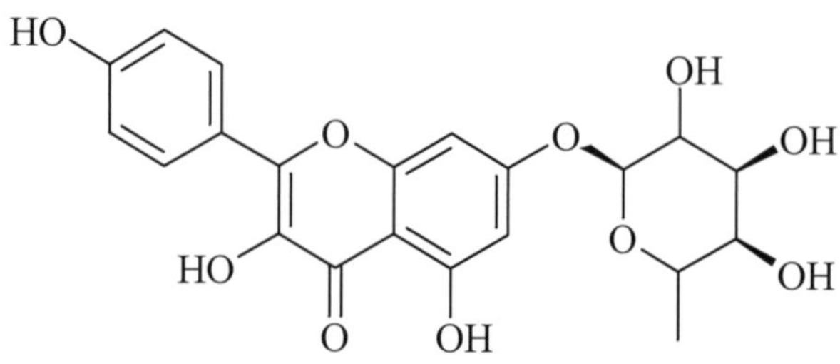

Kaempferol-7-rhamnoside (183)

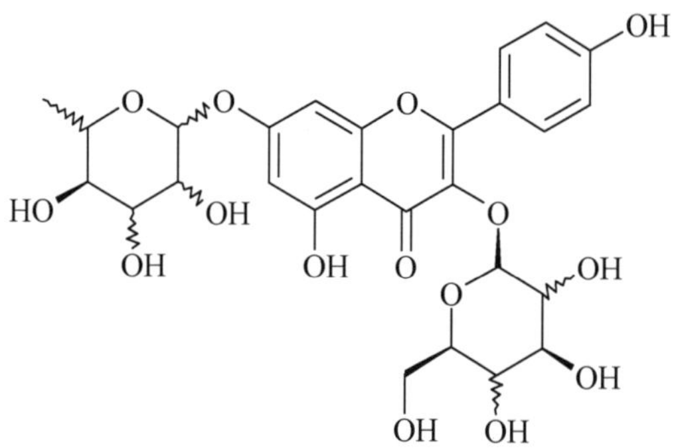

Kaempferol-3-glucoside-7-rhamnoside (184)

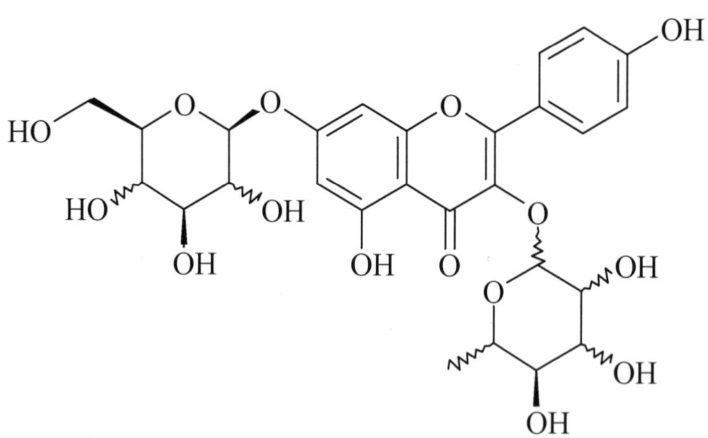

Kaempferol-3-rhamnoside-7-glucoside (185)

Contd...

Table 2.1–*Contd...*

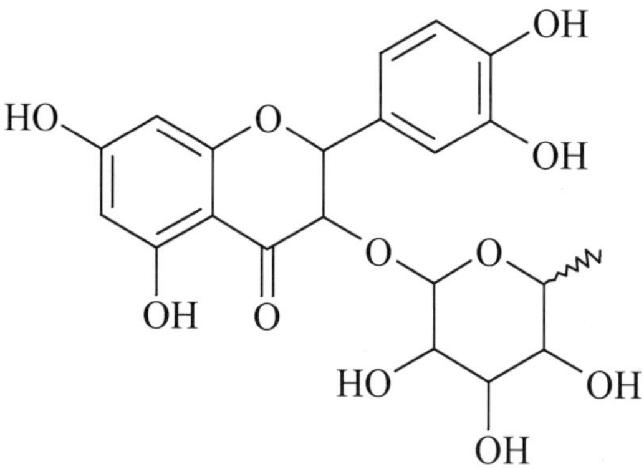

Quercetin-3-rhamnoside (186)

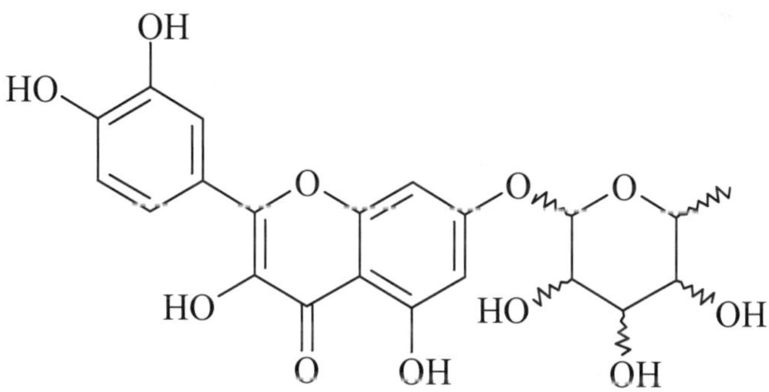

Quercetin-7-rhamnoside (187)

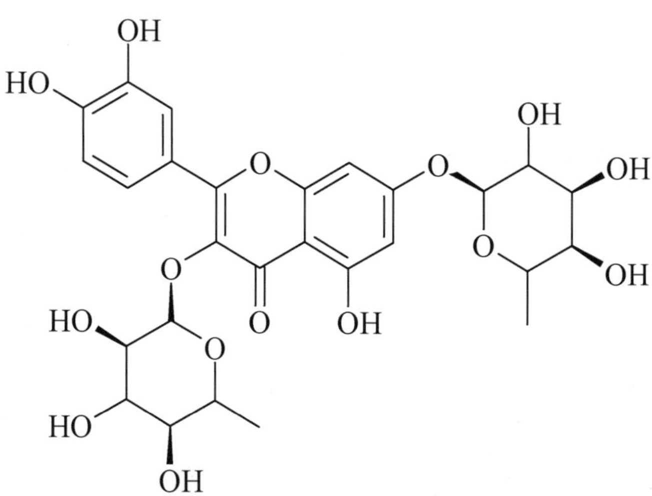

Quercetin-3,7-dirhamnoside (188)

Contd...

Table 2.1–*Contd...*

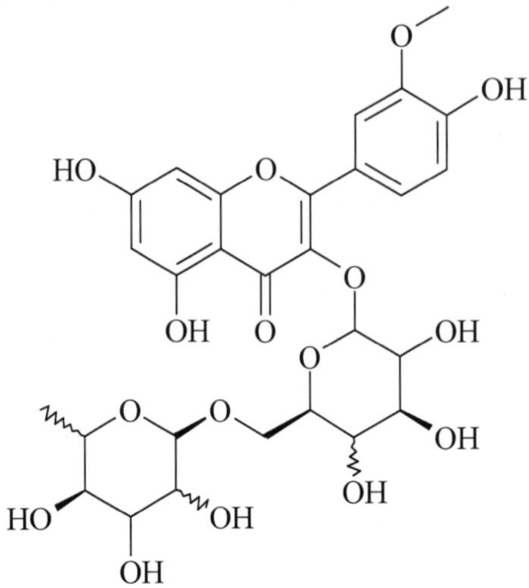

Isorhamnetin-3-rutinoside (189)

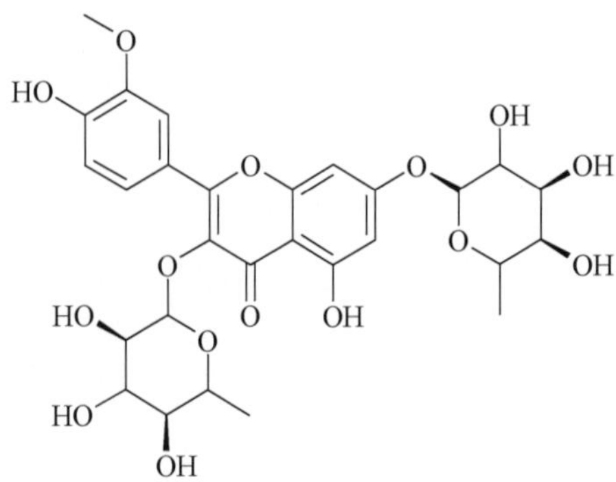

Isorhamnetin-3,7-dirhamnoside (190)

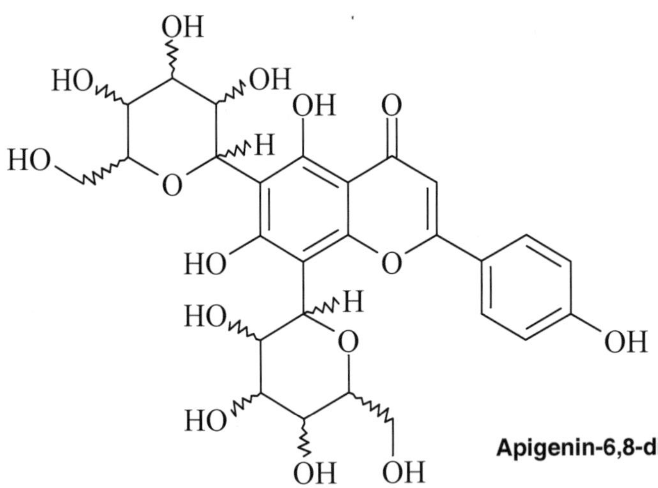

Apigenin-6,8-di-C-glucoside (191)

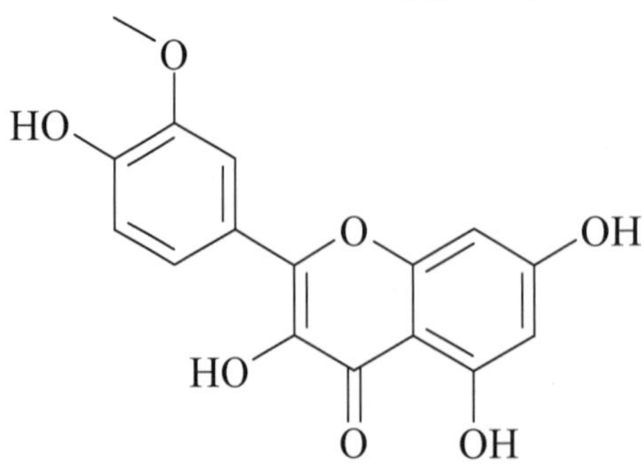

Isorhamnetin (192)

Contd...

Table 2.1–*Contd...*

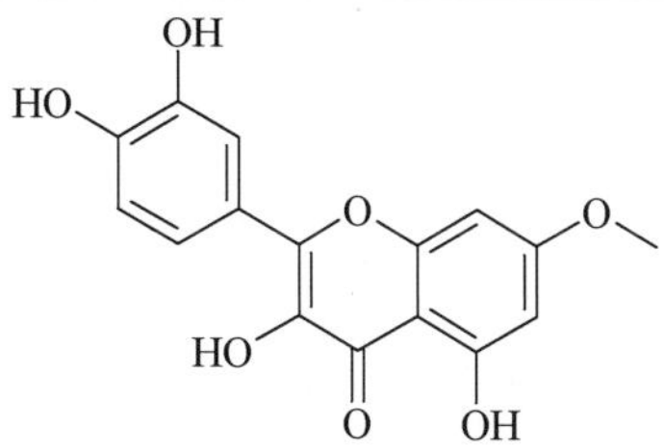

Rhamnetin (193)

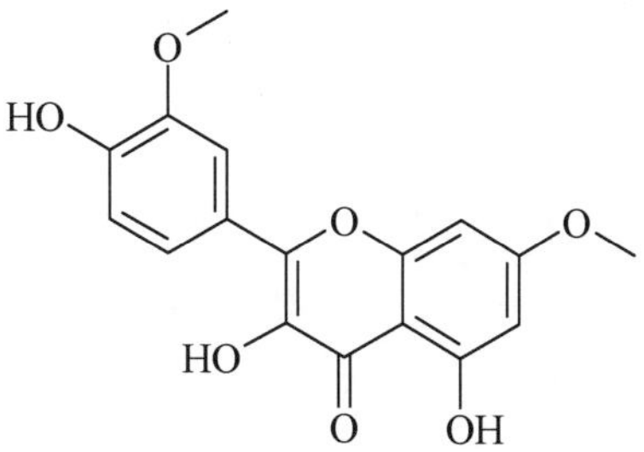

Rhamnozin (194)

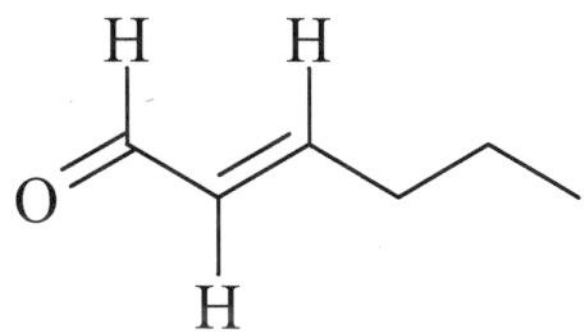

2-Hexenal (195)

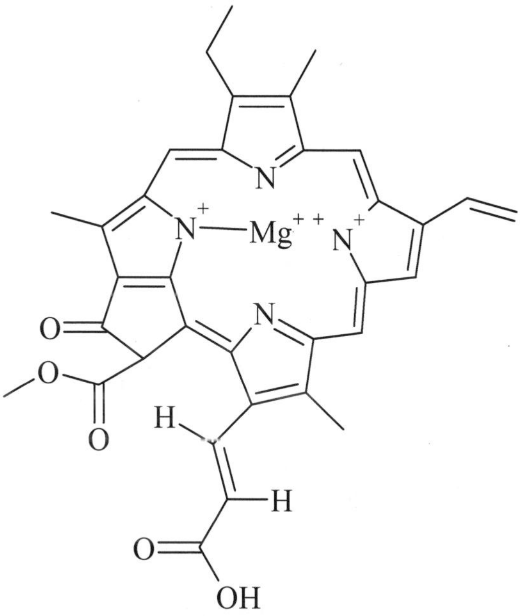

Chlorophyll (196)

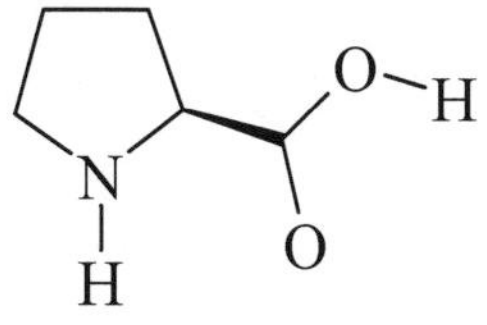

Proline (197)

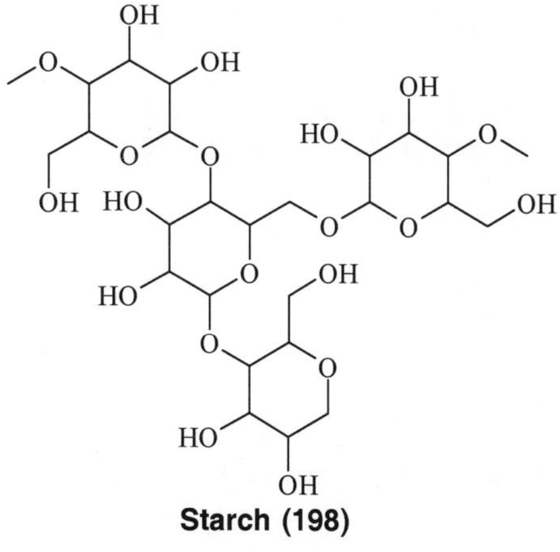

Starch (198)

Contd...

Table 2.1–*Contd...*

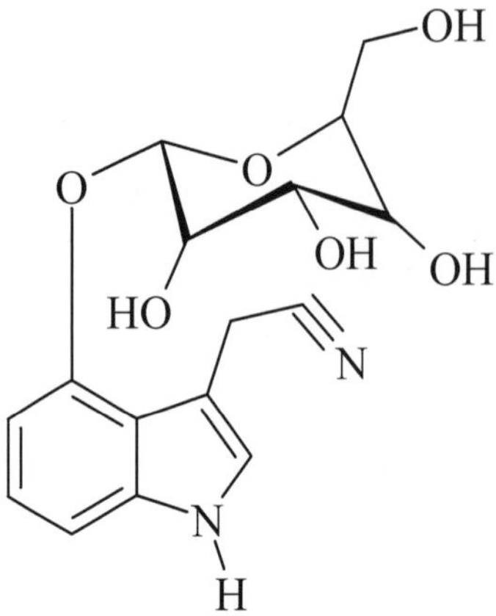

1H-Indole-3-acetonitrile glycoside (199)

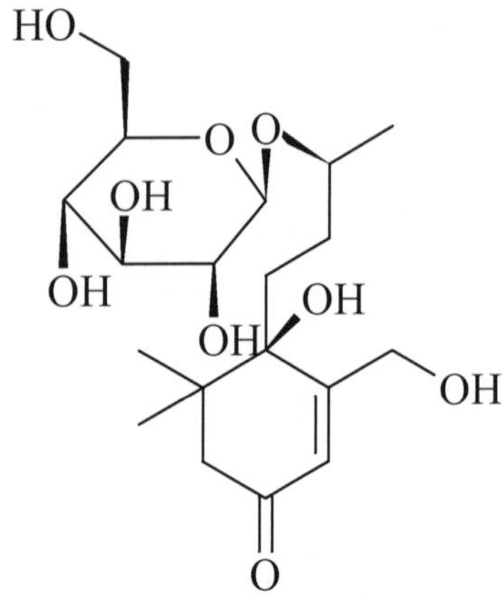

(9S)-Drummondol-9-O-β-D-glucoranoside (200)

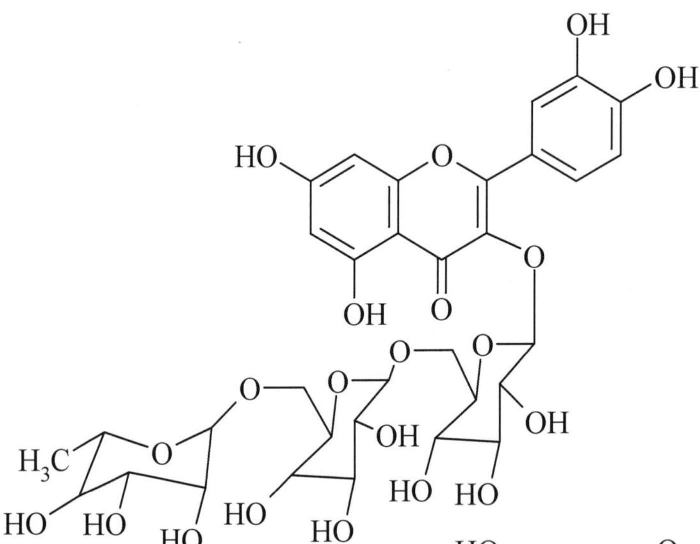

3-O-(6'''-α-L-rhamnosyl-6''-β-D-glucosyl)-β-D-glucoside (201)

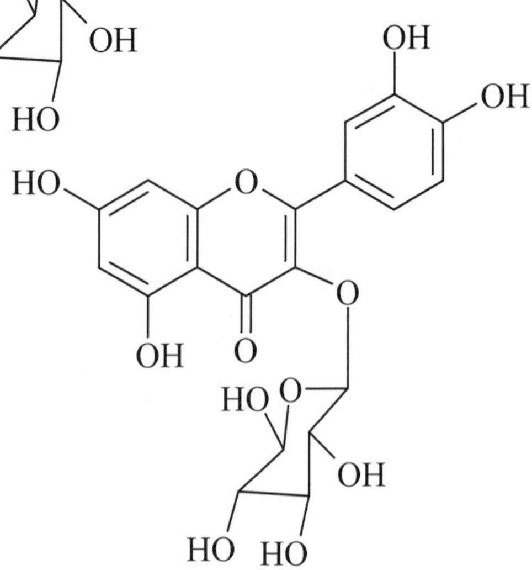

Quercetin-3-O-glucoside (202)

Contd...

Table 2.1–*Contd...*

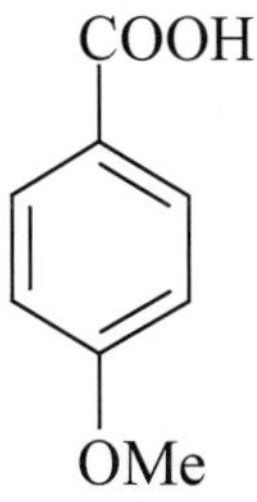

p-Methoxy benzoic acid (203)

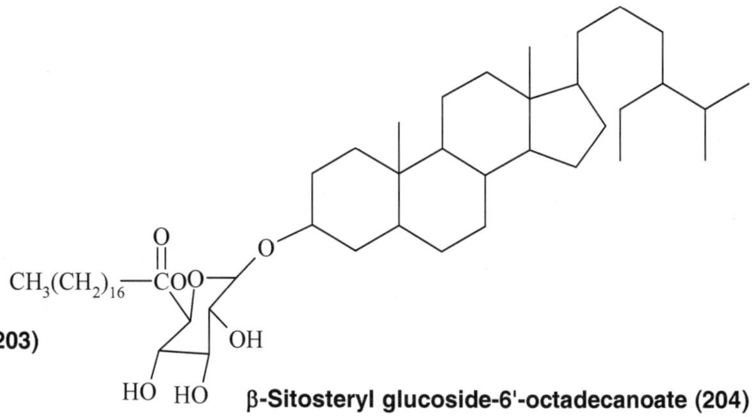

β-Sitosteryl glucoside-6'-octadecanoate (204)

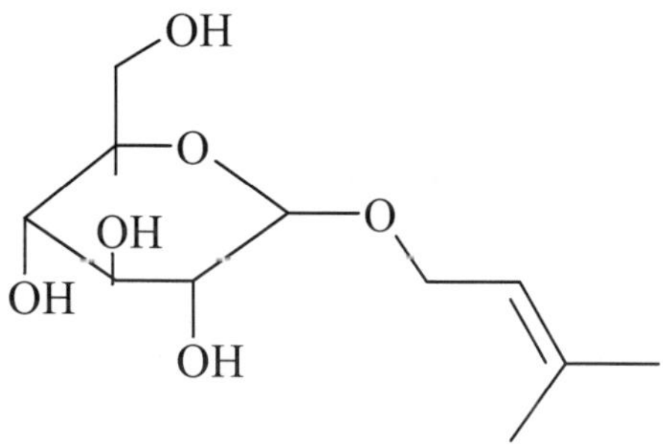

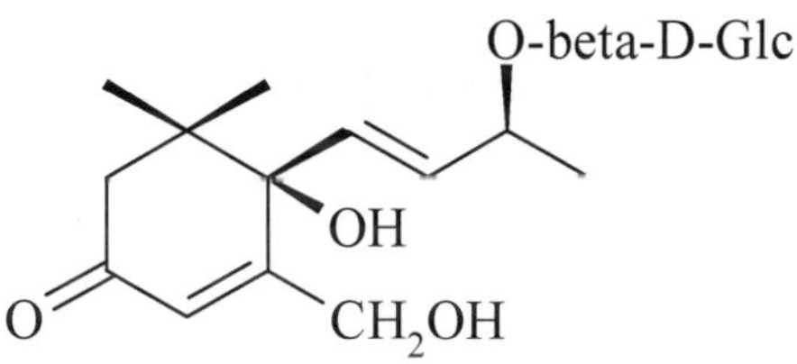

3-Methyl-2-butenyl-β-glycoside (205) **(6S)-Hydroxy-3-oxo-α-ionol glucosides (206)**

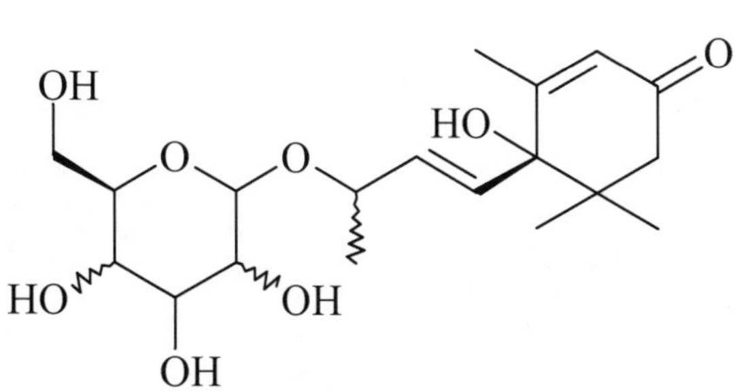

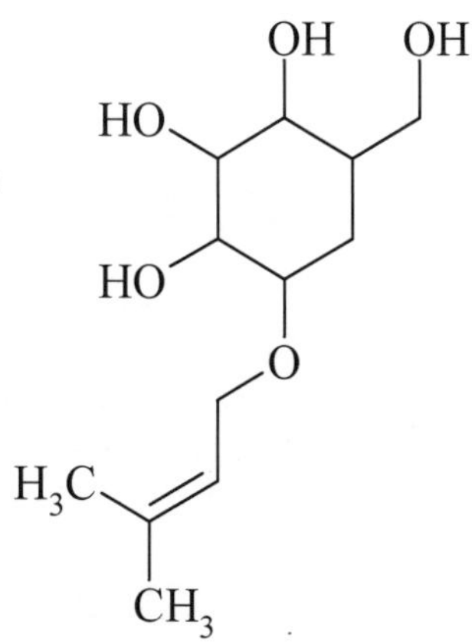

Corchoionoside C ((6S,9S)-roseoside) (207) **Prenyl glucoside (208)**

Contd...

Table 2.1–*Contd...*

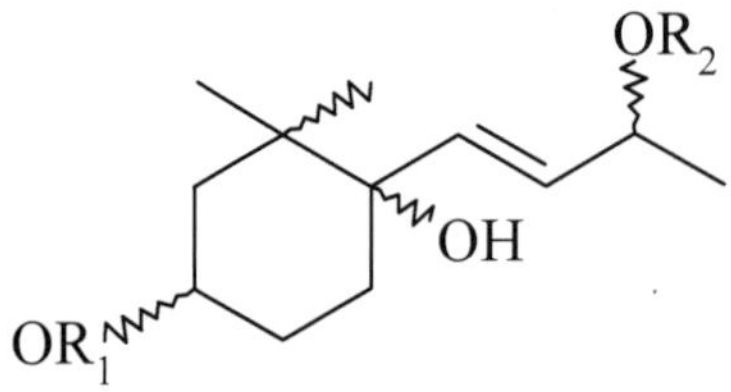

Ionol glycosides (209)

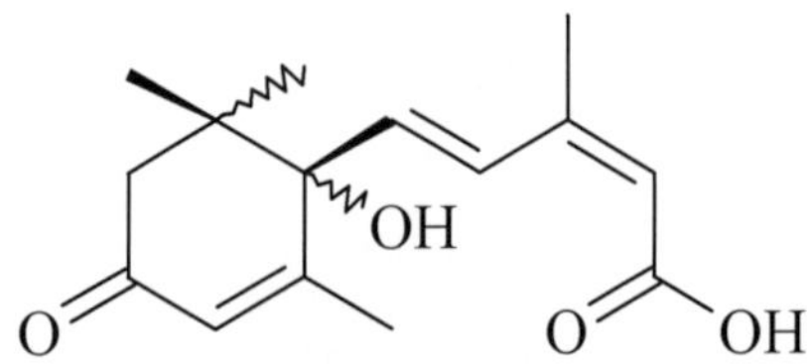

(+)-(S)-Abscisic acid (210)

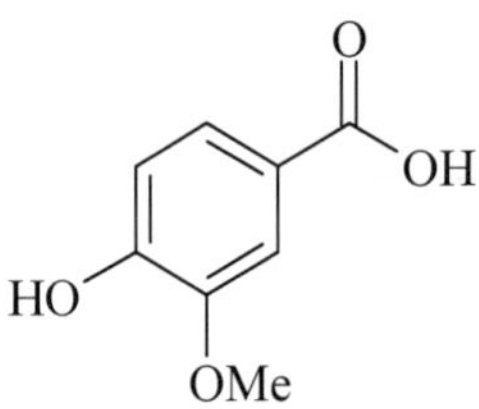

Vanillic acid (211)

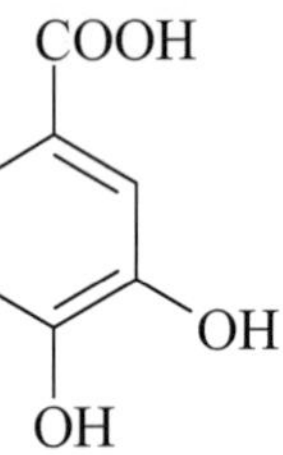

Protocatechuric acid (212)

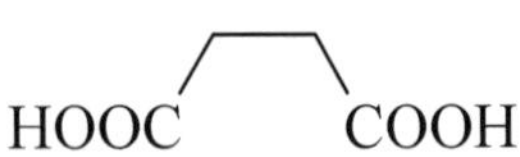

Butanedioic acid (213)

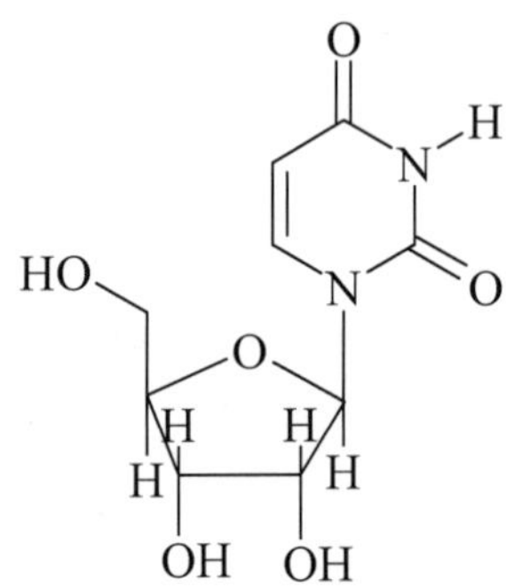

Uridine (214)

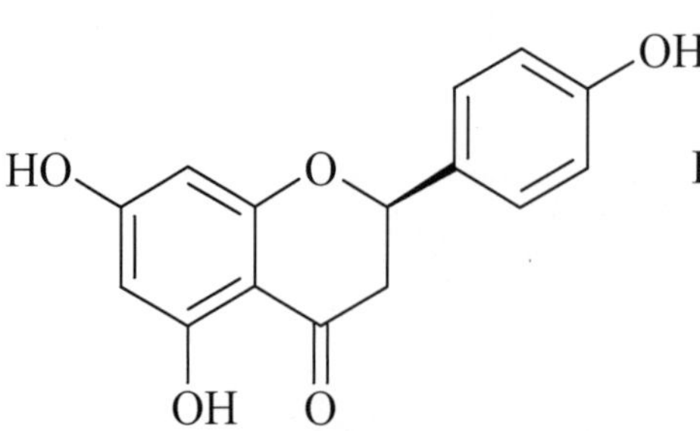

Flavonoids glycosides (215)

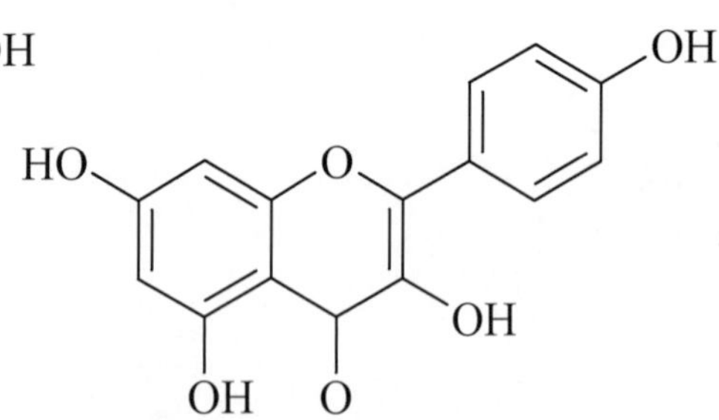

Kaempferol glycosides (216)

Contd...

Table 2.1–*Contd...*

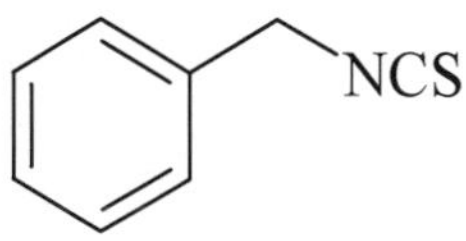

Benzyl isothiocyanate (217)

$C_{60}H_{98}O$

Cappaprenol-12 (218)

$C_{65}H_{106}O$

Cappapernol-13 (219)

$C_{70}H_{114}O$

Cappaprenol-14 (220)

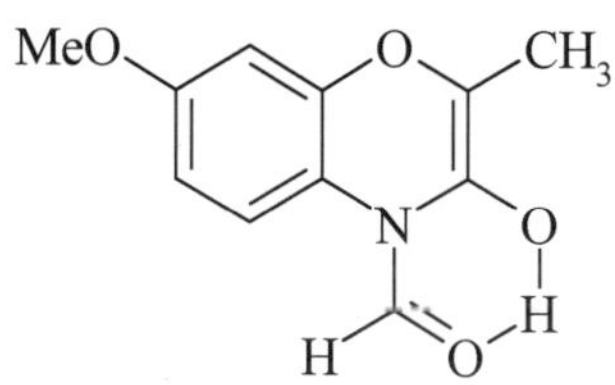

Cappamensin (221)

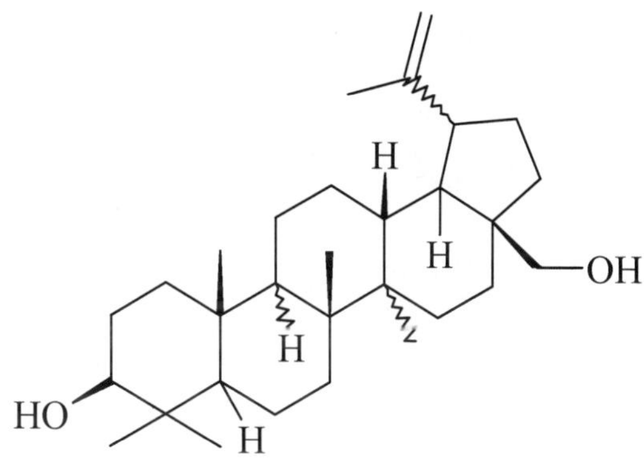

Betulin (222)

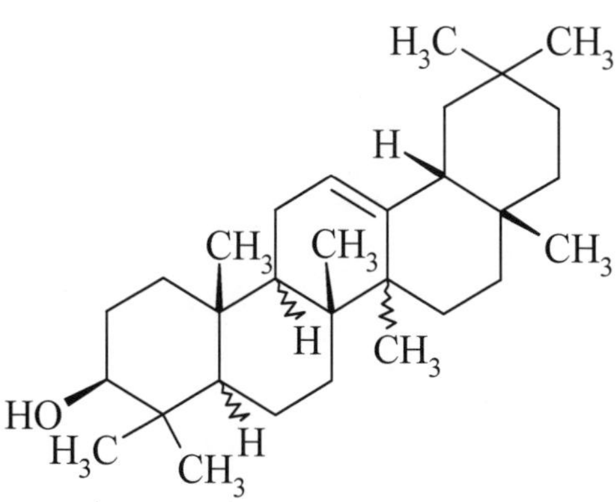

β-Amyrin (223)

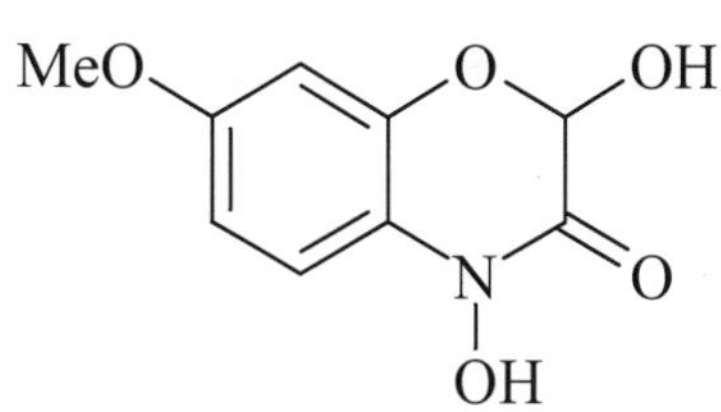

DIMBOA (2,4-dihydroxy-7-methoxy-2H-1,4-benzoxazin-3(4H)-one) (224)

Contd...

Table 2.1–*Contd...*

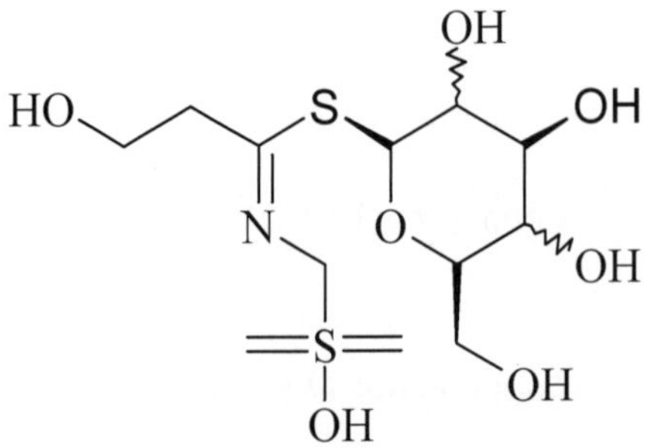

2-Hydroxyethyl-glucosinolate (225)

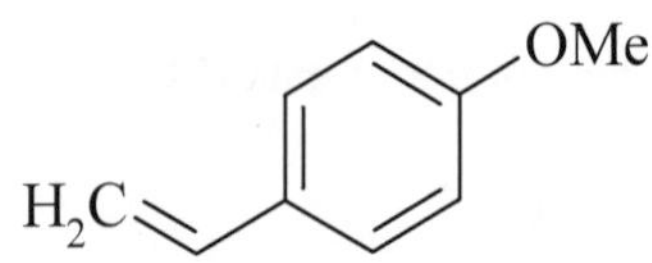

p-Methoxystyrene (226)

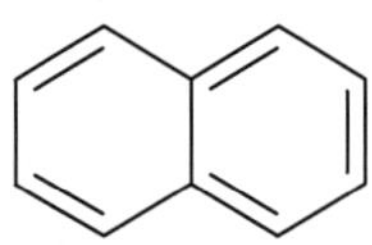

Naphthalene (227)

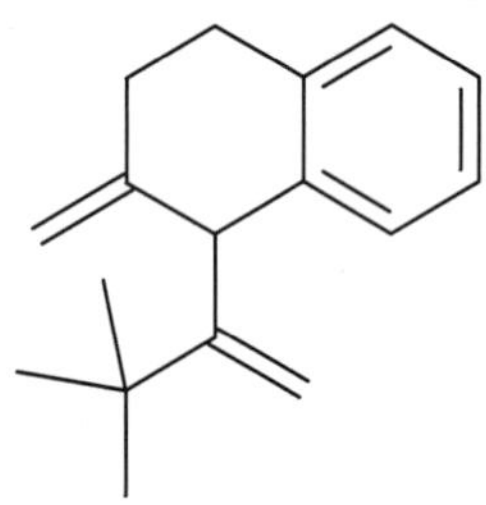

2-Naphthalenone (228)

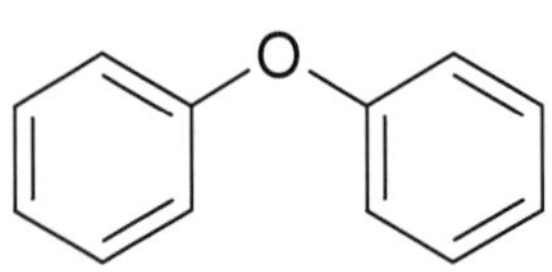

Diphenyl ether (229)

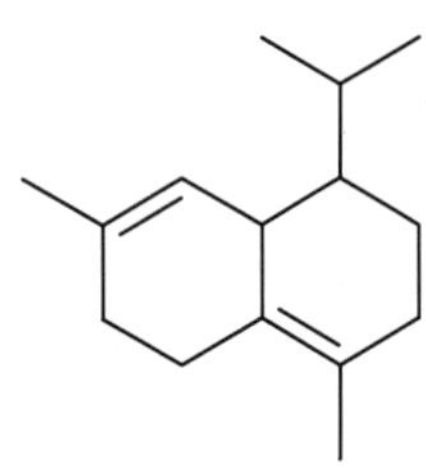

Sesquiterpenes (230)

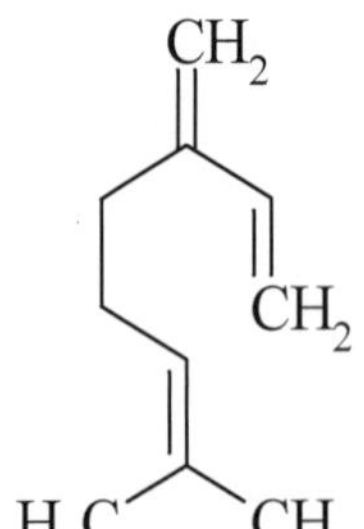

Monoterpenes (231)

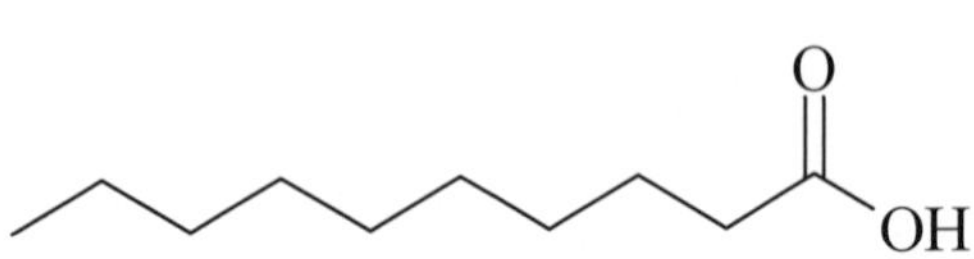

Capric acid (232)

Contd...

Table 2.1–*Contd...*

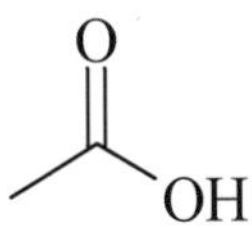

Acetic acid (233)

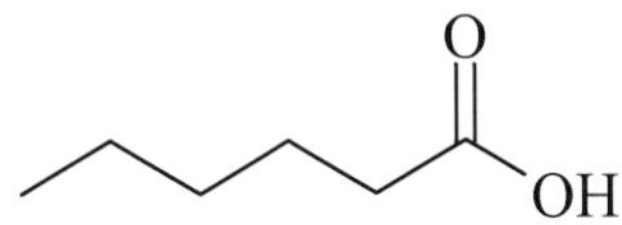

Hexanoic acid (234)

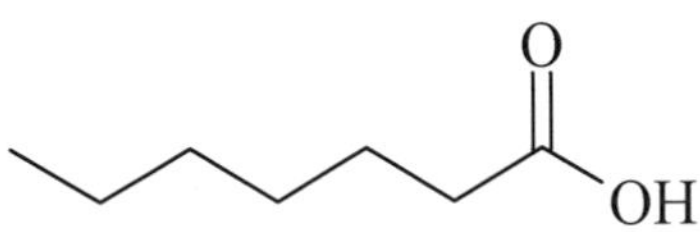

Heptanoic acid (235)

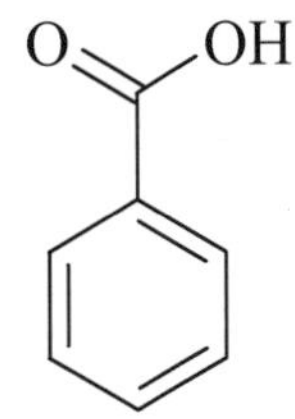

Benzoic acid (236)

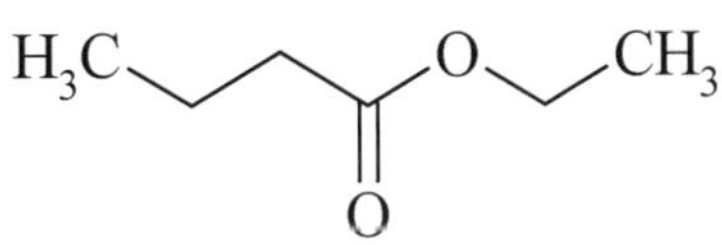

Ethyl butanoate (237)

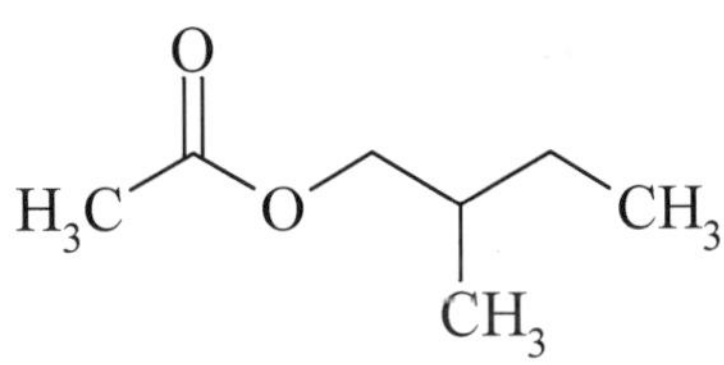

2-Methyl butyl acetate (238)

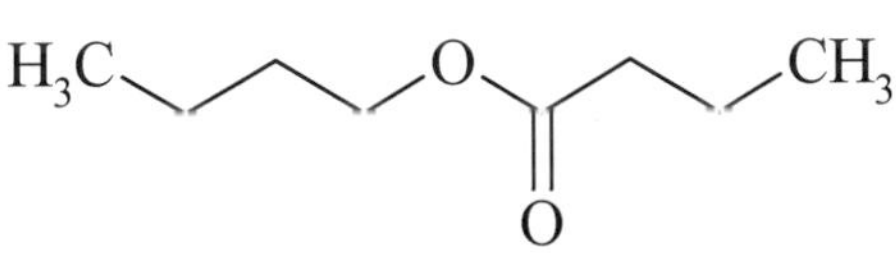

Butyl butanoate (239)

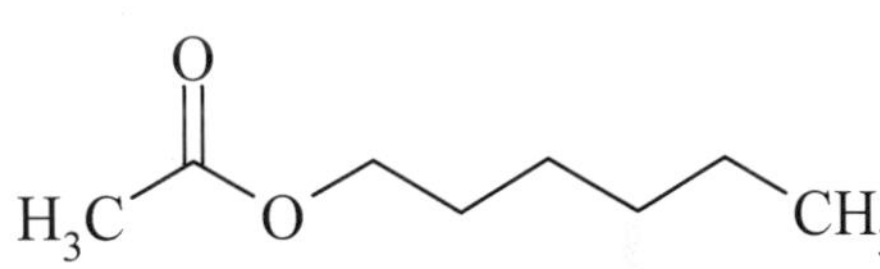

Hexyl acetate (240)

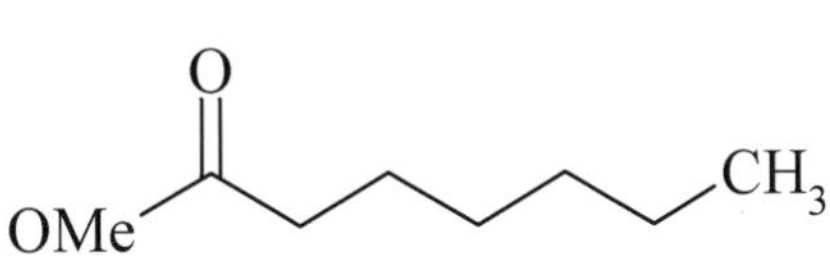

Methyl hepatonate (241)

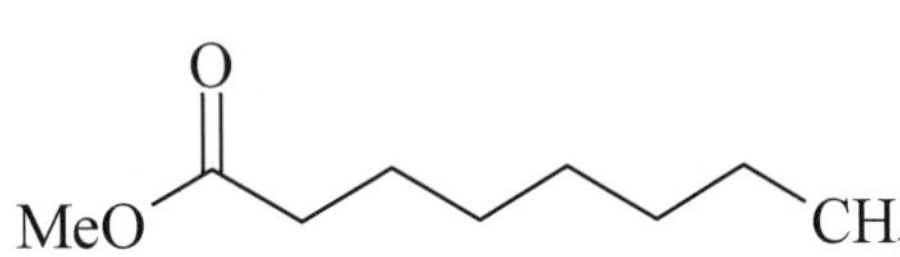

Methyl octanoate (242)

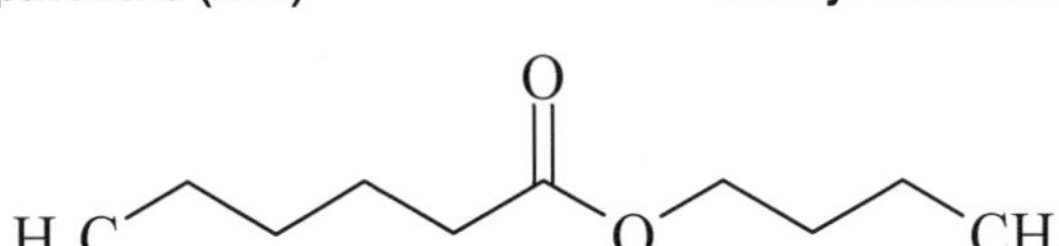

Butyl hexanoate (243)

Contd...

Table 2.1–*Contd...*

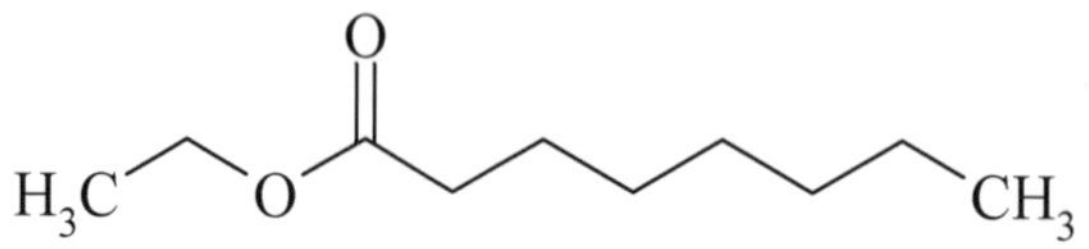

Ethyl octanoate (244)

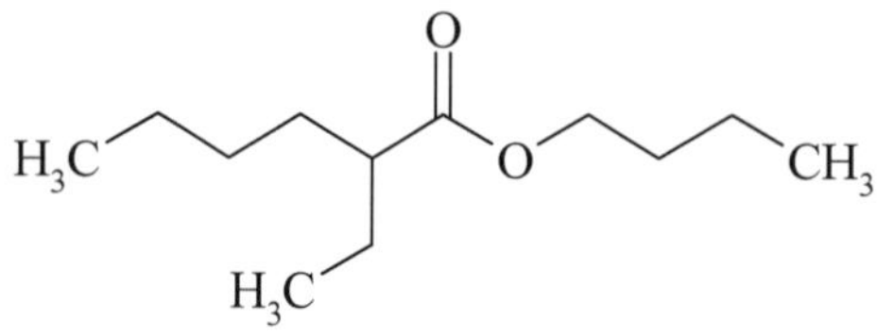

3-Ethyl butyl hexanoate (245)

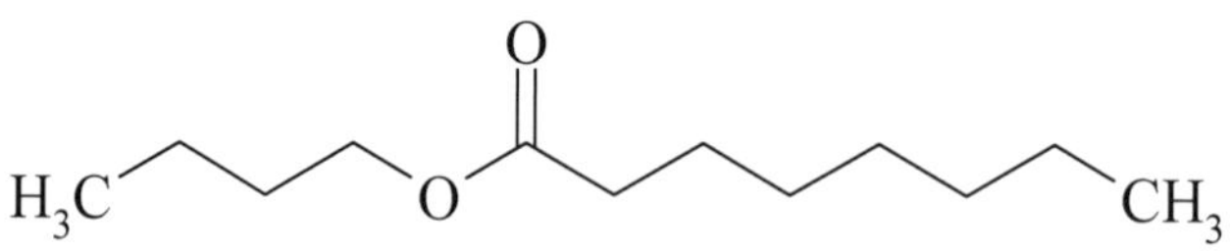

Butyl-octanoate (246)

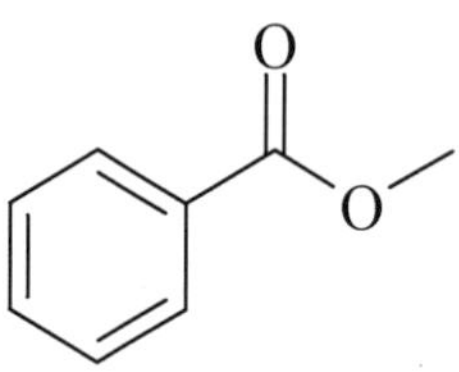

Methyl benzoate (247)

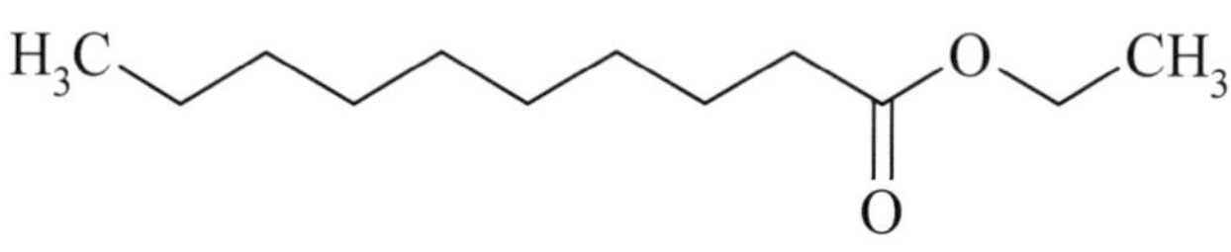

Ethyl decanoate (248)

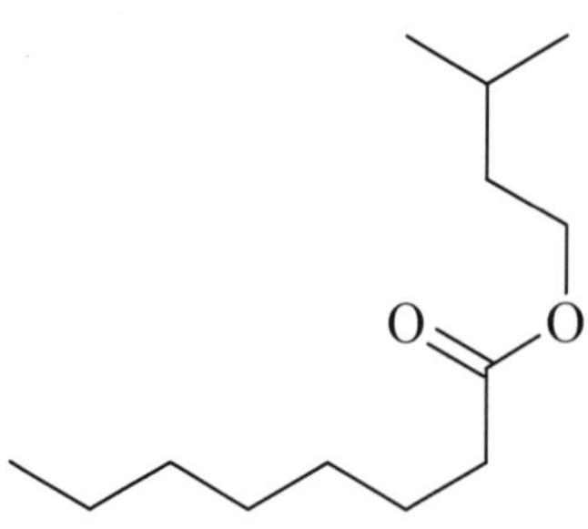

Isopentyloctanoate (249)

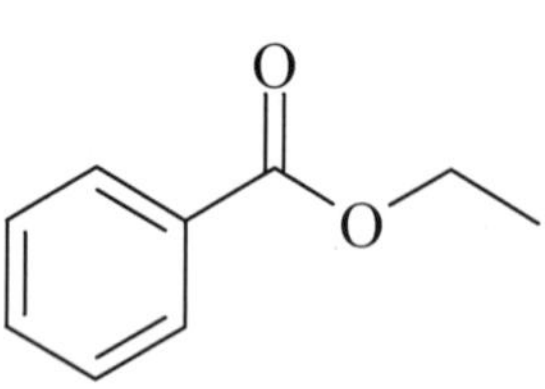

Ethyl benzoate (250)

Contd...

Table 2.1–*Contd...*

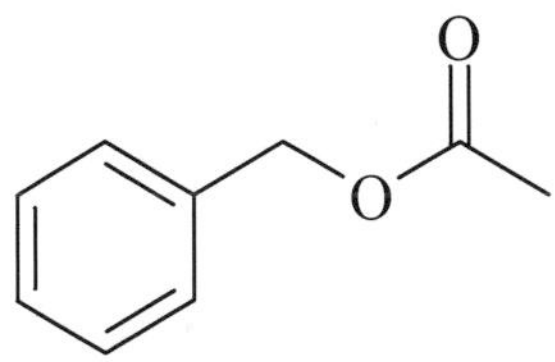

Benzyl acetate (251)

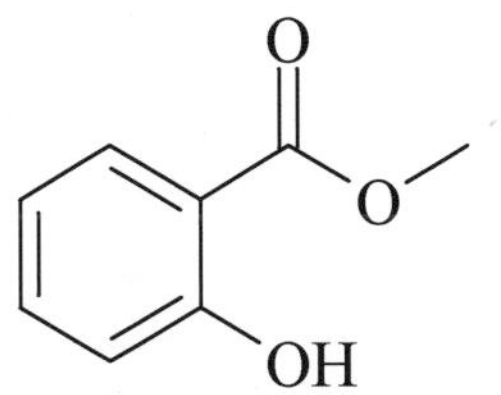

Methyl salicylate (252)

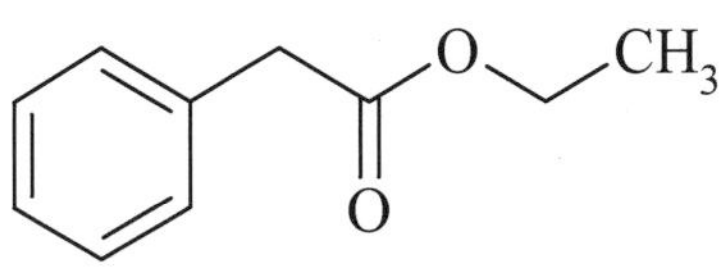

Ethyl phenylacetate (253)

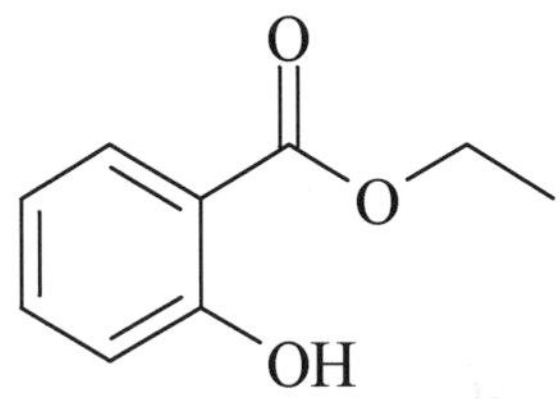

Ethyl salicylate (254)

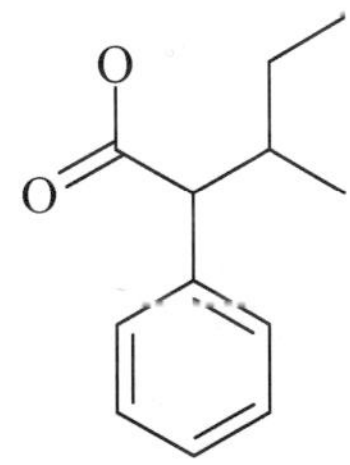

Phenyl methyl pentanoate (255)

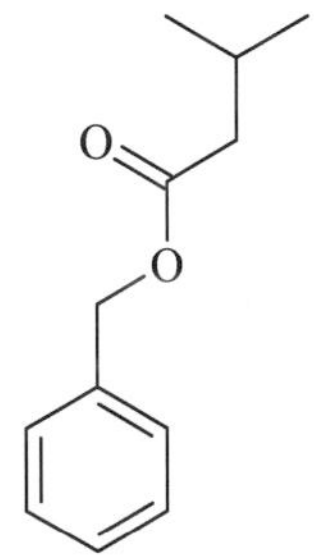

Benylisovalerate (256)

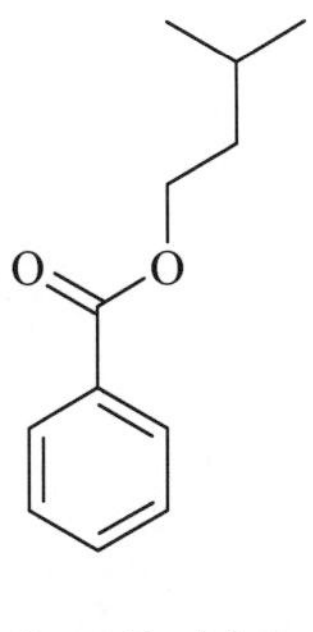

1-Butanol-3-methyl-benzoate (257)

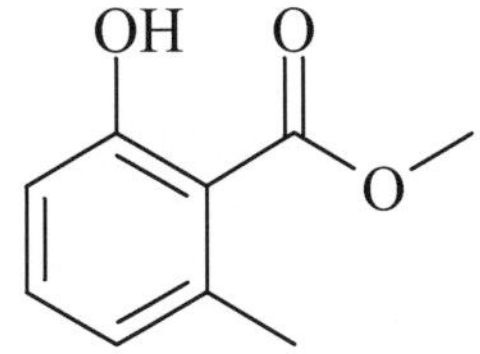

2,6-Cresotic acid methyl ester (258)

Contd...

Table 2.1–*Contd...*

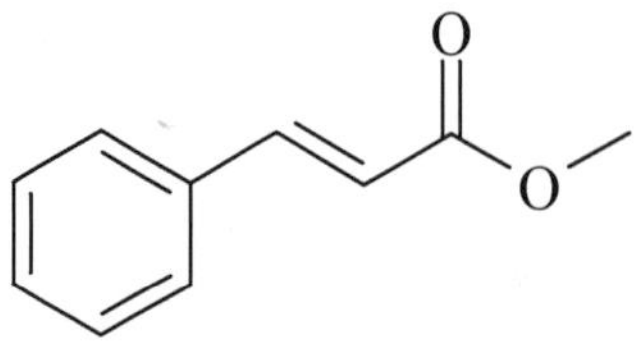

Methyl cinnamate (259)

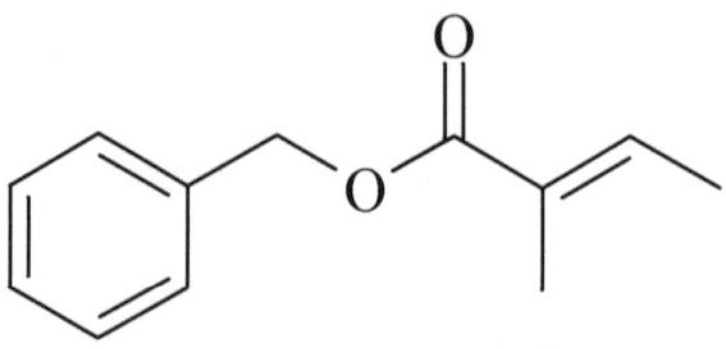

Benzyl tiglate (260)

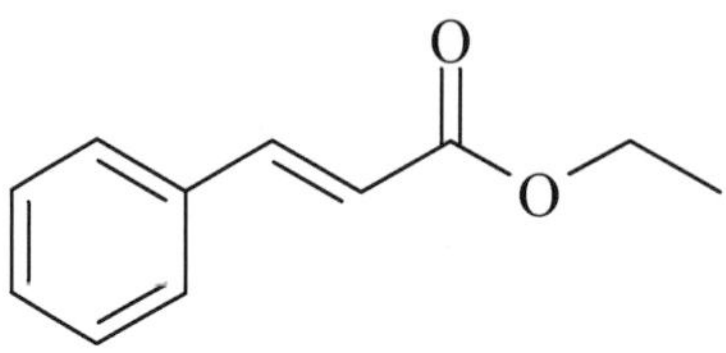

Ethyl cinnamate (261)

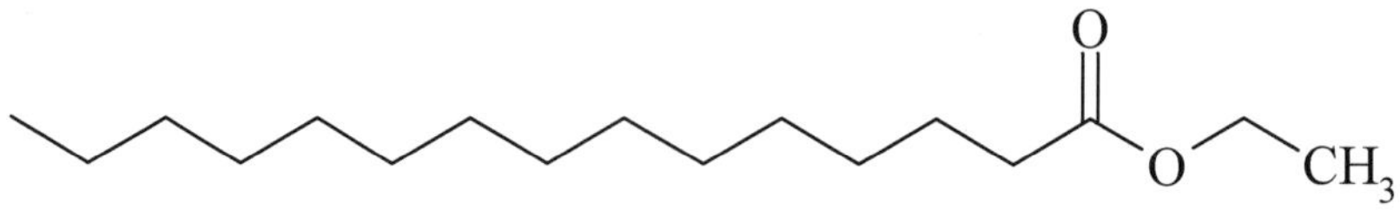

Ethyl pentadecanoate (262)

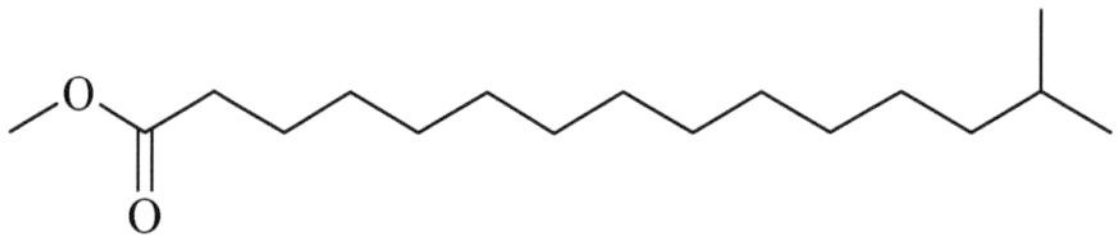

Methyl isohexadecanoate (263)

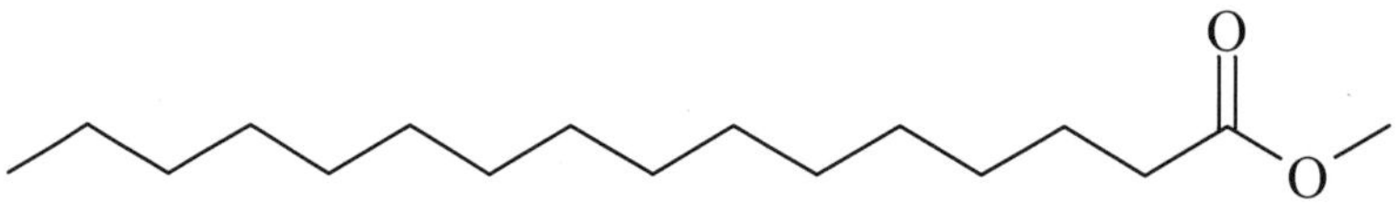

Methyl hexadecanoate (264)

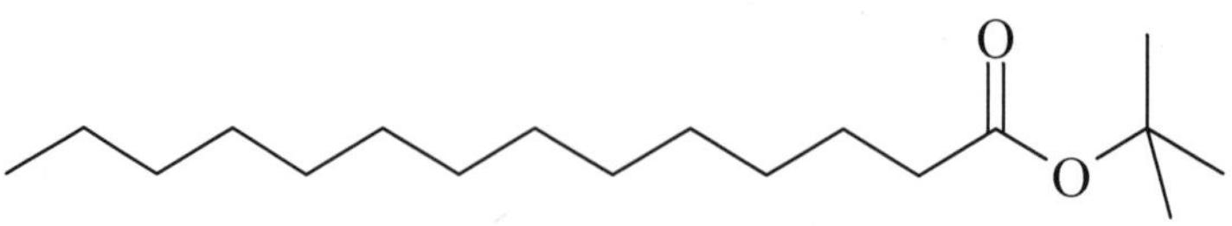

Butyl tetradecanoate (265)

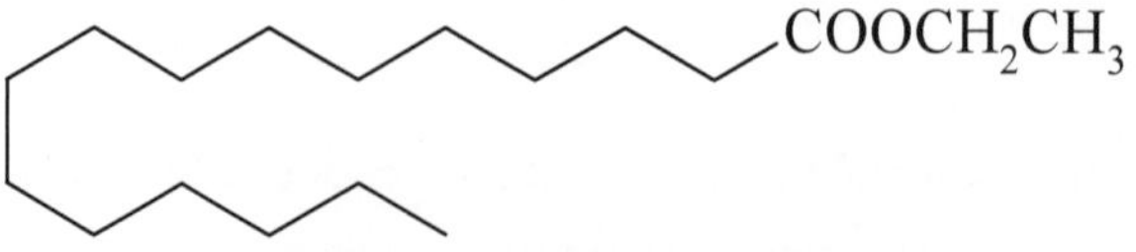

Ethyl hexadecanoate (266)

Contd...

Table 2.1–*Contd...*

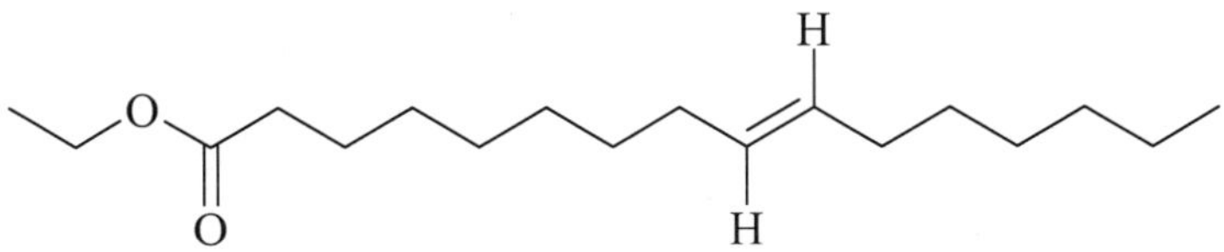

Ethyl-9-hexadecenoate (267)

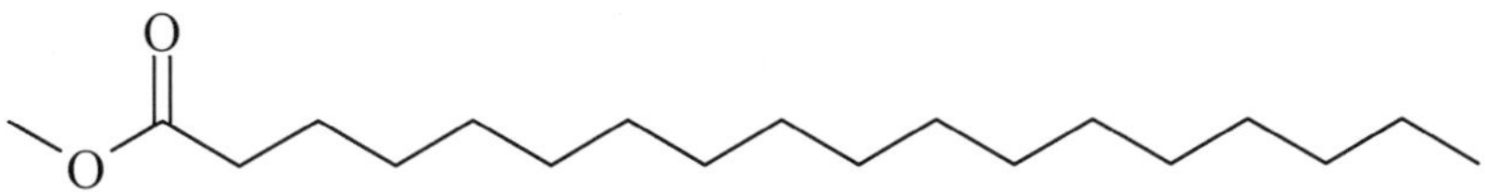

Methyl octadecanoate (268)

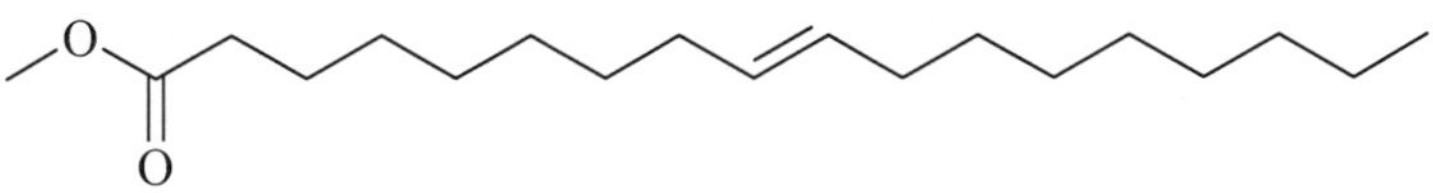

Methyl octadecenoate (269)

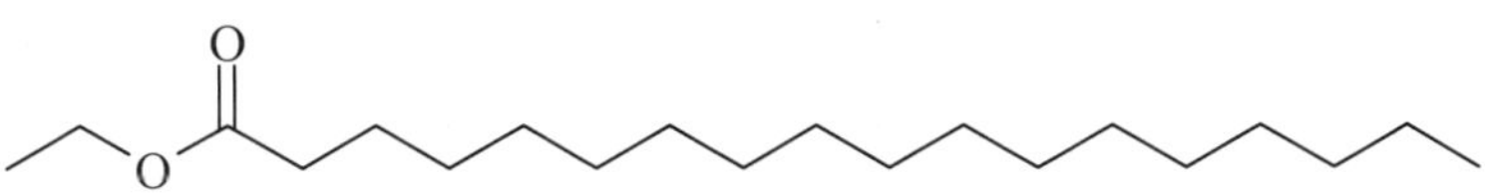

Ethyl octadecanoate (270)

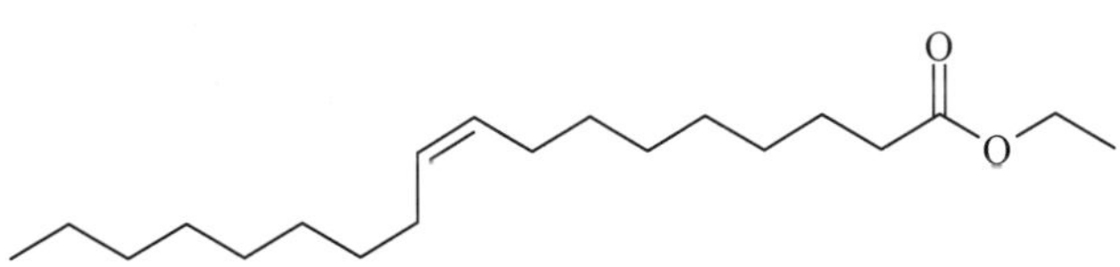

Ethyl 9-octadecenoate (271)

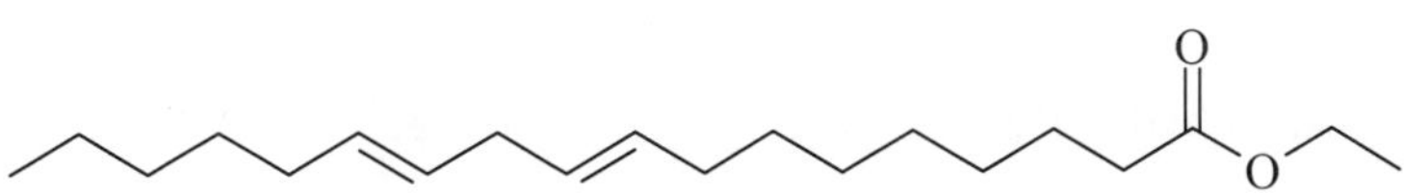

Ethyl 9,12-octadecadienoate (272)

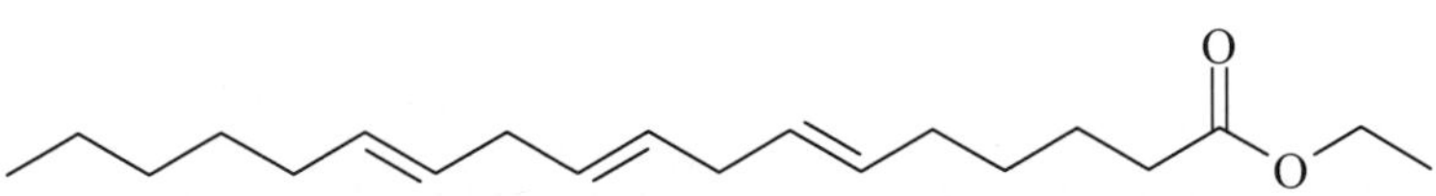

Ethyl 6,9,12-octadecatrienoate (273)

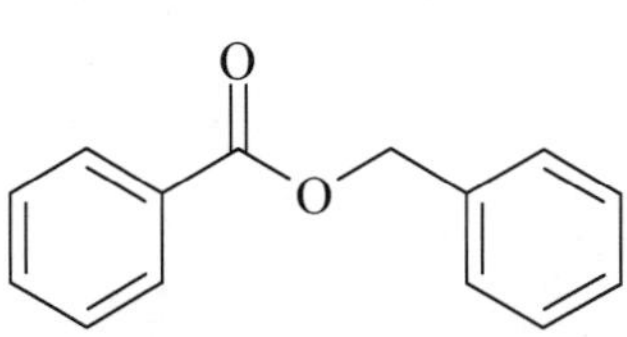

Benzyl benzoate (274)

Contd...

Table 2.1–*Contd...*

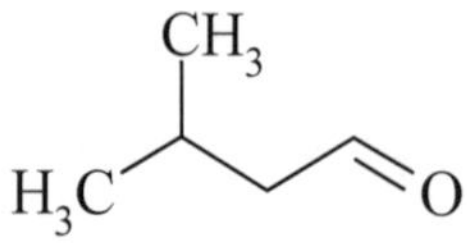

3-Methyl butane (275)

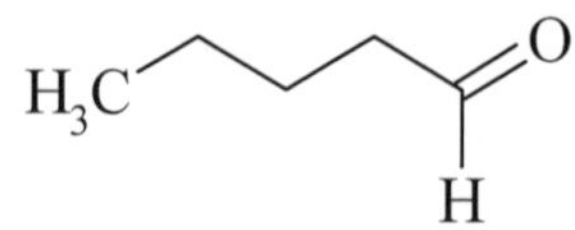

Pentanal (276)

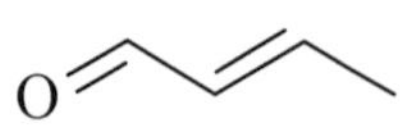

(E)-2-Butenal (277)

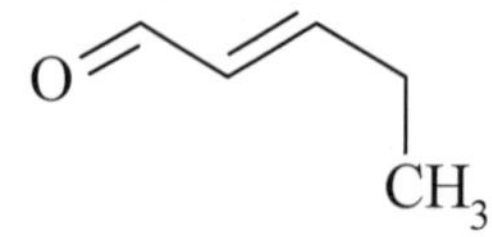

(E)-2-Pentenal (278)

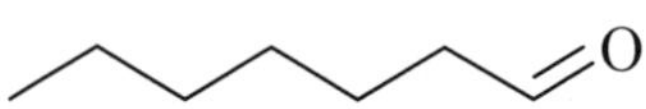

Heptanal (279)

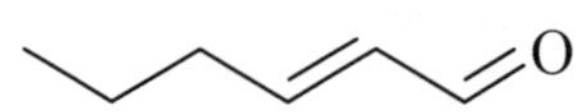

(E)-2-Hexenal (280)

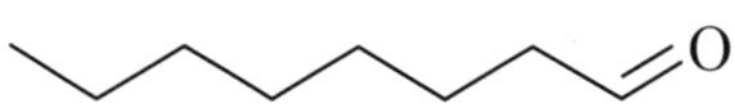

Octanal (281)

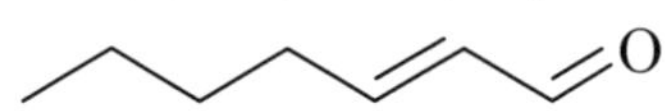

(E)-2-Heptenal (282)

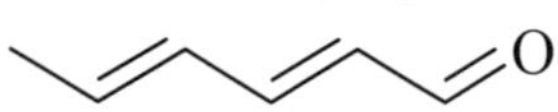

(E,E)-2,4-Hexadienal (283)

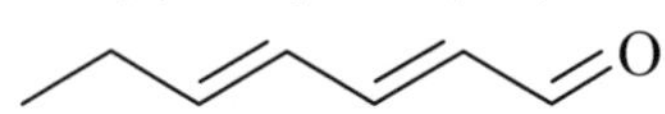

(E,E)-2,4-Heptadienal (284)

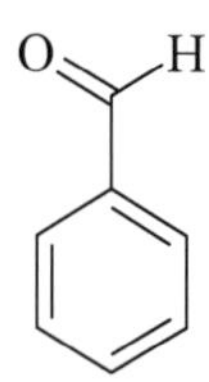

Benzaldehyde (285)

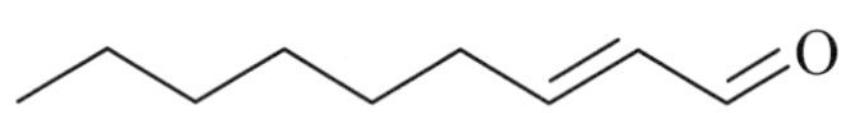

(E)-2-Nonenal (286)

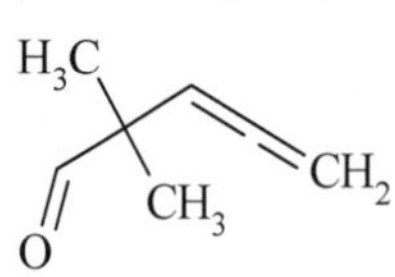

2,2-Dimethyl-3,4-pentadienal (287)

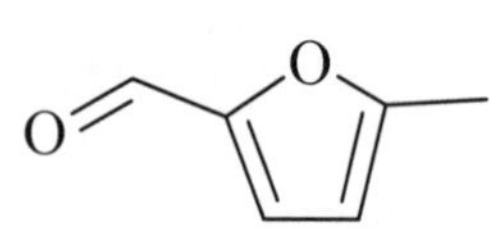

5-Methyl furan carboxaldehyde (288)

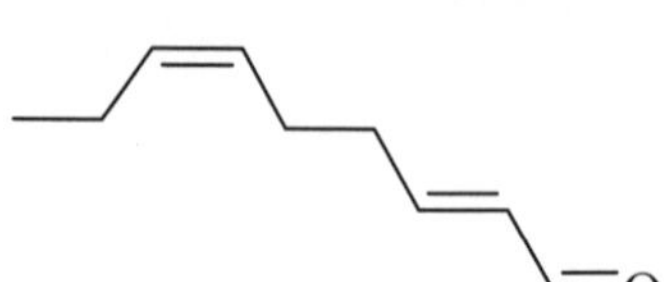

(E,Z)-2,6-Nonadienal (289)

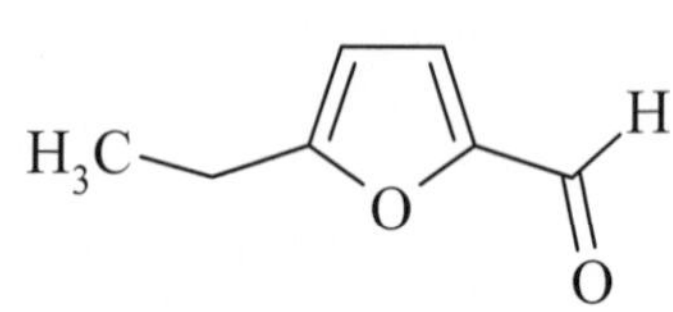

5-Ethyl-2-furaldehyde (290)

Contd...

Table 2.1–*Contd...*

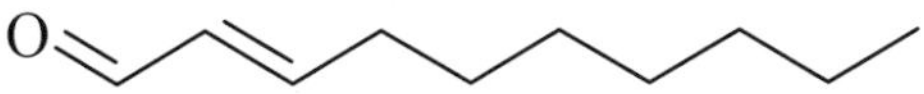

(E)-2-Decenal (291)

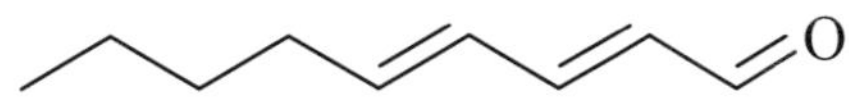

(E,E)-2,4-Nonadienal (292)

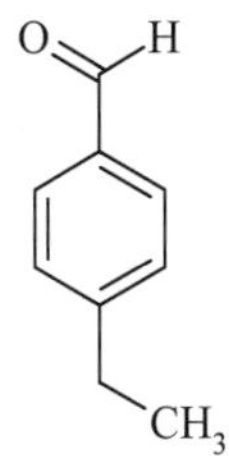

4-Ethyl benzaldehyde (293)

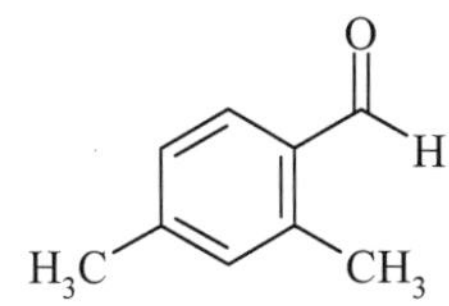

2,4-Dimethyl benzaldehyde (294)

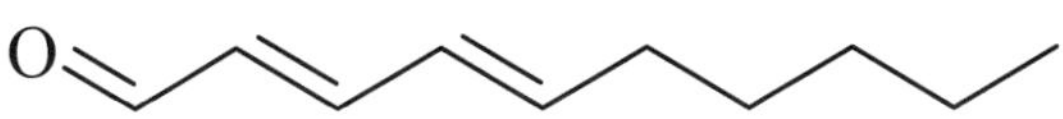

(E,E)-2,4-Decadienal (295)

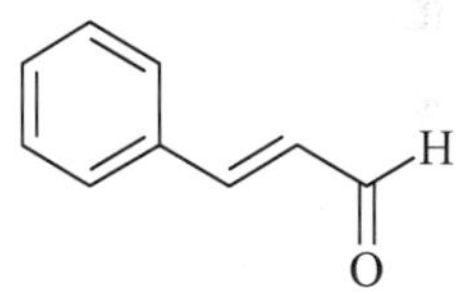

(E)-Cinnamaldehyde (296)

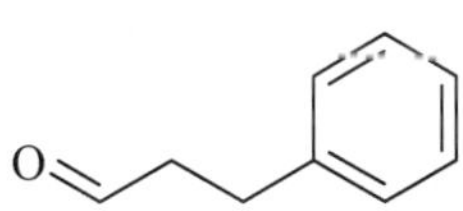

Benzylacetaldehyde (297)

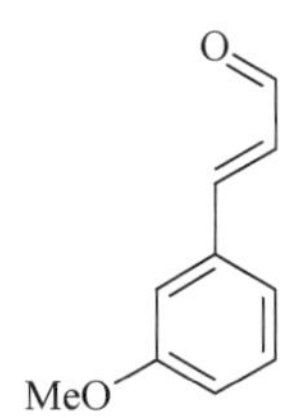

3-Methoxy cinnamaldehyde (298)

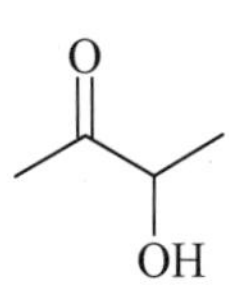

Acetoin (299)

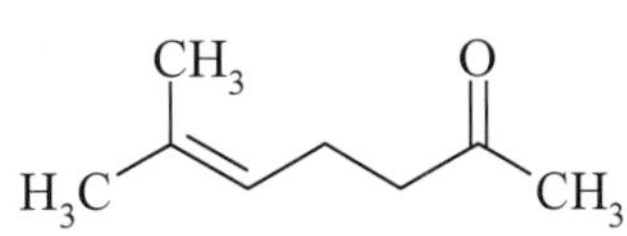

6-Methyl-5-hepten-2-one (300)

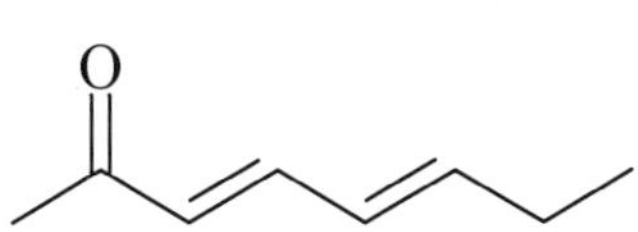

(E,E)-3,5-Octadiene-2-one (301)

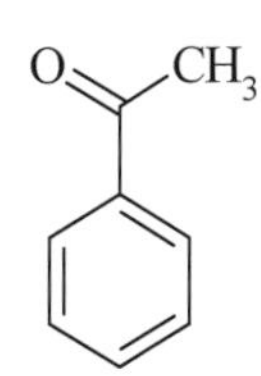

Acetophenone (302)

Contd...

Table 2.1–*Contd...*

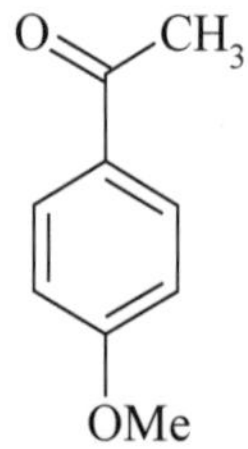

4'-Methoxy acetophenone (303)

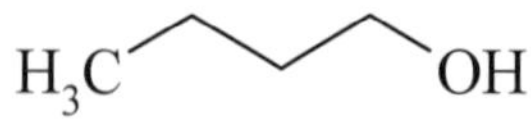

1-Butanol (304)

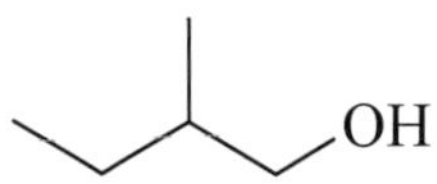

2-Methyl-1-butanol (305)

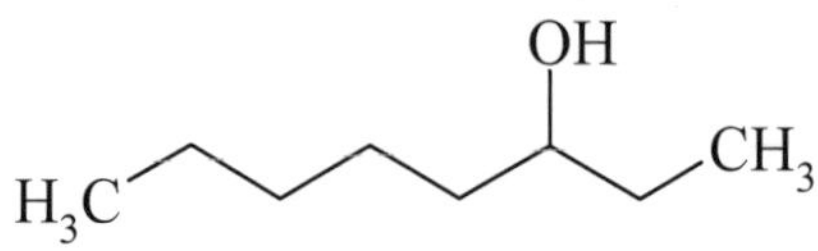

3-Octanol (306)

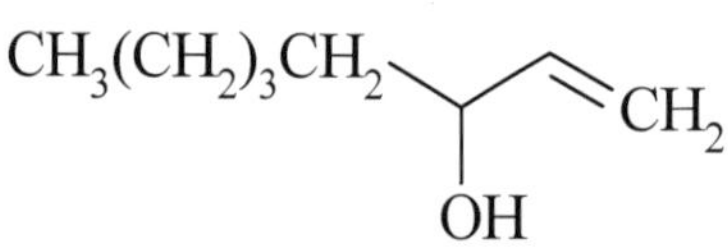

1-Octen-3-ol (307)

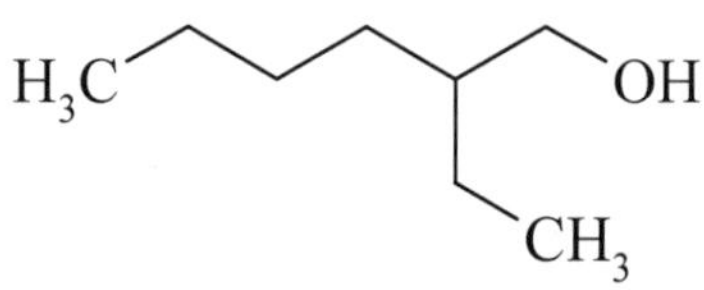

2-Ethyl-1-hexanol (308)

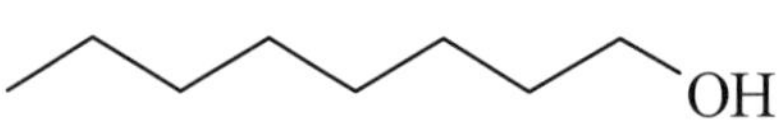

1-Octanol (309)

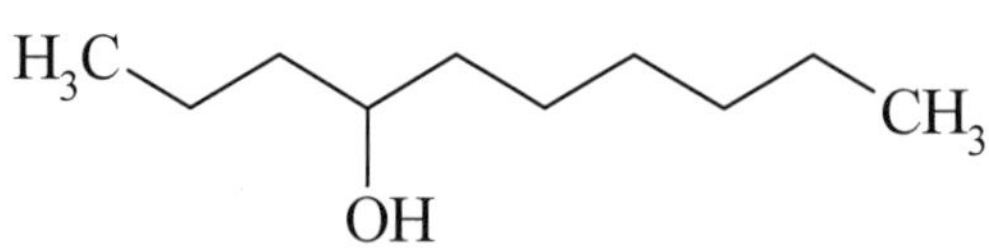

4-Decanol (310)

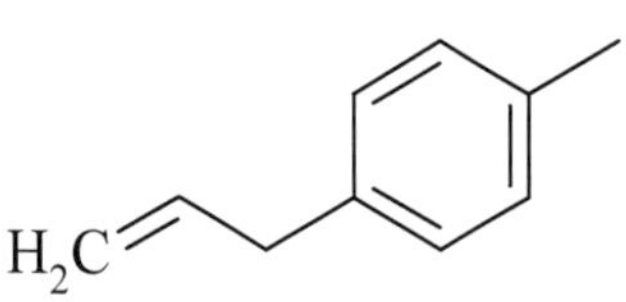

p-Allylanisole (311)

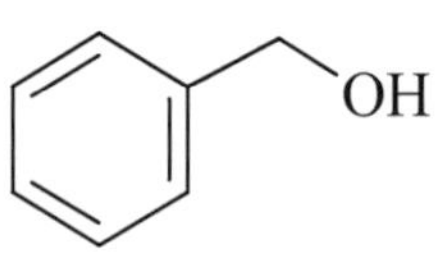

Benzyl alcohol (312)

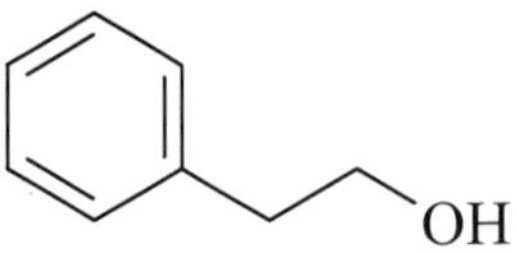

Phenyl ethyl alcohol (313)

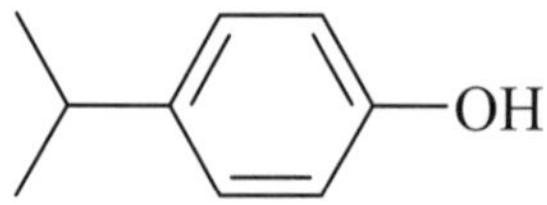

4-(1-Methyl propyl) phenol (314)

Contd...

Table 2.1–*Contd...*

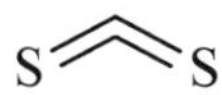

Carbon disulfide (315)

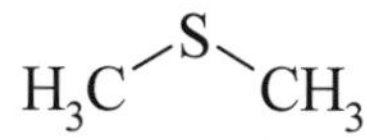

Dimethyl sulfide (316)

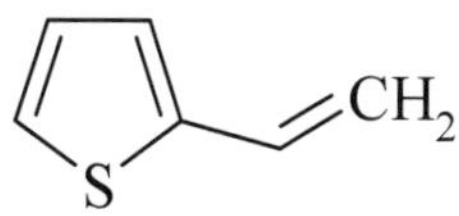

2-Ethyl thiophene (317)

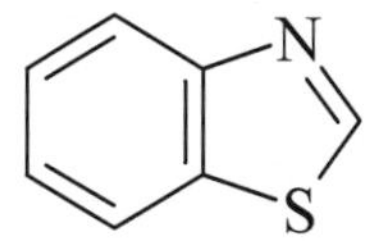

Benzothiazole (318)

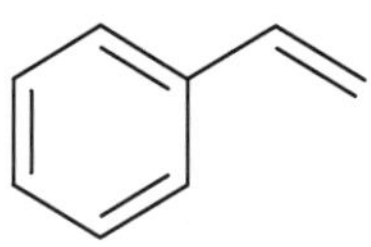

Styrene (319)

$H_3C—(CH_2)_{11}—CH_3$

Tridecane (320)

$H_3C—(CH_2)_{12}—CH_3$

Tetradecane (321)

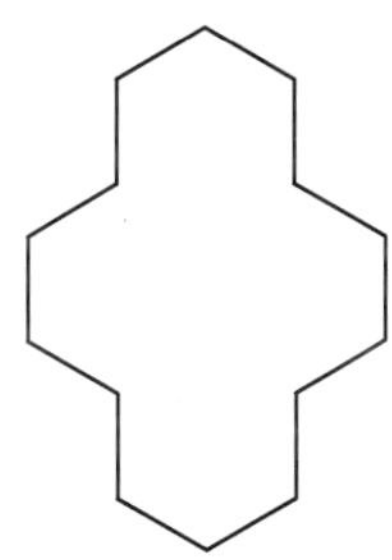

Cyclotetradecane (322)

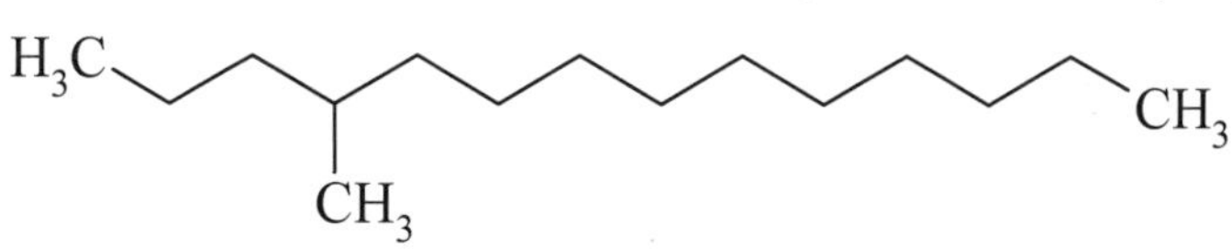

4-Methyl tetradecane (323)

$H_3C—(CH_2)_{13}—CH_3$

Pentadecane (324)

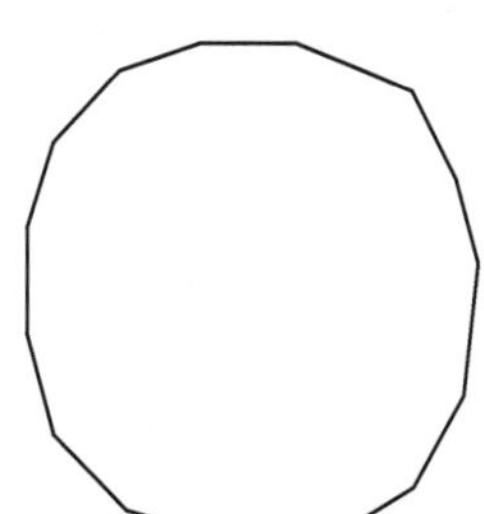

Cyclopentadecane (325)

Contd...

Table 2.1–*Contd...*

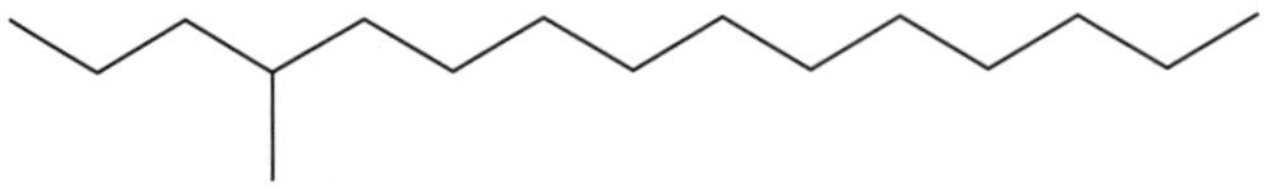

4-Methyl pentadecane (326)

$$H_3C-(CH_2)_{14}-CH_3$$

Hexadecane (327)

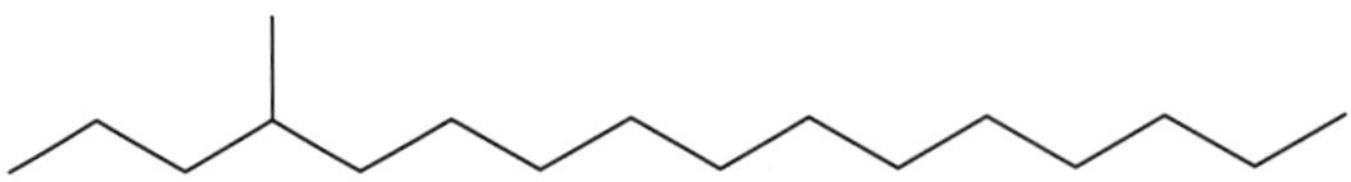

4-Methyl hexadecane (328)

$$H_3C-(CH_2)_{15}-CH_3$$

Heptadecane (329)

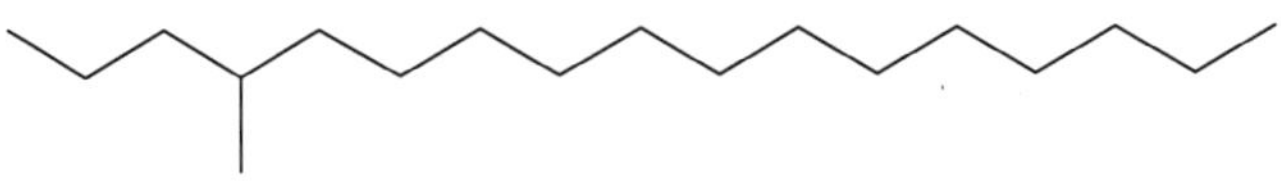

4-Methyl heptadecane (330)

$$H_3C-(CH_2)_{16}-CH_3$$

Octadecane (331)

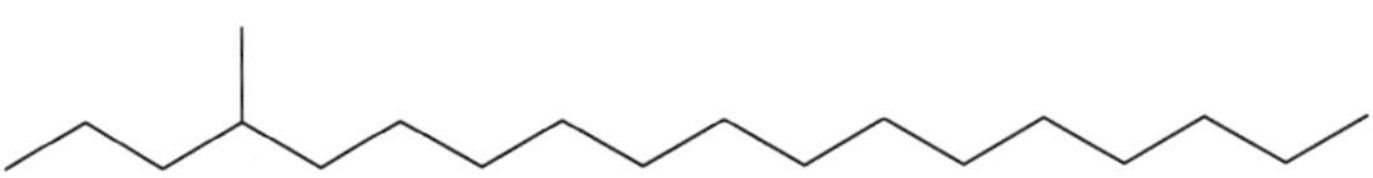

4-Methyl octadecane (332)

$$H_3C-(CH_2)_{17}-CH_3$$

Nonadecane (333)

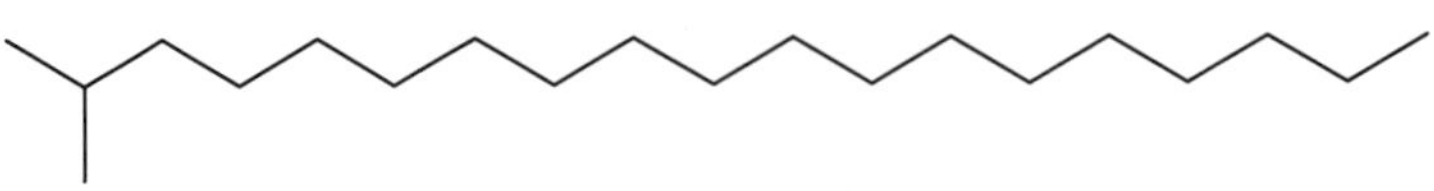

4-Methyl nonadecane (334)

$$H_3C-(CH_2)_{18}-CH_3$$

Eicosane (335)

$$H_3C-(CH_2)_{19}-CH_3$$

Heneicosane (336)

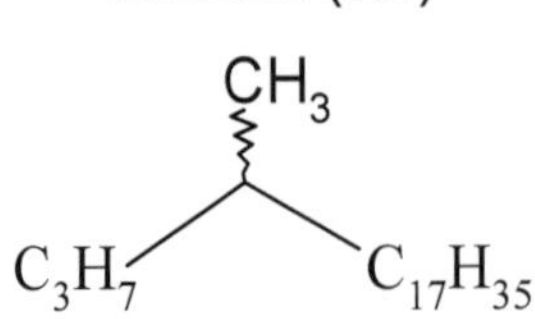

4-Methyl heneicosane (337)

$$H_3C-(CH_2)_{20}-CH_3$$

Docosane (338)

Contd...

Table 2.1–*Contd...*

$$H_3C—(CH_2)_{21}—CH_3$$

Tricosane (339)

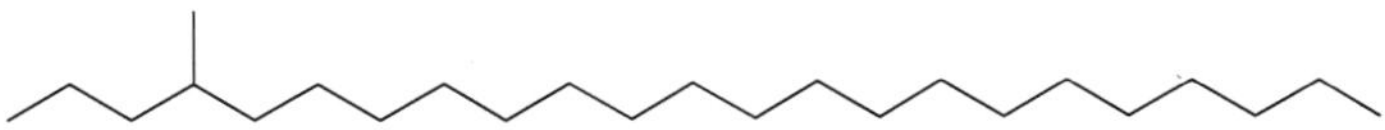

4-Methyl tricosane (340)

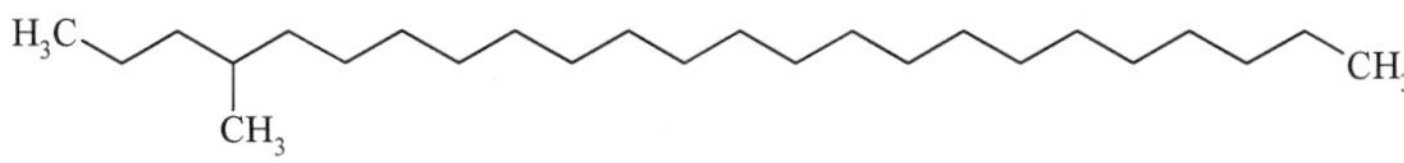

4-methyl tetracosane (341)

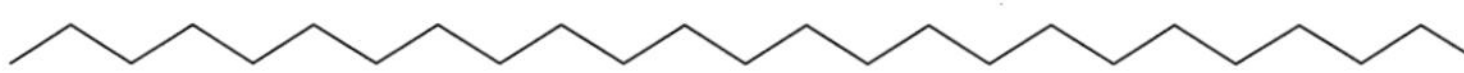

Pentacosane (342)

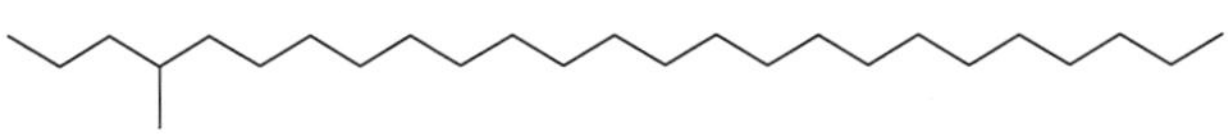

4-Methyl hexacosane (343)

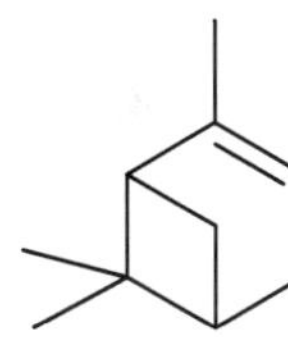

β-Pinene (344)

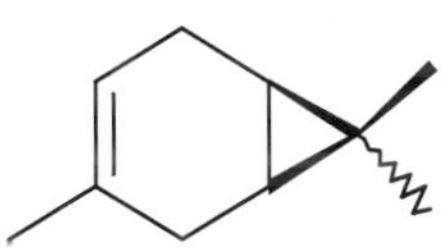

Δ-3-carene (345)

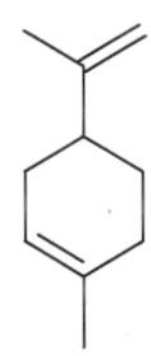

Limonene (346)

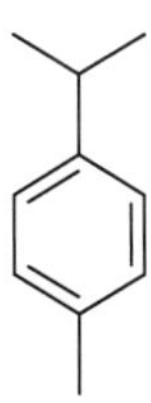

β-Cimene (347)

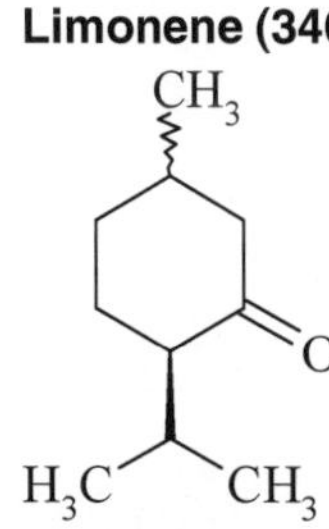

p-Menthone (348)

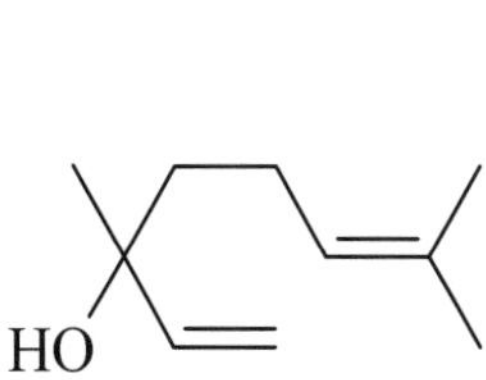

β-Linalool (349)

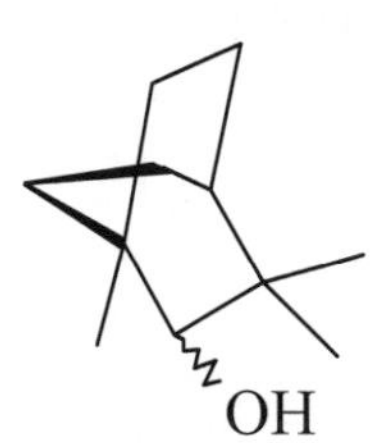

D-Fenchyl alcohol (350)

Contd...

Table 2.1–*Contd...*

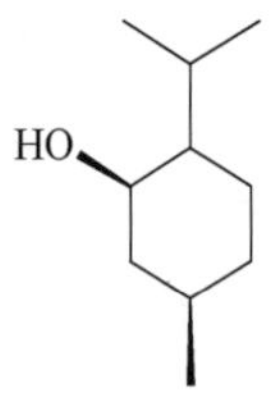

(-) Menthol (351)

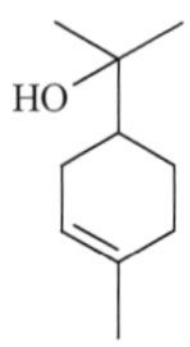

4-Terpineol (352)

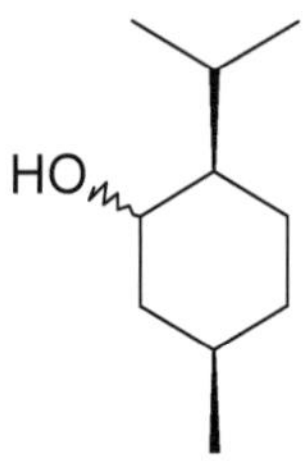

Isomenthol (353)

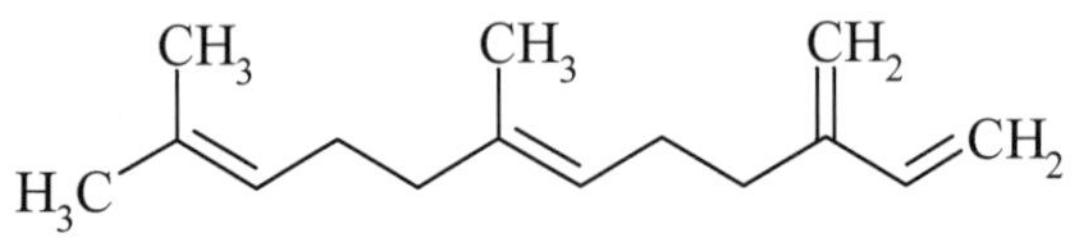

β-Farnesene (354)

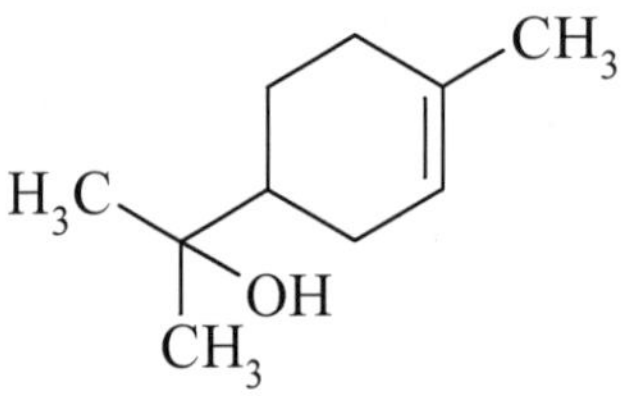

α-Terpineol (355)

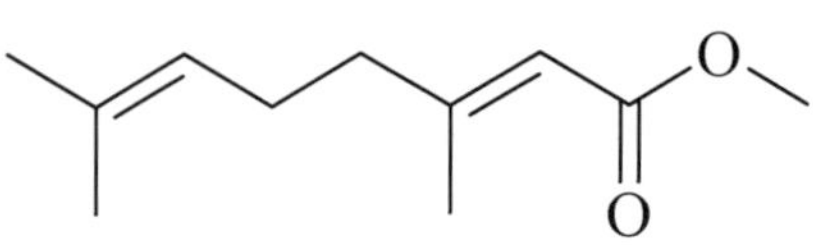

Methyl geranate (356)

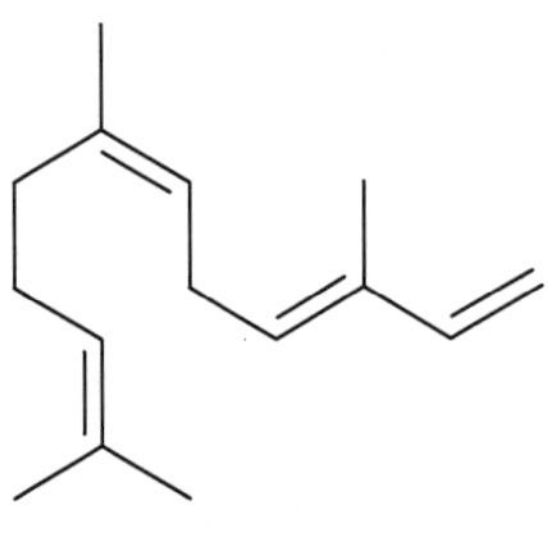

(E,Z)-α-Farnesene (357)

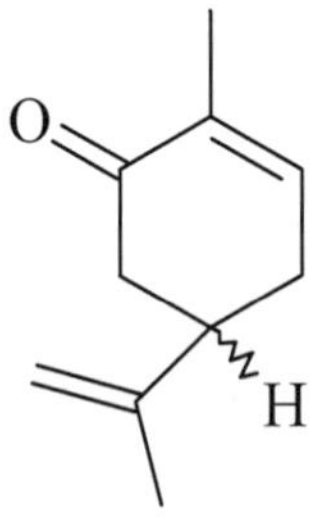

Carvone (358)

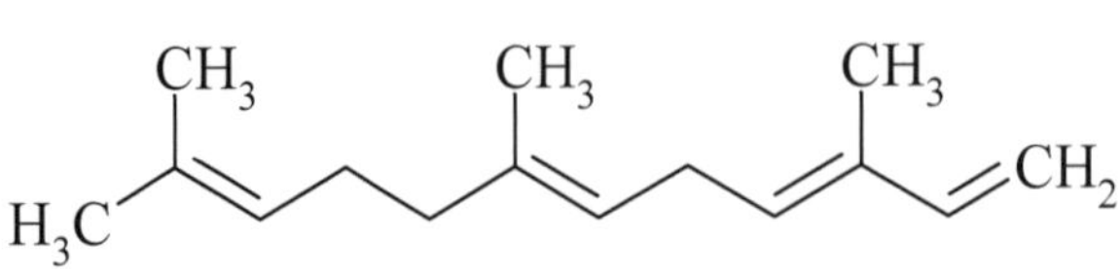

(E,E)-α-Farnesene (359)

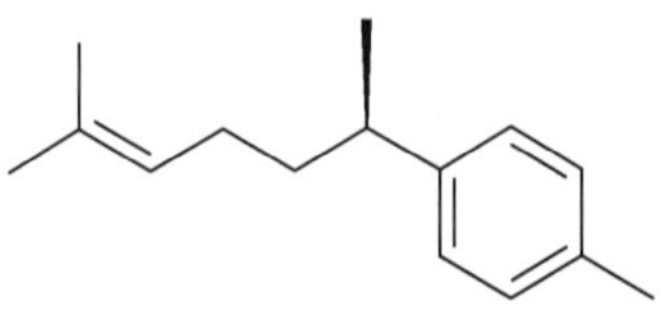

α-Curcumene (360)

Contd...

Table 2.1–*Contd...*

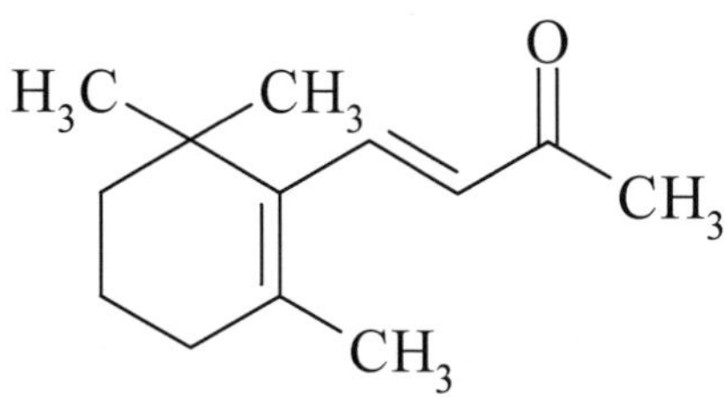

(E)-β-Ionone (361)

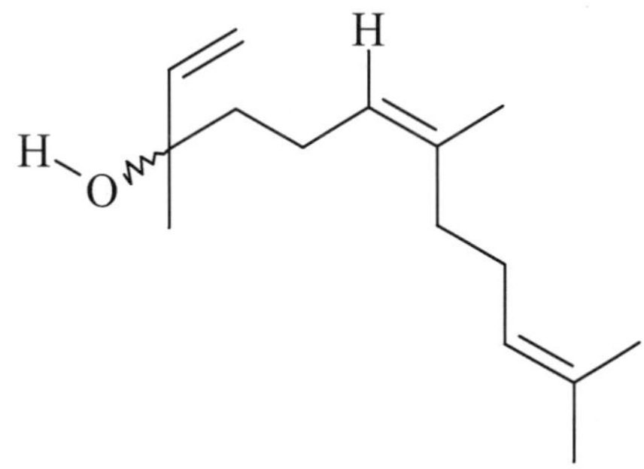

D-Nerolidol (362)

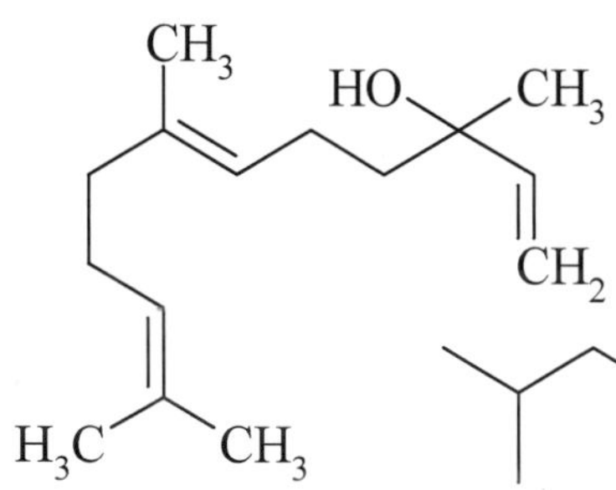

Trans-nerolidol (363)

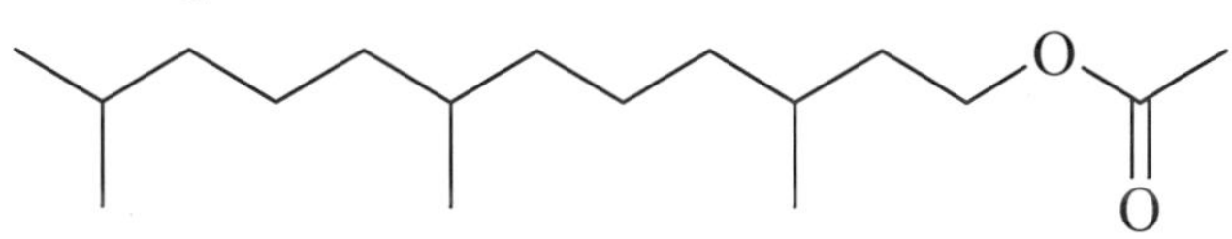

Hexahydrofarnesyl acetate (364)

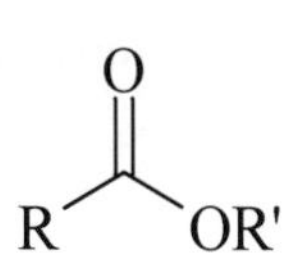

Esters (365)

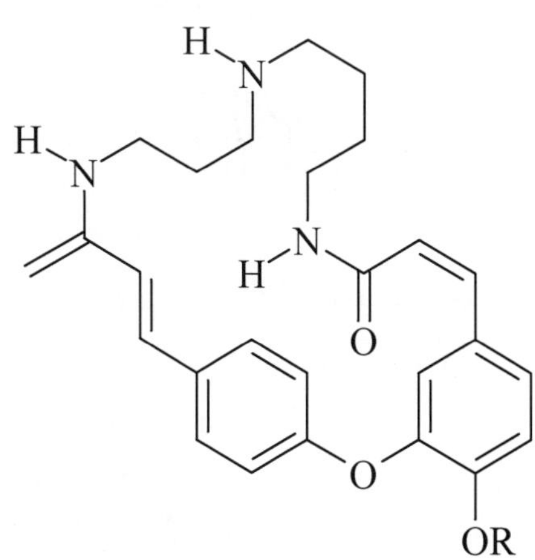

Capparispine (366)

Contd...

Table 2.1–*Contd...*

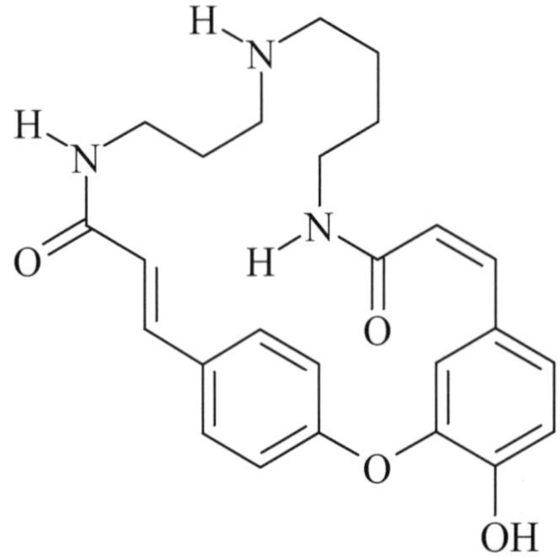

Capparispine-26-O-d-glucoside (367)

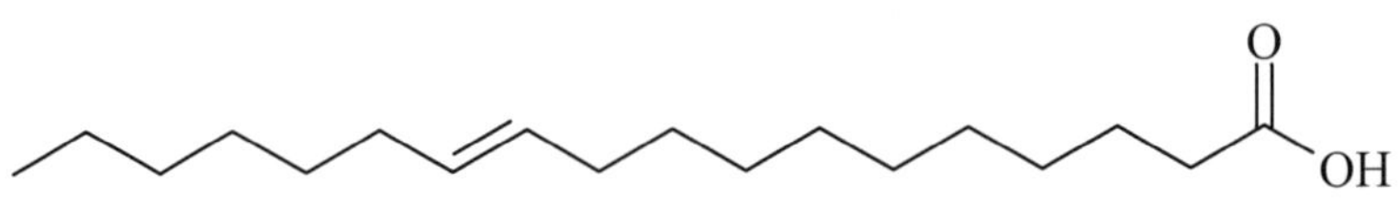

Vaccenic acid (368)

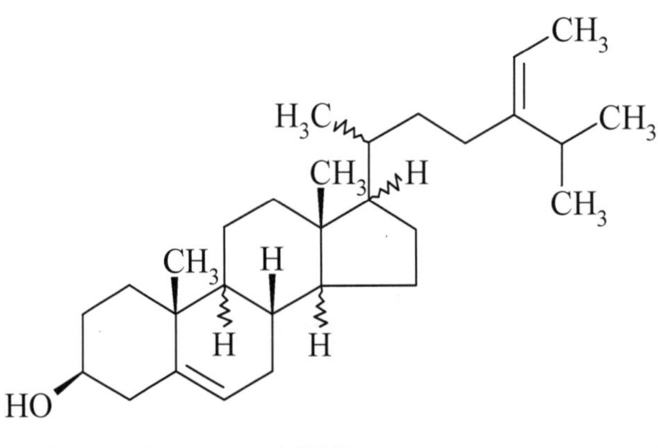

5-Avenasterol (369)

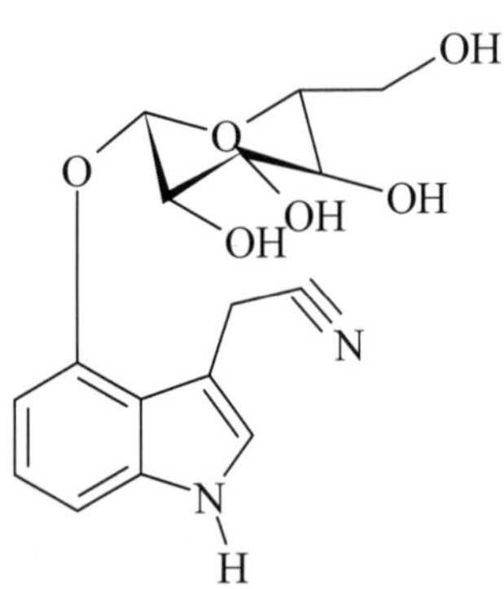

Cappariloside A (370)

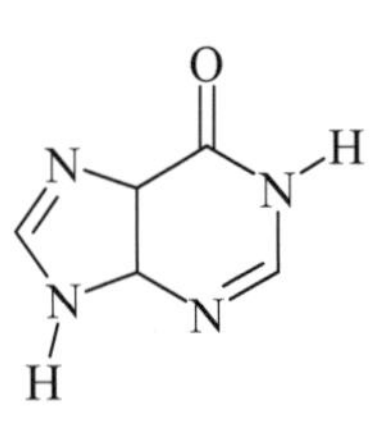

Hypoxanthine (371)

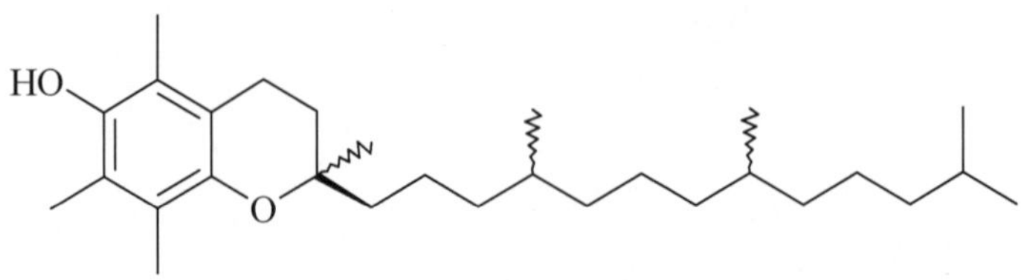

α-Tocopherol (372)

Contd...

Table 2.1–*Contd...*

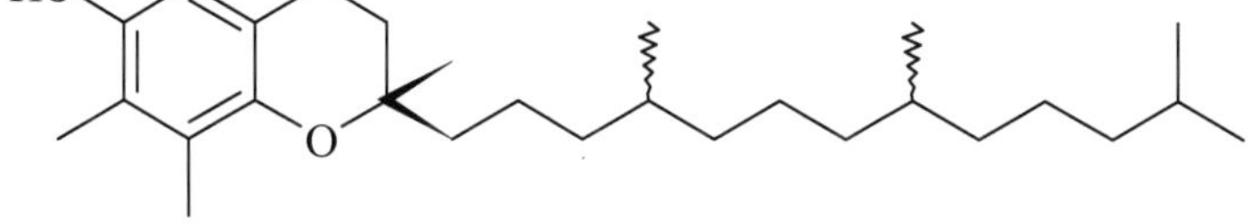

γ-Tocopherol (373)

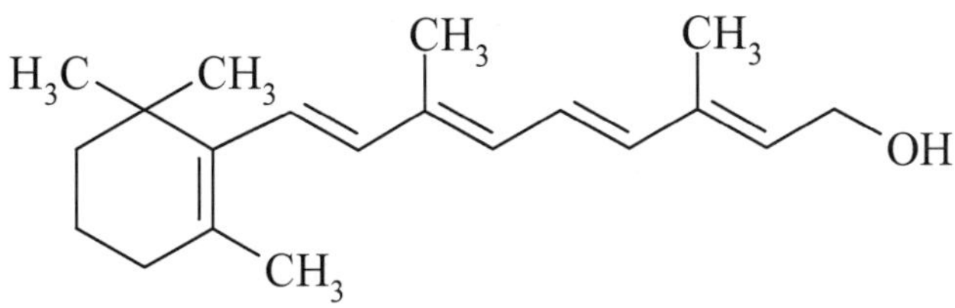

Vitamin A (374)

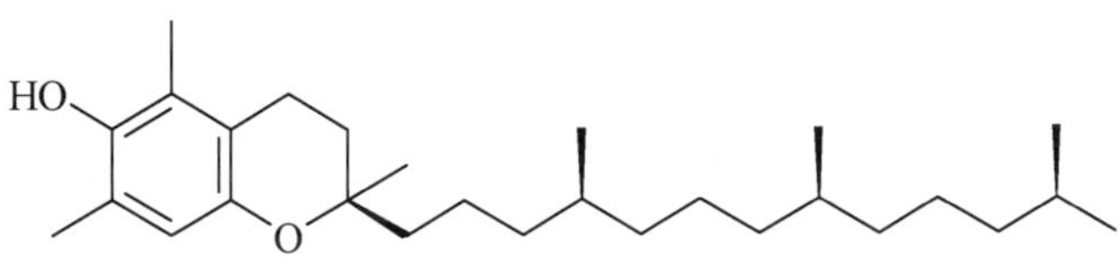

Vitamin E (375)

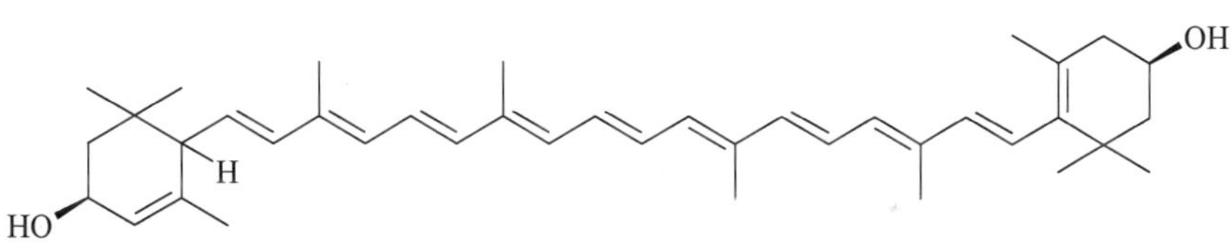

Lutein (376)

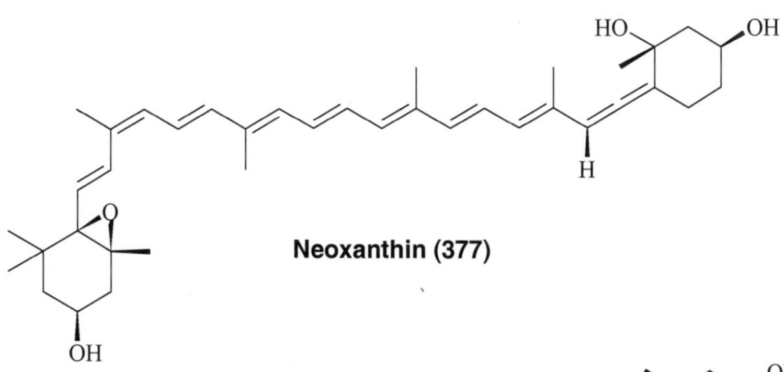

Neoxanthin (377)

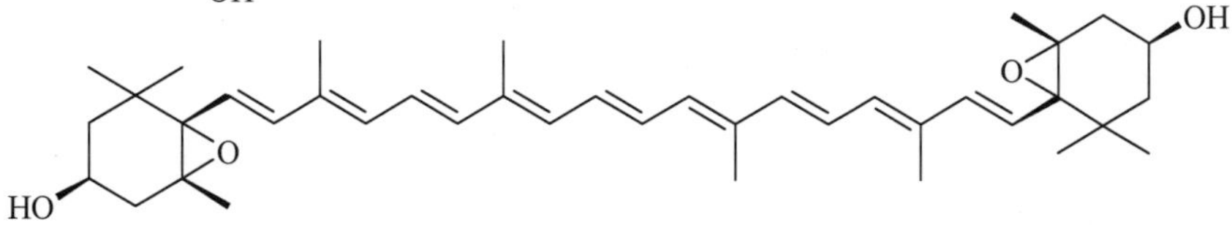

Violaxanthin (378)

Contd...

Table 2.1–*Contd...*

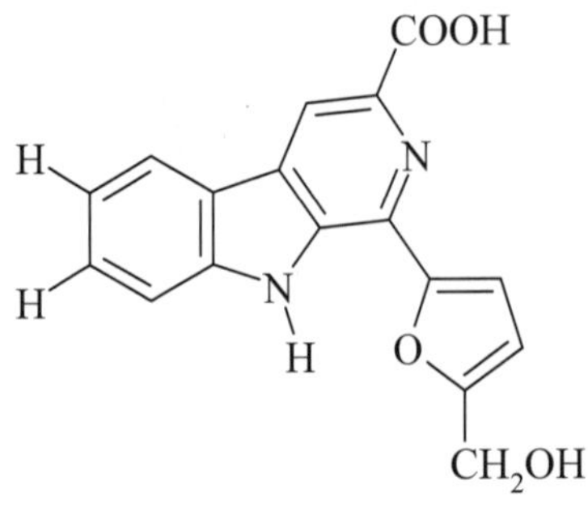

Flazin (379)

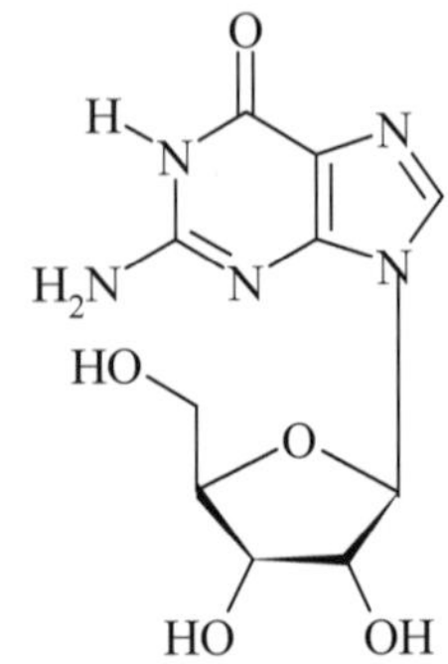

Guanosine (380)

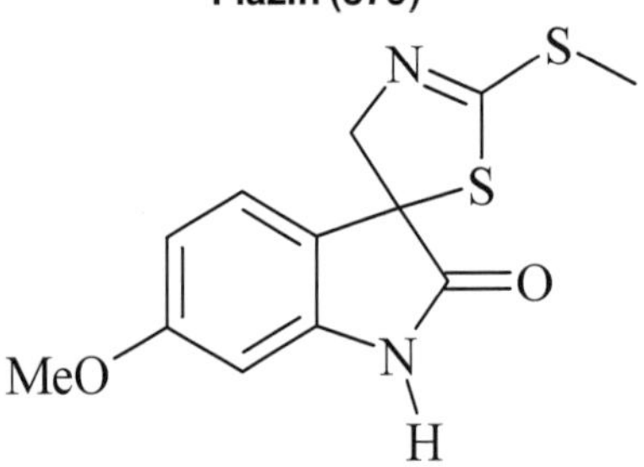

Capparine A (381)

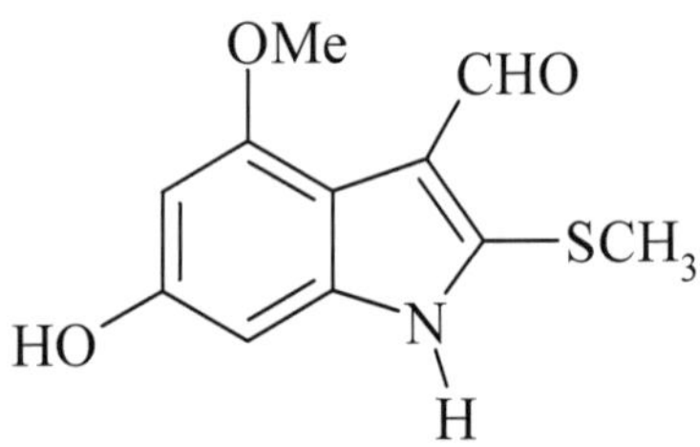

Capparine B (382)

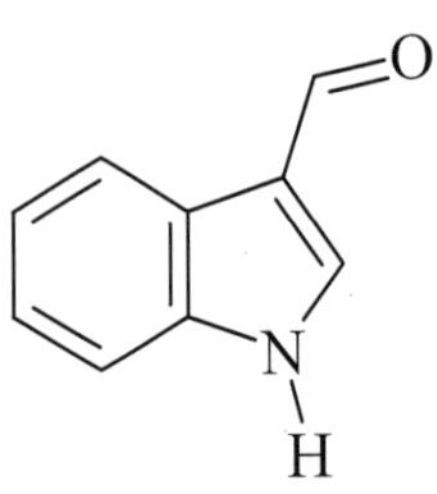

1H-Indole-3-carboxaldehyde (383)

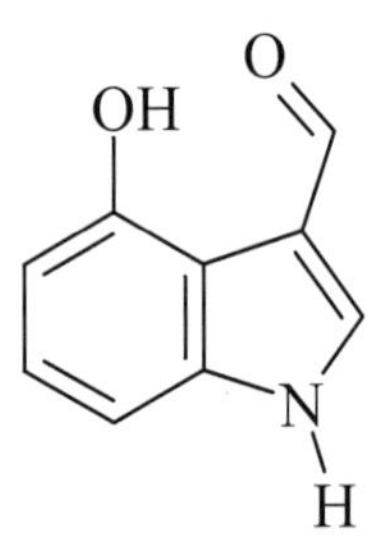

4-Hydroxy-1H-indole-3-carboxaldehyde (384)

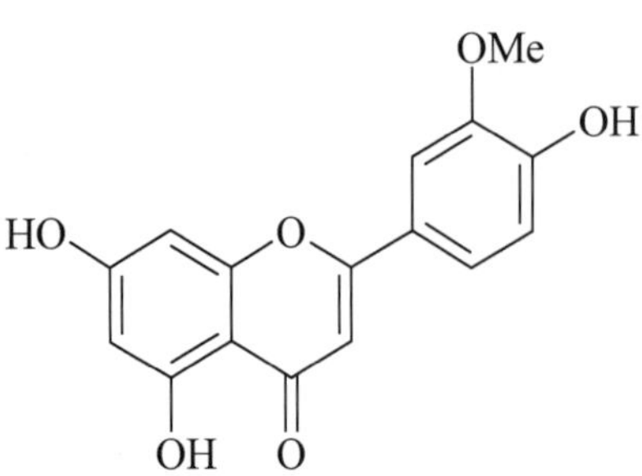

Chryxoeriol (385)

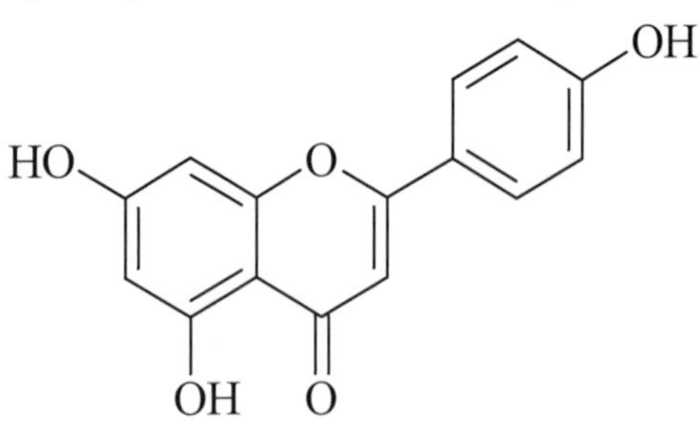

Apigenin (386)

Contd...

Table 2.1–*Contd...*

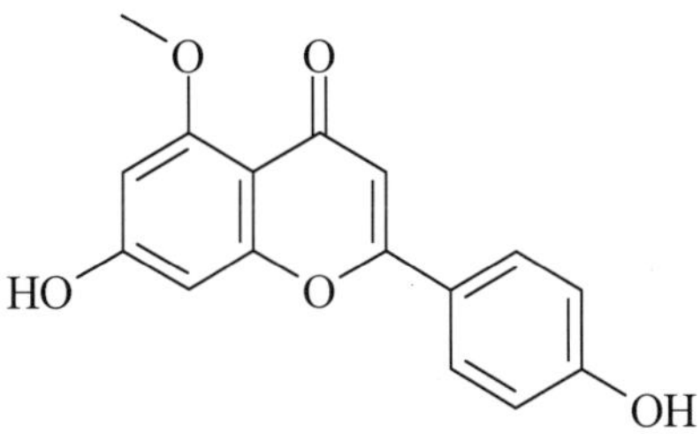

Thevetiaflavone (387)

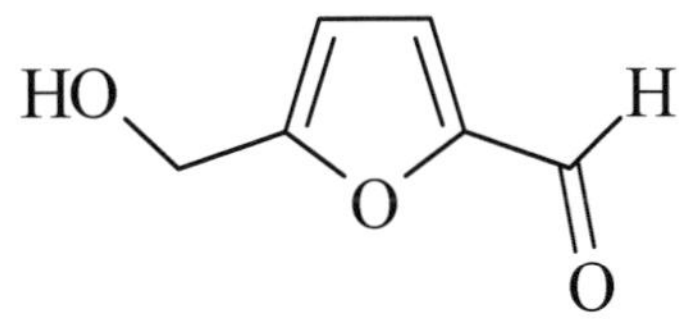

5-Hydroxymethyl furaldehyde (388)

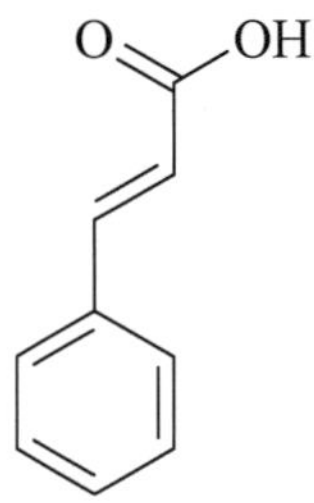

Cinnamic acid (389)

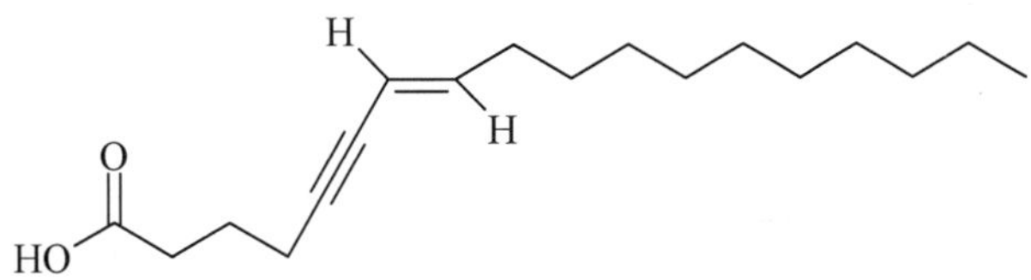

Octadec-7-en-5-ynoic acid (390)

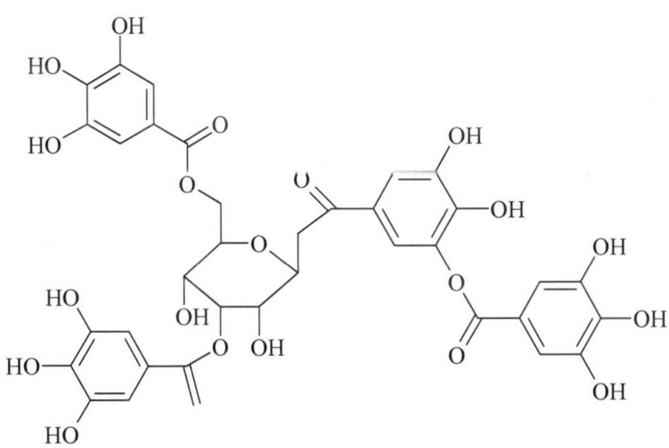

Tannins (391)

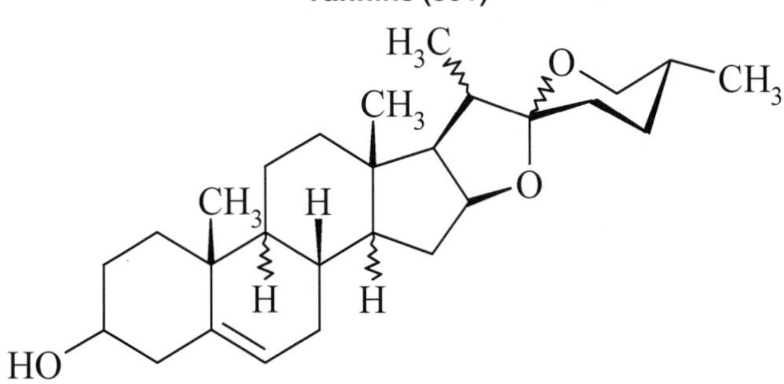

Saponins flavonoids (392)

Contd...

Table 2.1–*Contd...*

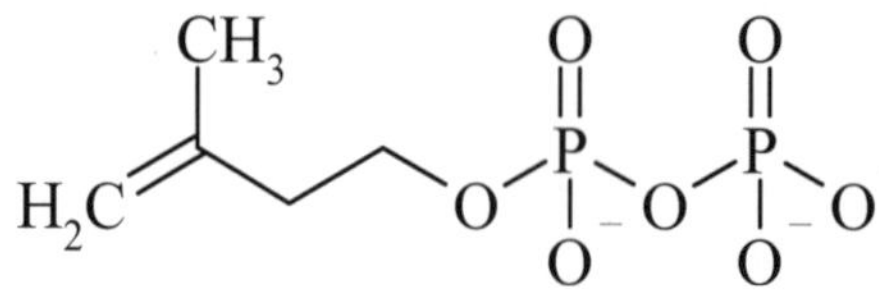

Terpenoids (393)

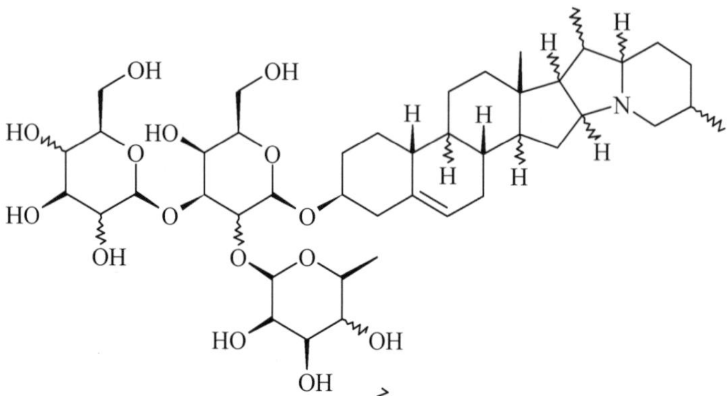

Saponins (394)

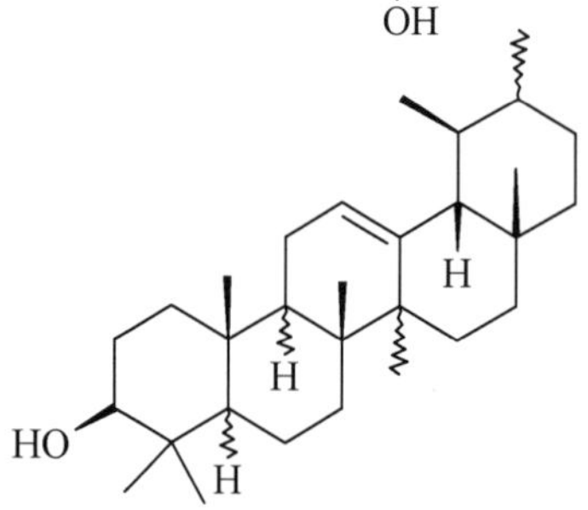

α-Amyrin (395)

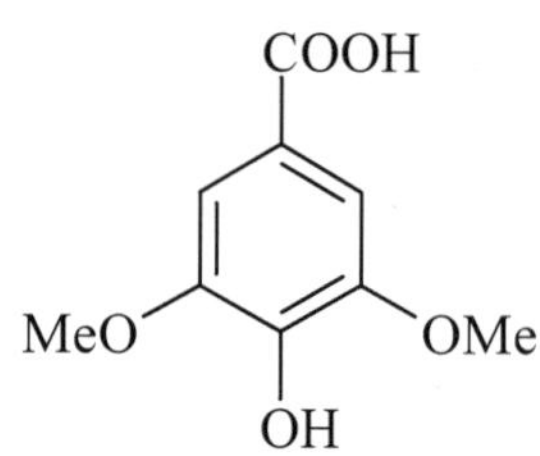

Syringic acid (396)

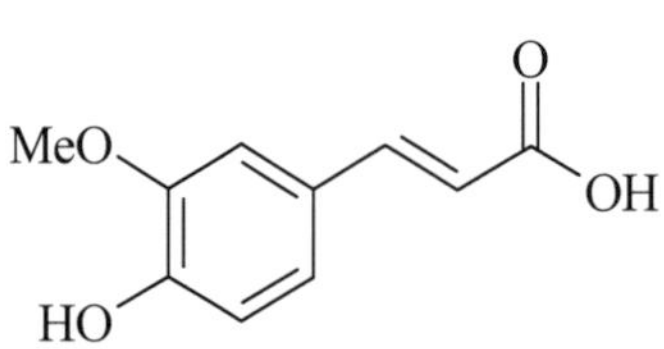

Ferrulic acid (397)

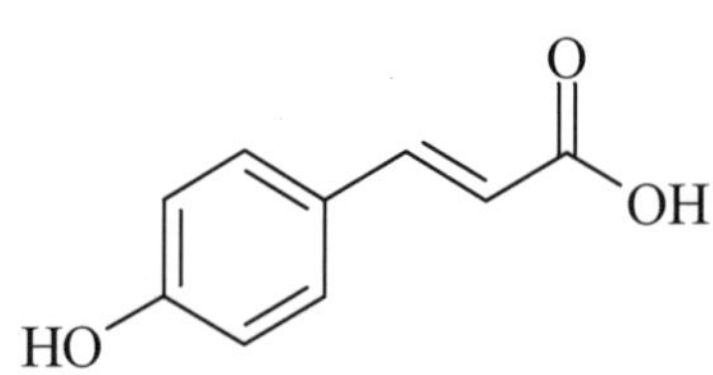

***p*-Coumanic acid (398)**

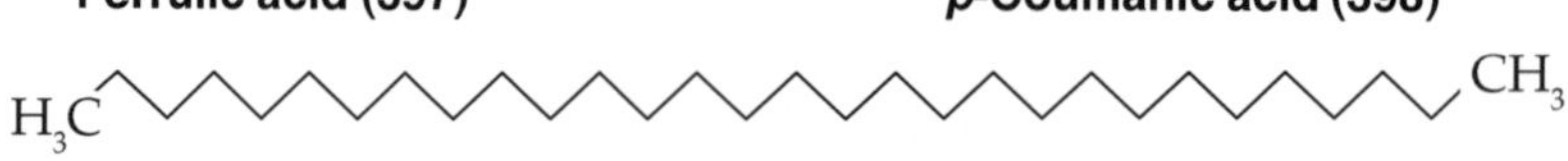

n-Trichontane (399)

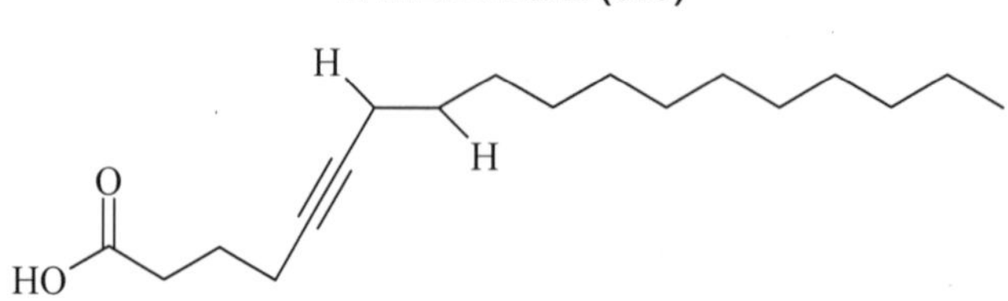

E-Octodec-7-enynoic acid (400)

The aerial parts of *Capparis spinosa* were investigated and reported for its flavonoids constituents and thirteen flavonoids glycosides *viz.*, quercetin-3-rutinoside **(62)**, quercetin-7-rutinoside **(170)**, quercetin-3-O-glucoside-7-O-rhamnoside **(171)**, kaempferol-7-rhamnoside **(183)**, kaempferol-3-glucoside-7-rhamnoside **(184)**, kaempferol-3-rhamnoside-7-glucoside **(185)**, quercetin-3-rhamnoside **(186)**, quercetin-7-rhamnoside **(187)**, quercetin-3,7-dirhamnoside **(188)**, isorhamnetin-3-rutinoside **(189)**, isorhamnetin-3,7-dirhamnoside **(190)** and apigenin-6,8-di-C-glucoside **(191)** (Sharaf *et al.*, 1997).

Table 2.2: Phytoconstituents Classification and its Chemical Nature of *Capparis* Genus

Phytoconstituents	*Number of Phytochemicals*
Alkaloids	16
Alkanes	34
Amino acids	3
Anthraquinones	5
Carbohydrate	7
Fats and fatty acids	115
Flavonoids	36
Glycosides	28
Phenolic compounds	65
Saponins	8
Steroids	11
Tannins	4
Triterpenoids	35
Vitamins	2
Colour pigments	7
Intermediate compounds	24
Total	**400**

The leaves of *Capparis spinosa* reported to possess phytochemicals such as quercetin **(65)**, kaempferal **(66)**, isorhamnetin **(192)** and their O-methyl derivative, thomnocitirin, rhamnetin **(193)** and rhamnozin **(194)** (Juan and Martinez, 1998). Other researches revealed and reported that the *C. spinosa* leaf oil composes of butyl isothiocyanate **(1)**, isopropyl isothiocyanates **(9)**, N-alkanes **(175)**, phenyl propanoid **(177)**, thymol **(180)**, 2-hexenal **(195)**, chlorophyll **(196)**, proline **(197)** and starch **(198)** (Afsharypuor *et al.*, 1998).

On the basis of spectral and chemical evidences 1H-indole-3-acetonitrile glycoside **(199)** has been isolated and reported from *Capparis spinosa* by (Calis *et al.*, 1999). In a later study, they isolated and reported three new glycosides compounds from caper berries as *C. spinosa*. They are 3 new glycosides ((+)-(6S,9S)-9-O-β-D-glucopyranosyloxy-6-hydroxy-3-oxo-α-ionol, (6S,9S)-roseoside), ((6S,9S)-6-

hydroxyinamoside,((-)-(6S,9S)-9-O-β-D-glycopyranosyloxy-6,13-dihydroxy-3-oxo-α-ionol)) and ((9S)-drummondol-9-O-β-D-glucoranoside) **(200)**.

Further studies have been reported on methanolic extract of the aerial parts of *Capparis spinosa* yielded a flavonoid and quercetin **(65)** such as 3-O-(6'''-α-L-rhamnosyl-6''-β-D-glucosyl)-β-D-glucoside **(201)**, rutin **(7)**, quercetin-3-O-glucoside-7-O-rhamnoside **(171)** and quercetin-3-O-glucoside **(202)** (Afsharypuor *et al.*, 1998). The p-methoxy benzoic acid **(203)** isolated from the methanolic fraction of the aqueous extract of *C. spinosa* was reported (Calis *et al.*, 1999). It was found to possess significant antihepatotoxic activity carbontetrachloride and paracetamol induced hepatotoxicity *in vivo* and thioacetamide and galactosamine induced hepatotoxicity in Wistar Albino rat hepatocytes by using *in vitro* technique (Gadgoli and Mishra, 1999).

In addition to rutin **(7)**, quercetin-3-O-glucoside-7-O-rhamnoside **(171)** and quercetin-3-O-glucoside **(202)** were reported in the methanolic extract of aerial parts of *Capparis spinosa* yielded a new flavonoid 3-O-(6'''-α-L-rhamnosyl-6''-β-D-glucosyl)-β-D-glucoside **(201)** (Sharaf *et al.*, 2000). The *Capparis spinosa* have been found and reported two new compounds, β-sitosteryl glucoside-6′-octadecanoate **(204)** and 3-methyl-2-butenyl-β-glycoside **(205)** (Khanfar *et al.*, 2002).

The (6S)-hydroxy-3-oxo-a-ionol glucosides **(206)**, together with corchoionoside C ((6S,9S)-roseoside) **(207)** and a prenyl glucoside **(208)** were reported from mature fruits of *Capparis spinosa*. The structures were established on the basis of spectroscopic, chiroptic and chemical evidence. In addition, the 13C resonance of 9C was reported to be of particular diagnostic value in assigning the absoluteconfiguration at that center in ionol glycosides **(209)**. The α-ionol derivative compounds are reported from metabolites of (+)-(S)-abscisic acid **(210)** (Ihsan Calis *et al.*, 2002).

Eight chemical compounds, β-sitosterol **(31)**, daucosterol **(167)**, uracil **(169)**, p-hydroxybenzoic acid **(203)**, vanillic acid **(211)**, protocatechuric acid **(212)**, butanedioic acid **(213)** and uridine **(214)** were reported from the fruit of *Capparis spinosa* by chromatographic methods and their structures were established and reported by spectroscopic methods (Yang *et al.*, 2006).

Besides rutin **(7)**, quercetin **(65)**, quercetin-3-O-glucoside-7-O-rhamnoside **(171)**, bitter quercetin3-O-[6'''-α-L-rhamnosyl-6''-β-Dglucosyl]-β-D-glucoside **(201)**, quercetin-3-O-glucoside **(202)**, flavonoid glycosides **(215)** (Sushila *et al.*, 2010) and kaempferol glycosides **(216)** reported from *Capparis spinosa.* Also the plant was reported the lipids content, methyl isothiocynate **(8)**, isopropyl isothiocyanate **(9)**, cadabicine (a 24-membered polyamine alkaloid) **(28)**, stachydrine (a pyridine alkaloid) **(29)** glucocapparin (methyl glucosinolate) **(34)**, sec-butyl isothiocyanate **(182)**, β-sitosterylglucoside-6′-octadecanoate **(204)**, benzyl isothiocyanate **(217)**, 3-methyl-2-butenyl-β-glycoside **(205)** and furthermore, homologous polyprenols namely; cappaprenol-12 **(218)**, cappaprenol-13 **(219)** and cappaprenol-14 **(220)** with 12, 13, and 14 isoprene units were also reported from the alcoholic extract of *C. spinosa* (Al-Said *et al.*, 1988 and Inocenico *et al.*, 2002).

The chemicals, rutin **(7)**, capparisinine **(23)**, capparidisine **(24)**, stachydrine **(29)**, β-sitosterol **(31)**, glucocapparin **(34)**, quercetin **(65)**, cappamensin A **(221)**, betulin **(222)**, β-amyrin **(223)**, DIMBOA (2,4-dihydroxy-7-methoxy-2H-1,4-benzoxazin-3(4H)-

one) **(224)**, quercetin-3-O-glucoside **(202)** and 2-hydroxyethyl-glucosinolate **(225)** were reported from the plant *Capparis spinosa* (Mishra *et al.*, 2007).

Miscellaneous compounds in the volatile fraction of pickled flower buds from *Capparis spinosa* such as p-methoxystyrene **(226)**, naphthalene **(227)**, 2-naphthalenone **(228)** and diphenyl ether **(229)** (Vincenza *et al.*, 2007).

In the volatile oils of *Capparis spinosa* 145 compounds were identified and reported, however, the major constituents were: aldehydes, esters and sulfur containing compounds. The presence of sesquiterpenes **(230)**, monoterpenes **(231)** and capric acid **(232)** was also reported (Arena *et al.*, 2008).

Acids in the volatile fractions of pickled flower buds from *Capparis spinosa* such as octanoic acid **(99)**, n-decanoic acid **(105)**, tetradecanoic acid **(111)**, acetic acid **(233)**, hexanoic acid **(234)**, heptanoic acid **(235)** and benzoic acid **(236)** were reported. Esters in volatile fractions such as ethyl butanoate **(237)**, 2-methylbutyl acetate **(238)**, butyl butanoate **(239)**, hexyl acetate **(240)**, methyl hepatonate **(241)**, methyl ocatanoate **(242)**, butyl hexanoate **(243)**, ethyl octanoate **(244)**, 3-ethylbutyl hexanoate (C6 isopentile) **(245)**, butyl-octanoate **(246)**, methyl benzoate **(247)**, ethyl decanoate **(248)**, isopentyl octanoate **(249)**, ethyl benzoate **(250)**, benzyl acetate **(251)**, methyl salicylate **(252)**, ethyl phenylacetate **(253)**, ethyl salicylate **(254)**, phenyl methyl pentanoate **(255)**, benyl isovalerate **(256)**, 1-butanol-3-methyl-benzoate **(257)**, 2,6-cresotic acid methyl ester **(258)**, methyl cinnamate **(259)**, benzyl tiglate **(260)**, ethyl cinnamate **(261)**, ethyl pentadecanoate **(262)**, methyl isohexadecanoate **(263)**, methyl hexadecanoate **(264)**, butyl tetradecanoate **(265)**, ethyl hexadecanoate **(266)**,ethyl-9-hexadecenoate **(267)**, methyl octadecanoate **(268)**, methyl octadecenoate **(269)**, ethyl octadecanoate **(270)**, ethyl 9-octadecenoate **(271)**, ethyl 9,12-octadecadienoate **(272)**, ethyl 6,9,12-octadecatrienoate **(273)** and benzyl benzoate **(274)** (Arena *et al.*, 2008).

Aldehydes in the volatile fractions of pickled flower buds from *Capparis spinosa* such as nonanal **(98)**, furfural **(165)**, 3-methyl butanal **(275)**, pentanal **(276)**, (E)-2-butenal **(277)**, (E)-2-pentenal **(278)**, heptanal **(279)**, (E)-2-hexenal **(280)**, octanal **(281)**, (E)-2-heptenal **(282)**, (E,E)-2,4-hexadienal **(283)**, (E,E)-2,4-heptadienal **(284)**, benzaldehyde **(285)**, (E)-2-nonenal **(286)**, 2,2-dimethyl-3,4-pentadienal **(287)**, 5-methyl furancarboxaldehyde **(288)**, (E,Z)-2,6-nonadienal **(289)**, 5-ethyl-2-furaldehyde **(290)**, (E)-2-decenal **(291)**, (E,E)-2,4-nonadienal **(292)**, 4-ethyl benzaldehyde **(293)**, 2,4-dimethyl benzaldehyde **(294)**, (E,E)-2,4-decadienal **(295)**, (E)-cinnamaldehyde **(296)**, benzylacetaldehyde **(297)** and 3-methoxycinnamaldehyde **(298)** (Arena *et al.*, 2008).

Ketones in the volatile fractions of pickled flower buds from *Capparis spinosa* such as acetoin **(299)**, 6-methyl-5-hepten-2-one **(300)**, (E,E)-3,5-octadiene-2-one **(301)**, acetophenone **(302)** and 4′-methoxy acetophenone **(303)** (Arena *et al.*, 2008).

Alcohols in the volatile fractions of pickled flower buds from *Capparis spinosa* such as 1-butanol **(304)**, 2-methyl-1-butanol **(305)**, 3-octanol **(306)**, 1-octen-3-ol **(307)**, 2-ethyl-1-hexanol **(308)**, 1-octanol **(309)**, 4-decanol **(310)**, p-allylanisole **(311)**, benzyl alcohol **(312)**, phenyl ethyl alcohol **(313)** and 4-(1-methyl propyl) phenol **(314)** (Arena *et al.*, 2008). Sulphur in the volatile fractions of pickled flower buds from *Capparis spinosa* such as methyl iosthiocyanate **(8)**, isopropyl thiocyanate **(9)**, benzyl isothiocyanate **(217)**, carbon disulfide **(315)**, dimethyl sulfide **(316)**, 2-ethyl thiophene **(317)** and benzothiazole **(318)** (Arena *et al.*, 2008).

Hydrocarbons in the volatile fractions of pickled flower buds from *Capparis spinosa* such as styrene **(319)**, tridecane **(320)**, tetradecane **(321)**, cyclotetradecane **(322)**, 4-methyl tetradecane **(323)**, pentadecano **(324)**, cyclopentadecane **(325)**, 4-methyl pentadecano **(326)**, hexadecane **(327)**, 4-methyl hexadecane **(328)**, heptadecane **(329)**, 4-methyl heptadecane **(330)**, octadecane **(331)**, 4-methyl octadecane **(332)**, nonadecane **(333)**, 4-methyl nonadecane **(334)**, eicosane **(335)**, heneicosane **(336)**, 4-methyl heneicosane **(337)**, docosane **(338)**, tricosane **(339)**, 4-methyl tricosane **(340)**, 4-methyl tetracosane **(341)**, pentacosane **(342)** and 4-methyl hexacosane **(343)** (Arena *et al.*, 2008).

Terpenes in the volatile fraction of pickled flower buds from *Capparis spinosa* such as β-pinene **(344)**, Δ-3-carene **(345)**, limonene **(346)**, β-cimene **(347)**, p-menthone **(348)**, β-linalool **(349)**, D-fenchyl alcohol **(350)**, (-) menthol **(351)**, 4-terpineol **(352)**, isomenthol **(353)**, β-farnesene **(354)**, α-terpineol **(355)**, methylgeranate **(356)**, (E,Z)-α-farnesene **(357)**, carvone **(358)**, (E,E)-α-farnesene **(359)**, α-curcumene **(360)**, (E)-β-ionone **(361)**, D-nerolidol **(362)**, trans-nerolidol **(363)** and hexahydrofarnesyl acetate **(364)** (Arena *et al.*, 2008).

The aldehyde **(178)**, sesquiterpenes **(230)**, ten monoterpenes **(231)** and esters **(365)** were reported; among sulphur compounds, methyl isothiocyanate **(8)** was the major one, followed by benzyl isothiocyanate **(217)** was reported. The application of this solvent free extraction technique combined with the GC-MS analysis, showed and reported its potential as a simple routine method for analyzing food flavour (Romeo *et al.*, 2007). Another study reported that new spermidine alkaloids **(19)** such as capparispine **(366)**, capparispine-26-O-d-glucoside **(367)** and cabadicine-26-O-d-glucoside hydrochloride from the roots of *Capparis spinosa* (Xiao *et al.*, 2008).

The dominating fatty acid of both species *Capparis spinosa* and *C. ovata* was linoleic acid **(60)**. Oleic acid **(59)** and its isomer vaccenic acid **(368)** were both found in the seed oils. The seed oils of both species were rich in τ-tocopherol **(91)**. The seed oils showed remarkably high contents of 5-avenasterol **(369)** (Matthaus and Ozcan, 2005). Two new (6S)-hydroxy-3-oxo-ionolglucosides **(206)**, together with corchoionoside C ((6S,9S)-roseoside) **(207)** and prenylglucoside **(208)**, were isolated and reported from mature fruits of *C. spinosa*. The 13C resonance of 9C was reported to be of particular diagnostic value in assigning the absolute configuration at that center in ionol glycosides **(229)** (Calis *et al.*, 1999).The known compounds stachydrine **(29)** and cappariloside A **(370)**, an adenosine nucleoside and for the first time from plants of the Capparidaceae family the known compounds uracil **(169)** and hypoxanthine **(371)** were isolated and reported from *C. spinosa* (Capparidaceae) fruit (Aisa *et al.*, 2011).

In addition to rutin **(7)**, quercetin-3-O-glucoside-7-O-rhamnoside **(171)** and quercetin-3-O-glucoside **(202)** the methanolic extract of the aerial parts of *Capparis spinosa* yielded the new flavonoidquercetin-3-O-(6'''-α-L-rhamnosyl-6''-β-D-glucosyl)-β-D-glucoside **(201)** (Sharaf *et al.*, 2000). More researches about capers proved that principal form of τ-tocopherol **(91)** detectedinleaves is α-tocopherol **(372)**. In bud sand flowers, there were both α-tocopherol **(372)** and γ-tocopherols **(373)**.The combined content of vitamin A **(374)** and vitamin E **(375)** in capers encourages researchers to more explore and find developments for this plant (Tlili *et al.*, 2009 and Moghaddasiane *et al.*, 2012).

The composition of carotenoid (β-carotene **(32)**, τ-tocopherol **(91)**, lutein **(376)**, neoxanthin **(377)** and violaxanthin **(378)**) was distinct in the leaves, buds, and flowers of *Capparis spinosa* as shown by using HPLC technique. Capers oil was found to contain Al, P, Na, Mg, Fe and Ca which are used in the evaluation of nutritional information. The heavy metal concentration was below the permissible limits defined (Ozcan, 2008). The *C. spinosa* oil was also investigated for its chemical composition and it was found to contain: τ-tocopherol **(91)**, fatty acid **(179)** and sterol as well as glucosinolates **(50)** (Hassan and Mohammad, 2010).

The phytochemicals namely, kaempferol **(66)**, vanillic acid **(211)**, flazin **(379)**, guanosine **(380)**, capparine A **(381)**, capparine B **(382)**, 1H-indole-3-carboxaldehyde **(383)**, 4-hydroxy-1H-indole-3-carboxaldehyde **(384)**, chryxoeriol **(385)**, apigenin **(386)**, thevetiaflavone **(387)**, 5-hydroxymethyl furaldehyde **(388)**, and cinnamic acid **(389)** were reported from aqueous extract of *Capparis spinosa* and also further reported to possess antiinflammatory activity (Haifeng *et al.*, 2010).

The *Capparis spinosa* was reported to determine diurnal change in rutin **(7)** content in different parts at fresh fruiting stage and subsequently assayed for rutin **(7)** content by HPLC analysis. Among different plant parts, floral buds and leaves were reported to be the principle organ for rutin **(7)**. Diurnal changes of rutin **(7)** were also observed and higher concentration of rutin **(7)** in whole plant was observed in the morning (Moghaddasian *et al.*, 2013).

The *Capparis spinosa* is a significant source of the treatment of a number of diseases and reported to reduce flatulence, antirheumatic and amenorrheaic plants (Baytop, 1984). In ayurvedic medicine, it is recorded as hepatic stimulant and protector by improving liver function (Handa *et al.*, 1986; Gadgoli and Mishra, 1995; Gadgoli and Mishra, 1999; Gez and Celik, 2000) and antiinflammatory effects (Alsaid *et al.*, 1988 and Rimbau *et al.*, 1996), infusions and decoctions from the root bark of *C. spinosa* have been reported in the treatment of dropsy, anemia, arthritis and gout and also *C. spinosa* contains great amounts of the antioxidant bioflavonoid rutin **(7)** (Bonina *et al.*, 2002). Their extracts and pulps are used in cosmetics, but there are some reports on contact dermatitis and sensitivity from their use. It is also determined that the risk of the death from coronary heart disease is reduced dramatically when the diet contains flavonoids (Inocencio *et al.*, 2000).

Further studies revealed and reported that antifungal activity in *Capparis spinosa* (Mahasneh *et al.*, 1996 and Mahasneh, 2002). The plant was agglutinated and killed the parasites of the Leishmania major disease (Alshtayeh and Abughdeib, 1999) and reported the activity mechanisms could be used by specific carbohydrates present in the plant. This indicates that lectins and toxins found in the tissue of *C. spinosa* may decrease the transmission of the parasite (Jacobsonand Schlein, 1999; Jacobson and Schlein, 2001). The *C. spinosa* extract has exhibited and reported potential acaricidal activity against the carmine spider mite (Mansour *et al.*, 2004).

This study was reported on evaluation the possible antihyperglycaemic and body weight reducing activities of the aqueous extract of both *Capparis spinosa* and *Chamaemelum nobile*. The study was reported the plant *C. spinosa* evoked potent antihyperglycemic and antiobesity effects (Lemhadri *et al.*, 2007).

The study was reported that ethanolic root bark extract of *Capparis spinosa* could afford significant dose-dependent protection against CCl_4 induced hepatocellular injury. The biochemical studies of blood samples of CCl_4 treated animals reported significant increase in the levels of serum enzyme activities, reflecting the liver injury caused by CCl_4 (Nasrin *et al.*, 2007).

The study reported that the antiviral and immunomodulatory properties of a methanolic extract of *Capparis spinosa* buds, rich in flavonoids including several quercetin **(65)** and kaempferol **(66)** glycosides. In particular the study has reported *in vitro* exposure of human peripheral blood mononuclear cell (PBMCs) to *C. spinosa* might inhibit the replication of HSV-2 and modulate the induction kinetics of IL-12, TNF-α and IFN-γ and up-regulating expression of peculiar proinflammatory cytokines; it is reported for the significant treatment of HSV-2 infections in immune compromised hosts (Arena *et al.*, 2007).

The study has been reported a protease was purified from capsules of *Capparis spinosa* and characterized. Ammonium sulphate fractionation and a CM Sephadex column were used for purification of the enzyme protease. The purification degree and the molecular mass of the enzyme were determined by SDS-PAGE and gel filtration chromatography. It was reported whether the purified and characterized protease could cause milk to congeal or digest chicken and cow meat and can be used for industrial production (Yasar *et al.*, 2008).

The *Capparis spinosa* flower buds aqueous extracts are reported in Turkey traditional medicine for their diuretic, antihypertensive, poultice, tonic and other properties. The reported study evaluates the genotoxic and antimutagenic effects of *C. spinosa* flower buds aqueous extract on the *Allium cepa* root tip meristem cells. The results of this study reported that *C. spinosa* buds aqueous extract is non-genotoxic. However, the study reveals that *C. spinosa* aqueous extract has reported to possess antimutagenic potential against EMS induced chromosomal aberrations (Aslantürk and Tulay, 2009).

The aims of study was to investigate the antimicrobial activity of the flower extract of *Capparis spinosa*, gel and leaf extract of *Aloe vera* were tested against isolated bacterial from skin infection *Staphylococcus aureus*, *Staphylococcus epidermidis*, *Streptococcus pyogenes*, *Pseudomonas aeruginosa* and *Escherichia coli*. The *Aloe vera* gel showed activity against gram negative and gram positive isolates. Also, it was reported that mixture containing of *Aloe vera*, *C. spinosa* showed prominent antibacterial activity against gram negative and positive. Also, reported that *in vivo* by study the effectiveness of flower extract of *C. spinosa* and gel of *Aloe vera* on the treatment of skin wounds inflamed by *S. aureus* suspension in rabbit. The mixtures were reported for the treatment of sun burns, rashes, burns, purulent wounds and other skin infections (Orooba, 2012).

The plant *Capparis spinosa* aerial part and root extracts in ethyl acetate reported to the highest concentration of phenolic compounds and flavonoids followed by the chloroform extract of roots. The enzymatic methods were realized by the production of uric acid and reduction of cytochrome C. The non enzymatic methods were conducted using *in vitro* techniques: In DPPH test, the radical scavenging activity for the root and aerial part extracts of *C. spinosa*. In general the aerial part extracts had reported an antioxidant activity through β-carotene-linoleate model system and ferric reducing ability greater than that of root part (Abderrahmane *et al.*, 2012).

The plant *Capparis spinosa* was used for the cytotoxic and cytogenetics effects in tumor cell lines as *in vitro* studies (Asaad *et al.*, 2012). The ethanolic and water extracts of aerial parts of *C. spinosa* reported as significant antihelminthic activity due to its previous studies phytochemicals (Fatin, 2012).

The study has been reported that consumption of Caper fruit *Capparis spinosa* extract lead to a significant decrease in blood sugar and also considerable decrease in blood triglycerides in diabetic rats, therefore it seems that Caper fruit consumption may has beneficial effects on blood sugar and lipid profile (Rasool *et al.*, 2013).

Capparis zeylanica

The crude extracts of *Capparis zeylanica* and a fatty acid **(179)**, octadec-7-en-5-ynoic acid **(390)**, from the root bark of *C. zeylanica* were screened for their antibacterial activities against Gram positive and negative bacteria. Among the crude extracts, chloroform extract reported significant activity against all pathogenic bacteria. The octadec-7-en-5-ynoic acid **(390)** isolated from chloroform extract exhibited antibacterial activities against test organisms except *E. coli*. The cytotoxic activities of crude extract and octadec-7-en-5-ynoic acid **(390)** were observed by brine shrimp bioassay value of the compound was reported (Haque *et al.*, 2008).

The plant *Capparis zeylanica* has been reported as a rasayana drug in the traditional Ayurvedic system of medicine. The *C. zeylanica* is reported to possess anti-oxidant, antipyretic, analgesic, antiinflammatory, antimicrobial and immunostimulant activity. Phytochemical screening of the plant *C. zeylanica* has reported the presence of fatty acid **(179)**, flavonoids, β-carotene **(32)**, alkaloids **(51)**, p-hydroxybenzoic acid **(164)**, vanillic acid **(211)**, octadec-7-en-5-ynoic acid **(390)**, tannins **(391)**, saponins glycosides **(392)**, terpenoids **(393)**, saponins **(394)**, α-amyrin **(395)**, syringic acid **(396)**, ferrulic acid **(397)** and *p*-coumanic acid **(398)** were reported (Amith Lather *et al.*, 2010).

The β-sitosterol **(31)**, β-carotene **(32)**, glucocapparin **(34)**, quercetin **(65)**, α-amyrin **(391)**, n-trichontane **(399)** and E-octodec-7enynoic acid **(400)** has been reported from root part of the plant *Capparis zeylanica* (Sunil Kumar and Singh, 2011).

The methanolic extract of *Capparis zeylanica* plant reported a significant dose dependent antipyretic effect in yeast induced elevation of body temperature in experimental rats (Amiya *et al.*, 2010).

The methanolic extracts of leaves of *Capparis zeylanica* are reported the immunomodulatory activity. It also produced a significant, dose related decrease in sheep erythrocyte specific heamagglutination antibody. The results reported

C. zeylanica to modulate the both cell mediated and humoral components of the immune system (Surendra *et al.*, 2010).

The methanolic extract of *Capparis zeylanica* root was reported for its wound healing potential in two different types of wound models *viz.*, incision and excision. There was better healing property observed significance while compared to povidone iodine ointment. It was reported through finding the percentage wound contraction, collegen content and DNA content (Chandan *et al.*, 2011).

The all parts of plant *Capparis zeylanica* being reported from the period of Susruta as anthelmintic, analgesic, antipyretic, antimicrobial, immunomodulatory effect. The different successive solvent extracts namely petroleum ether, ethanol and aqueous of *C. zeylanica* was reported for the *Pheretima posthuma* as test worms and reported to possess significant anthelmintic activity (Ravindra *et al.*, 2011). The *in vitro* antioxidant activity of the *C. zeylanica* extract reported to possess significant scavenging ability of hydroxyl peroxide radicals and DPPH (Sunil *et al.*, 2012).

Conclusion

Conclude the review on the *Capparis* genus was found and reported in this review chapter about 400 compounds from amino acids, carbohydrates, fatty acids, flavonoids, glycosides, phenolic compounds, triterpenoids, saponins, vitamins, colour pigments and intermediate compounds from different species as *Capparis aphylla, C. cartilaginea, C. deserti, C. decidua, C. grandiflora, C. humilis, C. ovata, C. orientalis, C. sicula, C. sepiaria, C. sikkimensis, C. spinosa* and *C. zeylanica*. The secondary metabolites such as β-sitosterol, capparisinine, cappriloside A, cappamensin, rutin *etc.*, compounds were reported from the above mentioned species. Also, the chapter reviewed the pharmacological and therapeutical applications of the reported compounds for various ailments and pharmacological activities. The chapter concluded that, reported *Capparis* genus consisting species having wide range of phytochemicals and its therapeutical applications will useful for the future research and development.

Abbreviations

TC: Total Cholesterol

TG: Triacyl Glycerol

LDL: Low Density Lipoprotein

HDL: High Density Lipoprotein

TLC: Thin Layer Chromatography

HPTLC: High Performance Thin Layer Chromatography

HPLC: High Performance Liquid Chromatography

GC-MS: Gas Chromatography - Mass Spectroscopy

GC-EI/MS: Gas Chromatography - Electro spectro Ionization - Mass Spectroscopy

IL-12: Interleukin-12

TNF-α: Tumor Necrosis Factor-α

IFN-γ: Interferon-γ

SDS-PAGE: Sodium Dodecyl Sulphate - Poly Acrylamide Gel Electrophoresis

References

Abderrahmane Baghiani., Djamila Ameni., Sabah Boumerfeg., Moufida Adjadj., Meriem Djarmouni., Noureddine Charef., Seddik Khennouf., and Lekhmici Arrar. (2012). Studies of Antioxidants and Xanthine Oxidase Inhibitory Potentials of Root and Aerial Parts of Medicinal Plant *Capparis spinosa* L. *American Journal of Medicine and Medical Sciences,* **2(1)**: 25-32.

Acharya, D. and Shrivastava, A. (2008). Indigenous Herbal Medicines: Tribal Formulations and Traditional Herbal Practices, Aavishkar Publishers Distributor, Jaipur- India. **pp.** 440.

Afsharypuor, S., Jeiran, K., and Arefian Jazy, A. (1998). First investigation of the flavour profiles of the leaf, ripe fruit and root of *Capparis spinosa* var. *mucronifolia* from Iran. *Journal of Pharmaceutica Acta Helvetiae,* **72**: 307-308.

Ahmad Sultan Abdullah Al-Shayeb. (2006). Chemical Composition of Essential Oil and Crude Extract Fractions and Their Antibacterial Activities of *Capparis spinosa* L. and*Capparis cartilaginea* Decne from Jordan. Thesis.

Ahmad, V.U., Arif, S., Amber, A.R., and Fizza, K. (1987a). Capparisinine, A New alkaloid from *Capparis decidua*. Liebigs. *Annals Chemistry,* 161-162.

Ahmad, V.U., Arif, S.A., Amber, R., Usamanghani, K., and Miana, G.A. (1985). A new spermidine alkaloid from *Capparis decidua*. *Heterocycles,* **23**: 3015-3020.

Ahmad, V.U., Ismail, N., Arif, S., and Amber, A.R. (1989). Isocodonocarpine from *Capparis decidua*. *Phytochemistry,* **28**: 2493-2495.

Ahmad, V.U., Ismail, N., Arif, S., and Amber, A.R. (1992). Two new N-acetylated spermidine alkaloids from *Capparis decidua*. *Journal Natural Products,* **55**: 1509-1512.

Ahmad, V.U., K. Fizza, A.U.R., Amber and S. Arif. (1987b). Cadabicine and cadabicine diacetate from *Crataeva nurvala* and *Cadaba farinose*. *Journal Natural Products,* **50**: 1186.

Ahmed R. Hamed., Khaled A. Abdel Shafeek., Nahla S. Abdel Azim., Shams I. Ismail andFaiza M. Hammouda. (2007). Chemical Investigation of Some *Capparis* Species Growingin Egypt and their Anti-oxidant Activity. *Electronic Complementary Alternative Medicines,* **4(S1)**: 25-28.

Ahmed, Z.F., Rizk, A.M., Hammouda, F.M., and Seif El-Nasr, M.M. (1972). Glucosinolates of Egyptian *Capparis* species. *Journal of Phytochemistry,* **11(1)**: 251-256.

Aisa XPFUHA., Abdurahim, M., Yili, A., Aripova, S.F., Tashkhodzhaev, B. (2007). Chemical composition of *Capparis spinosa* fruit. *Chemistry of Natural Compounds,* **43(2)**: 181-183.

Al-Said, M.S., Abdelsattar, E.A., Khalifa, S.I., and El Feraly, F.S. (1988). Isolation and identification of an anti-inflammatory principle from *Capparis spinosa*. *Pharmazie,* **43**: 640-641.

Al-Said, M.S., Abdelsattar, E.A., Khalifa, S.I., and El Feraly, F.S. (1988). Isolation and Identification of an Anti-inflammatory Principle from *Capparis spinosa*. *Pharmazie,* **43(9)**: 640-641.

Alshtayeh, M.S., and Abughdeib, S.I. (1999). Antifungal activity of Plant Extracts Against Dermatophytes. *Mycoses,* **42(11-12)**: 665-672.

Amit Lather., Chaudhary Amrendra Kumar., Gupta Vikas., Bansal Parveen., Bansal Renu. (2010). Phytochemistry and Pharmacological activities of *Capparis zeylanica*: An overview. *International Journal of Research in Ayurveda and Pharmacy,* **1(2)**: 384-389.

Amiya Ranjan Padhan., Anuj kumar Agrahari and Ashutosh Meher. (2010). A Study on Antipyretic Activity of *Capparis zeylanica* Linn. Plant Methanolic Extract. *International Journal of Pharma Sciences and Research,* **1(3)**: 169-171.

Arena, A., Bisifnano, G., Pavone, B., Tomaino, A., Bonina, F.P., Saija, A., Cristani, M., D'Arrigo, M., and Trombetta, D. (2008). Antiviral and immunomodulatory effect of a lyophilized extract of *Capparis spinosa* L. buds. *Phytotherapy Research,* **22(3)**: 313-317.

Arena, A., Bisignano, G., Pavone, B., Tomaino, A., Bonina, F.P., Saija, A., Cristani, M., Arrigo, M.D., and Trombetta, D. (2007). Antiviral and Immunomodulatory Effect of a Lyophilized Extract of *Capparis spinosa* L. Buds. *Phytotherapy Research,*

Asaad Abdulwahed B., AL-Asady., Khesar H. Khalil., and Saadi Saleh M. Barwari. (2012). Cytotoxic and Cytogenetics Effects of Aqueous, Methanolic and Secondary Metabolites Extracts of *Capparis spinosa* on Tumor Cell Lines *in vitro*. *Jordan Journal of Biological Sciences,* **5(1)**: 15-30.

Aslantürk Özlem Sultan., and Tülay A°kin Çelik. (2009). Genotoxic and Antimutagenic Effects of *Capparis spinosa* L. on the *Allium cepa* L. Root Tip Meristem Cells. *Caryologia,* **62(2)**: 114-123.

Baby Joseph., and Jini, D. (2011). A medicinal potency of *Capparis decidua* - A Harsh Terrain Plant. *Research Journal of Phytochemistry,* 1-13.

Baytop T. (1984). Therapy with medicinal plants. Istanbul University Publications. Istanbul.

Bonina, F., Puglia, C., Ventura, D., Aquino, R., Tortora, S., Sacchi, A., Saiija, A., Tomaino, A., and Pelegrino, M.L. (2002). *In vitro* Anti-oxidant and *in vivo* photoprotective effects of a lyophilized extract of Capparis *spinosa* L. Buds. *Jounral of Cosmetic Science,* **53(6)**: 321-335.

Calis, L., Kuruuzum, A., and Ruedi, R. (1999). 1H-Indole-3 acetonitrile glycosides from *Capparis spinosa* fruits. *Journal of Phytochemistry,* **50(7)**: 1205-1208.

Calis, L., Kuruuzum-Uz, A., Lorenzetto, P.A., and Ruedi, P. (2002). (6S)-hydroxy-3-oxo-ionol glucosides from *Capparis spinosa* fruits. *Journal of Phytochemistry,* **59**: 451-457.

Chandan Das., Sujit Dash., Durga Charana Sahoo., Abinash Kumar Sahu., Raghunandan Hota and Dolley Rout. (2011). *Journal of Chemical and Pharmaceutical Research,* **3(5)**: 15-19.

Cristina Inocencio., Diego Rivera., Francisco Alcaraz., Francisco A., and Tomas-Barberan. (2000). Flavonoid content of commercial capers (*Capparis spinosa, C. sicula* and *C. orientalis*) produced in mediterranean countries. *European Food Research Technology,* **212**: 70-74.

Dahot, M.U. (1993). Chemical evaluation of the nutritive value of flowers and fruits of *Capparis decidua*. *Journal of Chemical Society Pak.,* **15**: 78-81.

Dangi, K.S., and Mishra, S.N. (2011). Antioxidative and Cell Regeneration Effect of *Capparis aphylla* Stem Extract in Streptozotocin Induced Diabetic Rats. *Biology and Medicine,* **3(3)**: 82-91.

Fatin A., and Mustafa, A. (2012). *In vitro* Evaluation of *Capparis spinosa* against *Lumbricus terrestris* (Annelida). *PUJ.,* **5(2)**: 199-202.

Gadgoli C., and Mishra, S.H. (1995). Primarily Screening *Capparis spinosa* for Antihepatotoxic activity. *Fitoterapia,* **66**: 319.

Gadgoli, C., and Mishra, S.H. (1999). Antihepatotoxic activity of p-methoxy benzoic acid from *Capparis spinosa*. *Journal of Ethnopharmacology,* **66(2)**: 187-192.

Gaind, K.N. and Juneja, T.R. (1970). *Capparis decidua* Phytochemical study of flowers and fruits. *Research Bulletin Punjab Univ. Science,* **21**: 67-71.

Gez, S., and Celik, A. (2000). *Capparis Spinosa* in Analjezik ve Antimikrobial Etkileri yonunden Bir on Calisma. *Kocatepe Tip Dergisi.,* **3**: 169-172.

Gupta, J., and Ali, M. (1997). Oxygenated heterocyclic constituents from *Capparis decidua* root bark. *Indian of Journal Heterocycles Chemistry,* **6**: 295-302.

Haifeng Zhou., Renji Jian., Jie Kang., Xiaoling Huang., Yan Li., Changlong Zhuang., Fang Yang., Lele Zhang., Xiao Fan., Tong Wu., and Xianli Wu. (2010). Antiinflammatory effects of Caper (*Capparis spinosa* L.) Fruit Aqueous Extract and the Isolation of Main Phytochemicals. *Journal of Agricultural Food Chemistry,***58**: 12717-12721.

Handa, S.S., Sharma, A., and Chakraborti, K.K. (1986). Natural Products and Plants as Liver Protecting Drugs. *Fitoterapia,* **57**: 307-349.

Haque, M., Haqueme, Rahman, M.M., Khondkar, P., Rahman, M.M. (2008). Antibacterial and Cytotoxic Activities of *Capparis zeylanica* Linn Roots. *Ars Pharm.,* **49(1)**: 5-11.

Hassan Sher., and Mohammad N. Alyemeni. (2010). Ethnobotanical and pharmaceutical evaluation of *Capparis spinosa* L., validity of local folk and Unani system of medicine. *Journal of Medicinal Plants Research,* **4(17)**: 1751-1756.

Haydar Haciseferoбullari., Mehmet Musa Özcan., and Erman Duman. (2011). Biochemical and technological properties of seeds and oils of *Capparisspinosa* and *Capparis* ovata plants growing wild in Turkey. *Journal of Food Process Technology,* **2(6)**: 1-6.

Huxtable, R.J. (1992). The pharmacology of extinction. *Journal of Ethnopharmacology,* **37**: 1-11.

Ihsan Calis., Ayse Kuruuzum Uz., Piergiorgio A. Lorenzetto., and Peter Ruedi. (2002). (6S)-Hydroxy-3-oxo-α-ionol glucosides from *Capparis spinosa* fruits. *Phytochemistry,* **59**: 451-457.

Inocencio, C., Alcaraz, F., Calderon, F., Obon, C., and Rivera, D. (2002). The use of floral characters in *Capparis* sect. *Capparis* to determine the botanical and geographical origin of capers. *European Food Research Technology,* (Springer). **214(4)**: 335-339

Inocencio, C., Rivera, D., Alcaraz, F., and Tomas Barberan, F.A. (2000). Flavonoids content of Commercial capers (*Capparis spinosa, C. sicula* and *C. orientalis*) Produced in Mediterranean Countries. *European Food Research and Technology,* **212(1)**: 70-74.

Jacobson, R.L. and Schlein, Y. (1999). Lectins and Toxins in the Plants Diet of Phlebotomus Papatasi (Diptera: Psychodidae) Can Kill Leishmania Major Promastigotes in the Sandfly and in Culture. *Annals of Tropical medicines and Parasitology,* **93(4)**: 351-356.

Jacobson, R.L. and Schlein, Y. (2001). Phlebotomus Papatasi and Leishmania Major Parasites Express α-amylase and α-glucosidase. *Acta Tropica,* **78(1)**: 41-49.

Juan, P.P., and Del Pero Martinez, M.A. (1998). Flavonoid aglycones from Argentinian *Capparis* species (Capparaceae). *J. Biochemical Systematics and Ecology,* **26**: 577-580.

Jyotsna Shekhawat., and Naresh Vyas. (2013). Applied and Natural Science Foundation., Efficacy of *Capparis decidua* in control of *Lymnea acuminata* and their *Cercaria larvae* at Balsamand lake, Jodhpur. *Journal of Applied and Natural Science,* **5(1)**: 137-138.

Kapoor, B.B.S., and Mishra Raksha. (2013). Antimicrobial screening of Some Arid Herbal Plants of Rajasthan. *Universal Journal of Pharmacy,* **2(1)**: 110-112.

Kapoor, B.B.S., and Raksha Mishra. (2013). Capparidaceous Medicinal Plants of North-West Rajasthan: Good Sources of Ascorbic Acid. *Indian Journal of Pharmaceutical and Biological Research,* **1(1)**: 37-39.

Karanayil R. Sini., Barij N. Sinha., Aiyolu Rajasekaran., Mishal Thorakkattil., Dhanya Krishnan., and Mili K. Jose. (2011). Antimicrobial Activity of the Dried Root Powder of *Capparis grandiflora* Wall. Ex. Hook. F. and Thomson. *Asian Journal of Pharmaceutical and Clinical Research,* **4(2)**: 63-64.

Khanfar, M., Sabri, S., Abuzarga, M., Zeller, K.P. (2002). The chemical constituents of *C. spinosa* of Jordanian Origin. *Natural Product Research,* **17(1)**: 9-14.

Lai, P.K., and Roy, J. (2004). Antimicrobial and chemopreventive properties of herbs and spices. *Current Medicinal Chemistry,* **11(11)**: 1451-60.

Lemhadri, A., Mohamed Eddouks., Thierry Sulpice., and Remy Burcelin. (2007). Anti-hyperglycaemic and Anti-obesity Effects of *Capparis spinosa* and *Chamaemelum nobile* Aqueous Extracts in HFD mice. *American Journal of Pharmacology and Toxicology,* **2(3)**: 106-110.

Mahasneh, A.M. (2002). Screening of Some indigenuous Qatari medicinal Plants for Antimicrobial Activity. *Phytotherapy Research,* **16(8)**: 751-753.

Mahasneh, A.M., Abbas, J.A., and Eloglah, A.A. (1996). Antimicrobial activity of Extracts of herbal Plants used in the Traditional medicine of Bahrain. *Phytotherapy research,* **10(3)**: 251-253.

Manikandaselvi, S., and Brindha. P. (2014). Chemical standardization studies on *Capparis spinosa* L. *International Journal of Pharmacy and Pharmaceutical sciences,* **6(1)**: 47-54.

Mansour, F., Azalzeh, H., Saad, B., Tadmor, Y., Abo-moch, F., and Said, O. (2004). The potential of Middle Eastern flora as a source of new safe bio-acaroids to control *Tetranychus Cinnabarinus*. The Carmine spider mite. *Phytoparasitica,* **32(1)**: 66-72.

Matthaus, B., and Ozcan, M. (2005). Glucosinolates and fattyacid, sterol and tocopherol composition of seed oils from *Capparis spinosa* var. *spinosa* and *Capparis ovata* Desf. var. *canescens* (Coss.) Heywood. *Journal of Agricultural and Food Chemistry,* **53**: 7136-41.

Mishra, S.N., Tomar, P.C., and Lakra, N. (2007). Medicinal and Food Value of *Capparis* - A Harsh Terrain Plant. *Indian Journal of Traditional Knowledge,* **6(1)**: 230-238.

Moghaddasian Behnaz., Eradatmand Asli Davood., and Alaghemand Atena. (2013). Diurnal change in rutin content in *Capparisspinosa* growing wild in Tafresh/ Iran. *European Journal of Experimental Biology,* **3(3)**: 30-34.

Moghaddasian Behnaz., Eradatmand Asli., Davood., and Eghdami Anoosh. (2012). Caper the Mystique of the recent century. *International Journal of Agriculture and Crop Sciences,* **4(10)**: 604-608.

Mona S. Mohammed., Hassan S. Khalid., Muddathir A.K., Nasir A. Siddiqui., and Mohd Ali. (2012). A Novel Germacranolide Sesquiterpene Lactone with Anti-Inflammatory Effect From *Capparis decidua* (Forsk). *International Journal of Research in Pharmacy and Chemistry,* **2(4)**: 1073-1077.

Nasrin Aghela., Iran Rashidi., and Amir Mombeini. (2007). Hepatoprotective Activity of *Capparis spinosa* Root Bark Against CCl_4 Induced Hepatic Damage in Mice. *Iranian Journal of Phrmaceutical Research,* **6(4)**: 285-290.

Neelkamal Chahlia. (2009). Evaluation of Hypolipidaemic Activity of *Capparis decidua. International Journal of Biomedical Science,* **5(1)**: 70-73.

Orooba, M.S. Ibrahim. (2012). Evaluation of anti-bacterial activity of *Capparisspinosa* (Al-Kabara) and *Aloe vera* extracts against Isolates Bacterial Skin Wound Infections *in vitro* and *in vivo,* **3(2)**: 23-35.

Ozcan, M. (2005). Mineral composition of different parts of *Capparis ovata* Desf. Growing wild in Turkey. *Journal of Medicinal Food,* **8**: 405-407.

Pokharkar Raghunath, D., Funde Prasad, E., and Pingale Shirish, S. (2007). Aqueous Extract of *Capparis decidua* in Acute Toxicity Effects of the Rat by Use of Toothache Reliever Activity. *Pharmacologyonline,* **3**: 511-517.

Pradeep Singh., Garima Mishra., Sangeeta., Shruti Srivastava., Jha K.K. and Khosa, R.L. (2011). Traditional uses, phytochemistry and pharmacological properties of *Capparis decidua*: An Overview. *Der Pharmacia Letter,* **3(2)**: 71-82.

Raghunath D. Pokharkar., Prasad E. Funde., Shripad S. Joshi., and Shirish S. Pingale. (2008). Synthesis and Characterization of Fatty Acid Methyl Ester by *In-Situ* Transesterification in *Capparis* Deciduas Seed. *Leonardo Electronic Journal of Practices and Technologies,* **13**: 12-18.

Rai, S. (1987). Chemical examination of edible plants of Rajasthan desert with special reference to Capparadaceae. *Current Agriculture,* **11**: 15-23.

Rajesh, P., Latha, S., Selvamani, P., and Rajesh Kannan, V. (2010). *Capparis sepiaria* L. Pharmacognostical Standardization and toxicity Profile with Chemical Compounds Identification (GC-MS). *International Journal of Phytomedicine,* **2**: 71-79.

Rajesh, P., Latha, S., Selvamani, P., and Rajesh Kannan, V. (2010a). Phytochemical Screening and Toxicity Studies on the Leaves *Capparis sepiaria*L. (Capparidaceae). *Journal of Basic and Clinical Pharmacy,* **1(1)**: 41-46.

Rasool Rahmani., Mehdi Mahmoodio, Mehrnaz Karimi., Fateme hoseini., Rahim Heydari., Mohamadhosein Salchi., and Aliakbar Yousefi. (2013). Effect of Hydroalcoholic Extract of *Capparis spinosa* Fruit on Blood Sugar and Lipid Profile of Diabetic and Normal Rats. *Zahedan Journal of Research in Medical Sciences,* **15(11)**: 34-38.

Ravindra D. Bendgude., Manish S. Kondawar., Sandeep B. Patil., and Rupali V. Hirave. (2011). *In vitro* anthelmintic activity of roots of *Capparis zeylanica* Linn. *Journal of Advanced Pharmacy Education and Research,* **2**: 154-158.

Revathi, P., Vani, B., Sarathchandiran, I., Kadalmani. B., Prakash Shyam, K., and Palnivel, K. (2010). Reproductive toxicity of *Capparis aphylla* (Roth.) in male albino rats. *International Journal of Pharmaceutal and Biomedical Research,* **1(3)**: 102-112.

Rimbau, V., Risco, E., Canigueral, S., and Iglesias, J. (1996). Antiinflammatory activity of some extracts from plants used in the Traditional Medicine of North African countries. *Phytotherapy Research,* **10(5)**: 421-423.

Romeo, V., Ziino, M., Giuffrida, D., Condurso, C., and Verzera, A. (2007). Flavour profile of capers (*Capparis spinosa* L.) from the Eolian Archipelago by HS-SPME/ GC-MS. *Journal of Food Chemistry,* **101(30)**: 1272-1278.

Sharaf, M., Elansari, M.A., and Saleh, N.A.M. (1997). Flavonoids of Four Cleome and Three *Capparis* Species. *Biochemical systematic and Ecology,* **25(2)**: 161-166.

Sharaf, M., El-Ansari, M.A., and Saleh, N.A.M. (2000). Quercetin triglycoside from *Capparis spinosa*. *Fitoterapia,* **71**: 46-9.

Sharrif moghaddasi Mohammad., Hamed Haddad Kashani., and Zohre Azarbad. (2012). *Capparis spinosa* L. Propagation and Medicinal uses. *Life Science Journal,* **9(4)**: 684-686.

Sunil Kumar Mishra., and Singh, P.N. (2011). Ethnomedicinal, phytochemical and pharmacological review of *Capparis zeylanica* Linn. *Research Journal of Pharmaceutical, Biological and Chemical Sciences,* **2(2)**: 506-511.

Sunil Kumar Mishra., Singh, P.N., and Dubey, S.D. (2012). Evaluation of Antioxidant Activities in Ethanolic Extract of *Capparis zeylanica* L. root. *Rev. Latinoamer Quim.,* **41(1)**: 7-20.

Surendra S. Agarwal., Saurabh C. Khadase., and Goku S. Talele. (2010). Studies on Immunomodulatory activity of *Capparis zeylanica* leaf extracts. *International Journal of Pharmaceutical Sciences and Nanotechnology,* **3(1)**: 887-892.

Sushil Kumar., Ramavtar Sharma., Vinod Kumar., Govind K. Vyas., and Abhishek Rathore. (2013). Combining Molecular-marker and Chemical Analysis of *Capparis decidua* (Capparaceae) in the Thar Desert of Western Rajasthan (India). *Review of Biological Tropics,* **61(1)**: 311-320.

Sushil Kumar., Ramavtar Sharma., Vinod Kumar., Govind K. Vyas., and Abhishek Rathore. (2013). Combining molecular-marker and chemical analysis of *Capparis decidua* (Capparaceae) in the Thar Desert of Western Rajasthan (India). *International Journal of Tropical Biology,* **61(1)**: 311-320.

Sushila Rathee., Mogla, O.P., Permender Rathee., and Dharmender Rathee. (2010a). Quantification of β- Sitosterol using HPTLC from *Capparis decidua* (Forsk.). *Edgew. Der Pharma Chemica,* **2(4)**: 86-92.

Sushila Rathee., Permender Rathee., Dharmender Rathee., Deepti Rathee., and Vikash Kumar. (2010). Phytochemical and pharmacological Potential of Kair (*Capparis Decidua*). *International Journal of Phytomedicine,* **2**: 10-17.

Tapsell, L.C., Hemphill I. and Cobiac, L. (2006). Health benefits of herbs and spices: the past, the present, the future. *Medical Journal of Australia,* **185(4)**: S4-24.

Tlili, N., Nasri, N., Saadaoui, E., Khaldi, A., Triki, S. (2009). Carotenoid and tocopherol composition of leaves, buds and flowers of *Capparis spinosa* grown wild in Tunisia. *Journal of Agric Food Chemistry,* **24;57(12)**: 5381-5.

Upadhyay, R.K. (2012). Insecticidal Potential of *Capparis decidua* to *Rhizopertha dominica* (Fabr.) (Coleoptera: Bostrichidae). *World Journal of Agricultural Sciences,* **8(3)**: 269-279.

Verma, P.D., Dangar, R.D., Shah, K.N., Gandhi, D.M. and Suhagia, B.N. (2011). Pharmacognostical Potential of *Capparis decidua* Edgew. *Journal of Applied Pharmaceutical Science,* **1(10)**: 6-11.

Vincenza Romeo., Marisa Ziino., Baniele Giuffrida., Cettina Condurso., Antonella Verzera. (2007). Flavour Profile of Capers (*Capparis spinosa* L.) From the Eolian Archipelago by HS-SPME/GC-MS. Analytical, Nutritional and Clinical Methods., *Food Chemistry,* **101**: 1272-1278.

Xiao Pu Fu., Tao Wu., Miriban Abdurahim, M., Zhen Su., Xue Ling Hou., Haji Akber A., and Hankui Wu. (2008). New spermidine alkaloids from *Capparis spinosa* roots. *Phytochemistry Letters,* **1(1)**: 59–6

Xiaolu Feng., Jincai Lu., Hailiang Xin., Lei Zhang., Yuliang Wang., and Kexuan Tang. (2011). Anti-arthritic active fraction of *Capparis spinosa* Fruits and its chemical constituents. *Yakugaku Zasshi.,* 1**3(3)**: 423-429.

Yang Yu., Huiyuan Gao., Zhishu Tang., Xiaomei Song., and Lijun Wu. (2006). Several Phenolic acids from the Fruit of *Capparis spinosa. Asian Journal of Traditional Medicines,* **1(3-4)**: 1-4.R

Yasar Demir., Azize Alayli Güngor., Elif Duygu Duran., and Nazan Demir. (2008). Cysteine Protease (Capparin) from Capsulesof Caper (*Capparis spinosa*). *Food Technol. Biotechnol.,* **46(3)**: 286–291.

Zhong Hu., Jenny, A. lewis., Bryanhanley and Roger Fenwick, C.J. (1989). 2-hydroxyethyl glucosinolate from *Capparis masaikai* of Chinese origin. *Phytochemrstry,* **28(4)**: 1252-1254.

Bioactive Phytochemicals: Perspectives for Modern Medicine Vol. 3 (2015) *Pages* **93–119**
Editor: **V.K. Gupta**
Published by: **DAYA PUBLISHING HOUSE, NEW DELHI**

3

A Review on Pharmacology and Toxicology of Artesunate with its Antimalarial Profile

Papiya Bigoniya[1*], Sheetal Tiwari[1] and Alok Kumar Shukla[1]

ABSTRACT

Artesunate is part of the artemisinin group of drugs that treat malaria. It is a semi-synthetic derivative of artemisinin that is water-soluble and may therefore be given by injection. Artesunate is a potent and rapidly-acting blood schizontocide derived from the leaves of the chinese herb, Artemesia annua. Hepatotoxicity and hemotoxicity are associated with artesunate administration at both required and overdose conditions however these effects are magnified in overdose conditions. That artesunate at normal dose has a toxic effect on the liver cells and could be a potential hepatotoxic drug. Artemisinin and its derivatives are known to suppress reticulocyte production. This review article aims at compilation of pharmacological effect, toxicological reactions and antimalarial spectrum of artesunate.

Keywords: Artesunate, *Artemesia annua*, Pharmacological effects, Toxicological reactions, Antimalarial profile.

Introduction

Malaria is one of the commonly prevalent diseases in most parts of the world accounting for over a million deaths per year. 90 per cent of cases are in Sub-Saharan Africa, 85 per cent in children under five. For over 50 years the main drug for controlling the malaria parasite has been chloroquine, a synthetic derivative of the plant-based extract quinine. Chloroquine acts as both prophylactic and cure, and has the advantage of very low cost, but unfortunately in much of the population it is no

1 Radharaman College of Pharmacy, Fatehpur Dobra, Ratibad, Bhopal – 462 002, M.P., India

* *Corresponding author*: E-mail: p_bigoniya2@hotmail.com

longer effective due to the emergence of resistant strains of the malaria parasite. The best hope for a replacement treatment lies with drugs based on artemisinin group, the chemical compound extracted from the leaves of the plant *Artemisia annua.*

Its use in treating malaria has been known in China for over 2000 years. It had been forgotten for long, but was rediscovered in the 1970's, when the '*Chinese Handbook of Prescriptions for Emergency Treatments*' was found. A recipe for the use of *Artemisia* leaves as herbal infusion for treating "intermittent fever", dated to 168 BC, was found in a tomb excavated in Hunnan Province in 1972. Traditionally *Artemisia annua* leaves in China were collected from unimproved wild stands of the plant, and were used as herbal infusion to treat a range of diseases. In 1971, scientists demonstrated that the plant extracts had antimalarial activity. In 1972 the active ingredient *Artemisinin* was isolated and its chemical structure described and subsequently has been produced semi-synthetically as an antimalarial drug. The low water solubility of artemisinin made the infusion only marginally effective against malaria. Leaf yields were low in artemisinin content estimated as 0.03–0.3 per cent by weight. Artesunate is part of the artemisinin group of drugs that treat malaria. It is a semi-synthetic derivative of artemisinin that is water-soluble and may therefore be given by injection (Ellman, 2010).

During the Vietnam war *Artemisia* plantations were established in North Vietnam by the Vietcong using seed supplied by the Chinese Government, to combat a rapid rise in malaria cases among army personnel. In the mid-1980s *Artemisia* seed reached several European locations. Medicinal Plants Research Institute in Switzerland, Mediplant, scientists initiated an *Artemisia* hybridisation programme which by 1994 had resulted in a variety giving dramatically higher yields than the wild plants, up to 1.0–1.5 per cent artemisinin content (Mediplant, 1998). Hybrid seed of this variety was tested at several locations and now 5,000 small and large scale farmers are currently contracted to grow *Artemisia* for processing in factories in Kenya, Tanzania, Uganda and Madagascar. In 1993 artemisinin got approval as a medicine against Malaria and by 1997 introduced as first line anti-malaria drug to the Artemisinin-based combination treatment (ACTs) by the Ministries of Health in different countries. Over the last ten years as the worldwide demand for artemisinin has become apparent, Chinese, Vietnamese and Indian plant breeding institutes have developed high-yielding *Artemisia* hybrids. Pharmaceuticals are extracting artemisinin to manufacture anti-malarial drugs. The East African factories currently export artemisinin to pharmaceutical factories in India and Europe where the final products are made (WHO, 2005).

Artimesia annua

Biological source of artesunate is the unexpended flower heads of *Artemisia cina*, Berg., *Artemisia bevifolia* wall., *Artemesia maritime* Linn. and *Artemisia annua*, commonly known as sweet wormwood or sweet annie is a highly aromatic annual herb. It has fern-like alternate leaves dark green, bright yellow flowers and a camphor-like scent and tastes slightly bitter.

Family:	Compositae or Asteraceae.
Synonyms:	Santonica, worm seeds, Quinghoo
English:	Sweet wormwood, Chinese wormwood, Sweet Annie
French:	Absinthe chinoise, Armoise annuelle
Chinese:	Qinghao (pronounced ching how), Cao hao, Cao Qinghao, Cao Haozi, Chou Qinghao, Haoz, Kuhao, Xianghao, Xiang Qinghao, Xihehao
Japanese:	Kusoninijin Vietnamese: Than hao, Than cao hoa vang
Korean:	Chui ho, Hwang-hwa-ho, Gae-tong-sok
German:	Chinesischer Beifu

Geographic Source

A. annua occurs naturally as part of steppe vegetation in the northern parts of Chahar and Suiyuan provinces in China, at 1000 to 1500 m above sea level but able to grow in a wide range of sub-tropical and temperate environments. Now naturalized in many countries including the United States (Ferreira *et al.*, 1997). It found in kurran valley in Pakistan, Turkey and from Kashmir to kumaon in Himalayas, as well as in west Tibet upto altitude of 4000 meters. It is also found in Panjab, UP, And Haryana. The drug consists of yellowish or brownish flower-Heads, which are oval in shape. Flowers are fertile with tubular, corolla, calyx is absent. Collect on lat in spring or early in summer. *A. annua* is endemic to china and grows wild in Europe and America. Cultivated in Vietnam, China, Iran, Turkey and Australia. Cultivated on experimental bases in Gujarat, Jammu and Kashmir, Uttar Pradesh, Himachal Pradesh and Karnataka. CIMAP at Luck now has developed uniform and high yielding genetically improved plant and is being cultivated for the purpose of artemisin. Cultivation of *A. annua* in Africa has started after the World Health Organization recommended Artemisinin Combination Therapies (ACT) as a replacement of artemisinin monotherapy in the fight against multi-drug resistant *Plasmodium falciparum* malaria.

Macroscopic Characteristics

A. annua is a large shrub often reaching more than 2 meters in height, usually single-stemmed with alternate branches. Stems are longitudinal, cylindrical about 2-5 cm in diameter, 30-80 cm in length. Leaves are bipinnate compound and dark green in colour with strongly aromatic flavour and bitter in taste. The aromatic leaves are deeply dissected and range form 2.5 to 5 cm in length. Leaves and flowers contain both 10-celled biseriate trichomes and 5 cell filamentous trichomes. The nodding flowers (capitula), only 2 to 3 mm in diameter, are greenish-yellow enclosed by numerous, imbricated bracts. Capitula are displayed in loose panicles containing numerous central bisexual florets and marginal pistillate florets, the latter extruding stigmas prior to the central flowers. Both flowers have synpetalous tubular corolla with the top split into five lobes in the hermaphroditic florets and 2–3 lobes in the pistillate florets. Both florets and receptacle bear abundant 10-celled biseriate trichomes at the pedicel and bracts. The biseriate glandular trichomes sequester artemisinin as well as highly aromatic volatile oils (Lopes-Lutz *et al.*, 2008). The plant cannot tolerate drought and requires much care in cultivation. Good plants produce abundant small leaves, which are rich with *artemisinin*, which is very effective in treating malaria.

Chemical Constituents

A. annua contains approximately 150 different active components, many of them with anti-malarial activity. It contains artemisin, deoxy artemisin 1.0 per cent. It is sesquterpine lactone with an internal peroxide. Amyrin, lutealin, β-systosterol, stigmasterol are also repeated in this plant (Kokate *et al.*, 2007). It contains sesquterpenes (abscisic acid, artemisnic acid, dehydro-artemisinin, deoxyartemisinin), triterpenes (α-amylin, α-amyreron), courarins and flavanoid (scopolamine, apigenin chrysophenol, lutelin), sterols (β-sitosterol, stigmasterol) and essential oil (artemisia alcohol, artemisia ketone, camphene, caryophyllene oxide, 1,8- cineal, sabinene α and β-pinene, α-thujene camphor. Artemisinin, artemisinic acid, artether, artennuin B,(+)- deoxyartemisinin are some major constituents (Rajpal, 2005). There are at least 20 known sesquiterpenes including artemisinin (arteannuin A), arteannuin B, artemisitene, and artemisinin acid.

The essential oil up to 3 per cent of the leave weight is stored in the glandular trichomes of the leaf epidermis. Biseriate glandular trichomes are the source of highly aromatic volatile oils, mainly artemisia ketone, 1.8-cineole camphor; germacrene D, camphene hydrate, and α-pinene; β-caryophyllene, myrcene, and artemisia alcohol. Analyzed by GC-MS it contains camphor (44 per cent), germacrene D (16 per cent), transpinocarveol (11 per cent), β-selinen (9 per cent), β-caryophyllene (9 per cent), artemisia ketone (3 per cent) and around further 20 substances of which the content is less than 1 per cent (Juteau *et al.*, 2002). Further investigations with GC and NMR about the oil of A. vestita revealed the presence of around 15 compounds like α-terpinene, β-phellandrene, 1,4-cineole, β-thujone, nerol, α-phenanthrene, 1,8-cineole, citral, chamazulene and citronellal. These compounds are responsible for the characteristic odor and for the antibacterial activity (Liu *et al.*, 1989). Nonvolatile sesquiterpenes can be recovered from the plant by solvent extraction, some of which show high antimalarial activity. The main active ingredient is artemisinin, which is found in the leaves, stems, and inflorescences, and it is concentrated in the upper portions of plant within new growth. Artemisinin has been reported to be a potent plant inhibitor with potential as a natural herbicide (Zheng, 1994). Analysis of artemisinin is difficult because the compound is unstable, concentrations in the plant low, the intact molecule stains poorly, and other compounds in the crude plant extracts interfere in its detection. Most collections of artemisia derive from natural stands with highly variable artemisinin content, some as low of 0.01 per cent. Currently-used selections from Chinese, Swiss, and Brazilian origin vary from 0.3 to 1.5 per cent.

Pharmacological Uses

Artemisinin is a secondary or natural plant metabolite identified as a sesquiterpene lactone endoperoxide having potent anti malarial effect. Synthetic derivatives like artemether, arteether, artesunate, artenilic acid are effective anti malarial against the asexual forms of the erythrocytic stage of *P. falciparum* and *P. vivax* malaria (Chen *et al.*, 1987). Areether, artemther, artesunate are used as injectables in the treatment of malaria. Artemisic acid has antibacterial, antiinflammatory and cytotoxic activity. *A. annua* leaves (Zheng and Wang, 2001) and crude extracts have been reported to be a good source of antioxidants (Cai *et al.*, 2004). This high antioxidant capacity is probably due to the high content (Bilia *et al.*, 2006) and diversity of its leaf flavonoids, including the newly-reported C-glycosyl flavonoids as a possible component of the antioxidant and antiviral activity (Han *et al.*, 2008).

A. annua is believed to work as anticancer as, when artemisinin or any of its derivatives comes into contact with iron, a chemical reaction ensue spawning charged atoms called free radicals. Cells need iron to replicate DNA when they divide, and since cancer is characterized by out-of-control cell division, cancer cells have much higher iron concentrations than do normal cells. More aggressive cancers such as pancreatic and acute leukemia which are characterized by more rapid cell division and thus have higher iron concentrations may respond even better. Artemisia oil has inhibitory effects on the growth of bacteria, yeasts and dermatophytes.

Sixteen essential oils from tropical plants including *A. annua* were tested for their fungitoxicity. Five of them showed a strong activity against *Trichophytum rubrum*, *Microsporum gypseum* and other eight dermatophytes. An ointment made with artemisia oil was the most active to cure experimental ringworm infection of guinea pigs within 7 to 12 days (Kishore *et al.*, 1993). The essential oil of *A. annua* was tested for its repellent and inhibitory activity against two stored product insects, *Tribolium castaneum* and *Callosobruchus maculates*. Adult beetles, *T. castaneum* were repelled significantly by 1 per cent oil v/v of *A. annua* (Tripathi *et al.*, 2000). The essential oil of *A.annua* obtained by hydrodistillation was tested in animals in a psychopharmacological screening. The doses increased the latency time to convulsions induced by picrotoxin and pilocarpine, prevented the onset of pentylenotetrazol and strychnine induced seizures and caused marked inhibition in the Rota-rod assay. In addition, the essential oil has a high acute toxicity and a possible cholinergic reaction (Perazzo *et al.*, 2003). Many studies have shown that *A. annua* stimulates the immune system, increasing for example the monocyte count. This effect is probably due to other constituents than artemisinin: essential oils, flavonoids, coumarins, polysaccharides, saponins (Ogwang *et al.*, 2011).

Artesunate

Artesunate is recommended by the WHO in preference to quinidine for the treatment of severe malaria and has been used worldwide for many years. Artesunate is in the class of medications known as artemisinins, which are derivatives from the "quinghaosu" or sweet wormwood plant (*A. annua*). On June 21, 2007, the Food and Drug Administration (FDA) approved investigational new drug (IND) protocol entitled 'Intravenous Artesunate for Treatment of Severe Malaria in the United States'. This IND makes a new class of antimalarial medication, artemisinins, available in the United States for the first time. Artesunate must always be given with another antimalarial such as mefloquine (Dondorp *et al.*, 2005) or amodiaquine (Adjuik *et al.*, 2004) to avoid the development of resistance. The combination of artesunate and amodiaquine has been found to be equivalent to co-artemether (Oyakhirome *et al.*,

2007). For severe malaria during pregnancy, the World Health Organization (WHO) recommends artesunate or quinine during the first trimester and artesunate as the first-line therapy during the second and third trimesters (Rijken *et al.*, 2012).

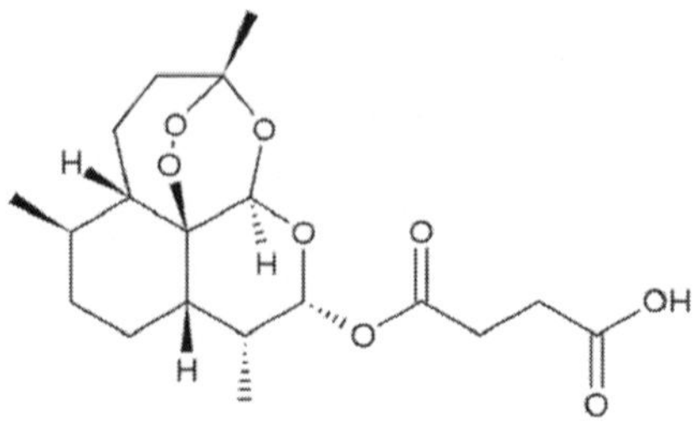

Figure 3.1: Chemical Structure of Artesunate.

Extraction Process

1. Top portion of *A. annua* herb constituting mainly of flowers and tender leaves and stems is crushed to a coarse powder.
2. The material is loaded in vertical extractors fitted with process pump for solvent circulation and transfer.
3. The extraction can also be done in rotator more efficiently or continuous solvent extraction systems can also be utilized for handling large bulk.
4. The n-hexane/benzene/ethylene dichloride is some of the solvent use for extraction.
5. TLC or HPTLC can monitor the extraction process.
6. On completion of extraction the marc is desolventized and micelle is taken for solvent recovery in vacuum distillation plant.
7. Suepending in methanol purifies the concentration obtained as greenish brown paste with aromatic odour.
8. The methanol soluble fraction is distilled under reduced pressure. This affords a greenish brown paste about 10.0 per cent (Kohler *et al.*, 1997; El-Sohly *et al.*, 1990; Christen and Veuthey, 2001; Fleming *et al.*, 2009).

Synthesis

Artesunate is prepared from dihydroartemisinin (DHA) by reacting it with succinic acid anhydride in basic medium. Pyridine as base solvent, sodium bicarbonate in chloroform and catalyst DMAP (N,N-dimethylaminopyridine) and triethylamine in 1,2-dichloroethane are used, with yields of up to 100 per cent. A large scale process involves treatment of DHA in dichloromethane with a mixture of pyridine, a catalytic amount of DMAP and succinic anhydride. The dichloromethane mixture is stirred for 6–9 hr to get artesunate in quantitative yield. The product is further re-crystallized from dichloromethane. α-artesunate is exclusively formed (M.P. 135–137 ^{0}C).

Mode of Action

Artesunate is a drug used to treat malaria, especially chloroquine resistant malaria. Artesunate is a potent and rapidly-acting blood schizontocide concentrated in parasitised erythrocytes. Artesunate is a potent blood schizonticide agent for *P. falciparum* but does not have hypozoiticidal activity. It is effective against *P. falciparum* resistant to all other antimalarial drugs. The exact mode of action is not clear but clinical studies have confirmed the effectiveness of artesunate in *P. vivax* and *P. falciparum* malaria. Artesunate has been reported to clear fever in patients with severe falciparum malaria in 16-25 hours after parenteral administration. Artesunate exerts its anti-malarial activity by generation of free radicals or reactive oxygen species (ROS), through iron-catalyzed cleavage of the endoperoxide bridge (Nontprasert *et al.*, 1998). The functional group responsible for antimalarial activity of artesunate is endoperoxide bond. It is converted to active metabolite dihydroartemesinin that then inhibits the sarcoplasmic/endoplasmic reticulum Calcium ATPase encoded by *P. falciparum* (Adebisi, 2007; Nosten and White, 2009). Artesunate binds tightly to parasite infected erythrocyte membrane (McGready *et al.*, 2006). Release of an active oxygen species from this bond kills the malaria parasite if accumulated in the erythrocytic cells. The ROS cause macromolecular damage by alkylating heme and several other proteins, such as translationally controlled tumor protein, histidine-rich protein and pfATP6 and the sarco/endoplasmatic reticulum calcium ATPase (Nontprasert *et al.*, 2000). Artesunate acts rapidly, stopping parasite development and preventing subsequent cytoadherence and rosetting. Artesunate may indirectly through generation of ROS or directly as toxin to the cells of the liver, affecting their cellular integrity and causing defect in membrane permeability and cell volume homeostasis. Artesunate has demonstrated the fastest clearance of all anti-malarials currently used and acts primarily on the trophozite phase, thus preventing progression of the malaria disease.

Dosing Schedule

Artesunate 50 mg tablets are used for the treatment of uncomplicated cases of malaria. Artesunate 50 mg is indicated only for attacks due to *Plasmodium falciparum*, against which the medicine is active. It reduces the number of malaria parasites in body.

Intravenous dose of IV artesunate for treatment of severe malaria:

- 2.4 mg/kg loading dose over 5 minutes
- 2.4 mg/kg dose 12 hours later
- 2.4 mg/kg once daily after that (WHOPAR, 2011).

Table 3.1 shows dosage quantity, frequency and related instructions related to use of artesunate in severe malaria in case of mono therapy and combination therapy. No data regarding the pediatric and neonatal dosages details of artesunate is available.

Table 3.2 shows artesunate dosing schedule for combination therapy in a treatment duration 3 days as recommended by WHO (2012).

Table 3.1: Dose Schedule of Artesunate

Dose	*Frequency*	*Route*	*Instructions*
2.4 mg/kg	As recommended	IM	Severe malaria: This dose is followed by 1.2 mg/kg at 12 and 24 hours then 1.2 mg/kg daily for 6 days. If the patient can swallow, the daily dose can be given orally.
2.4 mg/kg	As recommended	IV	Severe malaria: This dose is followed by 1.2 mg/kg daily until the patient can take orally artesunate or another effective antimalarial drug.
4.0 mg/kg	As recommended	PO	Monotherapy: 4 mg/kg loading dose on the first day followed by 2 mg/kg once a day for 6 days.
4.0 mg/kg	As recommended	PO	Combination therapy: 4 mg/kg once a day for 3 days plus mefloqine (15 mg or 25 mg of base per kg) as a single dose or split dose on the second and/or third day.

IM: Intramuscular; IV: Intravenous; PO: Per oral route of administration.

Table 3.2: Artesunate Dosing Scheme in Combination Therapy

Age	*No of Tablets per Day (Dose)*
1-6 years	1 tablet once daily (50 mg/day)
7-13 years	2 tablets once daily (100 mg/day)
Older than 13 years	4 tablets once daily (200 mg/day)

Artemisinin-Based Combination Therapy (ACT)

In combination therapy in adults and children, artesunate should be given at 4 mg/kg body weight once daily for three days (range 2-10 mg/kg; 200 mg per day in adults). Artesunate dosing scheme in combination therapy in a treatment duration 3 days (WHO, 2012).

In case of allergy, intolerance or contraindication to combination agents, artesunate can be used as single therapy:

- In adults a total dose of 600-800 mg should be given during five to seven days of treatment, and
- In children a total dose of 12 mg/kg body weight should be given during five to seven days of treatment.

Detailed dosing schedule for artesunate mono therapy is as recommended in Table 3.3.

Pharmacokinetics

Absorption and Bioavailability

Artesunate is rapidly absorbed after oral administration, well distributed and achieves high concentration in the intestines, liver and kidneys. Most of the artesunate is promptly biotransformed, mainly through plasma esterases, into the active metabolite dihydroartemisinin (DHA). Following 50 mg single dose administration

Table 3.3: Artesunate Dosing Scheme in Mono Therapy

Age	*No of Tablets per Day (Dose)*	
	Day 1	*Subsequent Days*
7-13 years	1 tablet twice daily (50 mg × 2)	1 tablet daily (50 mg × 1)
Older than 13 years	2 tablets twice daily (100 mg × 2)	1 tablet b.i.d (50 mg × 2)

in healthy volunteers, the C_{max} value was 1.94 µg/ml and the corresponding value for AUC was 3.55 µg.h/ml.

Distribution

DHA has been shown to substantially accumulate in *P. falciparum* infected erythrocytes. Artesunate is poorly protein bound.

Metabolism

Artesunate is extensively hydrolysed by plasma esterases and perhaps also by CYP2A6. Its main metabolite, DHA is presumed to account for most of the *in vivo* antimalarial activity. DHA is metabolised thorugh glucuronidation.

Elimination

Artesunate has a plasma half-life of 3-29 minutes. The active metabolite DHA has a plasma half-life of 40 to 95 minutes. Elimination half-life is about 45 min after IV administration. Only a small amount of artesunate is excreted in the urine and in the stools.

Adverse Effects

Adverse reactions of artesunate are transient and reversible reticulocytopaenia, drug fever, rash, headache, vomiting, diarrhea, abdominal pain, bradycardia, transient 1st-degree heart block and reversible elevation of serum transaminases (WHOPAR, 2011).

Contraindications

1. Hypersensitivity to the active substance or to any of the excipients.
2. Hepatic or renal insufficiency.
3. Pregnancy and lactation.

Drug Interaction

1. Potentiation of mefloquine, primaquine and tetracycline effect.
2. Additive effect with chloroquine.
3. Antagonist effect with pyrimethamine and sulphonamide (Minzi *et al.*, 2007).

Uses

1. Used as anti-malarial agent to alleviate fever, combination with other herbs to treat jaundice, headache and dizziness and nose bleeding.

2. Essential oil of plant is used in cosmetics and perfumes. The essential oil has been reported to have anti-microbial activity.
3. Used as anti-cancer agent. Have cytotoxic effect on leukemia.
4. Used in tratament of hemorrhoids.
5. Anti-HIV agent.
6. Have antioxidative activity.
7. Possess herbicidal property.

Biological Activities

Anticancer Activity

Artemisinin and the flavonoid quercetagetin 6, 7, 3′,4′-tetramethyl ether showed significant cytotoxicity against P-388, A-549, HT-29, MCF-7, and other human KB tumor cells (Zheng, 1994). Artesunate, a semisynthetic derivate of artemisinin was tested in 55 cell lines of the National Cancer Institute, USA and was found most active against leukemia and colon cancer cell lines. Compared with established antitumor drugs artesunate ranges in the same area (Effert *et al.*, 2001). Rats treated with a single dose of 50 mg/kg of 7,12-dimethylbenz(a) anthracene develop breast cancer. Rats provided with chow containing 0.02 per cent artemisinin for 40 weeks significantly delayed breast cancer development. An enriched sesquiterpene fraction of an ethanolic extract from *A. annua* aerial parts showed antiulcerogenic activity when administered orally to rats with indometacin induced ulcers (Dia *et al.*, 2001). Hepatocarcinoma cells (SMMC-7721) treated with essential oil of *A. annua* 100 µg/ml for induces apoptosis as verified by light and electronic microscopy and Giemsa stain (Li *et al.*, 2004). Artesunate inhibits the angiogenesis and VEGF production in chronic myeloid leukemia cells *in vitro. In vivo* the angiogenic effect was evaluated in chicken choriallantoic membrane neovascularization model. Artesunate decreased the angiogenic activity in a dose-dependant manner (Huan-huan *et al.*, 2004; Zhou *et al.*, 2007).

Cardiovascular Effect

Antimalarials can cause significant prolongation of the electrocardiograph QT interval, which can be associated with an increased risk of potentially lethal ventricular arrhythmias. High doses of artemether and artemotil have been associated with QT prolongation in dogs, raising the possibility of a class effect with the artemisinin derivatives. Serial electrocardiograms were recorded, and QTc interval was calculated before and after administration of artesunate by intravenous injection in patients with severe falciparum malaria in Bangladesh. The mean QTc interval was unaffected by bolus intravenous artesunate (2.4 mg/kg). No effect was observed on the JTc or PR interval, QRS width, blood pressure, or heart rate. Intravenous artesunate does not have significant cardiovascular effects in patients with severe falciparum malaria (Maude *et al.*, 2009). The histological effects of normal and double normal dose of artesunate on the heart in Wistar rats were studied by Izunya *et al.* (2011). The rats were treated with artesunate at 2, 4 and 8 mg/kg for 7 days. The histological findings of heart on 8th day showed normal histological features in all the groups. This study signifies that artesunate at normal and double normal dose has no effects on the histology of the heart in wistar rats.

Immunomodulatory Effect

Artesunate at 75 mg/kg, i.m. for 7 days decreased the humolysin-forming capacity and levels of serum IgG of mice sensitized with sheep red blood cell. Artesunate enhanced the PHA-induced lymphocyte transformation rate in mice and increased the weight of spleen but reduced that of thymus. Artesunate elevated the DNFB-induced delayed-type hypersensitivity and reduced the percentage of phagocytosis of peritoneal macrophages and the phagocytic index. Artesunate suppressed the humoral immune responses but enhanced the cell-mediated immunity (Lin *et al.*, 1995).

Artesunate (range 0.01-2 μg/ml) or dihydroartemisinin (range 0.01-8 μg/ml; DHART) were added to peripheral blood mononuclear cells (PBMC) or whole blood (WB) cultures before or simultaneously upon stimulation with phytohemagglutinin (PHA), a T cell mitogen. Lymphoproliferation was then measured by ^{3}[H]-thymidine incorporation, T cell activation was assessed by expression of CD69 or CD25 using flow cytometry. Artesunate concentrations between 0.1-1.5 μg/ml reduced lymphoproliferation in PHA-stimulated PBMC and WB cultures in a generally dose-dependent manner; inhibition by DHART was similar. Artesunate had little effect on qualitative cytokine mRNA levels in PHA-stimulated PBMC cultures. Artesunate and DHART may diminish some PBMC responses to immunologic stimuli (Veerusubramanian *et al.*, 2006).

Artesunate significantly increased the survival rate, body weight and blood leukocyte counts, and reduced the serum levels of antinuclear antibody and anti-double-stranded DNA, 24 h urinary protein, and serum creatinine in MRL/lpr murine model having systemic lupus erythematosus. Artesunate decreased MCP-1, major pro-inflammation cytokine, in serum, urine and kidney. The level of B cell activating factor was decreased in artesunate treated MRL/lpr mice. Artesunate can inhibit the progression of disease and reverse the pathologic lesion of lupus nephritis (Jin *et al.*, 2009).

Diuretic Effect

Sodium artesunate has been found to have diuretic and natriuretic effect. It causes renal vasodilatation and increase in renal blood flow leading to natriuresis. This action is due to increased nitric oxide synthesis and inhibitory effect on chloride transport across the cortical thick ascending loop of Henle (TALH) that suppresses tubuloglomerular feedback (Seguro and Campos, 2002). The principal site of action of artesunate in kidneys is supposed to be TALH, which has the highest concentration of the enzyme Na, K-ATPase per tubular length. The increase in the urinary excretion of sodium, chloride and potassium also suggests that this drug has a predominant effect on the proximal segments of the nephron *i.e.* proximal tubule and the TALH. Reduction in the reabsorption of sodium and an increase in the distal sodium delivery occurs with a consequent greater sodium reabsorption and potassium secretion in the collecting tubule (Campos *et al.*, 2001).

The diuretic effect of artesunate is a double-edged weapon that can modify the course of the acute renal failure in malaria. The increase urinary loss of water and electrolytes can worsen the renal failure in hypovolemic patients with pyrexia and tachypnea. However, the administration of artesunate can also be useful in the conversion of an oliguric renal failure to nonoliguric in patients with volume overload. In addition, rapid improvement in pulmonary function has been observed in a patient with respiratory distress syndrome due to the diuretic effect of artesunate (Zaki *et al.*, 2011).

Anticonvulsant Activity

Sanjana *et al.* (2012) explored the activity of artesunate in experimentally induced seizures in rodent models. Artesunate at doses 36.4 and 72.8 mg/kg respectively significantly reduced the duration of the hind limb extensions in the maximal electroshock-induced seizure model. However, no significant decrease was noted in the duration of clonic convulsions in a pentylenetetrazole-induced seizure model indicating lack of activity in petit mal epilepsy. The results indicated anticonvulsant activity of artesunate in the maximum electroshock-induced seizure model suggesting its potential utility in the management of generalized tonic-clonic seizures and parteal seizures.

Embriotoxicity

Many antimalarial drugs have been associated with male reproductive dysfunction. Artesunate has been reported to cause embryolethality and malformations when administered orally to rats during organogenesis. Pregnant rats were orally administered artesunate at 10, 17 or 30 mg/kg/day on single or multiple days of gestation. Embryolethality, cardiovascular malformations and a syndrome of skeletal defects were observed on 10 to 14 days postcoitum. The most sensitive day for the induction of malformations was day 10 postcoitum. Malformations tended to occur in parteally resorbed litters and included cardiovascular defects and bent and misshapen long bones and scapulae (White and Clark, 2008). In another study Clark *et al.* (2008) compared the developmental toxicity of structurally related artemisinins, dihdyroartemisinin, artemether and arteether to that of artesunate after oral administration to rats on Day 10 postcoitum. All artemisinins caused the same pattern of embryolethality and fetal cardiovascular and skeletal abnormalities as previously shown for artesunate. In the i.v. dose, marked postimplantation loss occurred at 1.5 and 3 mg/kg artesunate, but not at 0.75 mg/kg. An embryolethal dose of artesunate caused a 15 per cent decrease in maternal reticulocyte counts and no other hematologic effects.

Injectable artesunate cause fetal death and teratogenic effects in animals at levels below the human therapeutic dose. Similar toxicity has also been found for oral artemisinins in various animal species, but has not been found in humans. Li *et al.* (2008) performed tissue distribution (5 mg/kg) and toxicokinetics (30 mg/kg × 3) studies on pregnant and non-pregnant rats. Toxicokinetics profiles of artesunate showed that a daily single dose for 3 days has no change in plasma concentration in the pregnant animals, but a significant concentration decline was seen in the non-pregnant rats. Higher conversion rate of artesunate to dihydroartemisinin (DHA) was detected in the pregnant rats after both single and multiple dosing. The tissue/ blood partition coefficients demonstrated that the level of radiolabeled artesunate that was distributed into uterus, placenta, and ovary was 2-4-fold higher than in blood. This study showed that unchanged artesunate and DHA in the blood of pregnant rats was 1-4 folds higher in the pregnant animals, which all likely relate to the severe embryotoxicity even with a low-dosage regimen in pregnant animals.

Oral doses of 2 and 4 mg/kg artesunate was administered to pregnant rats from the 9th to the 11th day of gestation to follow the active osteogenic period in the animal. Records of litter size, number resorbed, dead, living or malformed foetuses were taken. The retrieved foetuses were weighed and morphological examinations were done to observe any distortion of a gross nature. Skeletal dysgenesis was seen as indicated by retarded calcification, severest in the 4 mg/kg treated group rats. These exhibited non-calcified palate, vertebrae, spine and arches; skull, sternabrae and ribs. Calcium and phosphorus content was low through out the foetal age. The mechanisms of its osteo-toxicity could not yet be ascertain presently; but it is possible that, like ethanol, artesunate could facilitate the action of the calcification inhibitors (Adebisi, 2002), that is, a family of inorganic pyrophosphatases, phosphonates and diphosphonates. These act normally to prevent calcium deposits from forming on soft tissues (Anderson, 1978). Although artesunate produced lesser assaults compared to other drugs, this work is indicative and confirms the adverse effect profiles of the artemisinin-based treatments, its toxicity cum teratogenicity (Clark *et al.*, 2004; Price *et al.*, 1999; Adebisi 2002, Taylor and White, 2004; Adebisi, 2005; White *et al.*, 2006; Clark *et al.*, 2006; Adebisi, 2008) hence, a caution in its use partecularly in early pregnancy (Nosten and White, 2009).

The effect of artesunate on male reproductive activities was studied using *in vivo* and *in vitro* experimental models. Artesunate did not cause any significant effects in short-term administration but significantly reduced the aforesaid parameters in long-term administration. There were visible lesions in the testicular and epididymal histological studies, although fertility was not significantly reduced. *In vitro* studies showed dose and duration dependent changes in sertoli cell viability and ds-DNA integrity (Olumide and Raji, 2011).

Liver Toxicity

Nwanjo (2007) studied the hepatotoxic potentials of artesunate in guinea pigs at 2, 4, 8 and 16 mg/kg dose orally for 7 days. The results showed significant increases of AST only at highest dose (16 mg/kg). The outcome suggests compromise of liver function and possible damage to the hepatocytes at the highest dose level tested. Hepatotoxicity and hemotoxicity are associated with artesunate administration at both required and overdose conditions (1, 2 and 4 mg/kg, oral) however these effects are magnified in overdose conditions. Hepatotoxicity was monitored in the rats as a function of changes in serum levels of aspartate transaminase (AST), alanine transaminase (ALT), alkaline phosphatase (ALP), total serum albumin and malondiadehyde (MDA) level. The hemolytic effect of this drug was monitored by changes in the packed cell volume (PCV), total bilirubin, conjugated bilirubin and

MDA levels of erythrocyte (Omotuyi *et al.*, 2008). An increased hepatocyte and erythrocyte malondiadehyde level was observed in 4 mg/kg group. The result also shows increased activities for the serum enzymes in 2 and 4 mg/kg treated groups. There is a clear indication that hepatotoxicity and hemotoxicity are associated with artesunate administration at both required and overdose conditions however these effects are magnified in overdose conditions.

Rats were orally administered with 2, 4 and 8 mg/kg of artesunate daily for 7 days. The histological findings after H and E method showed sinusoidal congestion with cytoplasmic vacuolation (hepatocyte oedema) and mild inflammation of the portal tracts. This study suggests that artesunate at normal dose has a toxic effect on the liver cells and could be a potential hepatotoxic drug (Lzunya *et al.*, 2010a). The effect of artesunate on the hematological indices, hepatotoxicity and histology of rat liver was investigated at 1, 2 and 5 mg/kg/day respectively for a period of 5 days. Hematological indices indicated insignificant difference in the RBC, WBC, while a significant dose dependent increase in PCV and hemoglobin content was observed. No changes were observed in the serum levels of AST, ALT and ALP among the groups. Histological examination of the liver revealed points of focal necrosis among the treated groups. The mild liver tissue damage was more evident among the over dosed group. Artesunate is thus safe, when administered within the therapeutic range. This suggests tonicity of the liver tissue in the treatment groups since elevation of the serum enzymes indigenous to liver is an indicator of hepatotoxicity. Transaminases are important useful markers of hepatocellular toxicity and damage. Points of focal necrosis were observed in the treatment groups though the extent of tissue damage amongst the various treated groups seemed almost the same (Hamman, 2011).

Nduka and Olufunso (2011) investigated the effect of varying doses of artesunate on function indices of rat kidney and liver at 2, 3, and 5 mg/kg. Result indicated an increased serum creatinine, L-γ glutamyl transaminase, sodium, potassium, chloride and bicarbonate levels in artesunate treated animals. Urea levels in serum of artesunate treated groups were significantly reduced. This study indicated alterations in biochemical parameters investigated with a more pronounced effect on kidney function than liver function tests. This suggests artesunate administration may adversely affect the functional capacities of the kidney and liver.

Neurotoxicity

Neurotoxicity in mammals has been associated partecularly with the use of intramuscular artemether or artemotil, which results in sustained blood concentrations, rather than oral administration of the same drugs, which are absorbed and eliminated rapidly by this route. The pattern of irreversible neuropathological damage in mammals is unusual selective damage is done to certain brain stem nuclei, partecularly to those associated with hearing and balance. In experimental mammal models, water-soluble artesunate given orally or parenterally is considerably less neurotoxic than is oil soluble artemether. These findings stimulated detailed prospective studies in humans none of which have led to findings of neurotoxicity. Case-control neurophysiological study on human brain pathology in a prospective clinical examination of a large series of patients with malaria treated with artemisinin derivatives sodium artesunate and dihydroartemisin, metabolites common to all artemisin analogues, were studied (Nontprasert *et al.*, 1998).

Intramuscular injections of high doses of the oil-soluble antimalarial artemisinin derivatives artemether and arteether produce an unusual pattern of selective damage to brain stem centers in experimental mammals, predominantly those involved in auditory processing and vestibular reflexes. The neurotoxic potential of the oral drugs was assessed and compared with the parenteral routes of administration. Once-daily oral administration of artesunate or artemether is relatively safe, presumably because the central nervous system is exposed transiently, whereas constant exposure either from depot intramuscular injection of oil-based drug or constant oral intake carries relatively greater neurontoxic potential (Nontprasert *et al.*, 2000). Intramuscular artemether (50-100 mg/kg/day for 28 days) caused dose-dependent neuropathologic damage to the brain stem. The neurons in the lower brain stem trapezoid nucleus, the gigantocellular reticular nucleus, and the inferior cerebellar peduncle were the most sensitive to the toxic effects of artemether. There was no pathologic evidence of neuronal death in mice receiving either oral artemether, or oral or intramuscular artesunate, in doses up to 300 mg/kg/day (Nontprasert *et al.*, 2002).

Reproductive Toxicity

Oral administration of artesunate at 2, 4 and 8 mg/kg for 7 day showed mild sloughing of germ cells from the basement membrane and varying degrees of reduced population of germ cells in testis. These findings suggest that artesunate at normal dose has a deleterious effect on the histology of the testis and could be a potential male antifertility agent. Long-term administration of artesunate could induce reversible infertility in rats which may act via distortion of blood–testis barrier formed by Sertoli cells (Izunya *et al.*, 2010b).

Genotoxicity

Artesunate acts both as an antimalarial agent and cytotoxically on tumor cells. Artesunate was administered by oral gavage at doses of 5, 50 and 100 mg/kg. Cytotoxicity was assessed by scoring 200 consecutive polychromatic and normochromatic erythrocytes (PCE/NCE ratio). The results demonstrate that artesunate induced significant DNA damage only in liver cells and high dose caused an increase in the mean number of micronucleated polychromatic erythrocytes. Artesunate showed weak genotoxic effects at low doses and clastogenic effects at high doses (Aquino *et al.*, 2011).

Nephrotoxicity

In a study conducted by Li *et al.* (2007) the acute toxicity of artesunate was illustrated as LD_{50} 488 mg/kg, following daily i.v. injection for 3 days in *Plasmodium berghei* infected rats. In uninfected rats, the LD_{50} values was 351 mg/kg after a single dose. This study showed vascular necrosis in 50 per cent of the animals at 42.8 mg/kg dose of artesunate. Animals also showed moderate signs of renal failure at 240 mg/kg dose (100 times higher than the therapeutic dose). At the same dose histopathological evaluation demonstrated mild to moderate tubular necrosis in uninfected rats, interestingly, fewer pathological lesions were observed in malaria-infected rats. Renal injury was reversible in all cases after 8 days of cessation of dosing.

Artesunate Combination Therapy

World Health Organization's strategy is to reduce malaria related mortality. The few available drugs might be safeguarded if combined with artesunate. The addition of artesunate to a standard antimalarial treatment substantially reduces treatment failure, recrudescence and gametocyte carriage. Artemisinin-based combination treatments (ACTs) are now generally accepted as the best treatments for uncomplicated falciparum malaria (Davis *et al.*, 2005; Nosten and White, 2009). The combination depending on the location and prevalence of malaria parasites could be: artesunate–mefloquine, artemether–lumefantrine, and dihydroartemisinin–piperaquine. They are rapidly and reliably effective. Efficacy is determined by the drug partnering the artemisinin derivative. Artesunate–sulfadoxine–pyrimethamine and artesunate–amodiaquine are effective in some areas, but in other areas, resistance to the partner precludes their use.

Artesunate-lamivudine

HIV-Malaria co morbidity frequently requires the co-administration of lamivudine and artesunate, in Malaria endemic areas where HIV is also a problem. This situation is a frequent occurrence in developing countries of the tropics, like Nigeria where the burden of Malaria and HIV is heavy. The co-administration of these drugs may result in interactions with possible physiologic and/or therapeutic consequences. Lamivudine-artesunate co administration have effect on body weight, relative organ weight and glucose tolerance. Glucose tolerance is altered with lamivudine-artesunate co-administration, and may be beneficial, as hypoglycaemia which is often a complication of Malaria therapy (Olurishe *et al.*, 2011; Olurishe *et al.*, 2012).

Artesunate-mefloquine

In prospective studies of acute uncomplicated, multidrug-resistant falciparum malaria on the western border of Thailand, the oral artemisinin derivatives used alone or in combination with mefloquine and mefloquine alone was used assessed. The combined regimens of mefloquine plus an artemisinin derivative were associated with more side effects than those with an artemisinin derivative alone *viz.* acute nausea, vomiting, anorexia and dizziness. Oral artesunate and artemether alone were very well tolerated. There was no difference in the incidence of possible adverse effects between the two drugs, and no evidence that either derivative caused allergic reactions, neurologic or psychiatric reactions, or cardiovascular or dermatologic toxicity (Price *et al.*, 1999).

Artesunate-amodiaquine

Artesunate-amodiaquine combination for the treatment of childhood malaria is one of the artemisnin combination therapies (ACTs) recommended by national authorities in many African countries. Effectiveness of artesunate plus amodiaquine combination is one Act recommended by the World Health Organization (WHO) for use in malaria control programmes and a first line treatment for African children with uncomplicated malaria data on this combination in young children in scarce (Oyakhirome *et al.*, 2007). Artesunate plus amodiaquine is a co-packaged product which is the most commonly used ACT. The incidence of experienced adverse reactions to the ACTs used for malaria treatment is generally mild and tolerable (Adisa *et al.*, 2008).

Otuechere *et al.* (2012) evaluated a subacute therapeutic dosing of artemether-lumefantrine and artesunate-amodiaquine on plasma cholesterol, renal antioxidants, and organ weights in rats. Rats were administered, twice daily, oral therapeutic doses of artemether-lumefantrine (1.14/6.86mg/kg/d) and artesunate-amodiaquine (2.86/8.58mg/kg/d), respectively, for seven days. The ACTs did not significantly alter catalase, superoxide dismutase, glutathione S-transferase, myeloperoxidase, total glutathione levels and relative organ weights. Plasma total cholesterol levels also decreased insignificantly. Artesunate-amodiaquine, but not artemether-lumefantrine, significantly increased lactate dehydrogenase activity and both ACTs increased lipid peroxidation. Artesunate-amodiaquine and artemether-lumefantrine may preserve renal antioxidants and organ weights *in vivo*. However, caution is required above therapeutic indications or in chronic doses as this may predispose to renal oxidative stress.

Artesunate-pyronaridine

Pyronaridine-artesunate is among the most promising novel artemisinin combination therapies for the treatment of malaria. Pyronaridine-artesunate demonstrated repeatedly high efficacy in the treatment of vivax and falciparum malaria and noninferiority was established compared to standard comparator regimens. An innovative paediatric drug formulation was developed in parallel to the tablet formulation for the treatment of young children. This combination is currently under evaluation by the European Medicines Agency - may become a preferred choice as first-line therapy in malaria endemic regions based on its low cost, long shelf-life, simplified once-daily dosing regimen, proven efficacy against falciparum and vivax malaria, and the parallel clinical development of a paediatric drug formulation (Boulanger *et al.*, 2007). A series of clinical phase II and III trials have been conducted for the indications of uncomplicated falciparum and vivax malaria in Africa and Asia. Pharmacokinetic analysis showed dose linearity, low interindividual variation and absence of a clinically important effect of food on the bioavailability of this drug combination (Kurth *et al.*, 2011). Artesunate, in addition to being a very effective treatment for uncomplicated malaria, can also sharply reduce the *S. haematobium* loads harboured by pre-school African children (Deen *et al.*, 2001).

Artesunate-sulfadoxine Pyrimethamine

The efficacy of artesunate (4 mg/kg. day, on days 0–2) plus sulfadoxine pyrimethamine (25 mg/kg, on day 0) for the treatment of uncomplicated *Plasmodium falciparum* malaria was investigated in four sentinel areas in Sudan, with different malaria transmission. A gametocytaemia were detected during the follow-up in one patient. Adverse drug effects detected like nausea and vomiting might influence the adherence to artesunate plus sulfadoxine pyrimethamine, especially science this therapy is only available in the oral form (Elamin *et al.*, 2005). No evidence of a teratogenic or otherwise harmful effect of gestational exposure to artesunate and sulfadoxine pyrimethamine. Treatment of a self-selected group of pregnant women with sulfadoxine pyrimethamine and artesunate during pregnancy was associated with a greater birthweight, which may have resulted from clearance of malaria parasites however, the influence of confounding factors cannot be excluded. Artesunate with sulfadoxine pyrimethamine is a promising antimalarial combination but few data are available on the safety of artemisinins when taken during pregnancy (Deen *et al.*, 2001).

Artesunate-sulfamethoxypyrazine/Pyrimethamine

A study was conducted to determine the efficacy of the antimalarial artemisinin-based combination therapy artesunate-sulfamethoxypyrazine/pyrimethamine, administered in doses used for malaria with *Schistosoma haematobium* in school aged children. The efficacy and safety of the antimalarial combination therapy artesunate-sulfamethoxypyrazine, administered in the doses used for the treatment of malaria, were compared to the efficacy and safety of pyrimethamine, the standard treatment for schistosomiasis, in children. Pyrimethamine was more effective than artesunate-sulfamethoxypyrazine for treating *S. haematobium*. However, the safety and tolerability profile of artesunate- sulfamethoxypyrazine was similar to that seen with pyrimethamine. Pyrimethamine was more efficacious to reduce haematuria during *S. haematobium* infections in comparison to artesunate-sulfamethoxypyrazine, administered in doses used for the treatment of malaria (Sissoko *et al.*, 2009).

Discussion

A number of herbal remedies made of *A. annua* dry leaves are suggested for the treatment and prevention of malaria. However, WHO does not recommend the use *A. annua* plant material in any form, including tea, for the treatment or the prevention of malaria. The content of artemisinin in the leaves is influenced by genetic, agricultural and environmental factors (Delabays *et al.*, 2001; Ferreira *et al.*, 2005; WHO 2006). Total recovery of artemisinin can vary from 0.01 to 1.4 per cent weight per cent of dry leaf mass (Liu *et al.*, 2006; Simonnet *et al.*, 2010). Harvesting season, drying procedures and storage conditions also influence the content in artemisinin (Simonnet *et al.*, 2008; Laughlin, 2002). Inadequate storage facilities causes loss of the artemisinin content when stored for a long period of time. In order to receive a dose equivalent to a 500 mg artemisinin tablet or capsule, patients would be required to drink as much as 5 litres of *A. annua* tea per day, for a minimum of seven consecutive days, making compliance to treatment difficult to achieve.

Artesunate an antimalarial drug was introduced by world health organization (WHO) to combat the problems of multi drug resistant *P. falciparum* malaria (Effert, 2001). Artesunate (AS), the most widely available of the artemisinin-related compounds, is a semi-synthetic hemisuccinate derivatives of dihydroartemisinin (DHA). Artesunate may be given parentrally, intravenously, intramuscularly, orally or rectally (Newton *et al.*, 2000). The artemisinin are potent antimalarial drugs that are remarkably well tolerated (Maude *et al.*, 2009). Artesunate and artemether rapidly degrade into dihydroartemisinin which is claimed by pharmaceutical companies to be 10 times more effective against malaria than artemisinin. Artemisinin itself does not metabolize into dihydroartemisinin and stays much longer in the plasma.

The derivatives of artemisinin are strong peroxides. They create radicals and reactive oxygen species which at high doses might damage cortical and brain stem neurons and are cytotoxic to many other cells (Schmuck *et al.*, 2002). Generally, Artesunate exert its anti-malarial activity by the generation of reactive oxygen species from its endoperoxide bond leading to lipid peroxidase. The reactive oxygen species cause macromolecular damage by alkylating heme and several other proteins. The recommended dose of artesunate is 2-10 mg/kg/day or maximum upto 200 mg/day in adult human body. Large clinical studies with malaria patients have shown that artesunate is well tolerated, with a few and insignificant side effects. However, several studies have showed evidence of toxicity on the brainstem, superior colliculus, stomach, testis and liver in artesunate treated rats. Moreover, Artesunate has been reported to destroy cancer cells and also reduces proliferation, interferes in DNA replication and cell cycle and enhance apoptosis through the intrinsic death pathway by ROS generation. It has been reported that artesunate is toxic to malaria parasites at nanomolar concentration, whereas micromolar concentration is required for toxicity in mammalian cells. Evidences show the neurotoxicity of artesunate at high doses (50-100 mg/kg/day oral and IM) in laboratory animals (Nontprasert *et al.*, 2000) including the cytotoxicity of Artesunate on tumor cell lines have been reported (Huan-huan *et al.*, 2004).

The genotoxicity of artesunate was studies in Brazil on mice (Aquino *et al.*, 2011). The artesunate was administered by oral gavage at doses of 5, 50 and 100 mg/kg. Artesunate showed weak genotoxic effects at low doses and severe (clastogenic effects) at high doses. Artesunate has been reported to cause embryo lethality and malformations when administered orally to rats during organogenesis. Artesunate also has teratogenic effect. Long term administration for six weeks at 2.9 mg/kg dose reduces reproductive efficiency of male rat and toxicity on development of fetus in female rats.

Artesunate induces hepatotoxicity when given at 4-8 mg/kg dose for 5-7 days along with adverse action on kidney, biochemical parameters of serum and hematological induces in rat. Artesunate at 8-16 mg/kg dose causes acute-toxicity in guinea pig when administered for 7 days. Artesunate at 4-8 mg/kg dose given into 7 day had no effect on the histology of the heart. The studies showed hepatotoxicity and hemolytic effects were clearly associated with artesunate. Literature citation showed that reported toxicity studies on artesunate was been mostly done following 7 days administration in a dose range of 2-10 mg/kg oral or I.P.). In humans hepatotoxicity can be particularly severe if artesunate is used in combination with HIV antiretroviral drugs (German *et al.*, 2007). Neurotoxicity and embriotoxicity were conducted on 15 days, 28 days and 42 days treatment schedule. 28 days I.P. administration at a dose of 7.5 mg/kg has been reported to have no adverse effect on kidney. The therapeutic dose of artesunate in adult human is minimum 50 mg/day to 200 mg/day.

Derivatives of artemisinin exhibit potent immunosuppressive activity (Wang *et al.*, 2007). Artesunate concentrations between 0.1-1.5 microg/ml reduced lymphocyte production in a generally dose dependant manner (Veerusubramanian *et al.*, 2006). Artesunate suppressed phagocytosis of peritoneal macrophage in mice (Lin *et al.*, 1995). Clinical trials in western Cambodia reduced neutrophil counts after 3 to 5 doses several patients required artesunate to be discontinued because of neutropenia (Bethell *et al.*, 2010). A high risk of neutropenia in HIV-infected children following treatment with artesunate was also noticed in Uganda (Gasasira *et al.*, 2008).

One of the side effects of the higher doses of artesunate is the dormancy effect induced in plasmodium. The parasite encapsulates itself against the aggressive peroxide artesunate and reawakens at the end of the treatment causing emergence of resistance. There is still uncertainty over the safety of artemisinin derivatives in the first trimester of pregnancy when they should not be used, unless there are no effective alternatives. Most malaria endemic countries have now adopted ACT as first-line treatment of falciparum malaria, but in most of these, only a minority of the patients that need ACT actually receive them. Effort should be made to encourage the use of ACT in the management of acute uncomplicated *P. falciparum* malaria. Because these drugs have not been evaluated extensively in early pregnancy in humans, they should be avoided in patients in the first trimester of pregnancy with uncomplicated malaria until more information is available. There is no evidence for adverse effects on the foetus exposed in the second and third trimesters, when these drugs are recommended depending on the safety profile of the partnering drug (Nosten and White, 2009). Future studies are also required to be done to assess the safety of this group of antimalarial drugs in vulnerable populations, therefore, be considered in order to generate a useful safety information and database to improve the quality of health care offered to the patient.

References

Adebisi, S.S. (2002). Effects of prenatal ingestion of alcohol and folic acid supplementation on foetal osteo-morphology: The Wistar rat model. *Journal of Tropical Biosciences* **2(1)**: 24-28.

Adebisi, S.S. (2005). Alcohol effects on embryonal bone growth. *Nigerian Journal of Surgical Research,* **7(1 – 2)**: 152 – 158.

Adebisi, S.S. (2007). Artesunate, A promising anti-malarial drug: A Review. *Ebonyi Medical Journal,* **6(2)**: 100-105.

Adebisi, S.S. (2008). The toxicity of artesunate on bone develpments: The Wistar rat animal model of malaria treatment. *The Internet Journal of Parasitic Diseases,* **4(1)**: Available online: http: / /ispub.com/IJPD/4/1/10327 accessed on May 2014.

Adisa, R., Fakeye, T.O., and Dike, D. (2008). Evaluation of adverse drug reactions to artemisinin based combination therapy in a Nigeria university community. *Tropical Journal of Pharmaceutical Research,* **7(2)**: 937-944.

Adjuik, M., Babiker, A., Garner, P., Olliaro, P., Taylor, W., and White N. (2004). International Artemisinin Study Group. Artesunate combinations for treatment of malaria: meta-analysis. *Lancet,* **363**: 9–17.

Anderson, H.C. (1978). Calcification of rachitic cartelage to study mature vesicles function. *Federation Proceedings*, **35**: 147.

Aquino, I., Perazzo, F.F. and Maistro, E.L. (2011). Genotoxicity assessment of the antimalarial compound artesunate in somatic cells of mice. *Food Chemistry and Toxicology*, **49(6)**: 1335-9.

Artemis, a high-yielding variety of *Artemisia annua*. Mediplant, Conthey, Switzerland, 1998

Bethell, D., Se, Y., Lon, C., Socheat, D., Saunders, D., Teja-Isavadharm, P., Khemawoot, P., Darapiseth, S., Lin, J., Sriwichai, S., Kuntawungin, W., Surasri, S., Lee, S.J., Sarim, S., Tyner, S., and Fukuda, M.M.(2010). Dose-dependent risk of Neutropenia after 7-Day courses of artesunate monotherapy in Cambodian patients with acute *Plasmodium falciparum* malaria. *Clinical Infectious Diseases*, **51(12)**: e105-e114. doi: 10.1086/657402.

Bilia, A.R., Melillo de Malgalhães, P., Bergonzi, M.C., and Vincieria, F.F. (2006). Simultaneous analysis of artemisinin and flavonoids of several extracts of *Artemisia annua* L. obtained from a commercial sample and a selected cultivar. *Phytomedicine*, **13**: 487-493.

Boulanger, D., Dieng, Y., Cisse, B., Remoue, F., Capuano, F., Dieme, J.L., Ndiaye, T., Sokhna, C., Trape, J.F., Greenwood, B., and Simondon, F. (2007). Antischistosomal efficacy of artesunate combination therapies administered as curative treatments for malaria attacks. *Transactions of the Royal Society of Tropical Medicine and Hygiene*, **101(2)**: 113-6.

Cai, Y., Luo, Q., Sun, M., and Corke, H. (2004). Antioxidant activity and phenolic compounds of 112 traditional Chinese medicinal plants associated with anticancer. *Life Sciences*, **74**: 2157–2184.

Campos, S.B., Rouch, L.H., and Seguro, A.C. (2001). Effects of sodium artesunate, a new antimalarial drug, on renal function. *Kidney International*, **59**: 1044–51.

Chen, P.K, Leather, G.R., and Klayman, D.L. (1987). Allelopathic effect of artemisinin and its related compounds from *Artemisia annua*. *Plant Physiology*, 83S: Abstr. 406.

Christen, P., and Veuthey, J.L. (2001). New trends in extraction, identification and quantification of artemisinin and its derivates. *Current Medical Chemistry*, **8**: 1827-1839.

Clark, R.L., Kumemura, M., Makori, M., Nkata, Y., Bernrad, F., White, T.E.K., and Arima, A. (2006). Artesunate developmental toxicity in monkeys. *Teratology Society Abstracts*: pp. 30.

Clark, R.L., White, T.E.A., Clode, S., Gaunt, I., Winstanley, P., and Ward, S.A. (2004). Developmental toxicity of artesunate and an artesunate combination in the rat and rabbit. Birth Defects Research. Part B. *Developmental and Reproductive Toxicology*, **71**: 380-394.

Davis, T.M., Karunajeewa, H.A., and Ilett, K.F. (2005). Artemisinin-based combination therapies for uncomplicated malaria. *Medical Journal of Australia*, **182**: 181–185.

Deen, J.L., Von Seidlein, L., Pinder, M., Walraven, G.E., and Greenwood, B.M. (2001). The safety of the combination artesunate and pyrimethamine-sulfadoxine given during pregnancy. *Transactions of the Royal Society of Tropical Medicine and Hygiene*, **95(4)**: 424-8.

Dia, P.C., Foglio, M.A., and Possenti, A. (2001). Antiulcerogenic activity of crude ethanol extract and some fractions obtained from aerial parts of *Artemisia annua*. *Phytotherapy Research*, **15(8)**: 670.

Dondorp, A., Nosten, F., Stepniewska, K., and Day, N. (2005). White N and group, South East Asian Quinine Artesunate malaria trial (SEAQUAMAT). Artesunate versus quinine for treatment of severe falciparum malaria: a randomised trial. *Lancet*, **366**: 717–725.

Effert, T., Dunston, H., and Sauerbrey, H. (2001). The antimalarial artesunate is also active against cancer. *International Journal of Oncology*, **18(4)**: 767-73.

Elamin, S.B., Malik, E.M., Abdelgadir, T., Khamiss, A.H., Mohammed, M.M., Ahmed, E.S., and Adam I. (2005). Artesunate plus sulfadoxine-pyrimethamine for treatment of uncomplicated *Plasmodium falciparum* malaria in Sudan. *Malaria Journal*, **4**: 41.

Ellman, A. (2010). Cultivation of *Artemisia annua* in Africa and Asia, *Outlooks on Pest Management*, DOI: 10.1564/21apr08.

El-Sohly, H.N., Croom, E.M., El-Feraly F.S., and El-Sherei M.M. (1990). A large-scale extraction technique of Artemisinin from *Artemisia annua*. *Journal of Natural Product*, **53(6)**: 1560–1564.

Ferreira, J.F.S. (2005). Cultivation and genetics of *Artemisia annua* L for increased production of the antimalarial artemisinin. *Plant Genetics Resources*, **3(2)**: 206-229.

Ferreira, J.F.S., Simon, J.E., and Janick, J. (1997). *Artemisia annua*: botany, horticulture, pharmacology (A Review). *Horticultural Reviews*, **19**: 319–371.

Fleming, A., Kooy, F.V.D., Liu, N.Q., Schuehly, W., and Freyhold, M.V. (2009). Novel commercial method for extracting artemisinin: Extracting *Artemisia annua* with ethanol and purifying ethanolic extracts. Available at: http: //www.mmv.org/sites/default/files/uploads/docs/artemisinin/06c_M_von_Freyhold_Presentation_Sept_09_ethanolic_Extraction_purification.pdf, accessed on 10 feb 2014.

Gasasira, A.F., Kamya, M.R., Achan, J., Mebrahtu, T., Kalyango, J.N., Ruel, T., and Charlebois, E. (2008). High risk of neutropenia in HIV-infected children following treatment with artesunate plus amodiaquine for uncomplicated malaria in Uganda. *Clinica Infectious Diseases*, **46**: 985-91.

German, P., Greenhouse, B., Coates, C., Dorsey, G., and Rosenthal, P.J. (2007). Hepatotoxicity due to a drug interaction between amodiaquine plus artesunate and efavirenz. *Clinical Infectious Diseases*, **44**: 889-891.

Hamman, W.O. (2011). Acute exposure to Artesunate and its effect on the hematological Indices, hepatotoxicity and histology of the liver of adult Wistar rats. *Asian Journal of Medical Sciences*, **3(4)**: 176-179.

Han, J., Ye, M., Qiao, X., Xu, M., Wang, B., and Guo, D. A. (2008). Characterization of phenolic compounds in the Chinese herbal drug *Artemisia annua* by liquid chromatography coupled to electrospray ionization mass spectrometry. *Journal of Pharmaceutical and Biomedical Analysis*, **47**: 516–525.

Huan-huan, C., Li-Li, Y., and Shang-Bin, L. (2004). Artesunate reduces chicken chorioallantoic membran neovascularization and exhibits antiangiogenic and apoptoic activity on human microvascular dermal endothelial cell. *Cancer Letter*, **21(2)**: 163-71.

Izunya, A.M. Nwaopara, A.O., Aigbiremolen, A., Odike, M.A.C., Oaikhena, G.A., and Bankole, J.K. (2010 a). Histological effects of oral administration of artesunate on the liver in Wistar rats. *Research Journal of Applied Science*, 2(4): 314-318.

Izunya, A.M., Nwaopara, A.O., Aigbiremolen, A.E. Odike, M.A.C., Oaikhena, G.A., and Bankole, J.K. (2010 b). Histological studies of the toxicity of artesunate on the testes in Wistar rats. *Biology and Medicine*, **2(2)**: 49-56.

Izunya, A.M., Nwaopara, A.O., Ayanwu, L.C, Odike, M.A.C., Oaikhena, G.A., Bankole, J.K., and Okhiai, O. (2011). Histological studies of the cardiotoxicity of artesunate in Wistar rats. *Archieves of Applied Science and Research*, **3(4)**: 1-6.

Jin, O., Zhang, H., Gu, Z., Zhao, S., Xu, T., Zhou, K., Jiang, B., Wang, J., Zeng, X., and Sun, L. (2009). A pilot study of the therapeutic efficacy and mechanism of artesunate in the MRL/lpr murine model of systemic lupus erythematosus. *Chinese Society of Immunology and University of Science and Technology of China*, **6**: 6.

Juteau, F., Masotti, V., and Bessire, J.M. (2002). Antibacterial and antioxidant activities of *Artemisia annua* essential oil. *Fitoterapia*, **73(6)**: 532-5.

Kishore, N., Mishra, A.K., and Chansouria, J.P. (1993). Fungotoxicity of essential oils against dermatophytes. *Mycoses*, **36(5)**: 211-15.

Kohler, M., Haerdi, W., Christen, P., and Veuthey, J.L. (1997). Extraction of artemisinin and artemisinic acid from *Artemisia annua* L. using supercritical carbon dioxide. *Journal of Chromatography A.*, **785(1-2)**: 353-60.

Kokate, C.K., Purohit, A.P., and Gokhale, S.B. (2007). Textbook of pharmacognosy. 39th ed. India: Nirali Prakashan. pp. 382-383.

Kurth, F., Belard, S., Basra, A., and Ramharter, M. (2011). Pyronaridine-artesunate combination therapy for the treatment of malaria. *Current Opinion in Infectious Diseases*, **24(6)**: 564-9. doi: 10.1097/QCO.0b013e32834cabdb.

Laughlin, J.C. (2002). Post-harvest drying treatment effects on antimalarial constituents of *Artemisia annua* L. *Hacta Horticulturae*, **576**: 315-320.

Li, O., Xie, L.H., Johnson, T.O., Si, Y., Haeberle, A.S., and Weina, P.J. (2007). Toxicity evaluation of artesunate and artelinate in *Plasmodium berghei* infected and uninfected rats. *Transactions of the Royal Society of Tropical Medicine and Hygiene*, **101(2)**: 104-12.

Li, Q., Si, Y., Smith, K.S., Zeng, Q., and Weina, P.J. (2008). Embryotoxicity of artesunate in animal species related to drug tissue distribution and toxicokinetic profiles. *Birth Defects Research. Part B, Developmental and Reproductive Toxicology*, **83(4)**: 435-45.

Li, Y., Li, M.Y., and Wang, L. (2004). Induction of apoptosis of cultured hepatocarcinoma cell by essential oil of *Artemisia annua*. *PMID.*, **15**: 181 - 829.

Lin, P., Feng, Z., Pan, J., Zhang, D., and Xiao, L. (1995). Effects of artesunate on immune function in mice. *Acta Pharmacologica Sinica*, **16**: 441-444.

Liu, C., Zhao, Y., and Wang, Y. (2006). Artemisinin: current state and perspectives for biotechnological production of an antimalarial drug. *Applied Microbiology Biotechnology*, **72**: 11-20.

Liu, K.C.S., Yang, S.L., and Roberts, M.F. (1989). The contribution of flavonoids to the antimalarial activity of *Artemisia annua*. *Planta Med.*,/ Abstr -P2-25.

Lopes-Lutz, D., Alviano, D.S., Alviano C.S., and Kolodziejczyk, P.P. (2008). Screening of chemical composition, antimicrobial and antioxidant activities of Artemisia essential oils. *Phytochemistry*, **69 (8)**: 1732-1738.

Maude, R.J., Plewes, K., Faiz, M.A., Hanson, J., Charunwatthana, P., Lee, S.J., Tarning, J., Yunus, E.B., Hoque, M.G., Hasan, M.U., Hossain, A., Lindegardh, N., Day, N.P., White, N.J., and Dondorp, A.M. (2009). Does artesunate prolong the electrocardiograph QT interval in patients with severe malaria. *American Journal of Tropical Medicine and Hygeine*, **80(1)**: 126-132.

McGready, R., Stepniewska, K., Ward, S.A., Cho, T., Gilveray, G., Looareesuwan, S., White, N.J., and Nosten, F. (2006). Pharmacokinetics of dihydroartemisinin following oral artesunate treatment of pregnant women with acute uncomplicated falciparum malaria. *European Journal of Clinical Pharmacology*, **62**: 367–371.

Minzi, O.M., Gupta, A., Haule, A.F., Kagashe, G.A., Massele, A.Y., and Gustafsson, L.L. (2007). Lack of impact of artesunate on the disposition kinetics of sulfadoxine/pyrimethamine when the two drugs are concomitantly administered. *European Journal of Clinical Pharmacology*, **63(5)**: 457-62.

Nduka, A.G., and Olufunso, O.O. (2011). Evaluation of selected biochemical parameters in renal and hepatic functions following oral administration of Artesunate to albino rats. *Researcher*, **3(7)**. Available at: http: // www.sciencepub.net/researcher accessed on 10 feb 2014.

Newton, P., Suputtamongkol, Y., Teja-Isavadharm, P., Pukrittayakamee, S., Navaratnam, V., Bates, I., and White, N. (2000). Antimalarial bioavailability and disposition of Artesunate in acute Falciparum Malaria. *Antimicrobial Agents and Chemotherapy*, **44(4)**: 972-977.

Nontprasert, A., Pukrittayakamee, S., Dondorp, A.M., Clemens, R., Looareesuwan, S., and White, N.J. (2002). Neuropathologic toxicity of artemisinin derivatives in a mouse model. *American Society of Tropical Medicine and Hygeine*, **67(4)**: 423-9.

Nontprasert, A., Pukrittayakamee, S., Nosten-bertrand, M., Vanijanonta, S., and White, N.J. (2000). Studies of the neurotoxicity of oral artemisinin derivatives in mice. *American Society of Tropical Medicine and Hygeine*, **62(3)**: 409–412.

Nontprasert. A., Nosten-Bertrand, M., Pukrittayakamee, S., Vanijanonta, S., Angus, B.J., and White, N.J. (1998). Assessment of the neurotoxicity of parenteral artemisinin derivatives in mice. *American Society of Tropical Medicine and Hygeine*, **59(4)**: 519-22.

Nosten, F., and White, N.J. (2009). Artemisinin-based combination treatment of falciparum malaria. *The American Society of Tropical Medicine and Hygiene*, Available at: http: //www.ajtmh.org accessed on 10 feb 2014.

Nwanjo, H.U. (2007). Acute hepatotocixity following administration of artesunate in guinea pigs. *The Internet Journal of Toxicology*, **4(1)**. DOI: 10.5580/15e2.

Ogwang, P.E., Ogwal, J.O., Kasasa, S., Ejobi, F., Kabasa, D., and Obua, C. (2011). Use of *Artemisia annua* L. infusion for malaria prevention: mode of action and benefits in a Ugandan community. *British Journal of Pharmaceutical Research*, **1(4)**: 124-132.

Olumide, S.A., and Raji, Y. (2011). Long-Term administration of artesunate induces reproductive toxicity in male rats. *Journal of Reproduction and Infertility*, **12(4)**: 249-260.

Olurishe, T.O., Kwanashie, H.O., Anuka, J., Muktar, H., and Bisalla, M. (2011). Histopathological effects of sub-chronic lamivudine-artesunate co-administration on the liver of diseased adult Wistar rats. *North American Journal of Medical Sciences*, **3(7)**: 325-28.

Olurishe. T., Kwanashie, H., Anuka, J., and Muktar, H. (2012). Lamivudine-artesunate co-administration affects glucose metabolism in healthy and diseased Wistar rats. *Pakistan Journal of Pharmaceutical Sciences*, **25(3)**: 543-547.

Omotuyi I. O., Nwangwu, S.C., Okugbo, O.T., Okoye, O.T., Ojieh, G.C., and Wogu, D.M. Hepatotoxic and hemolytic effects of acute exposure of rats to artesunate overdose. *African Journal of Biochemistry Research*, **2(5)**: 107-110.

Otuechere, C.A., Edewor, G., Kale, O.E., and Ekor M. (2012). Subacute therapeutic dosing of artemether-lumefantrine and artesunate-amodiaquine combination preserves plasma cholesterol, renal antioxidant status and organ weights in rats. *Malaria Research and Treatment*, 257986. doi: 10.1155/2012/257986.

Oyakhirome, S., Potschke, M., Schwarz, N.G., Dornemann, J., Laengin, M., Salazar, C.O., Lell, B., Kun, V., Kremsner, P.G., and Grobusch, M.P. (2007). Artesunate – amodiaquine combination therapy for falciparum malaria in young Gabonese children. *Malaria Journal*, **6**: 29-33.

Perazzo, F.F., Carvalho, J.C., Carvalho, J.E., and Rehder, V.L. (2003). Central properties of the essential oil and the crude methanol extract from aerial parts of *Artemisia annua* L. *Pharmacological Resarch*, **48(5)**: 497-502.

Price, R., Vugt, M.V., Phaipun, L., Luxemburger, C., Simpson, J., McGready, R., Kuile, F.T., Kham, A., Chongsuphajaisiddhi, White, N.J., and Noaten, F. (1999). Adverse effects in patients with acute falciparum malaria treated with artemisinin derivatives. *American Journal Tropical of Medicine and Hygiene*, **60(4)**: 547–555.

Rajpal, V. (2002). Standardization of botanicals: Testing and extraction methods of medicinal herbs. 2nd vol. India: Eastern Publishers. pp. 50-66.

Rijken, M.J., McGready, R., Boel, M.E., Poespoprodjo, R., Singh, N., Syafruddin, D., Rogerson, S., and Nosten, F. (2012). Malaria in pregnancy in the Asia-Pacific region. *Lancet Infectious Diseases*, **12(1)**: 75–88.

Sanjana, K., Shyamjith, M., Deepa, B., Rao, S.N., and Pai, P.G. (2012). Effect of artesunate on maximal electroshock and pentylenetetrazole-induced seizures in albino mice. *International Journal of Green Pharmacy*, **6**: 63-6. Available from: http: / /www.greenpharmacy.info / text.asp?2012 / 6 / 1 / 63 / 97132 accessed on 12 feb 2014.

Schmuck, G., Roehrdanz, E., Haynes, R.K., and Kahl, R. (2002). Neurotoxic mode of action of artemisinin. *Antimicrobial Agents and Chemotherapy*, **46(3)**: 821-827.

Seguro, A.C., and Campos, S.B. (2002). Diuretic effect of sodium artesunate in patients with malaria. *American Journal of Tropical Medicine and Hygiene*, **67**: 473-4.

Simonnet, X. and Rasamiharimanana, S. (2010). Comparison of different drying techniques in Madagascar. Artemisinin Conference / Madagascar. Medicines for Malaria Venture, Mediplant, Geneva.

Simonnet, X., Bouwmeester, H., Cutler, M. and Logan, J. (2008). *Artemisia annua* L. Harvest and post-harvest treatments. MMV Report 2007-2008. Medicines for Malaria Venture, Mediplant, Geneva.

Sissoko, M.S., Dabo, A., Traore, H, Diallo, M., Traore, B., Konate, D., Niare, B., Diakite, M., Kamate, B., Traore, A., Bathily, A., Tapily, A., Toure, O.B., Cauwenbergh, S., Jansen, H.F., and Doumbo, O.K. (2009). Efficacy of artesunate+ sulfamethoxypyrazine / pyrimethamine versus praziquantel in the treatment of *Schistosoma haematobium* in children 4(10), ODI: e6732PLoSONE.

Taylor, W.R., and White, N.J. (2004). Antimalarial drug toxicity: A review. *Drug Safety*, **27**: 25–61.

Tripathi, K., Prajapati, V. and Aggarwal, K.K. (2000). Repellency and toxicity of oil from Artemisia annua to certain stored-product beetles. *Journal Economic Entomology*. **93(1)**: 43-7.

Veerasubramanian, P., Gosi, P., Limsomwong, C. and Walsh, D.S. (2006). Artesunate and a major metabolite, dihydroartemisinin, diminish mitogen-induced lymphocyte proliferation and activation. *Southeast Asian Journal of Tropical Medicine and Public Health*, **37(5)**: 838–847.

Wang, J.X., Tang, W., Shi, L.P., Wan, J., Zhou, R., Ni, J., Fu, Y.F., Yang, Y.F., Li, Y., and Zuo, J.P. (2007). Investigation of the immunosuppressive activity of artemether on T-cell activation and proliferation. *British Journal of Pharmacology,* **150(5):** 652-661.

White, T.E., and Clark, R.L. (2008). Sensitive periods for developmental toxicity of orally administered artesunate in the rat. *Birth Defects Research. Part B, Developmental and Reproductive Toxicology,* **83(4)**: 407-17.

White, T.E., Bushdid, P.B., Ritter, S., Laffan, S.B., and Clark, R.L. (2006). Artesunate-induced depletion of embryonic erythroblasts precedes embryo lethality and teratogenicity *in vivo. Birth Defects Research. Part B, Developmental and Reproductive Toxicology,* **77**: 413–429.

WHO Position Statement. (2012). Effectiveness of non-pharmaceutical forms of *Artemisia annua* L. against malaria. World Health Oraganization, Geneva.

WHO. (2005). Monograph on good agricultural and collection practices (GACP) for *Artemisia annua*. World Health Oraganization, Geneva.

WHO. (2006). Monograph on good agricultural and collection practices (GACP) for *Artemisia annua* L., World Health Oraganization, Geneva.

WHOPAR, part 4. (2011). Summary of product characteristics. Artesunate 60 mg for injection. Guilin Pharmaceutical Co., Ltd., MA051. Available at: http: // apps.who.int/prequal/whopar/whoparproducts/MA051part4v1.pdf accessed on 13 march 2014.

Zaki, S.A., Shanbag, P., Lad, V., and Shenoy, P. Sodium artesunate-induced diuresis in a patient with malaria. *Indian Journal of Pharmacology,* **43(4)**: 472–473.

Zheng, G.Q. (1994). Cytotoxic terpenoids and flavonoids from *Artemisia annua. Planta Medica,* **60(1)**: 54-57.

Zheng, W., and Wang, Y. (2001). Antioxidant activity and phenolic compounds in selected herbs. *Journal of Agriculture and Food Chemistry,* **49(11)**: 5165–5170.

Zhou, H.J., Wang, W.Q., and Wu, G.D. (2007). Artesunate inhibits angiogenesis and down regulates vascular endothelial growth factor expression in chronic myeloid leukaemia K562 cells. *Vascular Pharmacology,* **47(2-3)**: 131-8.

Bioactive Phytochemicals: Perspectives for Modern Medicine Vol. 3 (2015) *Pages* **121–153**
Editor: **V.K. Gupta**
Published by: **DAYA PUBLISHING HOUSE, NEW DELHI**

4

Fractionation and Structural Characterization of Antimicrobials from *Woodfordia fruticosa* Kurz. (Lythraceae) Flowers

Yogesh Baravalia[1], Pooja Moteriya[2], Priyank Patel[2] and Sumitra Chanda[2*]

ABSTRACT

Increase in appearance of multi drug resistant organism necessitates or demands for the discovery of new antimicrobials for effective treatment. As a part of continuous search and considering the challenge of discovering potent antimicrobials the present study was carried out. Woodfordia fruticosa Kurz. (Lythraceae) flowers were selected for evaluation of its antimicrobial potential. Crude methanol extract was further fractionated into sub-fractions and were evaluated for their antimicrobial potential by agar disc diffusion technique against 5 Gram positive bacteria, 5 Gram negative bacteria and 5 fungal strains. An attempt was also done for characterization of the fractions showing best antimicrobial activity. Solvent-solvent partition of methanol extract yielded Fraction I and Fraction II, further column chromatography of these fractions yielded total of 67 and 66 sub-fractions respectively. TLC evaluation of these sub-fractions resulted in 9 and 8 major fractions respectively. The crude methanol extract and its fractions showed antibacterial activity for 9 bacteria. Fraction II and its sub-fractions showed more activity against Gram positive and Gram negative bacteria as compared to crude methanol extract, Fraction I and its sub-fractions. Amongst all the 20 fractions,

1 Department of Biochemistry, Saurashtra University, Rajkot – 360 005, Gujarat, India

2 Phytochemical, Pharmacological and Microbiological Laboratory, Department of Biosciences (CAS), Saurashtra University, Rajkot – 360 005, Gujarat, India

* *Corresponding author*: E-mail: svchanda@gmail.com

Fraction II-5 showed the most significant antibacterial activity. None of the fractions or subfractions or crude methanol extract showed antifungal activity. Total 18 peaks were obtained by GCMS analysis of Fraction II-4, Fraction II-5 and Fraction II-6. Specifically, Fraction II-4 showed 3 peaks, Fraction II-5 showed 9 peaks and Fraction II-6 showed 6 peaks and their mass spectra were recorded. The mass spectra were compared with the structures available in the structure library and previous findings reported. This finding of compounds may be useful as potential bio-control agents and afford efficient and safe antimicrobials which will certainly contribute to the ongoing search for new antimicrobial agents to fight against infectious diseases caused by antibiotic resistant strains.

Keywords: *Woodfordia fruticosa*, Solvent-Solvent Partition, Antibacterial activity, Column chromatography, GCMS analyses.

Introduction

Nature has always been a giant source of plants having medicinal values for hundreds of years. Plants are used medicinally in different countries and are a source of many potent and powerful drugs. Although chemical drugs are popular, however, herbal medicine is continued to be practiced due to richness of certain plants in varieties of secondary metabolites. A great number of modern drugs and its raw materials have been obtained from natural sources and will play a pivotal role in future. The use of plants by man to treat common ailments is time immemorial and many of the traditional medicines are still included as part of the habitual treatment of various maladies. Medicinal plants represent a rich source of antimicrobial agents; they are gifts of nature to cure limitless number of diseases among human beings. Plants generally produce many secondary metabolites which constitute an important source of microbicides, pesticides and many pharmaceutical drugs.

Plant derived natural products such as flavonoids, terpenes and alkaloids (Shukla *et al.*, 2010) have received considerable attention due to their diverse pharmacological properties including inflammatory, antipyretic and analgesic activities. Consumption of natural products reduces the risk of developing pathological conditions, including cancer, nervous system disorders, cardiovascular, genetic, epileptic, anti ulcer, inflammatory diseases, etc (Jurenka, 2009; Adediwura *et al.*, 2014; Hyuck-Ju *et al.*, 2014; Lily *et al.*, 2014; Makasana *et al.*, 2014). Plants contain numerous bioactive molecules that can improve the body's resistance to cellular stress and prevent the cytotoxicity of various agents since they are rich in antioxidant compounds (Hegazy and Ibrahium, 2012; Kaneria and Chanda, 2013; Chanda *et al.*, 2013; Kchaoua *et al.*, 2013; Ramirez *et al.*, 2014).

Natural products and their derivatives have traditionally been the most common sources of drugs, and still represent a fairly large percentage of the pharmaceutical market (Kirkpatrick, 2002). It has long been recognised that natural product structures have the characteristics of high chemical diversity, biochemical specificity and other molecular properties that make them favourable as lead structures for drug discovery (Okoye and Osadebe, 2010). According to World Health Organisation, infectious diseases are the major reason for the death worldwide with more than half of the death appearing in developing countries and estimated that 80 per cent of the population still relies on traditional medicines totally or partially, mostly plant based drugs for their primary healthcare needs. In these countries, treatment of infectious diseases is complicated due to occurrence of resistant microorganisms to commonly used antimicrobials and low income of the population (WHO, 2007; Kaur and Arora, 2009). The frequency of life-threatening infections caused by pathogenic microorganisms has increased worldwide and is becoming a main cause of morbidity and mortality in patients especially of backward countries (Li *et al.*, 2008a; Khan *et al.*, 2008a).

Development of Antimicrobials

Since antiquity mankind is searching for ways to deal with infectious diseases and disease causing microorganisms. The origin of anti-infective chemotherapy can probably be traced to about 3000 BC, when it is evident that early Chinese civilizations recognized the therapeutic properties of teas and herbs.

Antibiotics are low molecular weight natural substances or synthetic compounds with selective bactericidal and bacteriostatic effects that eliminate pathogens or slowdown their growth such that the host defence mechanisms can clear the infection. Antibiotics are classified mechanistically according to their site of action in the bacterial cell. Antibiotics are also classified on the basis of broad spectrum and narrow spectrum activity. Sometimes it is also put under limited spectrum where it is active only against specific organisms. Antimicrobial agents can be totally from biological entity (Antibiotics), partially from biological entity (Semi-synthetic antibiotics) or totally synthetic antibiotics (Chemotherapeutic agents).

Importance of Medicinal Plants in Discovery of New Drugs

Many medicinal plants have been used since long to treat various diseases and infections in traditional medicinal systems. Ayurveda and Siddha are the well known and the most ancient healthcare systems and are practiced widely all over the world (Shekhawat and Prasasd, 1971; Khanna and Chandra, 1972). Other classics that describe description of over thousands of herbs are Atharveda (around 1200 BC), Charak Samhita and Sushrut Samhita (100-150 BC) (Dash and Sharma, 2001; Chopra and Doiphode, 2002). Numerous studies have been reported with the extracts of various plants, screening antimicrobial activity as well as for the discovery of new antimicrobial compounds. The efficacy of the plants in curing various diseases and infections is well established and a large volume of work has been done in this field by the researchers all over the world (Muthuvelan and Raja, 2008; Li *et al.*, 2008a; Sharma and Patel, 2009; Bouzada *et al.*, 2009; Chanda and Baravalia, 2010; Vaghasiya and Chanda, 2010; Chanda *et al.*, 2012; Kaushik *et al.*, 2014). Antibacterial, antioxidant activities of *Melastoma malabathricum* leaves was reported by Alwash *et al.* (2014). *In vitro* antibacterial activity of *Emblica officinalis* and *Tamarindus indica* seed was reported by Ramanuj *et al.* (2014). Rakholiya *et al.* (2014a) reported mango pulp as a potential source of natural antimicrobial agent. In recent history, the use of plants as medicines has included the isolation of active compounds. Medicinal plant based drug discovery led to some key drugs such as digitoxin, cocaine, vinblastine, vincristine, silymarin, morphine, atropine, etc. (Butler, 2004; Van Der Heijden *et al.*, 2004).

Medicinal Plants as a Source of Antimicrobials

The increase in the occurrence of multiple drug resistance has opened up horizons for the search for new antimicrobials from alternative sources. Nature has blessed on us with a very rich botanical wealth and a great number of diverse types of plants that grow wild in different parts of the world. Herbs and spices with antibacterial activity have been widely used both traditionally and commercially (Chandarana *et al.*, 2005). The use of herbs as complementary and alternative medicine has increased dramatically in the last few years. It has been reported that natural compounds and their derivatives, analogues and intermediates represents over half of all drugs being used, with over 14-28 per cent of the total by higher plant derived substances (Ncube *et al.*, 2008). It is estimated that there are 2.5 to 5.0 lack species of plants on Earth, only 1 to 10 per cent of these are used as food by both humans and other animal species, leaving a huge potential for medicinal plant product development (Heinrich and Gibbons, 2001). The screening of plant extracts and plant products for antimicrobial activity has shown that plants represent a potential source of antimicrobials (Arora *et al.*, 2009; Chanda and Baravalia, 2010).

Any part of the plant may be a potential source of antimicrobics. All plant parts like seed, leaf, stem, bark, flower, peel, fruit rind, aerial parts, etc. are known to possess medicinal properties and can be a natural source of antimicrobics. For example, antibacterial and antiinflammatory activity of *Woodfordia fruticosa* flowers (Parekh and Chanda (2007a; Baravalia *et al.*, 2012), Antibacterial and antioxidant activities of *Schotia latifolia* stem bark (Oyedemi and Afolayan, 2011), anti ulcer and antibacterial activity of *Polyalthia longifolia* leaves (Chanda *et al.*, 2011), antimicrobial activity of *Mesua ferra* seed (Chanda *et al.*, 2013), antimicrobial activity of tamarind pulp (Das and Banerjee, 2014), antibacterial activity of fruit of date palm (Saleh and Otaibi, 2014), antimicrobial activity of *Morinda lucida* stem bark, leaf and root (Fakoya *et al.*, 2014), antibacterial activity of *Primula vulgaries* leaves and root Majid *et al.* (2014), antimicrobial activity of *Terminalia bellerica* leaf and stem (Chanda *et al.*, 2014), antibacterial activity of fruit and vegetable peels (Rakholiya *et al.*, 2014b), antibacterial activity of different parts of *Lagenaria siceraria* (Menpara *et al.*, 2014), etc.

Traditionally, people use crude extracts of plant parts as curative agents (Sanches *et al.*, 2005). The development of pharmaceuticals begins with isolation and identification of active constituents, detailed biological assays and dosage formulations, followed by clinical trials to establish safety, efficacy and pharmacokinetic profile of the new drug (Iwu *et al.*, 1999). Drug discovery from medicinal plants requires the pharmacognosists, phytochemists and other natural product scientists to continuously improve in the quality and quantity of compounds that can clear the drug development phase/trials (Butler, 2004). Bioassay-guided fractionation offers special advantages for identification of medicinal plant extracts. Most often, a desired biological response is not due to one component but rather due to a mixture of bioactive plant components. Therefore, crude extracts must be screened for biological activity and then any active extract should be fractionated with bioassays to exploit the bioactive compounds (Chanda and Baravalia, 2011). The search for bioactive constituents is one of the central subjects of industrial and academic natural products chemistry.

In some cases the isolated compound may not be potent enough to be drugs alone, but they can serve as pharmacophores (raw materials for pharmaceutical product), which often led to the potent and clinically useful drugs (Kingston *et al.*, 2000). The discovery of new antibiotics is now a matter of necessity and it is likely that future research will be preliminary concerned with the discovery of novel agents active against previously untapped bacterial targets (Chopra *et al.*, 1997). With the availability of several bacterial genome sequences, we are now in a good position to discover new antibiotics directed against novel targets (Moir *et al.*, 1999). In ethnopharmacology research the antimicrobial susceptibility test is used to determine the efficacy of potential antimicrobials from biological extracts against a number of microbial strains. In clinical research *in vitro* susceptibility tests are particularly important if an organism is suspected to belong to a strain that has shown resistance to frequently used antimicrobial agents.

The present study involves the fractionization and separation of crude methanol extract of *Woodfordia fruticosa* Kurz. flowers to its sub-fractions and evaluation of its antimicrobial potential.

Plant Description (Anjaria *et al.*, 2002)

Woodfordia fruticosa (Linn.) Kurz.

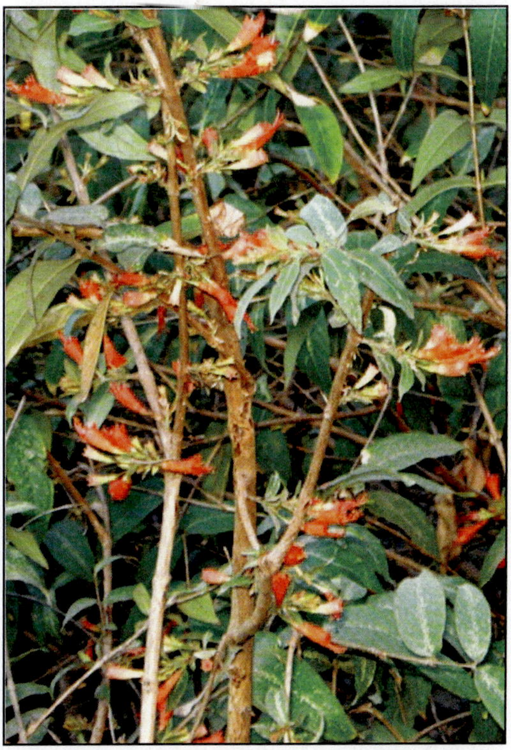

Family

Lythraceae

Habit

Deciduous leafy shrub; bark smooth, fissured.

Leaves

1.5 – 13 × 0.8 – 4 cm, sub-opposite, decussate, sometimes in whorls of 3, sessile.

Inflorescence

1.5 – 2.8 cm long, deep-red, axillary or extra axillary, 2 – 15 flowered, fascicled cymes.

Flower

Numerous, deep-red.

Calyx

1.5 cm long, sepals 6, gamosepalous, triangular acute.

Corolla

Petals 6

Androecium

Stamens 12, polyandrous, longitudinally.

Gynoecium

Bicarpellary; ovary sessile, stigma punctiform.

Fruit

Capsule 0.5 – 0.6 cm long, oblong.

Seeds

Minute, pale-brown, smooth, narrowly obconical-trigonous, base cuneate.

Distribution

Throughout India, but more abundant in North India upto 1600 m.

Vernacular Name

Dhavdi (Gujarati)

Parts Used

Flowers

Constituents

Tannin, sugar and naturally acquired Yeast microflora.

Action Uses

The flowers are astringent, acrid, refrigerant, stimulant, depurative, styptic, uterine sedative, anthelmintic, constipating, antibacterial, vulnerary, corrective of urinary pigments, alexeteric and febrifuge.

They are useful in vitiated conditions of kapha and pitta, leprosy, skin disease, burning sensations, haemorrhages, menorrhoea, diabetes, bilious fever, hepatopathy and verminosis. They are an important ingredient in *Aristam* and *Asavam* as they aid in fermentation; they are also highly valued as a stimulant in pregnancy.

Reported Activities

Woodfordia fruticosa Kurz is a much used medicinal plant in Ayurvedic and Unani system of medicines. The flowers are used in the preparation of Ayurvedic fermented drugs called "Aristhas" and "Asavas" (Sekar and Mariappan, 2008). It is also one of the ingredients of a preparation used to increase fertility of women (Dey, 1984). Antifertility activity was investigated by Khushalani *et al.* (2006).

Shome *et al.* (1981) investigated pharmacognosy of the flowers of *Woodfordia fruticosa*. Chapter described detail anatomy of the pedicel and various floral appendages, pollen ornamentation, seed with unusual mucilage hairs and embryo characters. Histochemical tests and fluorescence characteristics are also described. Other parameters include physicochemical constants, *e.g.* ash values, percentages of tannins, sugars and different extractive yields.

Antimicrobial activities of different parts of *Woodfordia fruticosa* were reported by Dabur *et al.* (2007); Parekh and Chanda (2007a); Bajracharya *et al.* (2008); Kaur and Kaur (2010). Kumaraswamy and Satish (2008) reported antioxidant activity of *Woodfordia fruticosa* flowers. Yoshida *et al.* (1990) and Kuramochi-Motegi *et al.* (1992) reported antitumor activity of isolated compound from *Woodfordia fruticosa* flowers. Kroes *et al.* (1993) reported immunomodularoty effect of fermented product from *Woodfordia fruticosa* flowers. Chandan *et al.* (2008) and Brindha and Geetha (2009) investigated hepatoprotective effect of *Woodfordia fruticosa* flowers against hepatic injury. Similarly, Shah and Juvenkar (2010) investigated immuno stimulatory effects. Baravalia and Chanda (2011) and Baravalia *et al.* (2011) reported hepatoprotective effect of *Woodfordia fruticosa* flowers against acetaminophen and diclofenac sodium induced hepatic toxicity in rats.

Materials and Methods

Collection and Identification of Plant Material

The fresh flowers of *W. fruticosa* were collected from Junagadh (Girnar region), Gujarat. The plant was compared with Voucher Specimen (No. PSN303) deposited at Department of Biosciences, Saurashtra University, Rajkot, Gujarat, India.

Extract Preparation

The flowers were washed under tap water, air dried, homogenized to fine powder and stored in air tight bottles. Ten grams of dried powder was first defatted with petroleum ether and then extracted with methanol by using Soxhlet apparatus (Lin *et al.*, 1999; Chanda and Parekh, 2010). The solvent was evaporated to dryness and the dried crude extract was stored in air tight bottle at 4°C in a refrigerator. The methanol extract of *W. fruticosa* was used for the entire study.

Separation and Isolation

Solvent-Solvent Partition (Tang *et al.*, 2010)

Five grams of crude methanolic extract of *W. fruticosa* was dissolved in hot methanol (200 ml). Slight precipitation was obtained and discarded as methanol insoluble matter. The methanol soluble fraction was filtered and collected. It was concentrated to about 50 ml volume and ethyl acetate was added till faint turbidity was obtained. Then it was kept in a refrigerator to settle down. The settled gelatinous reddish mass and supernatant was separated and collected separately. The supernatant was further concentrated and ethyl acetate step was repeated till reddish gelatinous mass obtained. All the settled mass was collected together and dissolved in methanol. It was concentrated further to dryness and designated as Fraction I. The collected supernatant was concentrated further to near dryness and then dissolved in methanol. Then chloroform was added and cooled. Light yellow waxy sediment was separated and light buff coloured supernatant was collected. This supernatant was concentrated further to dryness and designated as Fraction II.

Column Chromatography and Thin Layer Chromatography (Tang *et al.*, 2010)

Column chromatography is used as a purification technique, helps in the isolation of constituents from the mixture. Thin layer chromatography is used to determine the presence of mixture of constituents. In present study both techniques were used. 4.5 g of Fraction I and 3.0 g of Fraction II were coated onto silica gel (240-400 mesh) and chromatographed on a glass column packed with silica gel (240-400 mesh) (22 cm length). Columns were continuously eluted with hexane, hexane : ethyl acetate, hexane : ethyl acetate: methanol and ethyl acetate: methanol, gradients. The columns were finally eluted with methanol. All different fractions (each 10 ml) were collected and evaluated on TLC plate and based on their TLC profile, were combined to major fractions. After drying fractions were collected in air tight bottles and stored in a refrigerator.

Antimicrobial Susceptibility Test

Test Microorganisms

The microbial strains used are identified strains from National Chemical Laboratory, Pune, India. Five Gram positive bacteria (*Staphylococcus aureus* ATCC25923, *Staphylococcus epidermidis* ATCC12228, *Micrococcus flavus* ATCC10240, *Bacillus megaterium* ATCC9885, *Bacillus cereus* ATCC11778), five Gram negative bacteria (*Klebsiella pneumonia* NCIM2719, *Klebsiella aerogenes* NCIM2098, *Proteus vulgaris* NCIM2857, *Proteus morgani* NCIM2040, *Pseudomonas aeruginosa* ATCC27853) and five fungi (*Cryptococcus neoformans* NCIM3542, *Candida glabrata* NCIM3448, *Candida epicola* NCIM3367, *Candida albicans* NCIM3102, *Trichosporon beigelii* NCIM3404) were studied.

Preparation of Test Drug

Crude methanolic extract, Fraction I, Fraction II and all major fractions of *W. fruticosa* were dissolved in 100 per cent DMSO (dimethylsulfoxide) at a concentration of 20 mg/ml and 40 mg/ml. These were used as working stock.

Preparation of Inoculums

For antimicrobial assay active cultures were prepared by transferring a loopful of culture from stock slant to flasks of Muller Hinton Broth (MHB) for bacteria and Sabouraud Dextrose Broth (SDB) for fungi and were incubated at 37°C and 28°C for 24 hours respectively.

Antimicrobial Activity

Antimicrobial activity of the isolated fractions were assessed against 5 Gram positive bacteria, 5 Gram negative bacteria and 5 fungal strains using agar disc diffusion method (Bauer *et al.*, 1966; Nair and Chanda, 2007). Petriplates were prepared by pouring 200 ml of sterilized molten Muller Hinton Agar (MHA) in 200 mm × 20 mm sized plates seeded with 1 ml of test culture. Plates were allowed to solidify. Sterile filter paper discs (HiMedia Sterile disc, 6 mm) were impregnated with 20 µl of each fraction (400 µg/disc and 800 µg/disc) and allowed to saturate for 30 min. Then they were placed on the surface of the solidified agar; which had previously been inoculated with tested microorganisms. All plates were incubated at 37°C and 28°C for bacteria and fungi respectively for 24 hours. Results were recorded by measuring the zone of inhibition appearing around the discs. All the tests were performed in triplicate and the mean values are presented with standard error of mean values. 100 per cent DMSO was used as a control.

Gas Chromatography Mass Spectroscopy (GCMS)

GCMS analyses of active fractions (Fraction II-4, Fraction II-5 and Fraction II-6) were performed in a GCMS-QP-2010 equipped with glass column SGE BPX5 and capillary dimensions 30 m × 0.25 mm × 0.25 µ. The oven temperature was programmed from 80-260°C respectively. Carrier gas was He (Helium) at a flow of 1.0 ml/min. Ion source temperatures were maintained at 200°C and spectra were measured.

Results and Discussion

Extraction of plant materials used pharmaceutically involves the separation of active metabolites from plant tissues by using selective solvents with appropriate extraction technique. The quality of an extracts are mainly influenced by i) Plant part used, ii) Solvent used for extraction and iii) Extraction technique used, etc (Ncube *et al.,* 2008).

Extractive Yield

There are several reports that water, acetone, ethanol, methanol, dichloromethane, ethyl acetate, petroleum ether, hexane are used as solvents for the extraction, and these extracts showed antimicrobial activity (Hazra *et al.,* 2007; Lawrence *et al.,* 2009; Vaghasiya and Chanda, 2010). However, the most commonly used solvents for investigating antimicrobial activity in plants are methanol, ethanol and water (Parekh *et al.,* 2005; Rojas *et al.,* 2006). It is reported that methanol act as a better solvent for the consistent extraction of antimicrobial substances from medicinal plants as compared to other polar and non-polar solvents (Sengul *et al.,* 2005; Kaneria *et al.,* 2009; Kuete *et al.,* 2011). Hence, in the present study, methanol was used as a solvent for extraction. The extractive yield of *Woodfordia fruticosa* flowers in methanol using Soxhlet apparatus technique was 36 per cent.

Crude methanol extract of *Woodfordia fruticosa* flowers have been reported for antimicrobial activity against a range of human pathogenic bacteria as well as against standard bacterial strains (Parekh and Chanda, 2007a; Kumaraswamy *et al.,* 2008), However, fractionation and isolation of active constituents can be more effective even in smaller quantities. Bisignano *et al.* (2000) studied antimicrobial activity of methanol extract of *Mitracarpus scaber,* further methanol extract was partitioned between water and ç-Butanol and evaluated for antibacterial and antifungal activities and found 10 times higher activity of fractioned compound than crude methanol extract.

Isolation of active constituents (fractions) depends on composition of the crude extract extracted in a particular organic solvent. The strategy used to separate and identify plant constituents containing antimicrobial activity was to fractionate it using different techniques.

Solvent-Solvent Partition

In order to fractionate and isolate, crude methanol extract was first partitioned using solvent-solvent partition technique into the Fraction I and Fraction II. Fresh or dried plant material can be used as a source of secondary plant components. However, most scientists have tended to use dried plant material, because differences in water content may affect solubility of subsequent separation by liquid-liquid extraction and the secondary metabolites stability, especially if it is used as an antimicrobial agent (Cork and Krochenberger, 1991; Baris *et al.*, 2006).

Column Chromatography and Thin Layer Chromatography

Fraction I and Fraction II were further separated to its sub-fractions using silica gel column chromatography technique. To determine the presence of mixture of constituents, thin layer chromatography technique was used.

Fraction I

Fraction I (4.5 g) was coated onto silica gel (240-400 mesh) and chromatographed on a silica gel (240-400 mesh) column (22 cm length); eluted continuously with hexane, hexane : ethyl acetate, hexane : ethyl acetate : methanol and ethyl acetate : methanol, gradients. The column was finally eluted with methanol. A total of 67 fractions (each 10 ml) were collected. The eluted fractions were evaluated by TLC and combined to 9 major fractions (Fraction I-1 - Fraction I-9) based on similar TLC profile. They were screened for antibacterial and antifungal activity using disc diffusion method.

These major fractions after drying were collected in air tight bottles and stored at 4°C in a refrigerator. Fraction I-1 to Fraction I-4 did not dry completely, possibly due to presence of oil content.

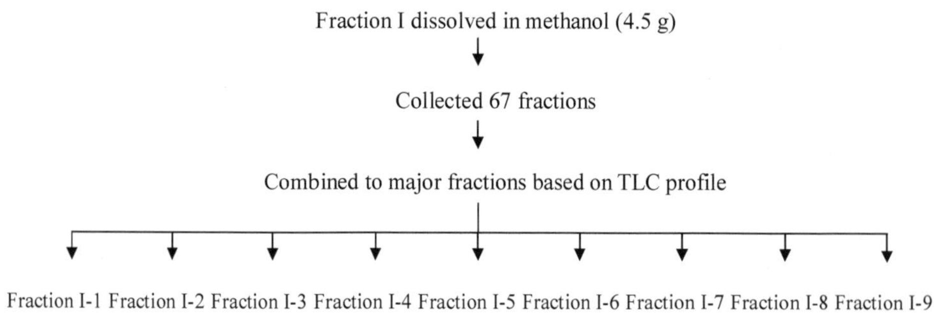

Table 4.1: Dry Weight of Isolated Major Fractions from Fraction I

Plant	*Extract*	*Silica Used*	*Solvents Used*	*Major Fractions Obtained*	*Dry Weight of Fractions (mg)*
Woodfordia fruticosa Kurz. Flower	Fraction I (4.5 g)	240-400 mesh	Hexane, Ethyl acetate, Methanol	Fraction I-1	162
				Fraction I-2	195
				Fraction I-3	273
				Fraction I-4	178
				Fraction I-5	410
				Fraction I-6	360
				Fraction I-7	202
				Fraction I-8	223
				Fraction I-9	303

Fraction I-5 showed transparent crystals but failed to show antimicrobial activity.

Fraction II

Fraction II (3.0 g) was coated onto silica gel (240-400 mesh) and chromatographed on a silica gel (240-400 mesh) column (22 cm length); eluted continuously with hexane : ethyl acetate, hexane : ethyl acetate : methanol and ethyl acetate : methanol, gradients. The column was finally eluted with methanol. A total of 66 fractions (each 10 ml) were collected. The eluted fractions were evaluated by TLC and combined to 8 major fractions (Fraction II-1 – Fraction II-8) based on similar TLC profile. They were screened for antibacterial and antifungal activity using disc diffusion method.

These major fractions after drying were collected in air tight bottles and stored at 4°C in a refrigerator.

Fraction II dissolved in methanol (3.0 g)

↓

Collected 66 fractions

↓

Combined to major fractions based on TLC profile

↓

Fraction II-1 Fraction II-2 Fraction II-3 Fraction II-4 Fraction II-5 Fraction II-6 Fraction II-7 Fraction II-8

Table 4.2: Dry Weight of Isolated Major Fractions from Fraction II

Plant	*Extract*	*Silica Used*	*Solvents Used*	*Major Fractions Obtained*	*Dry Weight of Fractions (mg)*
Woodfordia fruticosa Kurz. Flower	Fraction II (3.0 g)	240-400 mesh	Hexane, Ethyl acetate, Methanol	Fraction II-1	37
				Fraction II-2	414
				Fraction II-3	300
				Fraction II-4	414
				Fraction II-5	486
				Fraction II-6	1000
				Fraction II-7	115
				Fraction II-8	192

In a similar study conducted by Lee *et al.* (2008), $CHCl_3$-MeOH step gradient systems with increasing polarity; from 2 per cent to 7 per cent, 10 per cent and 15 per cent MeOH was used to elute the different fractions of EtOH extract. The author had reported eluting nine fractions in their study.

Further, the fractionation of ethanol fraction of *Cryptomeria japonica* reported by Li *et al.* (2008b) yielded 16 sub-fractions, which is comparatively higher than in the present study. The variation in the number of fractions in the present study could be due to the type of extract, solvent system and the technique adopted.

Antimicrobial Activity

All the 20 fractions *i.e.* crude methanol extract, Fraction I, Fraction II, Fraction I-1 to Fraction I-9 and Fraction II-1 to Fraction II-8 were screened against five Gram positive bacteria, five Gram negative bacteria and five fungal strains by disc diffusion method. For antimicrobial activity assessment; two concentrations of all fractions were used (*i.e.* 400 µg/disc and 800 µg/disc).

Crude methanol extract, Fraction I, Fraction II, Fraction II-2, Fraction II-4, Fraction II-5, Fraction II-6, Fraction II-7 and Fraction II-8 showed activity for 7 bacteria at both the concentrations tested. Fraction I-7, Fraction I-8 and Fraction I-9 showed activity for 5 bacteria at both the concentrations tested and 2 bacteria at higher concentration. None of the fractions or crude methanol extract showed activity against any of the fungal strains used.

Antimicrobial Activity against Gram Positive Bacteria

Antimicrobial activity of *W. fruticosa* fractions against *Staphylococcus aureus* and *Staphylococcus epidermidis* is shown in Figure 4.1. Fraction I showed positive activity against *S. aureus* and *S. epidermidis*. None of the sub-fractions of Fraction I showed activity against both the organism at either concentration; except Fraction I-7, Fraction I-8 and Fraction I-9. These three fractions showed activity but only at higher concentration. Crude methanol extract inhibited the growth of *S. aureus* and *S. epidermidis*. Fraction II and its sub-fractions showed higher activity as compared to crude methanol extract. Fraction II-3 did not show activity at both the concentrations.

Antimicrobial activity of *W. fruticosa* fractions against *M. flavus, B. megaterium* and *B. cereus* is shown in Figure 4.2. Fraction I, Fraction I-7, Fraction I-8 and Fraction I-9 inhibited *M. flavus* and *B. megaterium* at both the concentrations tested; Fraction I-6 inhibited the growth only at higher concentration. Fraction II showed more activity than crude methanol extract. Amongst all the sub-fractions of Fraction II; Fraction II-5 showed highest activity against *M. flavus* followed by Fraction II-4, Fraction II-7, Fraction II-6, Fraction II-8 and Fraction II-2 respectively. Fraction I, and none of its sub-fractions showed antibacterial activity against *B. cereus*, except Fraction I-2. Crude methanol extract and Fraction II and many of its sub-fractions did not show activity against *B. cereus*.

Amongst 20 fractions tested on five Gram positive bacteria; only Fraction I, Fraction I-7 to Fraction I-9, crude methanol extract, Fraction II, Fraction II-2, Fraction II-4 to Fraction II-8 showed antibacterial activity against 3 Gram positive bacteria *viz. S. aureus, S. epidermidis* and *M. flavus*. The Gram positive bacterium *B. megaterium* was not inhibited by Fraction II-1, Fraction II-3, Fraction II-5 to Fraction II-7. *B. cereus* on the other hand resistant to crude methanol extract, Fraction I, Fraction II and their sub-fractions *i.e.* it did not show any activity. The most susceptible bacterium was *M. flavus* followed by *S. epidermidis* and *S. aureus* respectively and the least susceptible bacterium was *B. cereus*. Contrasting to these findings, Vaghasiya and Chanda (2007) reported antimicrobial activity of methanol extracts of several plants against *B. cereus*. Nair and Chanda (2008) reported that methanol extract of *P. betel* showed maximum activity against *S. aureus* and *B. cereus*. Sarac and Ugar (2007) reported that *S. epidermidis* was most susceptible amongst Gram positive bacteria. Vaghasiya and Chanda (2010) reported that *M. flavus* was most susceptible to *Mangifera indica* methanol extract followed by *B. cereus, S. epidermidis* and *S. aureus* respectively which is supportive to the present findings. It is reported that Gram positive bacteria are

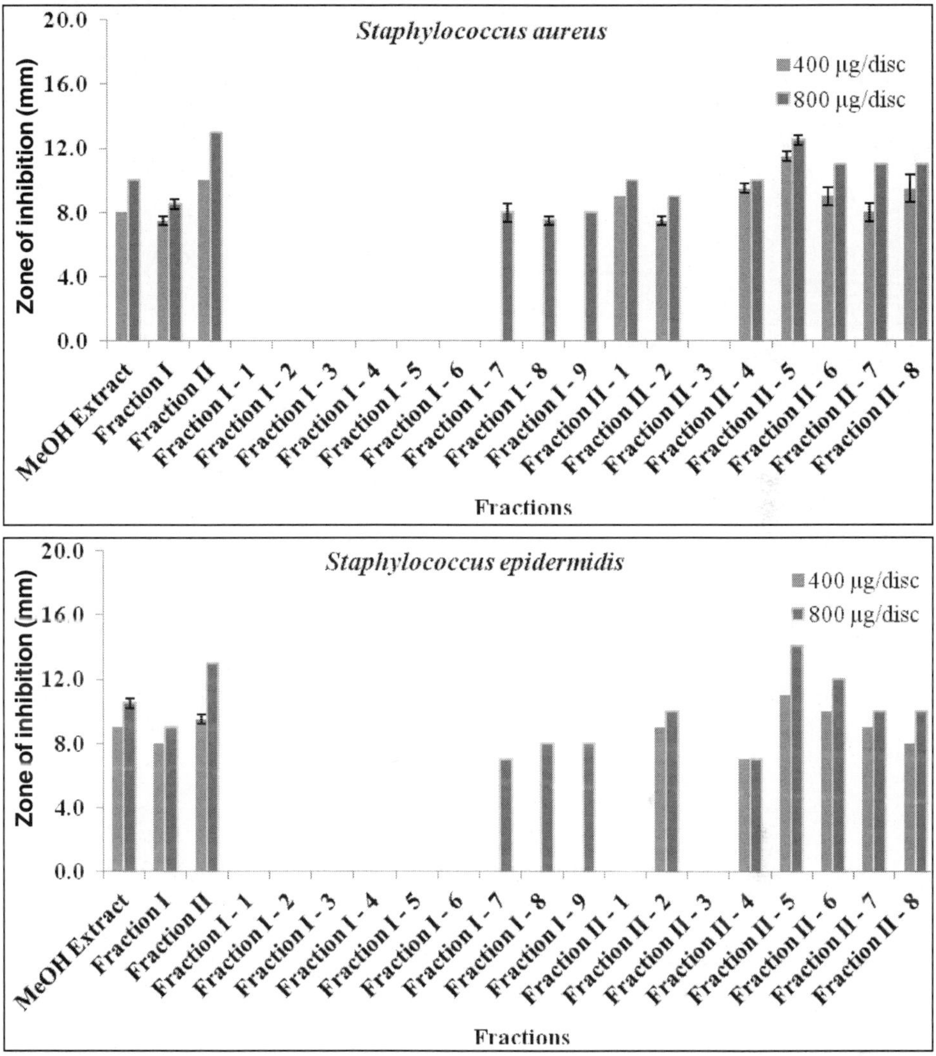

Figure 4.1: Antimicrobial Activity of *Woodfordia fruticosa* Fractions against *S. aureus* and *S. epidermidis.*

more susceptible to plant extracts than Gram negative bacteria this might be ascribed to the differences in their morphology.

Antimicrobial Activity against Gram Negative Bacteria

Antimicrobial activity of *W. fruticosa* fractions against *K. pneumoniae* and *K. aerogenes* is shown in Figure 4.3. Crude methanol extract, Fraction I, I-3, I-7 and I-9 showed activity against *K. pneumoniae* at both the concentrations. Fraction II with all its sub-fractions showed activity against *K. pneumoniae*, except Fraction II-3. Highest activity was shown by Fraction II-5. Activity against *K. pneumoniae* was found to be concentration dependent. Fraction I and its sub-fractions: Fraction I-7 and Fraction

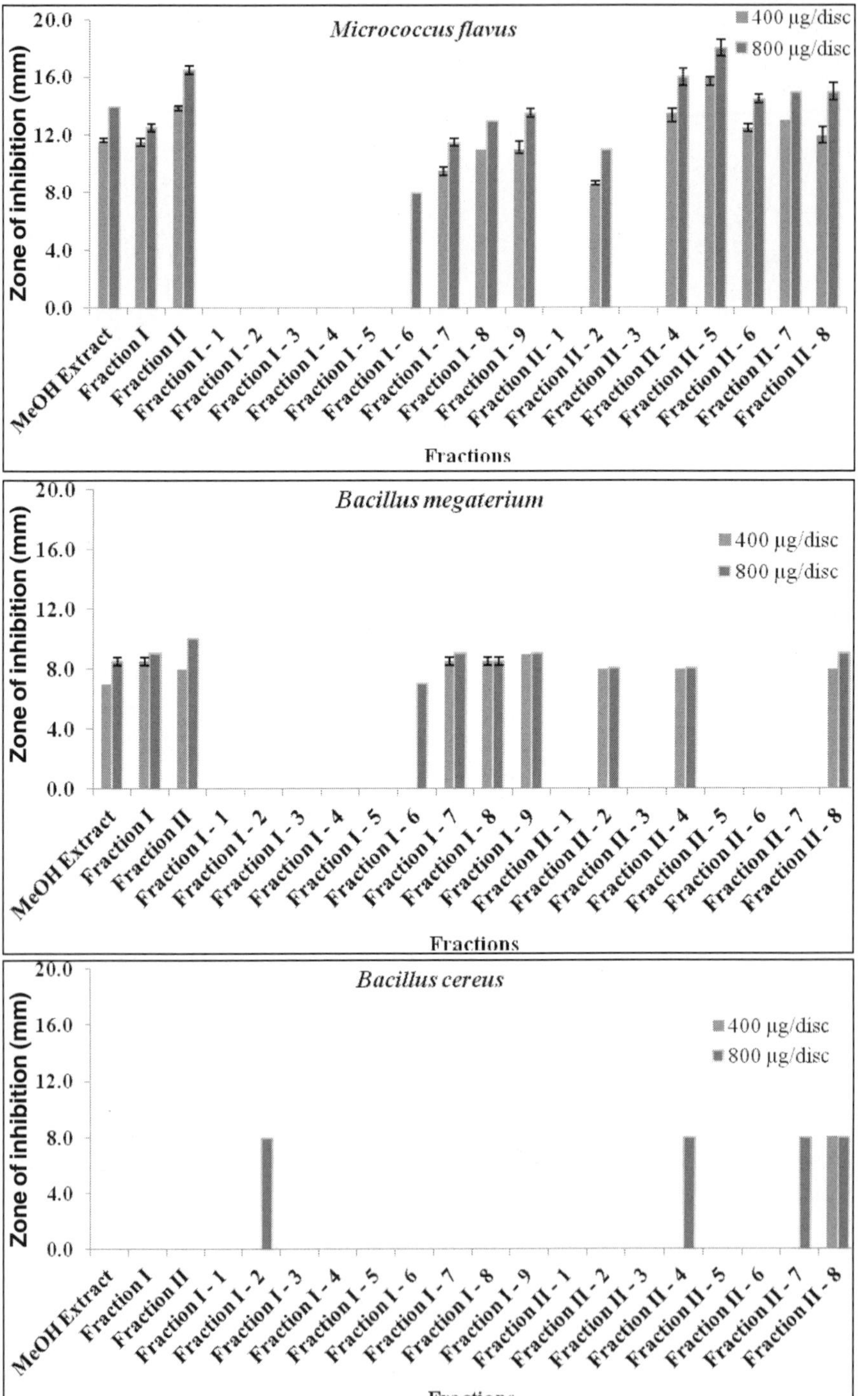

Figure 4.2: Antimicrobial Activity of *Woodfordia fruticosa* Fractions against *M. flavus, B. megaterium* and *B. cereus.*

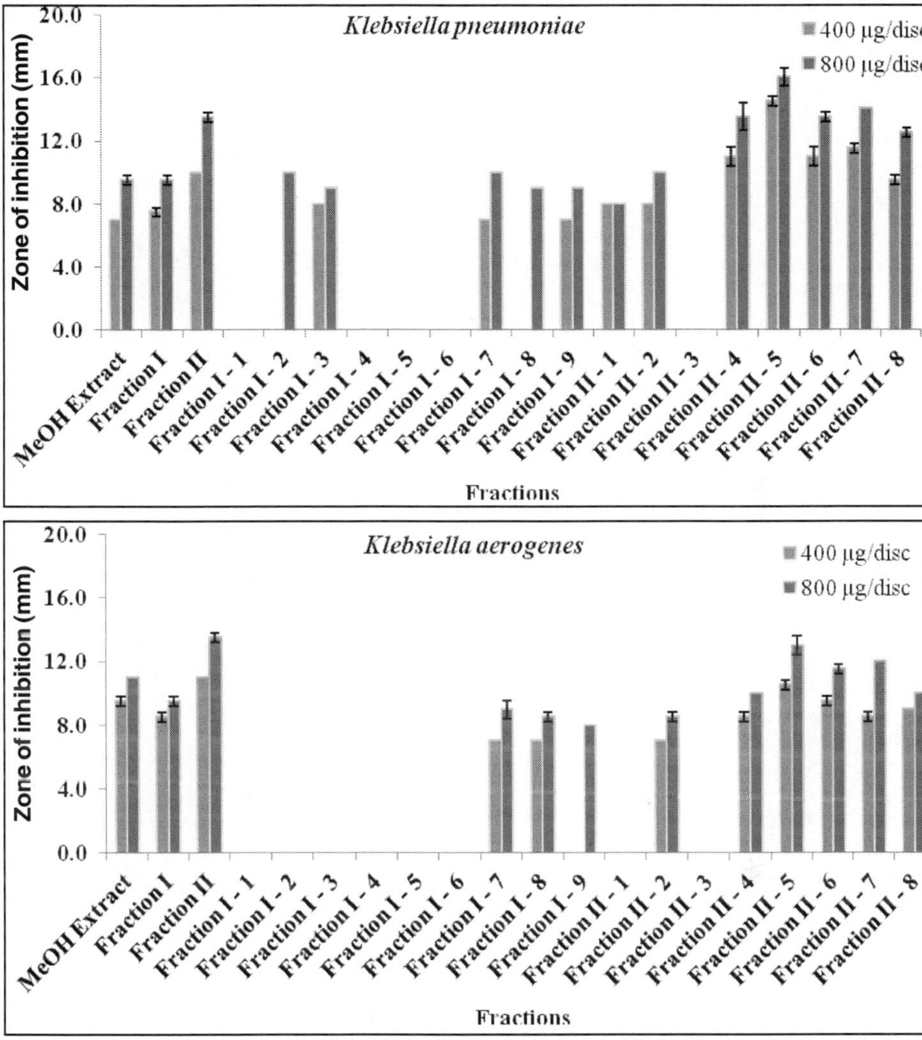

Figure 4.3: Antimicrobial Activity of *Woodfordia fruticosa* Fractions against *K. pneumoniae* and *K. aerogenes.*

I-8 at both the concentrations and Fraction I-9 only at higher concentration showed activity against *K. aerogenes*. Highest activity was shown by Fraction II and II-5.

Antimicrobial activity of *W. fruticosa* fractions against *P. vulgaris* and *P. morgani* is shown in Figure 4.4. Fraction I and its sub-fractions: Fraction I-7, Fraction I-8, Fraction I-9 showed activity against *P. vulgaris* and *P. morgani* at both the concentrations. Remaining sub-fractions did not show any activity. Crude methanol extract, Fraction II and its sub-fractions showed activity except fraction II-1 and II-3 against both organisms.

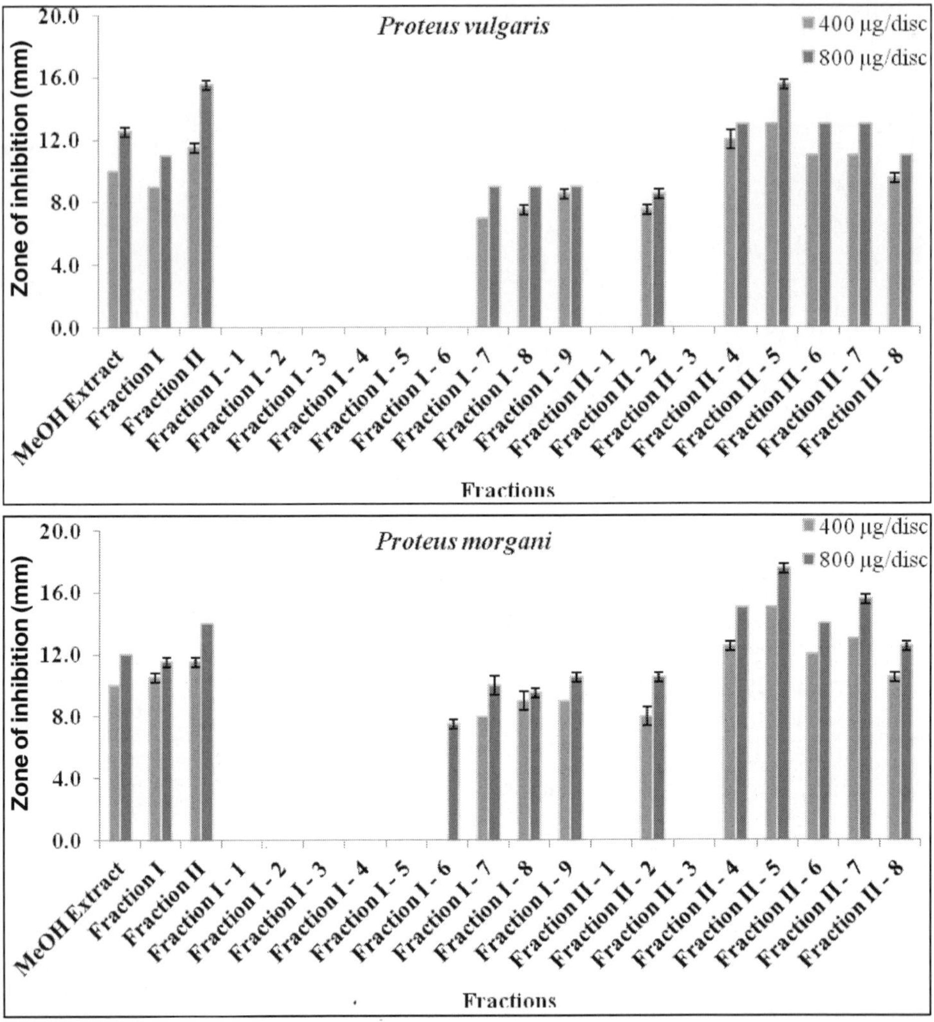

Figure 4.4: Antimicrobial Activity of *Woodfordia fruticosa* Fractions against *P. vulgaris* and *P. morgani*

Amongst 20 fractions tested on five Gram negative bacteria; only Fraction I, I-7, I-8, I-9, crude methanol extract, Fraction II, II-2, II-4, II-5, II-6, II-7 and II-8 showed antibacterial activity against 4 Gram negative bacteria *viz. K. pneumoniae, K. aerogenes, P. vulgaris* and *P. morgani*. Additionally Fraction II-1 and Fraction II-3 did not show any activity against Gram negative bacteria. The most susceptible bacterium was *P. morgani* followed by *K. pneumoniae, P. vulgaris and K. aerogenes* respectively. Amongst 20 fractions tested none of the fractions showed activity against *P. aeruginosa*. Similar results were reported by Vaghasiya and Chanda (2007) and Boussaada *et al.* (2008).

It is popular belief that Gram negative bacteria are more resistant to herbal extracts (Prashanth kumar *et al.*, 2006; Khan *et al.*, 2008b; Marin-Loiza *et al.*, 2008), but few researchers also reported that Gram negative bacteria were inhibited more by plant extracts than that of Gram positive bacteria (Delaquis, 2002; Chanda *et al.*, 2010; Djeussi *et al.*, 2013, Menpara *et al.*, 2014). In the present study, maximum activity was seen against Gram negative bacteria.

In the present study, amongst 20 fractions tested on five fungal strains *viz. Cryptococcus neoformans, Candida glabrata, Candida epicola, Candida albicans* and *Trichosporon beigelli*; none of the fractions showed activity. Martinez *et al.* (1996) reported that 23 extracts of 12 Cuban plants, used in traditional medicine failed to inhibit growth of yeast. Karaalp *et al.* (2009) reported that flower head extract of *Achillea* species showed selected activity against the tested bacterial isolates, but did not show activity against *C. albicans*. Parekh and Chanda (2006) reported *Cyperus rotundus* and *Trapa natans* possess good antibacterial activity, but they turned out to be poor antifungal agents. Ogundare *et al.* (2006) reported that the plant extracts were more active against bacterial strains than the fungal strains. The resistance of fungi to plant extracts can be explained by chitinous structure of the cell wall, which disallows easy penetration of bioactive substances. Doughari (2006) reported that stem bark and leaf extract of *Tamarindus indica* demonstrated activity against both Gram positive bacteria and Gram negative bacteria, but did not show any antimycotic activity. Parekh and Chanda (2007b) reported that the aqueous extract of *Terminalia chebula* was more active against Gram positive bacteria than Gram negative bacteria, but did not show any antifungal activity. Chakraborthy (2008) reported that extracts exhibited *in vitro* antibacterial activity against Gram positive and Gram negative bacteria, but did not show any antifungal activity. Abdoul-Latif *et al.* (2010) investigated that the essential oil and methanol extract of *Jasminum sambac* showed better activity against bacterial species than against yeast. Shihabudeen *et al.* (2010) reported that methanol extracts of *Eugenia jambolana* and *Cassia auriculata* showed antibacterial activity against all the bacteria, but did not show antifungal activity.

In the present study also crude methanol extract and separated fractions of *W. fruticosa* exhibited significant antibacterial activity. The extent of inhibition was greater in separated fractions than that of the crude extract. The crude methanol extract, Fraction I, Fraction II and sub-fractions of Fraction II showed broad spectrum antibacterial activity; whereas remaining sub-fractions showed narrow spectrum or limited spectrum activity. Similar results were reported by Khanna and Kannabiran (2008). Contrasting to these findings, Akerele *et al.* (2008) reported that antimicrobial activity of the seeds of *Garcinia kola* crude ethanol extract has broad spectrum of activity, while the fractions exhibited narrow spectrum of activity.

Gas Chromatography Mass Spectroscopy (GCMS) Analysis

Fraction II-4, Fraction II-5 and Fraction II-6 being active, were further analyzed for its chemical structure and biological characterization.

There are some reports on the structural characterization of the secondary metabolites of this plant. The compounds identified are predominantly phenolics, particularly hydrolysable tannins and flavonoids. A few of such diverse structures are shown in Figures 4.5–4.8 (Das *et al.*, 2007).

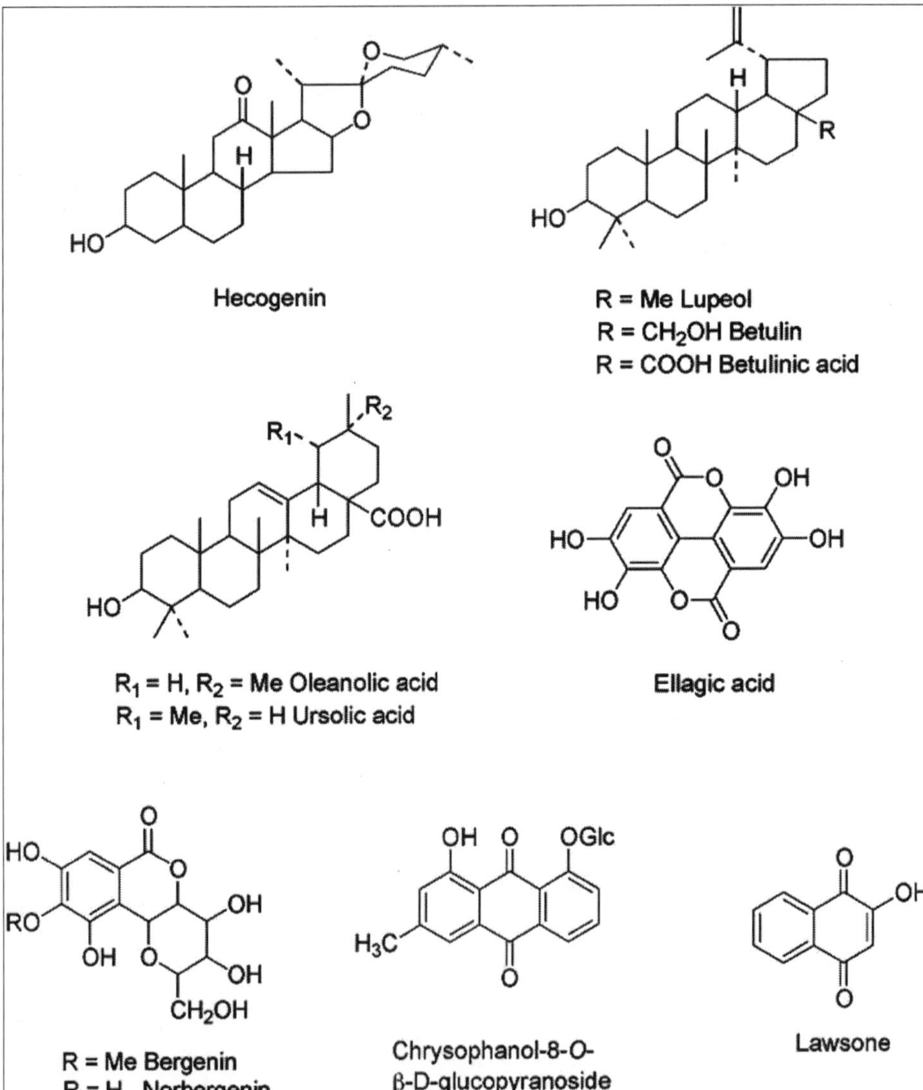

Figure 4.5: Some Non-tannin, Non-flavonoid Constituents of *Woodfordia fruticosa*.

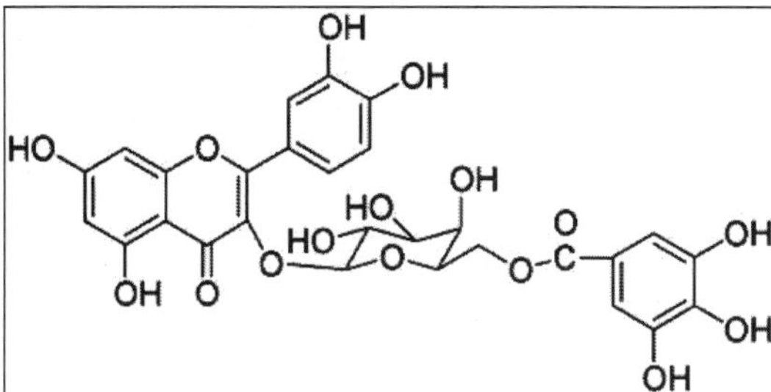

Quercetin 3-*O*-(6''-galloyl)-β-D-galactopyranoside

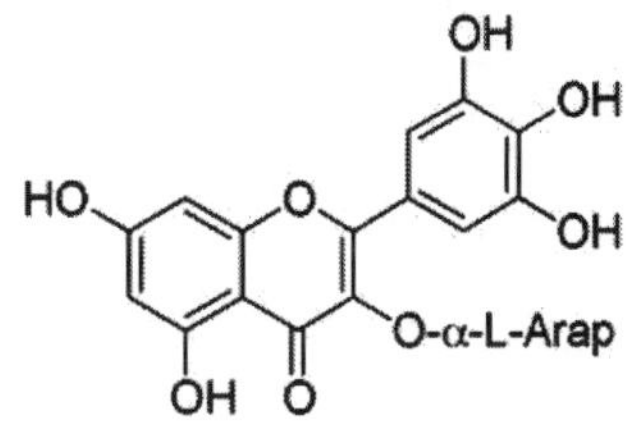

Myricetin 3-*O*-α-L-arabinopyranoside

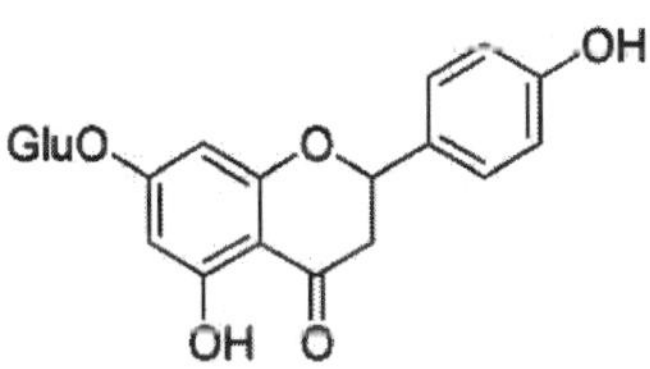

Naringenin 7-glucoside

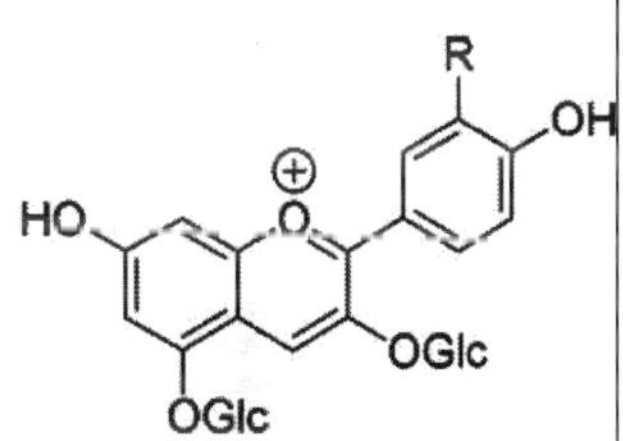

R = H Pelargonidin 3,5-diglucoside
R = OH Cyanidin 3,5-diglucoside

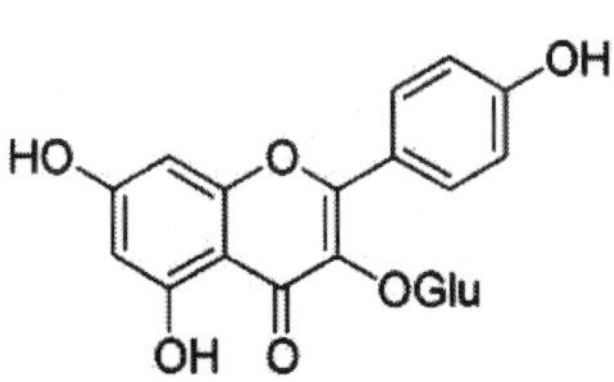

Kaempferol 3-*O*-glucoside

Figure 4.6: Selected Flavonoid Constituents of *Woodfordia fruticosa*.

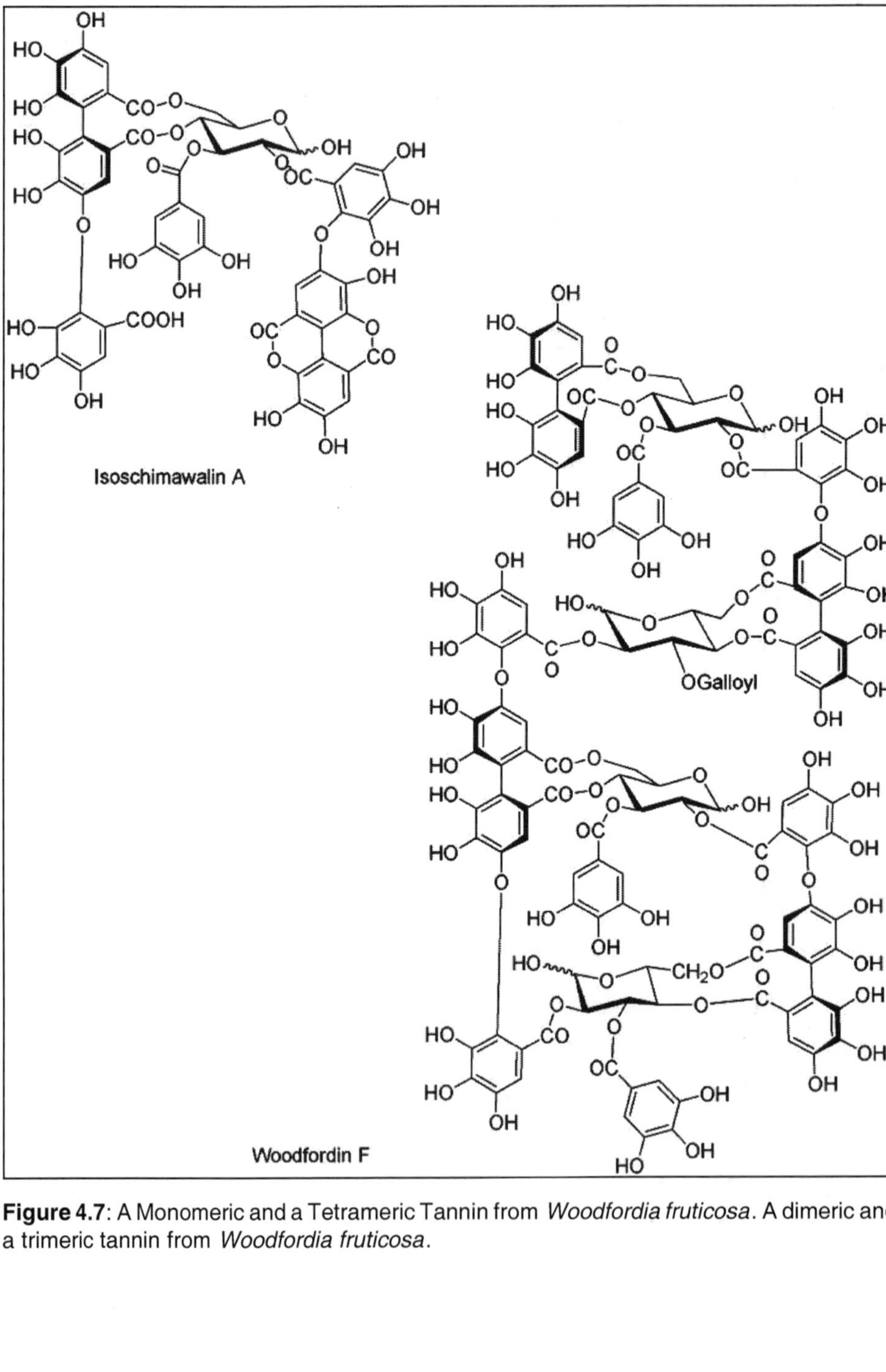

Figure 4.7: A Monomeric and a Tetrameric Tannin from *Woodfordia fruticosa*. A dimeric and a trimeric tannin from *Woodfordia fruticosa*.

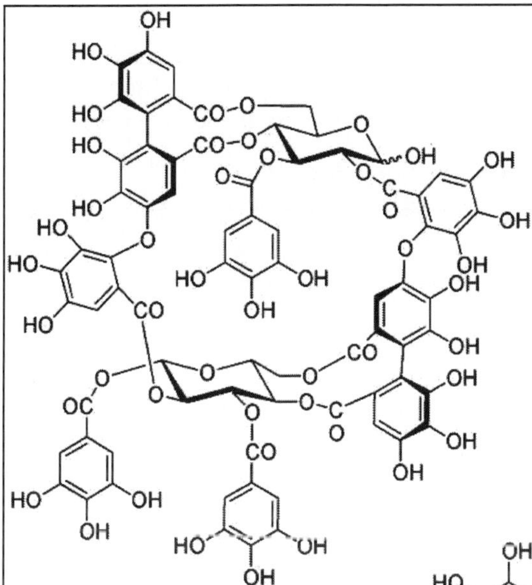

Woodfordin C

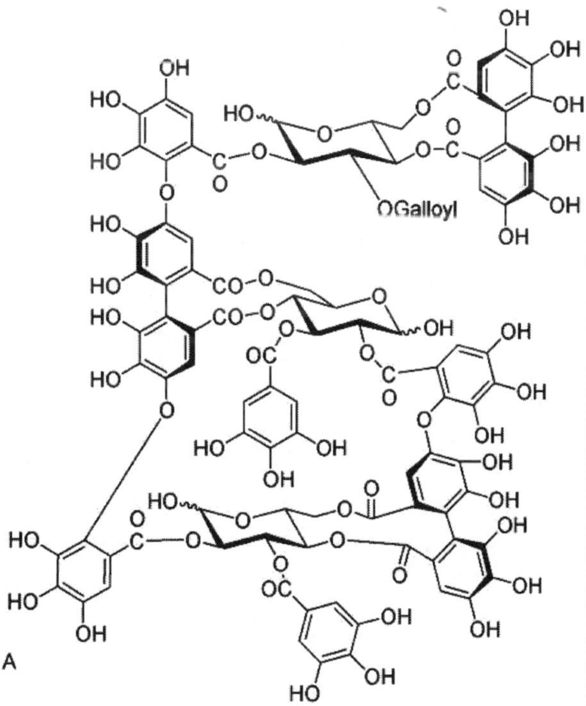

Oenothein A

Figure 4.8: (Continued).

We have attempted to elucidate the structure from library search after GCMS analysis, but unfortunately we could not succeed to find out relevant structure. Further work in this direction will be carried out.

The bioactive compounds present in Fraction II-4 were analysed by GCMS at different retention time as shown in the chromatogram. The maximum area was covered at 15.292 minutes and the area covered was 50.57 per cent as shown in peak report TIC. GCMS data showed three peak, further their mass spectra were recorded.

Fraction II-4: Chromatogram/GCMS Solution/Data

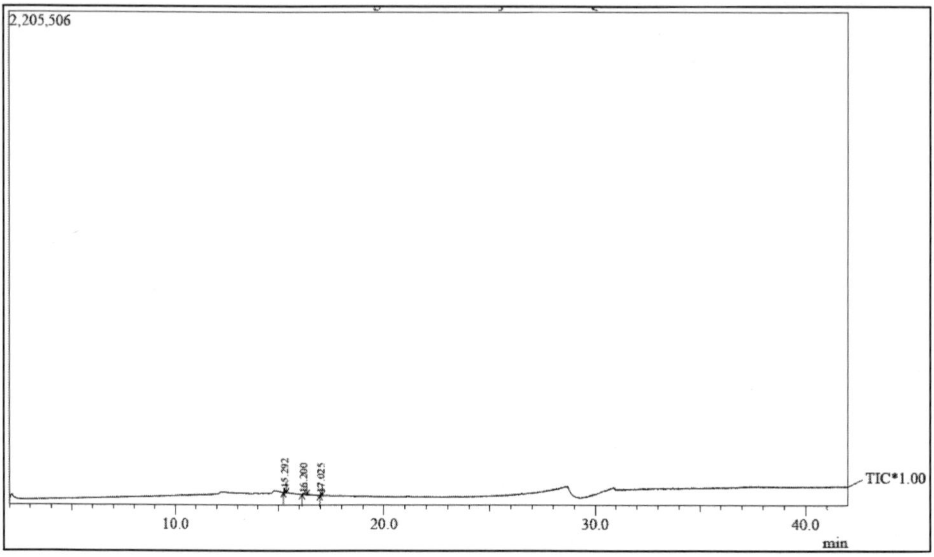

Peak Report TIC

Peak#	R.Time	Area	Area%	Height	Name
1	15.292	61007	50.57	20059	
2	16.200	35136	29.12	6158	
3	17.025	24500	20.31	11524	
		120642	100.00	37741	

The bioactive compounds present in Fraction II-5 were analysed by GCMS at different retention time as shown in the chromatogram. The maximum area was covered at 10.917 minutes and the area covered was 62.47 per cent as shown in peak report TIC. GCMS data showed nine peak, further their mass spectra were recorded.

Fraction II-5: Chromatogram/GCMS Solution/Data

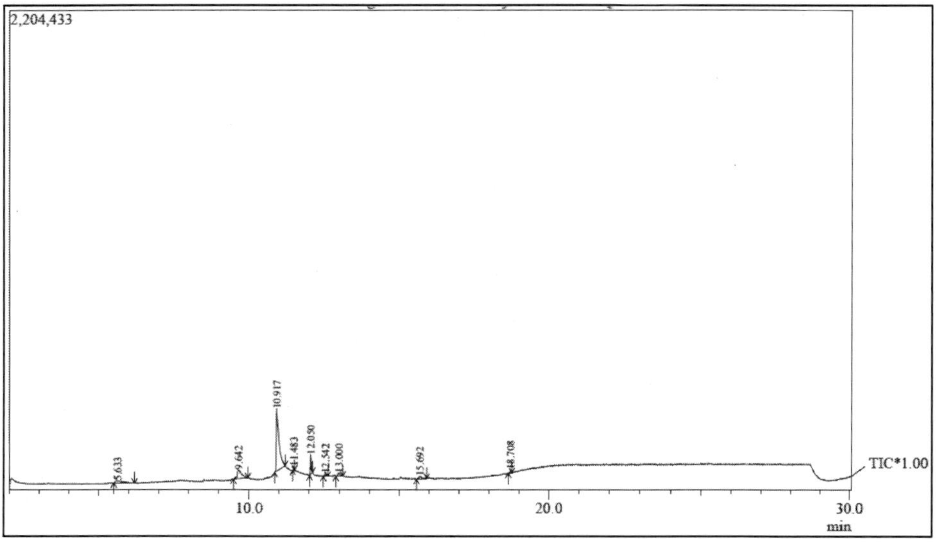

Peak Report TIC

Peak#	R.Time	Area	Area%	Height	Name
1	5.633	189877	6.95	10772	
2	9.642	389975	14.28	40621	
3	10.917	1705767	62.47	284735	
4	11.483	26121	0.96	18772	
5	12.050	217003	7.95	90913	
6	12.542	19514	0.71	13540	
7	13.000	73727	2.70	15110	
8	15.692	77121	2.82	12259	
9	18.708	31520	1.15	16181	
		2730624	100.00	502903	

The bioactive compounds present in Fraction II-6 were analysed by GCMS at different retention time as shown in the chromatogram. The maximum area was covered at 9.542 minutes and the area covered was 58.12 per cent as shown in peak report TIC. GCMS data showed six peak, further their mass spectra were recorded.

Fraction II-6: Chromatogram/GCMS Solution/Data

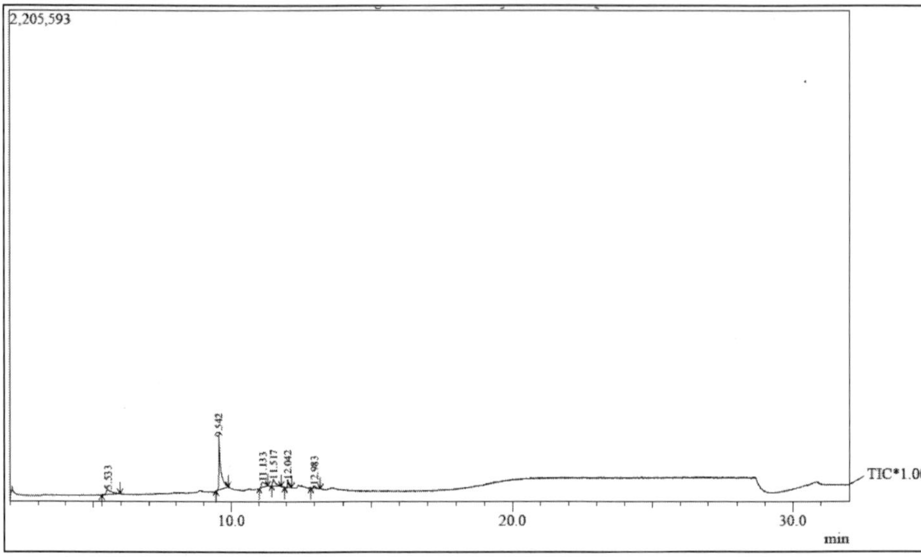

Peak Report TIC

Peak#	R.Time	Area	Area%	Height	Name
1	5.533	283626	13.47	21775	
2	9.542	1224014	58.12	235435	
3	11.133	216230	10.27	23532	
4	11.517	208169	9.89	27714	
5	12.042	112975	5.36	35010	
6	12.983	60885	2.89	11675	
		2105898	100.00	355141	

Conclusion

Woodfordia fruticosa Kurz. flowers extract showed extractive yield 36 per cent. Solvent-solvent partition of methanol extract yielded Fraction I and Fraction II, further column chromatography of these fractions yielded total of 67 and 66 sub-fractions respectively. TLC evaluation of these sub-fractions resulted in 9 and 8 major fractions respectively. The crude methanol extract and its fractions showed antibacterial activity for 9 bacteria. Fraction II and its sub-fractions showed more activity against Gram positive and Gram negative bacteria as compared to crude methanol extract, Fraction I and its sub-fractions. Amongst all the 20 fractions, Fraction II-5 showed the most significant antibacterial activity. None of the fractions or subfractions or crude methanol extract showed antifungal activity. Total of 3, 9 and 6 peaks were obtained by GCMS analysis of Fraction II-4, Fraction II-5 and Fraction II-6 respectively and their mass spectra were recorded.

This finding of compounds may be useful as potential bio-control agents and afford efficient and safe antimicrobials which will certainly contribute to the ongoing search for new antimicrobial agents to fight against infectious diseases caused by antibiotic resistant strains.

References

Abdoul-Latif, F., Edou, P., Eba, F., Mohamed, N., Ali, A., Djama, S., Obame, L.C., Bassole, I., and Dicko, M. (2010). Antimicrobial and antioxidant activities of essential oil and methanol extract of *Jasminum sambac* from Djibouti. *African Journal of Plant Science*, **4**: 38-43.

Adediwura, A., Fred-Jaiyesimi, Oluwatosin, F., and Ogunjobi. (2013). Antiepileptic activities of the extract and fractions of *Mondia whitei* (Hook f.) Skeel leaves. *Pharmacognosy Journal*, **5**: 256-258.

Akerele, J.O., Obasuyi, O., Ebomoyi, M.I., Oboh, E., Osamuyi, and Uwumarongie, H. (2008). Antimicrobial activity of the ethanol extract and fractions of the seeds of *Garcinia kola* Heckel (Guttiferae). *African Journal of Biotechnology*, **7**: 169-172.

Alwash, M.S., Ibrahim, N., Yaacob, W.A., and Din, L.B. (2014). Antibacterial, antioxidant and cytotoxicity properties of traditionally used *Melastoma malabathricum* Linn leaves. *Advance Journal of Food Science and Technology*, **6(1)**: 6-12.

Anjaria, J., Parabia, M., and Dwivedi, S. (2002). Ethnovet heritage Indian ethnoveterinary medicines. An overview. 1st edition, Pathik Enterprise, Ahmedabad, India.

Arora, D.S., Kaur, G.J., and Kaur, H. (2009). Antibacterial activity of tea and coffee: Their extracts and preparations. *International Journal of Food Properties*, **12**: 286-294.

Bajracharya, A.M., Yami, K.D., Prasai, T., Basnyat, S.R., and Lekhak, B. (2008). Screening of some medicinal plants used in Nepalese traditional medicine against enteric bacteria. *Scientific World*, **6**: 107-110.

Baravalia, Y., and Chanda, S. (2011). Protective effect of *Woodfordia fruticoza* Kurz. flowers against acetaminophen induced hepatic toxicity in rats. *Pharmaceutical Biology*, **49(8)**: 826-832.

Baravalia, Y., Vaghasiya, Y., and Chanda, S. (2012). Brine shrimp cytotoxicity, anti-inflammatory and analgesic properties of *Woodfordia fruticosa* Kurz flowers. *Iranian Journal of Pharmaceutical Research*, **11(3)**: 851-861.

Baravalia, Y., Vaghasiya,Y., and Chanda, S. (2011). Hepatoprotective effect of *Woodfordia fruticosa* Kurz flowers on diclofenac sodium induced liver toxicity in rats. *Asian Pacific Journal of Tropical Medicine*, **1**: 342-346.

Baris, O., Gulluce, M., Sahin, F., Ozer, H., Kilic, H., Ozkan, H., Sokmen, M., and Ozbek, T. (2006). Biological activities of the essential oil and methanol extract of *Achillea Biebersteinii* Afan. (Asteraceae). *Turkish Journal of Biology*, **30**: 65-73.

Bauer, R.W., Kirby, M.D.K., Sherris, J.C., and Turck, M. (1966). Antibiotic susceptibility testing by standard single disc diffusions method. *American Journal of Clinical Pathology*, **45**: 493-496.

Bisignano, G., Sanogo, R., Marino, A., Aquino, R., D'Angelo, V., Germano, M.P., Pasquale, R.D., and Pizza, C. (2000). Antimicrobial activity of *Mitracarpus scaber* extract and isolated constituents. *Letters in Applied Microbiology*, **30**: 105-108.

Boussaada, O., Chriaa, J., Nabli, R., Ammar, S., Saidana, D., Mahjoub, M.A., Chraeif, I., Helal, A., and Mighri, Z. (2008). Antimicrobial and antioxidant activities of methanol extracts of *Evax pygmaea* (Asteraceae) growing wild in Tunisia. *World Journal of Microbiology and Biotechnology*, **24**: 1289-1296.

Bouzada, M.L.M., Fabri, R.L., Nogueira, M., Konno, T.U.P., Duarte, G.G., and Scio, E. (2009). Antibacterial, cytotoxic and phytochemical screening of some traditional medicinal plants in Brazil. *Pharmaceutical Biology*, **47**: 44-52.

Brindha, D., and Geetha, R. (2009). Evaluation of the protective efficacy of *Woodfordia fruticosa* on phenytoin induced liver damage in rats. *Journal of Cell and Tissue Research*, **9**: 1981-1984.

Butler, M.S. (2004). The role of natural product chemistry in drug discovery. *Journal of Natural Products*, **67**: 2141-2153.

Chakraborthy, G.S. (2008). Antimicrobial activity of the leaf extracts of *Calendula officinalis* (Linn.). *Journal of Herbal Medicine and Toxicology*, **2**: 65-66.

Chanda, S. and Parekh, J. (2010). Assessment of antimicrobial potential of *Manilkara hexandra* leaf. *Pharmacognosy Journal*, **2**: 448-455.

Chanda, S., and Baravalia, Y. (2010). Screening of some plant extracts against some skin diseases caused by oxidative stress and microorganisms. *African Journal of Biotechnology*, **9**: 3210-3217.

Chanda, S., and Baravalia, Y. (2011). Brine shrimp cytotoxicity of *Caesalpinia pulcherrima* aerial parts, antimicrobial activity and characterisation of isolated active fractions. *Natural Product Research*, **25**: 1955-1964.

Chanda, S., Baravalia, Y., and Kaneria, M. (2011). Protective effect of *Polyalthia longifolia* var. pendula leaves on ethanol and ethanol/HCl induced ulcer in rats and its antimicrobial potency. *Asian Pacific Journal of Tropical Medicine*, **4(9)**: 673-679.

Chanda, S., Baravalia, Y., Kaneria, M., and Rakholiya, K. (2010). Fruit and vegetable peels – strong natural source of antimicrobics. In A. Mendez-Vilas (Ed.) Current Research, Technology and Education Topics in Applied Microbiology and Microbial Biotechnology, Formatex, Spain, 444-450.

Chanda, S., Kaneria, M, and Baravalia, Y. (2012). Antioxidant and antimicrobial properties of various polar solvent extracts of stem and leaves of four *Cassia* species. *African Journal of Biotechnology*, **11(10)**: 2490-2503.

Chanda, S., Menpara, D., and Desai, D. (2014). Antimicrobial activity of *Terminalia bellerica* leaf and stem collected from two different sites. *American Journal of Phytomedicine and Clinical Therapeutics*, **1(9)**: 721-733.

Chanda, S., Rakholiya, K., and Parekh, J. (2013). Indian medicinal herb: Antimicrobial efficacy of *Mesua ferrea* L. seed extracted in different solvents against infection causing pathogenic strains. *Journal of Acute Disease* **2(4)**: 277-281.

Chanda, S., Rakholiya, K., Dholakia, K., and Baravalia, Y. (2013). Antimicrobial, antioxidant and synergistic property of two nutraceutical plants: *Terminalia catappa* L. and *Colocasia esculentum* L. *Turkish Journal of Biology*, **37**: 81-91.

Chandan, B.K., Saxena, A.K., Shukla, S., Sharma, N., Gupta, D.K., Singh, K., Suri, J., Bhadauria, M., and Qazi, G.N. (2008). Hepatoprotective activity of *Woodfordia fruticosa* Kurz flowers against carbon tetrachloride induced hepatotoxicity. *Journal of Ethnopharmacology*, **119**: 218-224.

Chandarana, H., Baluja, S., and Chanda, S.V. (2005). Comparison of antibacterial activities of selected species of *Zingiberaceae* Family and some synthetic compounds. *Turkish Journal of Biology*, **29**: 83-97.

Chopra, A., and Doiphode, V. (2002). Ayurvedic medicine: core concept, therapeutic principles and current relevance. *Medical Clinics of North America*, **86**: 75-89.

Chopra, I., Hodgson, J., Metcalf, B., and Poste, G. (1997). The search for antimicrobial agents effective against bacteria resistant to multiple antibiotics. *Antimicrobial Agents and Chemotherapy*, **41**: 497-503.

Cork, S.J., and Krockenberger, A.K. (1991). Methods and pitfalls of extracting condensed tannins and other phenolics from plants: insights from investigations on Eucalyptus leaves. *Journal of Chemical Ecology*, **17**: 123-134.

Dabur, R., Gupta, A., Mandal, T.K., Singh, D.D., Bajpai, V., Gurav, A.M., and Lavekar, G.S. (2007). Antimicrobial activity of some Indian medicinal plants. *African Journal of Traditional Complementary and Alternative Medicines*, **4**: 313-318.

Das, A.P.M., and Banerjee, A. (2014). Extraction of tamarind pulp and its antimicrobial activity. *Pelagia Research Library*, **4(2)**: 47-49.

Das, P.K., Goswami, S., Chinniah, A., Panda, N., Banerjee, S., Sahu, N.P., and Achari, B. (2007). *Woodfordia fruticosa*: Traditional uses and recent findings. *Journal of Ethnopharmacology*, **110**: 189-199.

Dash, B., and Sharma, B.K. (2001). Charak Samhita. Chaukhamba Sanskrit Series Office, Varanasi, India.

Delaquis, P.J., Stanich, K., Girard, B., and Mazza, G. (2002). Antimicrobial activity of individual and mixed fractions of dill, cilantro, coriander and eucalyptus essential oils. *International Journal of Food Microbiology*, **74**: 101-109.

Dey, K.L. (1984). The indigenous drugs of India. International Book Distributors, Dehradun, India, p. 311.

Djeussi, D.E., Noumedem, A.K.J., Seukep, A.J., Fankam, G.A., and Voukeng, K.I. (2013). Antibacterial activities of selected edible plants extracts against multidrug-resistant Gram-neagative bacteria. *BMC Complementary and Alternative Medicine*,**13**: 164.

Doughari, J.H. (2006). Antimicrobial activity of *Tamarindus indica* Linn. *Tropical Journal of Pharmaceutical Research*, **5**: 597-603, 2006.

Fakoya, A., Owojuyigbe, O.S., Fakoya, S., and Adeoye, S.O. (2014). Possible antimicrobial activity of *Morinda lucida* stem bark, leaf and root extracts. *African Journal of Biotechnology*, **13(3)**: 471-475.

Hazra, K.M., Roy, R.N., Sen, S.K., and Laskar, S. (2007). Isolation of antibacterial pentahydroxy flavones from the seeds of *Mimusops elengi* Linn. *African Journal of Biotechnology*, **6**: 1446-1449.

Hegazy, A.E., and Ibrahium, M.I. (2012). Antioxidant activities of orange peel extracts. *World Applied Science Journal*, **18(5)**: 684-688.

Heinrich, M., and Gibbons, S. (2001). Ethnopharmacology in drug discovery: an analysis of its role and potential contribution. *Journal of Pharmacy and Pharmacolology*, **53**: 425-432.

Hyuck-Ju, K., Yon-Suk, K., Jin-Woo, H., Chul, Y.K., Sang-Hoon, L., Sang-Ho, M., Byong-Tae, J., Pyo-Jam, P. (2014). Isolation and identification of an anticancer compound from the bark of *Acer tegmentosum* Maxim. *Process Biochemistry*, **49**: 1032–1039.

Iwu, M.W., Duncan, A.R., and Okunji, C.O. (1999). New antimicrobials of plant origin. In Janick J (Ed.) Prospectives on new crops and new uses, ASHS Press, Alexandria, 457-462.

Jurenka, J.S. (2009). Anti-inflammatory properties of curcumin, a major constituents of *Curcuma longa*: a review of preclinical and clinical research. *Alternative Medicine Review*, **14**: 141-153.

Kaneria, M. and Chanda, S. (2013). The effect of sequential fractionation technique on the various efficacies of pomegranate (*Punica granatum* L.). *Food Analytical Methods*, **6**: 164-175.

Kaneria, M., Baravalia, Y., Vaghasiya, Y., and Chanda, S. (2009). Determination of antibacterial and antioxidant potential of some medicinal plants from Saurashtra region, India. *Indian Journal of Pharmaceutical Sciences*, **71**: 406-412.

Karaalp, C., Yurtman, A.N., and Yavasoglu, N.U.K. (2009). Evaluation of antimicrobial properties of *Achillea L.* flower head extracts. *Pharmaceutical Biology*, **47**, 86-91.

Kaur, G.J., and Arora, D.S. (2009). Antibacterial and phytochemical screening of *Anethum graveolens*, *Foeniculum vulgare* and *Trachyspermum ammi*. *BMC Complementary and Alternative Medicine*, **9**: 30-39.

Kaur, R., and Kaur, H. (2010). The antimicrobial activity of essential oil and plant extracts of *Woodfordia fruticosa*. *Archives of Applied Science Research*, **2**: 302-309.

Kaushik, S., Tomar, R.S., Shrivastava, V., Shrivastav, A., and Jain, S.K. (2014). Antimicrobial efficacy of essential oils of selected plants and vaccine design against meca protein of methicillin resistant *Staphylococcus aureus*. *Asian Journal of Pharmaceutical and Clinical Research*, **7**: 52-56.

Kchaoua, W., Abbèsa, F., Bleckerb, C., Attia, H., and Besbesa, S. (2013). Effects of extraction solvents on phenolic contents and antioxidant activities of Tunisian date varieties (*Phoenix dactylifera* L.). *Industrial Crop and Production*, **45**: 262–269.

Khan, A., Rahman, M., and Islam, M.S. (2008a). Antibacterial, antifungal and cytotoxic activities of Amblyone isolated from *Amorphophallus campanulatu*. *Indian Journal of Pharmacology*, **40**: 41-44.

Khan, R., Islam, B., Akram, M., Shakil, S., Ahmad, A., Ali, S.M., Siddiqui, M., and Khan, A.U. (2008b). Antimicrobial activity of five herbal extracts against multi drug resistant (MDR) strains of bacteria and fungus of clinical origin. *Molecules*, **13**.

Khanna, K.K., and Chandra, S. (1972). Antifungal activity of some plant extracts. Proceedings of the National Academy of Sciences of India, Section A, **42B**: 111.

Khanna, V.G., and Kannabiran, K. (2008). Antimicrobial activity of saponin fractions of the leaves of *Gymnema sylvestre* and *Eclipta prostrata*. *World Journal of Microbiology and Biotechnology*, **24**: 2737-2740.

Khushalani, H., Tatke, P., and Singh, K.K. (2006). Antifertility activity of dried flowers of *Woodfordia fruticosa* Kurz. *Indian Journal of Pharmaceutical Sciences*, **68**: 528-529.

Kingston, I.T., Nakabayashi, T., and Kida, H. (2000). Screening of various plant extracts used in ayurvedic medicine for inhibitory effects on human immunodeficiency virus type-1 (HIV-1) protease. *Phytotherapy Research*, **9**: 180-184.

Kirkpatrick, P. (2002). Stitching together naturally. *Nature Reviews Drug Discovery*, **1**: 748.

Kroes, B.H., van den Berg, A.J.J., Abeysekera, A.M., De Silva, K.T.D., and Labadie, R.P. (1993). Fermentation in traditional medicine: the impact of *Woodfordia fruticosa* flowers on the immunomodulatory activity, and the alcohol and sugar contents of Nimba arishta. *Journal of Ethnopharmacology*, **40**: 117-125.

Kuete, V., Kamga, J., Sandjo, L.P., Ngameni, B., Poumale, H.M.P., Ambassa, P. and Ngadjui, B.T. (2011). Antimicrobial activities of the methanol extract, fractions and compounds from *Ficus polita* Vahl. (Moraceae). *BMC Complementary and Alternative Medicine*, **11**: 6.

Kumaraswamy, M.V., and Satish, S. (2008). Free radical scavenging activity and lipoxygenase inhibition of *Woodfordia fructicosa* Kurz and *Betula utilis* Wall. *African Journal of Biotechnology*, **7**: 2013-2016.

Kumaraswamy, M.V., Kavitha, H.U., and Satish, S. (2008). Antibacterial potential of extracts of *Woodfordia fruticosa* Kurz on human pathogens. *World Journal of Medical Sciences*, **3**: 93-96.

Kuramochi-Motegi, A., Kuramochi, H., Kobayashi, F., Ekimoto, H., Takahashi, K., Kadota, S., Takamori, Y., and Kikuchi, T. (1992). Woodfruticosin (woodfordin C), a new inhibitor of DNA topoisomerase II. Experimental antitumor activity. *Biochemical Pharmacology*, **44**: 1961-1965.

Lawrence, R., Tripathi, P., and Jeyakumar, E. (2009). Isolation, purification and evaluation of antibacterial agents from *Aloe vera*. *Brazilian Journal of Microbiology*, **40**: 906-915.

Lee, J., Lee, J., Lim, J., Sim, S. and Park, D. (2008). Antibacterial effects of *S*-(-)-tulipalin B isolated from *Spiraea thunbergii* Sieb. on *Escherichia coli*, a major food borne pathogenic microorganism. *Journal of Medicinal Plants Research*, **2**: 59-65.

Li, A., Zhu, Y., He, X., Tian, X., Xu, L., Ni, W., and Jiang, P. (2008a). Evaluation of antimicrobial activity of certain Chinese plants used in folkloric medicine. *World Journal of Microbiology and Biotechnology*, **24**: 569-572.

Li, W.H., Chang, S.T., Chang, S.C., and Chang, H.T. (2008b). Isolation of antibacterial diterpenoids from *Cryptomeria japonica* bark. *Natural Product Research*, **22**: 1085-1093.

Lilly, B.A., Aarrthy, M.A., Kantha, D.A., Sathesh, K.A., and Kalaivani, A.K. (2014). *In vivo* anti-ulcer, anti-stress, anti-allergic, and functional properties of Gymnemic Acid Isolated from Gymnema sylvestre R Br. *BMC Complementary and Alternative Medicine*, **14(70)**: 1-11.

Lin, J., Opoku, A.R., Geheeb-Keller, M., Hutchings, A.D., Terblanche, S.E., Jager, A.K., and van Staden, J. (1999). Preliminary screening of some traditional zulu medicinal plants for anti-inflammatory and antimicrobial activities. *Journal of Ethnopharmacology*, **68**: 267-274.

Majid, A., Hassan, S., Hussain, W., Khan, A., Hassan, A., Khan, A., Khan, T., Ahmad, T., Rehman, M.U. (2014). *In vitro* approaches of *Primula vulgaries* leaves and root extraction against human pathogenic bacterial strains. *World Applied Sciences Journal*, **30(5)**: 575-580.

Makasana, A., Ranpariya, V., Desai, D., Mendpara, J., and Parekh, V. (2014). Evaluation for the anti-urolithiatic activity of *Launaea procumbens* against ethylene glycol-induced renal calculi inrats. *Toxicology Reports*, **1**: 46–52.

Marin-Loaiza, J.C., Avila, J.G., Canales, M., Hernandez, T., and Cespedes, C.L. (2008). Antifungal and antibacterial activities of endemic *Pittocaulon*. spp. from Mexico. *Pharmaceutical Biology*, **46**: 66-71.

Martinez, M.J., Betancourt, J., Alonso-Gonzalez, N., and Jauregui, A. (1996). Screening of some Cuban medicinal plants for antimicrobial activity. *Journal of Ethnopharmacology*, **52**: 171-174.

Menpara, D., Desai, D., Rathod, T., and Chanda, S. (2014). Evaluation of nutraceutical bottle gourd (*Lagenaria siceraria*) as a potential source of natural antimicrobial agent. *American Journal of Phytomedicine and Clinical Therapeutics*, **2(3)**: 375-389.

Moir, D.T., Shaw, K.J., Hare, R.S., and Vovis, G.F. (1999). Genomics and antimicrobial drug discovery. *Antimicrobial Agents and Chemotherapy*, **43**: 439-446.

Muthuvelan, B., and Raja, R.B. (2008). Studies of the efficiency of different extraction procedure on the antimicrobial activity of selected medicinal plants. *World Journal of Microbiology and Biotechnology*, **24**: 2837-2842.

Nair, R., and Chanda, S. (2007). Antibacterial activities of some medicinal plants of the western region of India. *Turkish Journal of Biology*, **31**: 231-236.

Nair, R., and Chanda, S. (2008). Antimicrobial activity of *Terminalia catappa, Manilkara zapota* and *Piper betel* leaf extract. *Indian Journal of Pharmaceutical Sciences*, **70**: 390-393.

Ncube, N.S., Afolayan, A.J., and Okoh, A.I. (2008). Assessment techniques of antimicrobial properties of natural compounds of plant origin: current methods and future trends. *African Journal of Biotechnology*, **7**: 1797-1806.

Ogundare, A.O., Adetuyi, F.C., and Akinyosoye, F.A. (2006). Antimicrobial activities of *Vernonia tenoreana*. *African Journal of Biotechnology*, **5**: 1663-1668.

Okoye, F.B.C., and Osadebe, P.O. (2010). A new anti-inflammatory flavonol glycoside from *Alcornea floribunda* leaves. *Natural Product Research*, **24**: 266-273.

Oyedemi, S.O., and Afolayan, A.J. (2011). Antibacterial and antioxidant activities of hydroalcoholic stem bark extract of *Schotia latifolia* Jacq. *Asian Pacific Journal of Tropical Medicine*, **4(12)**: 952-958.

Parekh, J., and Chanda, S. (2006). *In-vitro* antimicrobial activities of extracts of *Launaea procumbens* Roxb. (Labiateae), *Vitis vinifera* L. (Vitaceae) and *Cyperus rotundus* L. (Cyperaceae). *African Journal of Biomedical Research*, **9**: 89 -93.

Parekh, J., and Chanda, S. (2007a). *In vitro* antibacterial activity of the crude methanol extract of *Woodfordia fruticosa* Kurz. flower (Lythraceae). *Brazilian Journal of Microbiology*, **38**: 204-207

Parekh, J., and Chanda, S. (2007b). Evaluation of antimicrobial activity of *Terminalia chebula* Retz. fruit in different solvents. *Journal of Herbs, Spices and Medicinal Plants*, **13**: 107-116.

Parekh, J., Jadeja, D., and Chanda, S. (2005). Efficacy of aqueous and methanol extracts of some medicinal plants for potential antibacterial activity. *Turkish Journal of Biology*, **29**: 203 210.

Prashanth kumar, V., Chauhan, N.S., Padh, H., and Rajani, M. (2006). Search for antibacterial and antifungal agents from selected Indian medicinal plants. *Journal of Ethnopharmacology*, **107**: 182-188.

Rakholiya, K., Kaneria, M., and Chanda, S. (2014b). Inhibition of microbial pathogens using fruit and vegetable peel extracts. *International Journal of Food Science and Nutrition*, **65(6)**: 733-739.

Rakholiya, K.D., Kaneria, M.J., and Chanda S.V. (2014a). Mango pulp: A potential source of natural antioxidant and antimicrobial agent. In: Medicinal Plants: Phytochemistry, Pharmacology and Therapeutics – Ed. Gupta VK, Daya Publishing House, New Delhi, 3: 253-284.

Ramanuj, K., Kothari, V., and Kothari, D.R. (2014). *In vitro* antibacterial activity of *Emblica officinalis* and *Tamarindus indica* seed extracts against multidrug resistant *Acinetobacter baumannii*. *International Journal of Epidemiology and Infection*, **2(1)**: 1-6.

Ramirez, L.A.O., Garcia, I.R., Leyva, J.M., Valenzuela, M.R.C., Espinoza, B.A.S., Aguilar, G.A.G., Siddiqui, M.W., and Zavala, J.F.A. (2014). Potential of Medicinal Plants as Antimicrobial and Antioxidant Agents in Food Industry: A Hypothesis. *Journal of Food Science*, **79**: R129-R137.

Rojas, J.J., Ochoa, V.J., Ocampo, S.A., and Munoz, J.F. (2006). Screening for antimicrobial activity of ten medicinal plants used in Colombian folkloric medicine: A possible alternative in the treatment of non-nosocomial infections. *BMC Complementary and Alternative Medicine*, **6**: 2.

Saleh, F.A., and Otaibi, M.M. (2013). Antibacterial activity of Date palm (*Pheonix dectylifera* L.) fruit at different ripening stage. *Journal of Food Process Technology* **4 (12)**: 1-6.

Sanches, N.R., Cortez, D.A.G., Schiavini, M.S., Nakamura, C.V., and Filho, B.P.D. (2005). An evaluation of antibacterial activities of *Psidium guajava* (L.) *Brazilian Archives of Biology and Technology*, **48**: 429-436.

Sarac, N., and Ugar, A. (2007). Antimicrobial activities and usage in folkloric medicine of some Lamiaceae species growing in Mugla, Turkey. *EurAsian Journal of Biosciences*, **4**: 28-37.

Sekar, S., and Mariappan, S. (2008). Traditionally fermented biomedicines, *arishtas* and *asavas* from Ayurveda. *Indian Journal of Traditional Knowledge*, **7**: 548-556.

Sengul, M., Ogutcu, H., Adiguzel, A., Sahin, F., Kara, A.A., Karaman, I., and Gulluce, M. (2005). Antimicrobial effects of *Verbascum georgicum* Bentham extract. *Turkish Journal of Biology*, **29**: 105-110.

Shah, A.S., and Juvekar, A.R. (2010). *In vitro* and *in vivo* immunostimulatory activity of *Woodfordia fruticosa* flowers on non-specific immunity. *Pharmaceutical Biology*, **48**: 1066-1072.

Sharma, A., and Patel, V.K. (2009). *In-vitro* screening of the antibacterial activity and identification of bioactive compounds from plants against selected *Vibrio* spp. pathogens. *Turkish Journal of Biology*, **33**: 137-144.

Shekhawat, P.S., and Prasad, R. (1971). Antifungal properties of some plant extracts against dermatophytes and related keratinophilic fungi. *Current Advances in Plant Science*, **10**: 249-251.

Shihabudeen, H.M.S., Priscilla, D.H., and Thirumurugan, K. (2010). Antimicrobial activity and phytochemical analysis of selected Indian folk medicinal plants. *International Journal of Pharma Sciences and Research*, **1**: 430-434.

Shome, U., Mehrotra, S., and Sharma, H.P. (1981). Pharmacognostic studies on the flower of *Woodfordia fruticosa* Kurz. *Proceedings of Indian Academy Science* (Plant Science), **90**: 335-351.

Shukla, S., Mehta, A., Mehta, P., Vyas, S.P., Shukla, S., and Bajpai, V.K. (2010). Studies on anti-inflammatory, antipyretic and analgesic properties of *Caesalpinia bonducella* F. seed oil in experimental animal models. *Food and Chemical Toxicology*, **48**: 61-64.

Tang, J., Meng, X., Liu, H., Zhao, J., Zhou, L., Qiu, M., Zhang, X., Yu, Z., and Yang, F. (2010). Antimicrobial activity of Sphingolipids isolated from the stems of Cucumber (*Cucumis sativus* L.). *Molecules*, **15**: 9288-9297.

Vaghasiya, Y., and Chanda, S. (2007). Screening of methanol and acetone extracts of fourteen Indian medicinal plants for antimicrobial activity. *Turkish Journal of Biology*, **31**: 243-248.

Vaghasiya, Y., and Chanda, S. (2010). Antimicrobial and free radical scavenging activity of different solvent extracts of *Mangifera indica* L. seeds. *Research Journal of Microbiology*, **5**: 1207-1212.

Van Der Heijden, R., Jacobs, D.I., Snoeijer, W., Hallard, D., and Verpoorte, R. (2004). The *Catharanthus* alkaloids: pharmacognosy and biotechnology. *Current Medicinal Chemistry*, **11**: 607-628.

World Health Organization (2007). WHO guidelines for assessing quality of herbal medicines with reference to contaminants and residues. World Health Organization.

Yoshida, T., Chou, T., Nitta, A., Miyamoto, K., Koshiura, R., and Okuda, T., Woodfordin, C. (1990). A macro-ring hydrolyzable tannin dimer with antitumor activity, and accompanying dimers from *Woodfordia fruticosa* flowers. *Chemical and Pharmaceutical Bulletin*, **38**: 1211-1217.

Bioactive Phytochemicals: Perspectives for Modern Medicine Vol. 3 (2015) *Pages* **155–175**
Editor: **V.K. Gupta**
Published by: **DAYA PUBLISHING HOUSE, NEW DELHI**

5

Exocyclic-Nitrogen Alkaloids in Herbalism as Sources of New Drugs

Sunday J. Ameh[1*], Nneka N. Ibekwe[1], Magaji Garba[1,2], Peace C. Babalola[3] and Karniyus S. Gamaniel[4]

ABSTRACT

Alkaloids are naturally occurring nitrogen-containing organic compounds that are mostly basic and have diverse and important biological effects on animals. Alkaloids are small molecules (molecular weight < 900 daltons; diameter < 1nm) produced by all forms of life, especially plants. In some alkaloids (cyclic-nitrogen alkaloid) the basic nitrogen is part of a cyclic system, but in others called "exocyclic-nitrogen alkaloid" (ENA) the basic nitrogen occurs outside the ring system. Many seed-producing plants (spermatophytes) generate secondary metabolites (phytochemicals) classifiable as ENAs. Outstanding ENAs produced by such are: ephedrine, pseudoephedrine, norephedrine and norpseudoephedrine, by Ephedra, which grows in temperate zones; and cathine and cathinone, by Catha species, which grow in the Tropics. The well-known therapeutic actions of ENAs are based largely on their abilities to modulate the release or actions of adrenalin and noradrenalin (adrenal medulla hormones) and dopamine (a neurotransmitter). Owing to the ways in which these ENAs influence adrenal and nervous functions, they are described as having one or more of the following dose-dependent effects, especially humans, in whom they may be used as: i) anorectic, nootropic, stimulant, and thermogenic (i.e., medical uses); and ii) empathogenic, entactogenic, entheogenic, and hallucinogenic (i.e., recreational/religious uses). History revealed that the current

1 Department of Medicinal Chemistry and Quality Control, National Institute for Pharmaceutical Research and Development (NIPRD), Abuja, Nigeria

2 Department of Pharmaceutical and Medicinal Chemistry, Ahmadu Bello University, Zaria, Nigeria

3 Department of Pharmaceutical Chemistry, University of Ibadan, Ibadan, Nigeria

4 Department of Pharmacology and Toxicology, NIPRD, Abuja, Nigeria

* *Corresponding author*: E-mail: sjitodo@yahoo.com

medicinal uses of ENAs arose from their ancient religious uses. ENAs are relatively easy to modify chemically, and currently hundreds of such modified ENAs are in use worldwide for various recreational/spiritual purposes. Evidence suggests that it is relatively easy to discover or create newer drugs from ENAs or plants associated with herbalism. Among such plants are: Ephedra sinica (Ephedraceae) – a Gymnosperm; and several Angiosperms, such as Catha edulis (Celastraceae). The ENAs found in these and other plants are outlined with their structures and key attributes. The comments/discussionare on the prospects developing new drugs from such ENAs.

Keywords: Alkaloid, Cyclic-nitrogen, Exocyclic-nitrogen, Herbalism, New drug, Spermatophyte.

Introduction

A Definition of Alkaloids

Alkaloids are organic compounds containing one or more basic nitrogen atoms. This definition includes compounds with nitrogen as part of a heterocyclic system and those in which the nitrogen is exocyclic. In such compounds the basic nitrogen is said to exist in a negative oxidation (Grycova *et al.*, 2007). Alkaloids are mostly naturally occurring, and they are basic because the lone pair of electrons on a basic nitrogen atom attracts a proton.

Occurrence and Biochemical Importance

The occurrence of alkaloids in nature is widespread. Their key biological importance stems from the fact that, irrespective of origin, alkaloids have diverse and dramatic biological effects on humans and other animals. Alkaloids occur in all forms of life, but primarily in plants, in which over 3,000 types have been identified as secondary plant metabolites (phytochemicals) in about 4,000 plant species, especially among certain families of flowering plants (Angiosperms). In general, a given species contains only a few types, but some families such as the amaryllis (Amaryllidaceae), buttercups (Ranunculaceae), opium poppy (Papaveraceae) and nightshade (Solanaceae) may each contain scores of different alkaloids. The role of alkaloids may vary from plant to plant, and may include one or more of the following:

- Protect some plants from destruction by certain insect species
- Protect some plants from consumption by mammalian herbivores
- Signal specific events, *e.g.* seed formation (when alkaloid levels rise) and seed ripening (when alkaloid levels fall)
- Serve as a means of excreting nitrogenous waste

Two categories of non-plant alkaloid deserve mentioning: i) ergot and a few other fungi produce a group of secondary metabolites called ergot alkaloids; and ii) a few types of alkaloids, most probably derived from plant diet, occur in some animals, *e.g.* poison-dart frogs (*Phyllobates*) sequester and secrete lipophilic alkaloids through their skin as a defense against predation. Epibatidine, one of such alkaloids, is 200x as potent as morphine (Prince and Sine, 2008).

Key Chemical Feature of Alkaloids

The chemical structures of alkaloids are extremely variable. But all alkaloids contain at least one nitrogen atom in an amine-type formation, ie: RNH_2, R_2NH, R_3N or R_4N^+ derived from NH_3. This or another nitrogen atom can be active as a base in acid-base reactions, just as alkalis and other inorganic bases do, hence this N is deemed basic or alkali-like ("alkaloid").

Cyclic-N versus Exocyclic-N Alkaloids

Most alkaloids have one or more basic-N atoms as part of a ring structure called a "heterocycle". Examples of such cyclic-N alkaloids include morphine, nicotine, quinine, strychnine, and others. Fewer, but nevertheless important, alkaloids have their basic-N outside a cyclic structure. Such exocyclic-N alkaloids include colchicine, ephedrine, pseudoephedrine and cathine and others.

Nomenclature and Classification Schemes

Alkaloid names generally end in the suffix "-ine", signifying their classification as "amines". In pure form most alkaloids are colorless, nonvolatile, and crystalline. Some may appear oily, especially if impure. They also tend to have a bitter taste. Alkaloids can be classified in many ways. Two of the commonest are:

- ☆ Based on type of cyclic-N ring structure. For example, alkaloids that contain a N-cyclic structure called indole are known as indole alkaloids. On this basis, the principal classes of N-cyclic alkaloids are: pyrrolidines, pyridines, tropanes, pyrrolizidines, isoquinolines, indoles, quinolines, and the terpenoids and steroids.
- ☆ Alternatively, alkaloids can be classified according to the biological system in which they occur. For example, the opium alkaloids occur in Papaveraceae, the nightshade alkaloids occur in Solanaceae, and the vinca and iboga alkaloids occur in Apocynaceae.

This dual classification system is instructive and helpful because there is a rough correlation between the chemical types of alkaloids and their biological occurrence or distribution.

An Overview of Alkaloids in Medicine

Interest in alkaloids dates to antiquity and stems from the wide range of pharmacological and toxicological effects that they produce in humans. Their diverse medicinal attributes are exemplified as follows:

- ☆ Cocaine (from *Erythroxylon coca*) is a potent local anesthetic, but is addictive
- ☆ Codeine is also analgesic/antitussive, but causes constipation
- ☆ Coniine may be used clinically, but is the chief toxicant of hemlock (*Conium maculatum*)
- ☆ Ephedrine, from *Ephedra*, acts as anticholinergic to reduce catarrhal symptoms

- Ergonovine, from *Claviceps*, is used as a vasoconstrictor to reduce uterine hemorrhage
- Mescaline, from *Anhalonium*; and psilocybin, from *Psilocybe* are illicit hallucinogens
- Lobeline, from *Lobelia inflata*, is a safe respiratory stimulant, but not always effective
- Morphine is a powerful narcotic/analgesic, but it is addictive
- Nicotine, from *Nicotiana tabacum*, is the chief addictive alkaloid of tobacco
- Quinidine, from *Cinchona*, is used to treat arrhythmias
- Quinine, from *Cinchona*, remains a powerful and strategic antimalarial, but it is ototoxic
- Strychnine, from *Strychnos*, is a powerful stimulant/nootropic, but toxic for clinical use
- Morphine and lysergic acid derivatives, heroin and LSD, are useful, but too addictive
- Tubocurarine is a useful muscle relaxant, but can be toxic even in low doses
- Vincristine/vinblastine are anticancer, but cause aplastic anemia/other serious effects

The Aim of This Review

Given the foregoing diversities in the types and sources/distribution of alkaloids and their multiple biological attributes, this review focused on medicinal/ economically importance exocyclic-N alkaloids that occur in select Angiosperms, particularly those used in folk medicine worldwide. The focus was on the state of pertinent knowledge, the methodologies applicable, and the prospects of discovering or developing new drug molecules based on exocyclic-N alkaloids that occur in select Angiosperms used in herbal medicine worldwide.

A Survey of ENAs in Spermatophytes Commonly Used in Herbalism

Exocyclic-nitrogen alkaloids (ENAs) are sometimes called "protoalkaloids" or "biological amines", and because they are actually benzyl or phenyl entities bearing an N-alkyl group, they are also called "phenylalkylamines". In this section, some of themost outstanding, medicinally important ENAs in spermatophytes used in herbalism around the globe are mentioned.

Ephedra Alkaloids

Ephedra plants, typified by *Ephedra sinica*, are a genus of Gymnosperms that have a long history of use in Traditional Chinese Medicine (as "ma huang" for various conditions, especially asthma), India (as "soma" – a drink used in Vedic religious rituals), Persia (as "haoma - a drink used in Zoroastrian rituals) and North America (formerly as Indian Tea by Amerindians and latterly as Mormon Tea because some earlier Latter-Day Saints in the US popularized its use). *Ephedra*, which is mostly a temperate genus, is used as above because it contains up to 4 or 6 psychoactive compounds called ephedra alkaloids (Ephedrinediet, 2014; Das, 1985; Botany of Haoma, 2014). *Ephedra sinica*, for example, contains ephedrine, pseudoephedrine and 4 other alkaloids, constituting 0.02-3.4 per cent w/w of the aerial parts (Abourashed *et al.*, 2003).These alkaloids are "phenylalanine" derivatives, and include ephedrine, pseudoephedrine, norephedrine (phenylpropanolamine), and norpseudoephedrine (cathine). Today, one or more of these alkaloids are incorporated in many contemporary medicines and "health" products that are patronized worldwide. A careful inspection of the compounds indicated in Table 5.1, may suggest that each can be modified to accentuate, fine-tune, or tune-down a particular pharmacological or toxicological attribute.

Table 5.1: Structures and Attributes of Ephedra Alkaloids (Chemically modifiable)

Ephedra Alkaloid	*Attributes*	*Pertinent comments*
Ephedrine 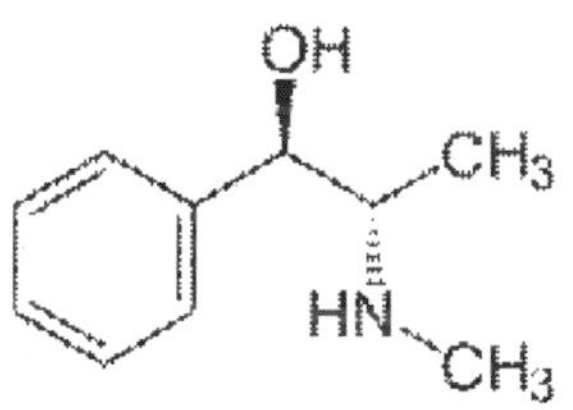 Ephedrine is an alkaloid with a phenethylamine skeleton found in various plants in the genus *Ephedra* (family Ephedraceae). It is similar to phenylpropanolamine, methamphetamine, and epinephrine (adrenalin). **Pseudoephedrine** 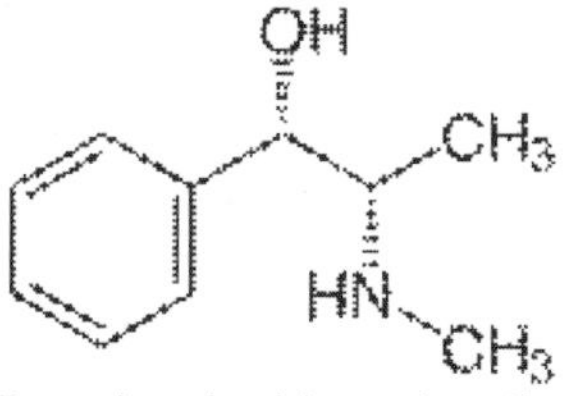 Pseudoephedrine is the diastereomer of ephedrine. It is used similarly to ephedrine (Hodges *et al.*, 2006). It is readily reduced to the more potent methamphetamine or oxidized to methcathinone, which is also bioactive.	Ephedrine is a sympathomimetic, stimulant, anorectic, nootropic, decongestant, and usable to treat hypotension due to anaesthesia. The mode of action relies on indirect stimulation of adrenergic receptors of the sympathetic nervous system (*SNS*). It increases action of noradrenaline at the post-synaptic α- and β-receptors (EPHEDrine, 2014). **Ephedrine vs. Adrenaline** **Ephedrine** 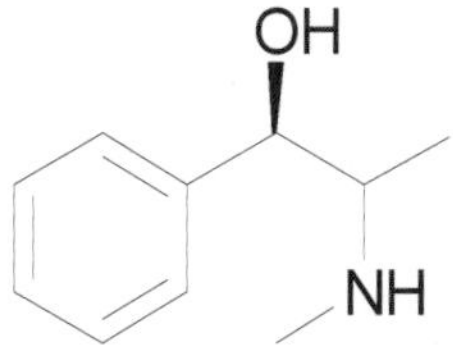 Ephedrine is a phytochemical. **Adrenaline** 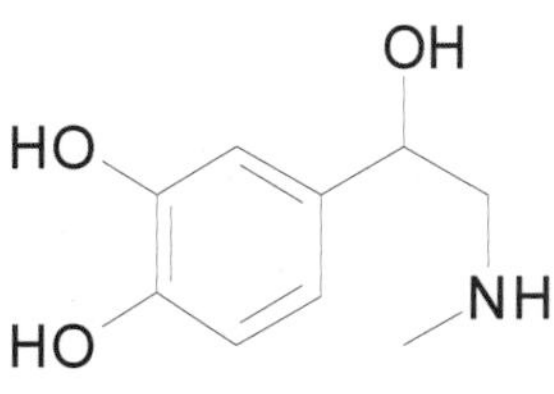	Ephedrine exhibits optical isomerism and has two chiral centres, giving rise to four stereoisomers. By convention the pair of enantiomers with the stereochemistry (1R,2S and 1S,2R) is designated ephedrine, while the pair of enantiomers with the stereochemistry (1R,2R and 1S,2S) is called pseudoephedrine. It is key to note that ephedrine binds better than *N*-methylephedrine, which has an additional methyl group at the N-atom. Also the steric orientation of the OH group is essential for receptor binding and bioactivity (Guoyi *et al.*, 2007).

Contd...

Table 5.1–*Contd...*

Ephedra Alkaloid	*Attributes*	*Pertinent comments*
	Adrenaline (epinephrine) is an adrenal hormone produced by human and other animals	
Norephedrine and Norpseudoephedrine Phenylpropanolamine 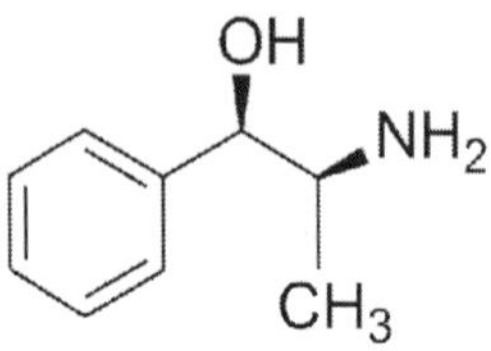 Phenylpropanolamine (PPA) covers both stereoisomers: norephedrine and norpseudoephedrine, which unlike ephedrine or pseudoephedrine lack "CH_3"	**Norephedrine vs. Noradrenaline Norephedrine** 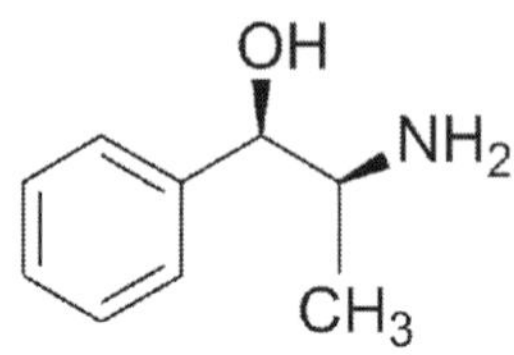 Norephedrine is a phytochemical produced by plants for various ecophysiological purposes **Noradrenaline** 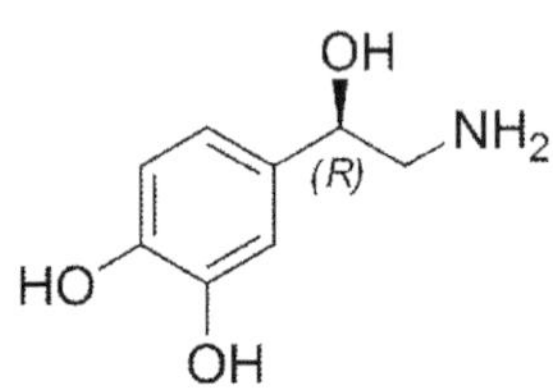 Noradrenaline (norepinephrine) is an adrenal hormone.	Norephedrine and norpseudoephedrine, occur also in *Catha edulis*, along with their isomers. They can easily cross the blood brain barrier, and act like ephedrine and pseudoephedrine. Both are CNS stimulants similar to amphetamines, but less pronounced. Each these compounds can be modified with changes in bioactivity

Table 5.1: The presence of an *N*-methyl group decreases binding affinities at α-receptors, compared with norephedrine. Ephedrine is a substituted amphetamine and a structural methamphetamine analogue. It differs from methamphetamine only by the presence of a hydroxyl (OH). Amphetamines, however, are more potent and have additional biological effects. The isomer which is marketed is (–)-(1R,2S)-ephedrine (Martindale, 1989).

Khat Alkaloids

It is unknown when *Catha edulis* (Celastraceae) – a tropical Angiosperm, popularly called "Khat", began to be used by humans. However, its medicinal uses were first described in the 13th Century by the Islamic physician, Naguibed-Din, who used it to treat depression (Thepoisongarden, 2014). Khat contains cathine and cathinone, and other alkaloids, such as some ephedra alkaloids. These alkaloids are psychoactives and similar to the amphetamines. Khat is a popular stimulant in Africa and the Arabian Peninsula, where it is known by various names – "Abyssinian tea",

"African salad", "African tea", "Arabian tea", and "Yemen tea", among others. Khat's effects are like those of ephedra or amphetamine, and include euphoria, increased alertness and excitement, ability to concentrate, confidence, sociability, contentment and flow of ideas (Thepoisongarden, 2014). Unlike *Ephedra*, which is an only genus of Ephedraceae, an only Gymnosperm family, *Catha* belongs to an Angiosperm family (Celastraceae, "staff vine" or "bittersweet") of about 100 genera (APG, 2009). Table 5.2 shows the structures and attributes of khat alkaloids. Khat alkaloids, like ephedra's, are relatively easy to modify to yield newer drugs.

Use of Ephedra, Khat and other ENAs in "Clandestine Chemistry" and Products

"Clandestine chemistry" refers to chemical production or related activities carried out in secret, make-shift laboratories. Some of the most common products of "clandestine chemistry" are controlled substances, especially amphetamines and other hallucinogens derived from ENAs like those of ephedra, khat, peyote and other

Table 5.2: Structures and Attributes of Khat Alkaloids (chemically modifiable)

Khat Alkaloid	*Attributes*	*Pertinent comments*
Cathine 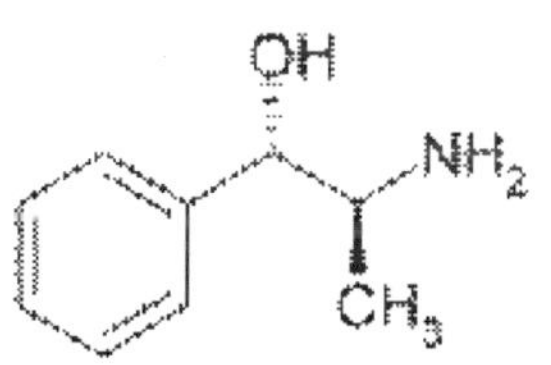 Cathine is an isomer of norpseudoephedrine. It is designated "d-norpseudoephedrine". It is a phenylethylamine, psychoactive, and similar to the amphetamines which act as stimulants. It occurs naturally and commonly in *Catha edulis* (khat) with cathinone, and other ephedra-like alkaloids.	Being like the amphotamines and ephedra-like alkaloids, cathine, acts as a releasing agent of noradrenaline and adrenaline. It also acts as a dopamine releasing agent (DRA) to a lesser extent, which may make it useful in Parkinsonism and related syndromes. **Cathine versus Noradrenaline** **Cathine** – phytochemical 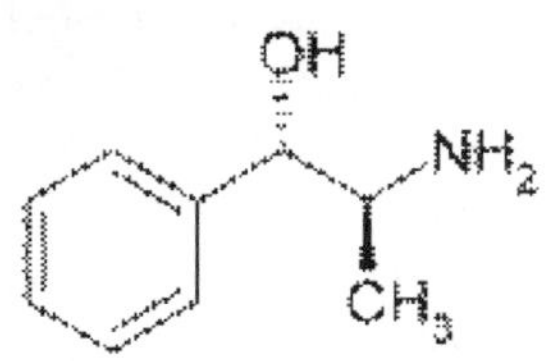 **Noradrenaline** – animal hormone 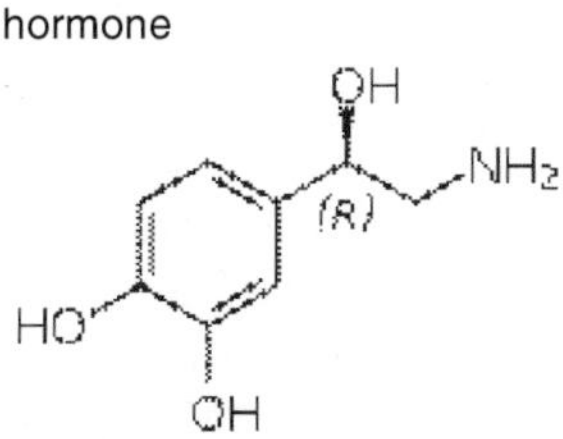	Cathine is one of several optical isomers of phenylpropanolamine (PPA). **Cathine vs. Phenylpropanolamine** **Cathine** 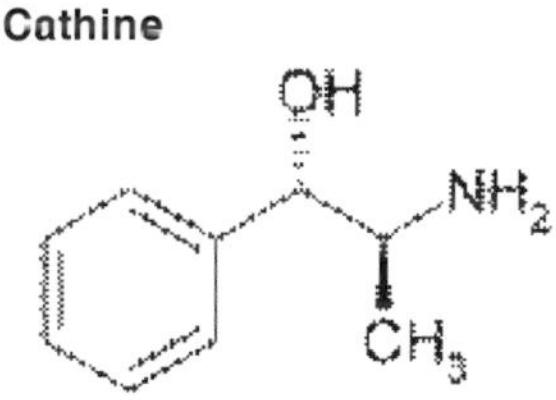 **Phenylpropanolamine** 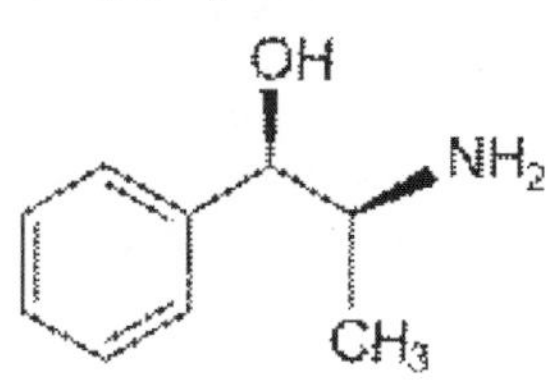 PPA is used to control urinary incontinence in dogs.

Contd...

Table 5.2–*Contd...*

Ephedra Alkaloid	*Attributes*	*Pertinent comments*
Cathinone 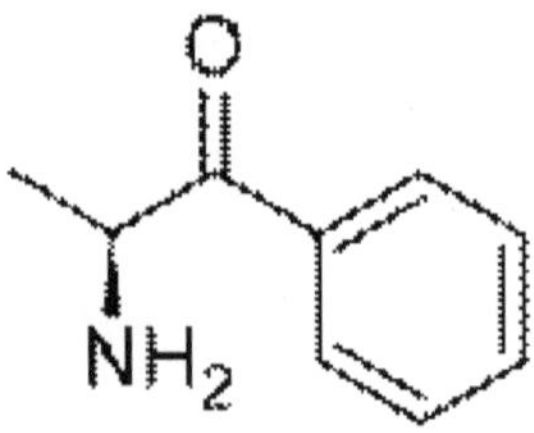 Cathinone is a β-ketone-amphetamine. It occurs in khat, and is similar to ephedrine, cathine, methcathinone and other amphetamines. The differences/similarity of cathinone to related drugs/stimulants are indicated in the middle column.	Cathinone is a key contributor to the stimulant effect of khat. It can induce the release of dopamine from preparations labeled with dopamine (Kalix, 1981).[3] **Cathinone vs. Bupropion and Methcathinone** **Bupropion** 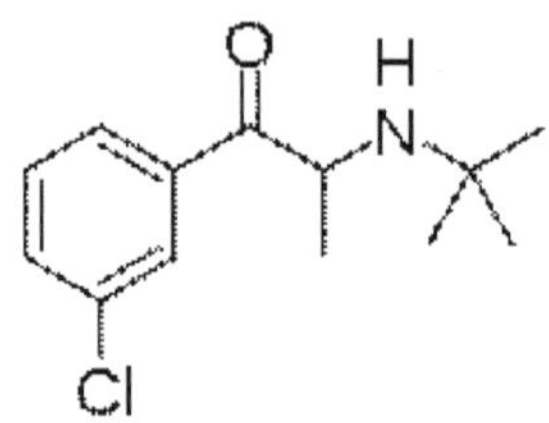 **Methcathinone** 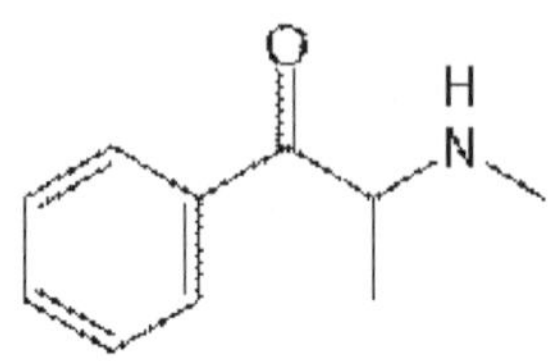 Like cathinone, both bupropion - a clinically important antidepressant, and methcathinone – a stimulant, are synthetic and have a ketone group each.	Cathinone is related to methcathinone, in same way as amphetamine is related to methamphetamine. Cathine, the corresponding alcohol of cathinone is a less potent stimulant than the ketone. Conversion of cathinone to cathine leads to potency loss, which is why fresh leaves have higher ratios f cathinone to cathine than dry ones.

Table 5.2: Over 100 ecstasy-type molecules, eg: MDMA, or 3,4-methylenedioxy-*N*-methylamphetamine (popularly called "ecstasy") have been produced by "Clandestine Chemistry" alone in the last few years DHSFS (2014). "Clandestine Chemistry" is extremely active and vibrant in the USA (DEA, 2012; DEA, 2014). The very large numbers of modified and modifiable ENAs would indicate the immense possibilities that exist for creating newer therapeutic entities from ENA associated with herbalism worldwide.

Spermatophytes or fungi. In some countries, especially in the Americas, such activities or labs are rampant and usually run by organized outfitsthat produce for distribution on the black market "drugs-of-abuse" orother controlled substances. The term "Clandestine Chemistry" or "clandestine lab" is used in any circumstance involving the production of controlled substances, regardless of whether the principle or the facility used for such activities qualify to be called"chemistry" or "laboratory".

Colchicine - a *Colchicum* Alkaloid

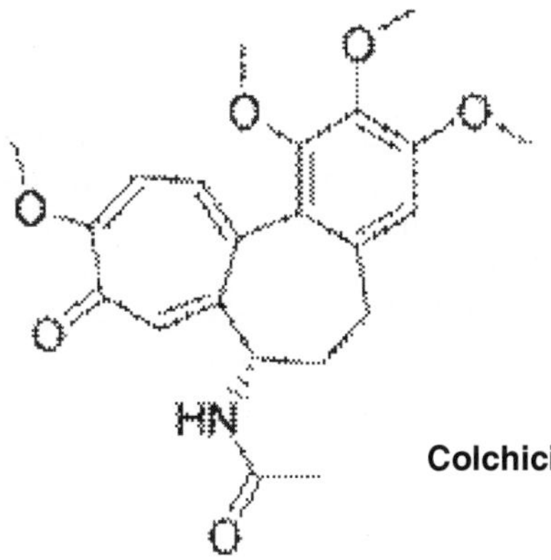

Colchicine – Note that the N is exocyclic

Colchicine is a pale-yellow crystalline alkaloid extracted from seeds or corms of a *Colchicum* species, such as, the "autumn crocus" - *Colchicum autumnale* (Colchicaceae). There are some 160 species of *Colchicum*, among which is *Colchicum melanthioides* - the commonest tropical species (Manning *et al.*, 2007). Colchicine is used in the treatment of Behçet's disease, Mediterranean fever, pericarditis, rheumatism, and especially gout. It is also recommended for its cathartic and emetic effects, but it is toxic. In agriculture, biochemistry, botany and molecular biology colchicine is highly valued for its ability to create polyploid plants by inhibiting chromosome separation during meiosis. Colchicine's use as a medicine dates to antiquity (Hartung, 1954). Colchicine is a tricyclic ENA, and both its pain-relieving and anti-inflammatory effects have been linked to its structure/biochemical attributes (Cocco *et al.*, 2010), namely:

- Colchicine inhibits both meiosis and mitosis by binding to tubulin, which prevents microtubule polymerization – a key event in chromosomal separation and cell division
- Colchicine also inhibits neutrophil motility and activity, leading to a net anti-inflammatory effect.

Colchicine, whose structure is given above, is considered a plant hormone. Its empirical formula and molecular weight are: $C_{22}H_{25}NO_6$ and 399 daltons (Colchicine database, 2014).

Use of a Pro-Drug of Colchicine as Anticancer Treatment

As might be expected from its antimitotic effect, a congener of colchicine designated ZD6126, or ANG453, has been a candidate antitumor drug under development by a UK concern, Angiogene.

The congener, or pro-drug, is a water-soluble phosphate of N-acetylcolchinol, which has a "potential for antiangiogenesis and antineoplastic activities". It is converted *in vivo* to N-acetylcolchinol, which acts by binding selectively to tubulin cytoskeleton of cells of blood vessels that nourish cancerous tissues. The drug also selectively binds the tubulin cytoskeleton of cancer cells. These bindings ultimately result disruption of supplies, apoptosis, and necrosis of both the supply network and the cancer cells (NCI-DD, 2014).

Peyote alkaloids

Peyote - *Lophophora williamsii* (Cactaceae)is a spineless cactus (Lophophora williamsii-GRIN, 2014) from which 5 psychoactive alkaloids (mescaline, anhalonidine, anhalonine, lophophorine, and pellotine) have been isolated (Bruhn *et al.*, 1978; Gabermann, 1978). Of these, only mescaline, which is the most active, is an ENA. All the other 4 are cyclic-N alkaloids (CNA). It is thought that peyote, native to the shrub and desert areas of Texas (USA) and Mexico, had been used by Amerindians for entheogenic purposes since 3,500 BC or earlier (El-Seedi *et al.*, 2005).

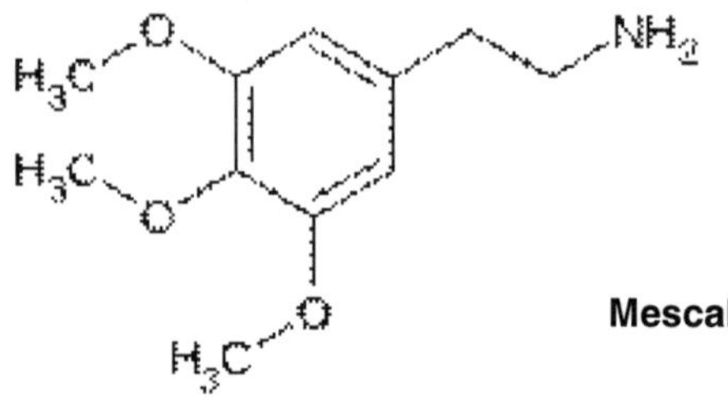

Mescaline – an exocyclic N-alkaloid (ENA)

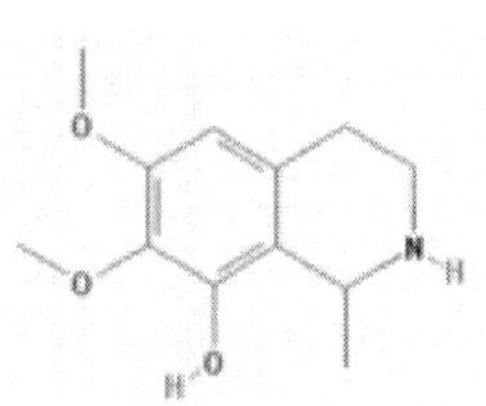

Anhalonidine – a cyclic-N alkaloid (CNA)

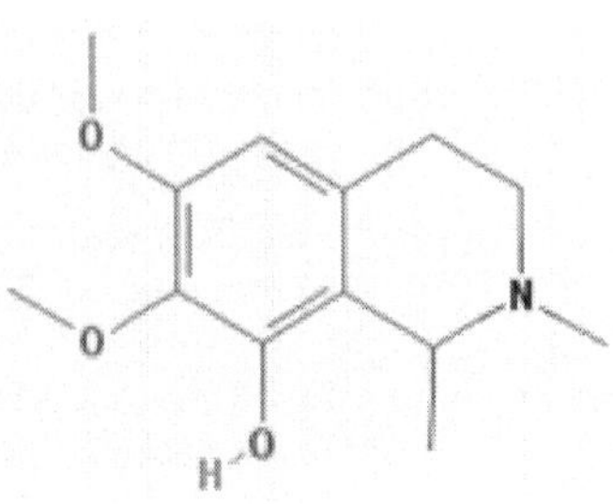

Pellotine – a cyclic-N alkaloid (CNA)

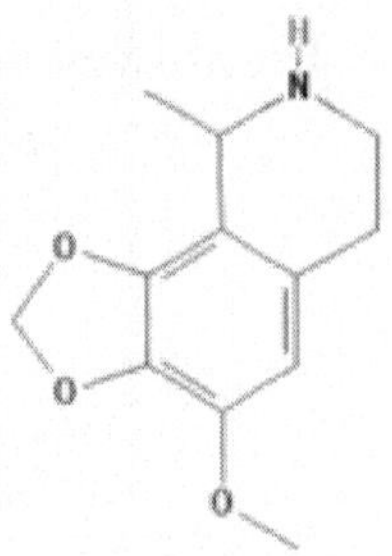

Anhalonine – a cyclic-N alkaloid (CNA)

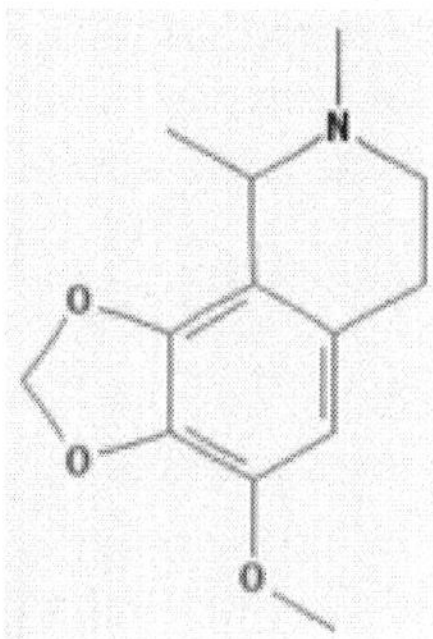

Lophophorine – a cyclic-N alkaloid (CNA)

It may be discerned from the structures above that mescaline has a relatively simple structure that can be modified to yield newer entities with modified pharmacological and toxicological properties. Today peyote, its alkaloids, or their synthetic derivatives are used in many developed countries in America, Asia and Europe as entheogens, supplement to spiritual practices, psychonautics and psychedelic therapeutics, often with little scientific/regulatory backing.

Hordenine – an ENA in many Spermatophytes

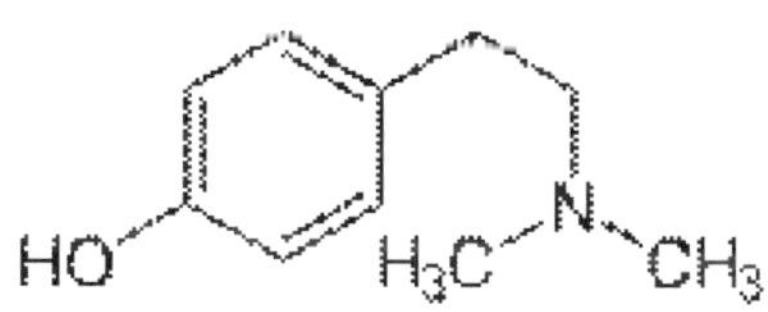

Hordenine – a weak adrenergic stimulant and MAO inhibitor

Pharmacology and Toxicology

Hordenine is an ENA in the class of phenylethylamine that occurs in many plants. It is so called because it occurs in *Hordeum* species (barley). It can be derived from tyrosine, or tyramine, with which it shares some properties (Reti, 1953; Wheaton and Stewart, 1970; Smith, 1977; Poocharoen, 1983; Lundstrom, 1989), namely:

- ☆ Provoking nausea in rabbits.
- ☆ Producing CNS paralysis in frogs.
- ☆ In horse intravenous injection increased respiratory and heart rates and sweating but not temperature or behaviour. But the same dose given orally produced no such effects.
- ☆ In dogs and rats hordenine increased systolic and diastolic blood pressure, and increased the volume of peripheral blood flow. But gut movements were inhibited.
- ☆ Hordenine promoted gastrin release in the rats.
- ☆ Hordenine's LD50 in animals varied very widely from lab to lab. For example, it is: >100 mg/kg in mice by IP; 300 mg/kg in dog by IV; 2000 mg/kg in dog by PO; 250 mg/kg in rabbit by IV; 300 mg/kg in guinea pig by IV; 2000 mg/kg in guinea pig by SC; and ~ 1000 mg/kg in rat by SC.

These findings are variously interpreted to support the view that hordenine act as a weak adrenergic stimulant, ie: acts as an agent that exert its pharmacological effects by promoting the release of stored norepinephrine (Hapke and Strathmann,1995). Hordenine also acts as an MAO-B inhibitor. MAO is an enzyme that breaks down the neurotransmitters phenylethylamine and dopamine among others (Nootriment.com/hordenine, 2014).

Sources among Spermatophytes

Hordenine is present in a fairly wide range of Angiosperms, namely: bitter orange (Sander *et al.*, 2008), cacti (Wheaton and Stewart,1970), and in the seedlings of grasses, such as *Hordeum vulgare* (~ 0.2 per cent w/w), *Panicum miliaceum* (~ 0.2 per cent w/w), and *Sorghum vulgare* (~0.1 per cent). But the richest source of hordenine is the cactus, *Echinopsis candicans*, which was found to contain 0.5-5 per cent of the alkaloid (Reti, 1953; Smith, 1977).

Use of Hordenine

The use of hordenine as a CNS stimulant and promoter of weight loss, by enhancing metabolism, has been criticized on the following ground: In experimental animals, given large doses by injection, hordenine does produce an increase in blood pressure, and other stressful effects on cardio-vascular, respiratory and nervous systems, but these effects were mostly not reproduced by oral administration. Moreover, there is a dearth of data on the effects of hordenine in humans (Reti, 1953; Smith, 1977). Despite this drawback hordenine's molecular simplicity and ready availability make it a useful research tool for structure activity relations.

Comment on the Recent Discovery of a Synthetic ENA in *Nauclea latifolia* (Rubiaceae)

"The analgesic tramadol has been isolated from the root bark of *N. latifolia*, an African medical plant. This finding is a rare example of a common synthetic drug that occurs at considerable concentrations in nature." Boumendjel and co-workers (2013).Tramadol is described as "a centrally-acting opioid analgesic used to treat moderate to severe pain". However, from a structural point of view it is an "exocyclic-N alkaloid (ENA)". The structures of tramadol and morphine (a cyclic and opioid alkaloid) are shown below:

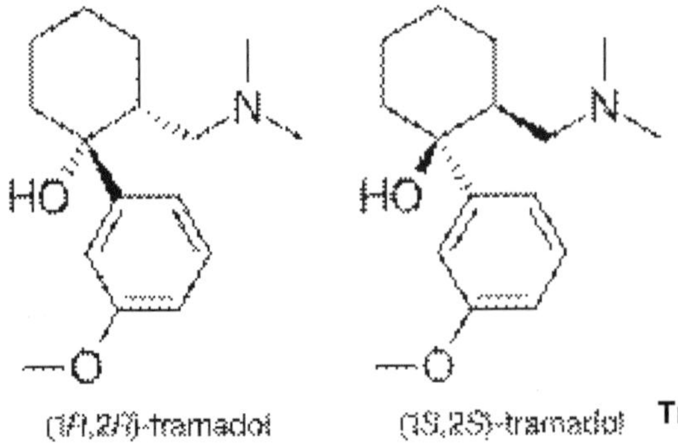

Tramadol: an exocyclic-N alkaloid

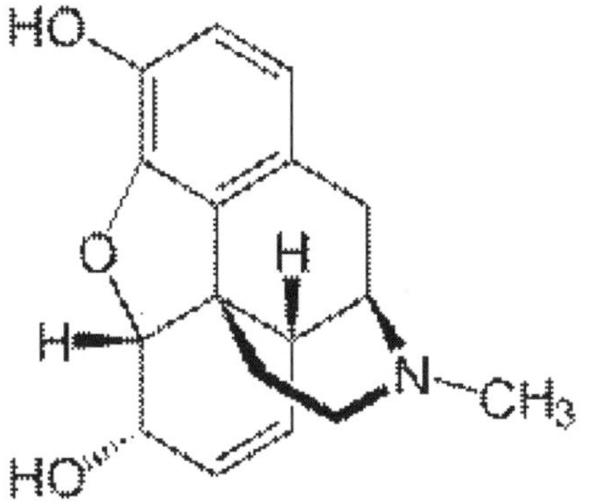

Morphine: a cyclic-N alkaloid

Tramadol was initially launched and marketed as "Tramal" by Grünenthal GmbH in 1977 in the then West Germany. It is marketed as a racemic mixture of both R and S stereoisomers (Martindale, 2014). This is because the two isomers complement each other's analgesic activity. It is often combined with paracetamol (acetaminophen) as this is known to improve the efficacy of tramadol in relieving pain (Martindale, 2014). Tramadol is a reuptake inhibitor of noradrenaline (norepinephrine) and serotonin (5-HT) and a weak μ-opioid receptor agonist (Reimann and Schneider, 1998; Gobbi *et al.*, 2002). It is metabolized to O-desmethyltramadol, a significantly more potent opioid (Martindale, 2014). Until a few months ago, biomedical scientists, chemists, herbalists, and physicians thought that the molecular entity called "Tramadol" was a purely "synthetic opioid" (Martindale, 2014). No one imagined that nature already had this entity, which is from one of NIPRD's pet plants - *Nauclea latifolia* (Rubiaceae) – the "herbal substance" of Niprd-AM1 (Gamaniel, 2008; Ameh *et al.*, 2010a, 2013, 2014).

Outline of Methods Used in Drug Discovery from Herbalism

Herbalism and Ethnobotanical Research

Herbalism, herbal medicine, or phytotherapy is the study and/or use of plant materials to prevent and treat ill health or promote wellness (Ameh *et al.*, 2010b). It dates to antiquity and is the backbone of ethnomedicine or traditional medicine (TM) worldwide. TM was formally defined and recognized in 1978 by the World Health Assembly at Alma-ata (WHO, 1978). Various WHO publications (WHO, 1993; WHO, 1998; WHO, 2000) provide guidelines and methodologies for research and regulation of herbalism (Ameh *et al.*, 2010b). WHO does not delve into advance research in herbalism, but provides guidelines that underpin drug discovery research and clinical trials (WHO, 1995; Ameh *et al.*, 2011, 2012). Drug discovery and clinical trials are largely undertaken in the industrialized countries of America, Asia and Europe, by the research and development divisions of large drug and biotechnology firms in collaboration with universities, and regulated by State institutions like the US-Drug Administration (US-FDA).

Drug Discovery and Development from Plants used in Herbalism

While herbal medicine (HM) uses crude or marginally processes plant parts, conventional medicine (CM) mostly uses highly purified chemical entities. Such entities, if obtained from plants, partly or wholly, may be called "phytomedicines" but not "herbal medicines". A phytomedicine may be a single chemical or a mixture of several, including synthetics. In the following sections drug discovery and development will focus on the search for a single chemical entity that accounts for a defined bioactivity or pharmacological effect of an herbal medicine, and the development of that entity into a new product, referred to hereafter as "new drug" (ND). Most of what will follow is generic, but where possible, will focus on ENAs occurring in defined extracts of defined plants from defined locations.

Extraction/Isolation of Alkaloid Fraction/Bioactivity/Structure Elucidation/Optimization

Special methods have been developed for isolating economically useful alkaloids. The general procedure is as follows:

- ✰ In most cases, plant tissue is processed to obtain aqueous solutions of the alkaloids.
- ✰ The alkaloids are then recovered from the solution by any of several extraction processes such pH-dependent precipitation with select bases, followed by dissolution/extraction with a water-immiscible solvent such as diethylether or chloroform.
- ✰ Column or other types of chromatography can separate/purify select alkaloids from mixtures.
- ✰ Suitable biological tests (*e.g.* antimicrobial, enzymological, or pharmacological) can be conducted on fractions to determine their levels of activity.
- ✰ The extent of fractionation or purification can followed by continual determination of bioactivity, a process termed "bioactivity guided fractionation"– a common approach for both pharmacologic (Huang *et al.*, 2011) and antimicrobial agents (Boligon *et al.*, 2013).

Drug discovery may also involve more elaborate steps/procedures, including:

- ✰ Use of high through put (HTP) screening procedures, in which larges number of samples are rapidly analyzed to identify fractions or compounds with the desired bioactivity (hits).
- ✰ Subjection of such hits to detailed chemical studies to establish its profile as a drug molecule. These may, for example, involve:
- ✰ Wet chemistry, TLC, and simple physicochemical studies.
- ✰ Application of a suitable hyphenated technique such as liquid or gas chromatography-mass spectrometry (LC-MS or GC-MS), which allows compounds to be identified based on their mass/charge ratio, after ionization.

- ✰ Nuclear magnetic resonance (NMR) spectroscopy is a key technique used to determine the characteristics of individual hydrogen and carbon atoms within the molecule, thereby allowing detailed reconstruction of the molecule's structure.
- ✰ Optimization of hits so as to increase their drug-likeness requires that the structures be known. The aim of optimization is to increase, if necessary, the candidate drug's drug-likeness, *i.e.,* to increase its: i) affinity and selectivity for the target receptor (to reduce potentials of side effects); ii) efficacy or potency and metabolic stability (to increase efficiency and duration of action); and oral bioavailability, if necessary, for convenience.

Once a hit, *i.e.,* a compound that fulfills these requirements has been identified, it may then commence the often perilous process of "drug development" prior to "clinical trials".

In some scenarios, where the compound of interest is known, such is simply isolated, with the aim of modifying it chemically to generate a new candidate drug that may, if needs be, undergo further "development" prior to "clinical trials". Other scenarios may involve application of techniques, such as, combinatorial chemistry libraries and computer-aided drug design. Usually the "candidate drug" or the eventual "new drug" is envisaged to be a "small molecule" (length or diameter ≤1nm; molecular weight ≤900 Dalton).

Comments on Drug Discovery and Development Outside Herbalism

Although drug discovery using chemical libraries of synthetic small molecules is modern and laudable and has recorded successes, the process is still not only uncertain voyage but can prove to be a wild-goose chase and a financial Russian roulette. For this reason, only a few, rich and privileged companies worldwide actually and fully engage in it. Some 5 years ago, the cost of discovering and developing a new drug was estimated to be 1.8 billion USD (Paul *et al.,* 2010), up from about 800 million in 2005. Thus, drug discovery and development from outside herbalism is extremely capitalist, as the real end product is a "patent". Thereafter, the prospective drug commences another costly voyage through Phase I, II and III clinical trials, which most fail. Therefore, to minimize risks and costs, the venture from chemical libraries that may be a success, involves complex interplays between a firm with a strong R&D, academia, patent laws, competent and transparent regulators, a vibrant polity, and a huge capital outlay. By contrast, the venture from herbalism requires far less capital, and entails far less risks. This is because the long use of TM plants provides reasonable assurances of efficacy or tolerability or both, and hence a brighter chance of success.

Combinatorial Chemistry and Herbalism as Sources of New Drugs

Despite the rise of combinatorial chemistry and computer-aided drug design in drug discovery and development, phytochemicals discovered from herbalism continue to play the major or critical role as starting materials for drug discovery (Feher and Schmidt, 2003). Of the 974 small molecule new chemical entities that featured in 1981-2006 as prospective drugs 63 per cent were natural products or their derivatives (Newman and Cragg, 2007). For those in the classes of antimicrobials, antineoplastics, antihypertensive and anti-inflammatory drugs, the percentages were even higher than 63 per cent. Moreover, in most instances the phytomedicines were discovered from herbalism. On the whole, a comparison of combinatorial library synthetics with natural products from herbalism reveals the following(Feher and Schmidt, 2003):

- Synthetics cover only a limited and uniform chemical space, whereas existing drugs and natural products exhibit greater diversity and distribution within a greater chemical space
- Structure rigidity/number of chiral centers are much higher in natural compounds
- Heterocycles with O and N are more common in natural products
- Non-aromatic unsaturation is more common in natural products

Since structure rigidity and chirality are both well-established to enhance compounds specificity and efficacy as drugs, it may be concluded that natural products still offer the better opportunities for drug discovery and development than do combinatorial chemistry libraries.

Conclusion

While developing countries like Nigeria and research institutions like the Nigerian Institute for Pharmaceutical Research and Development (NIPRD) should pursue relevant research in any area in which they have a comparative advantage and capability, it seems from the foregoing that priority and focus should be given to the following:

- Rigorous documentation of all traditional herbal remedies and identification of the most promising
- Development of promising herbal remedies with a view to modernizing and maximizing their traditional usage
- Rigorous and detailed study of medicinal plants with respect to their cultivation, the types of phytochemicals they produce, the factors that cause them to produce particular phytochemicals, and how best to extract/process such phytochemicals
- Liaise with registered herbalists, select universities andteaching hospitals, industries, and the national drug regulatory agency, with a view to:
    - Developing herbal medicines based on proven traditional herbalism
    - Developing phytomedicines, phytopharmaceuticals, and synthetics based natural product scaffolds.

Such an approach will make for greater productive and efficiency in resource utilization, which should at any rate include a suitably staffed and equipped Advanced Biology-Chemistry Laboratory (ABC-Lab).

References

Abourashed, E. A., El-Alfy, A. T., Khan, I. A., and Walker, L. (2003). Ephedra in perspective – a current review.*Phytotherapy Research,***17**: 703–712.

Ameh,S. J., Obodozie, O. O., Gamaniel, S.K., Abubakar, M. S., and Garba, M (2010a). Physicochemical variables and real time stability of the herbal substance of Niprd-AM1®- an antimalarial developed from the root of *Nauclea latifolia* S.M. (Rubiaceae). *International Journal of Phytomedicine*, **2**: 332-340.

Ameh, S. J., Obodozie, O. O., Inyang, U. S., Abubakar, M. S., and Garba, M. (2010b). Current phytotherapy - a perspective on the science and regulation of herbal medicine. *Journal of Medicinal Plants Research*, **4(2)**: 072-081.

Ameh, S. J., Obodozie, O. O., Chindo, B. A., Babalola, P. C., and Gamaniel, K. S. (2012). Herbal clinical trials-historical development and application in the 21st century. *Pharmacologia*, **3**: 121-131.

Ameh, S. J., Obodozie, O. O., Babalola, P. C., and Gamaniel, K. S. (2011). Medical herbalism and herbal clinical research: *A Global Perspective. British Journal of Pharmaceutical Research*, **1(4)**: 99-123.

Ameh Sunday, Mujtaba Abubakar, Aminu Ambi, Patrick Ikokoh, Obiageri Obodozie, Magaji Garba and Herbert Cocker (2013). Phytochemical, physicochemical and chromatographic profiling in quality control systems for select herbal medicines (Conavir and Niprd-AM1).*British Journal of Pharmaceutical Research*, **3(1)**: *13-36.*

Ameh, S. J., Ibekwe, N., Ambi, A., Obodozie, O., Abubakar, M., Garba, M., Cocker, H., and Gamaniel, K. S. (2014). Standardization of *Andrographis paniculata*, *Mitracarpus scaber*, and *Nauclea latifolia* herbal preparations as per European and Nigerian Drug Regulations. *European Journal of Medicinal Plants*, **4(4)**: 413-443.

APG (2009). Angiosperm Phylogeny Group (2009). An update of the Angiosperm Phylogeny Group classification for the orders and families of flowering plants: APG III. *Botanical Journal of the Linnean Society*, **161 (2)**: 105–121.

Boligon, A. A., Kubica, T. F., Mario, D. N., de Brum, T. F., Piana, M., Weiblen, R., Lovato, L., Alves, S. H., Santos, R. C. V., Alves, C. F. S., and Athayde, M. L. (2013). Antimicrobial and antiviral activity-guided fractionation from *Scutia buxifolia* Reissek extracts. *Acta Physiologiae Plantarum*, **35(7)**: 2229-39.

Botany of Haoma (2014). *Encyclopædia Iranica*. http: //www.iranicaonline.org/ articles/haoma-i Accessed 2014 April 15

Boumendjel, A., Sotoing, T. G., Ngo, B. E., Chabrol, T., Beney, C., Sinniger, V., Haudecoeur, R., Marcourt, L., Challal, S., Ferreira,Q. E., Souard, F., LeBorgne, M., Lomberget, T., Depaulis, A., Lavaud, C., Robins, R., Wolfender, J. L., Bonaz, B., and DeWaard, M. (2013). Occurrence of the synthetic analgesic tramadol in an African medicinal plant.*Angewandte Chemie International Edition*, **52 (45)**: 11780–11784.

Bruhn, J. G., Linggren, J. E., Homstedt, B., and Adovasio, J. M. (1978). Peyote Alkaloids: Identification in a Prehistoric Specimen of *Lophophora* from Coahuila, Mexico. *Science 31 March 1978: 199(4336): 1437-1438.DOI: 10.1126/science.199.4336.1437*

Cocco, G., Chu, D. C. C., and Pandolfi, S. (2010). Colchicine in clinical medicine.A guide for internists. *European Journal of Internal Medicine,* **21 (6)**: 503. doi: 10.1016/ j.ejim.2010.09.010. PMID 21111934.

Colchicine database (2014). Colchicine: Biotoxin. Emergency Response Safety Database. National Institute for Occupational Safety and Health (NIOSH) http: //www.cdc.gov/niosh/

Das, R. P. (1985). "On the Identification of a Vedic Plant" in Meulenbeld, G. J. and Wujastyk, D. eds., *Studies on Indian Medical History: Papers Presented at the International Workshop on the Study of Indian Medicine Held at the Wellcome Institute for the History of Medicine, 2-4 Sept.* 1985, Groningen Oriental Studies 2, Groningen, 1987, pp. 19-42.

DEA (2012). Methamphetamine Lab Incidents 2004-2012. http: //www.justice.gov/ dea/resource-center/meth-lab-maps.shtml Accessed 2014 April 18

DEA (2014). DEA Domestic Drug Seizures ('Methamphetamine' column). http: // www.justice.gov/dea/resource-center/statistics.shtml##seizuresAccessed 2014 April 18

DHSFS (2014).Methylenedioxymethamphetamine (MDMA, Ecstasy).Drug and Human Society Fact Sheet. http: //www.nhtsa.gov/people/injury/research/ job185drugs/methylenedioxymethamphetamine.htm

El-Seedi, H. R., De Smet, P. A., Beck, O., Possnert, G., and Bruhn, J. G. (2005). Prehistoric peyote use: alkaloid analysis and radiocarbon dating of archaeological specimens of Lophophora from Texas. *J Ethnopharmaco.*, **101(1–3)**: 238–42.

Ephedrine (2014).Ephedrine.Merck Manuals. www.merckmanuals.com/ professional/lexicon/ephedrine.html Accessed 2014 April 15.

Ephedrinediet (2014). What Are The Ephedra Alkaloids? http: //ephedrinediet.org/ ephedra-alkaloids/#sthash.ug7p4OJz.dpuf Accessed 2014 April 13.

Feher, M., and Schmidt, J. M. (2003). Property distributions: differences between drugs, natural products, and molecules from combinatorial chemistry. *J. Chem. Inf. Comput. Sci.,* **43 (1)**: 218–27.

Gabermann, V. (1978). Estimation of mescaline and pellotine in Lophophora coulter plants (Cactaceae) by means of the oscillographic polarography. *Biokhimiia (Moscow, Russia)*, **43(2)**: 246–51. PMID 647075.

Gamaniel, K. (2008). A comparative randomized clinical trial of NIPRD AM1 against a chloroquine and sulphadoxine/pyrimethamine combination in symptomatic but uncomplicated malaria. *African Journal of Traditional, Complementary and Alternative medicines (AJTCAM), Abstracts of the World Congress on Medicinal and Aromatic* Plants, Cape Town, November 2008.

Gobbi M, Moia M, Pirona L, Ceglia, I., Reyes-Parada, M., Scorza, C., and Mennini, T. (2002). "p-Methylthioamphetamine and 1-(m-chlorophenyl) piperazine, two non-neurotoxic 5-HT releasers in vivo, differ from neurotoxic amphetamine derivatives in their mode of action at 5-HT nerve endings in vitro". *Journal of Neurochemistry,* **82(6)**: 1435–43. doi: 10.1046/j.1471-4159.2002.01073.x. PMID 12354291.

Grycová, L., Dostál, J., and Marek, R. (2007). Quaternary protoberberine alkaloids. *Phytochemistry,* **68(2)**: 150-175.

Guoyi, M., Bavadeka, S. A., Davis, Y. M., Lalchandani S. G., Nagmani R., Schaneberg, B. T., Kan, I. A., and Feller, D. R. (2007). Pharmacological effects of ephedrine alkaloids on human {α}1- and {α}2-adrenergic receptor subtypes. *J. Pharmacol. Exp. Ther.,* **322(1)**: 214-221.

Hapke, H. J., and Strathmann, W. (1995). "Pharmacological effects of hordenine." *Dtsch. Tierarztl.Wochenschr.,* 1**02**: 228-232.

Hartung, E. F. (1954). History of the Use of Colchicum and related Medicaments in Gout. *Ann Rheum Dis.,* 1**3 (3)**: 190–200. doi: 10.1136/ard.13.3.190

Hodges, K., Hancock, S., Currel, K., Hamilton, B., and Jeukendrup, A. E. (2006). Pseudoephedrine enhances performance in 1500-m runners. *US National Library of Medicine National Institutes of Health,* **38 (2)**: 329–33. doi: 10.1249/01.mss.0000183201.79330.9c. PMID 16531903.

Huang, L. Z., Huang, B. K., Ye, Q., and Quin, L. P. (2011). Bioactivity-guided fractionation for anti-fatigue property of *Acanthopanax senticosus. J. Ethnopharmacol.,* **133(1)**: 213-9.

Johnson, T. M., and Sargent, C. F. (1996). Ethnopharmacology: The Conjunction of Medical Ethnography and the Biology of Therapeutic Action. *Medical Anthropology: Contemporary Theory and Method*. Westport, Connecticut: Praeger Publishers.

Kalix, P. (1981). Cathinone, an alkaloid from khat leaves with an amphetamine-like releasing effect. *Psychopharmacology* (*Berl.*),**74 (3)**: 269–70. doi: 10.1007/BF00427108. PMID 6791236. Accessed 2014 April 17

Lophophora williamsii-GRIN (2014). *Lophophora williamsii* information from NPGS/GRIN.*GRIN* taxonomy for plants. http: //www.ars-grin.gov/cgi-bin/npgs/html/taxon.pl?22667 Accessed 2014 April 22

Lundstrom, J. (1989). β-Phenethylamines and ephedrines of plant origin. In *The Alkaloids, Vol. 35 (A. Brossi, Ed.) pp. 77-154.*

Manning, J., Forest, F., and Vinnersten, A. (2007), The genus *Colchicum* L. redefined to include *Androcymbium* Willd. based on molecular evidence. *Taxon,* **56**: 872-882.

Martindale (1989). *Martindale: The complete drug reference* 29th Ed. By Reynolds JEF, ed.London: Pharmaceutical Press. ISBN 0-853690-6.

Martindale (2013). Tramadol Hydrochloride. *Martindale: The Complete Drug Reference.* Edited by Brayfield, A. Pharmaceutical Press.

NCI-DD (2014).ZD6126. Code ANG453. NCI Drug Dictionary.National Cancer Institute website.http: //www.cancer.gov/drugdictionary?CdrID=3531532014 April 19

Newman, D. J., and Cragg, G. M. (2007).Natural products as sources of new drugs over the last 25 years. *J. Nat. Prod.*, **70 (3)**: 461–77.

Nootriment.com/hordenine (2014) http: //nootriment.com/hordenine/ #sthash.EsThIm5g.dpuf Accessed 2014 April 24.

Paul, S. M., Mytelka, D. S., Dunwiddie, C. T., Persinger, C. C., Munos, B. H., Lindborg, S. R., and Schacht, A. L. (2010). How to improve R and D productivity: the pharmaceutical industry's grand challenge. *Nat Rev Drug Discov.*, **9(3)**: 203–14. doi: 10.1038/nrd3078. PMID 20168317.

Poocharoen, B. (1983). Determination of selected secondary and tertiary amine alkaloids in barley malt. PhD Thesis, Oregon State University. http: // ir.library.oregonstate.edu/xmlui/handle/1957/27227

Prince, R. J., and Sine, S. M. (2008). Epibatidine activates muscle acetylcholine receptors with unique site selectivity. *Biophysical Journal*, **75(4)**: 1817–27. doi: 10.1016/ S0006-3495(98)77623-4. PMC 1299853.PMID 9746523

Qi, Z. (2014). Traditional Medicine: Definitions. Traditional and Complementary Medicine. WHO/Geneva. http: //www.who.int/medicines/areas/ traditional/definitions/en/

Reimann, W., and Schneider, F. (1998). Induction of 5-hydroxytryptamine release by tramadol, fenfluramine and reserpine.*European Journal of Pharmacology*, **349(2–3)**: 199–203. doi: 10.1016/S0014-2999(98)00195-2. PMID 9671098.

Reti, L. (1953). In *The Alkaloids*, Vol. III, (R. H. F. Manske and H. L. Holmes, Eds.), pp. 313-338, New York: Academic Press.

Sander, L.C., Putzbach, K., Nelson, B.C., Rimmer, C.A., Bedner, M., Thomas, J.B., Porter, B.J., Wood, L.J., Schantz, M.M., Murphy, K.E., Sharpless, K.E., Wise, S.A., Yen, J.H., Siitonen, P.H., Evans, R.L., Nguyen Pho, A., Roman, M.C., and Betz, J.M. (2008). Certification of standard reference materials containing bitter orange. *Anal Bioanal Chem.*, **391(6)**: 2023-34.

Smith, T. A. (1977). Phenethylamine and related compounds in plants.*Phytochem.*, **16**: 9-18.

Thepoisongarden (2014). Catha edulis, khat.THE POISON GARDEN website http: / /www.thepoisongarden.co.uk/atoz/catha_edulis.htm Accessed 2014 April 16.

Wheaton, T. A., and Stewart, I. (1970). The distribution of tyramine, N-methyltyramine, hordenine, octopamine, and synephrine in higher plants. *Lloydia*, **33(2)**: 244-54.

WHO (1978). Declaration of Alma-Ata. International Conference on Primary Health Care, Alma-Ata, USSR, 6-12 September 1978. WHO/Geneva. http: // www.who.int/publications/almaata_declaration_en.pdf

WHO (1993). Research Guidelines for Evaluating the Safety and Efficacy of Herbal Medicines.WHO/Geneva.http: //apps.who.int/medicinedocs/en/d/Jh2946e/5.3.2.html

WHO (1995).Guidelines for good clinical practice (GCP) for trials on pharmaceutical products. WHO Technical Report Series, No. 850, 1995, Annex 3. WHO/Geneva.http: //apps.who.int/medicinedocs/collect/medicinedocs/pdf/whozip13e/whozip13e.pdf

WHO (1998). Quality Control Methods for Medicinal Plant Materials. World Health Organization, Geneva, 1998. 128 p.

WHO (2000). General guidelines for methodologies on research and evaluation of traditional medicine (Document WHO/EDM/TRM/2000.1). 2000. World Health Organization, Geneva. p. 184.

Bioactive Phytochemicals: Perspectives for Modern Medicine Vol. 3 (2015) *Pages* **177–199**
Editor: **V.K. Gupta**
Published by: **DAYA PUBLISHING HOUSE, NEW DELHI**

6

Naringin: A Citrus Flavonone Inhibits the Benzo[a]pyrene (BaP)-Induced Forestomach Carcinogenesis in Mice

Ganesh Chandra Jagetia[1]*

ABSTRACT

The chemopreventive activity of 1, 2.5, 5, 10, 25, 50, 100 or 250 mg/kg b. wt. naringin (NIN), a citrus flavonone was studied on the benzo[a]pyrene (BaP)-induced forestomach carcinoma in female Swiss albino mice. NIN was given before (pre-treatment), after (post-treatment) or both (pre-post-treatment) orally or intraperitoneally to mice receiving BaP for the induction of chemical carcinogenesis. The optimum chemopreventive dose was found to be 10 mg/kg p.o. and oral administration was more effective than the intraperitoneal treatment. A maximum chemopreventive activity of NIN was observed when it was given during and after the termination of BaP treatment. The tumor incidence and tumor multiplicity were reduced in a NIN dose dependent manner, and a highest reduction of 78 per cent in tumor multiplicity was observed at 10 mg/kg, where a 20 per cent reduction in tumor incidence was also observed. However, a reduced chemopreventive effect was observed when NIN was given either before or after chemically induced carcinogenesis. These observations were further confirmed by PCNA labeling where NIN pretreatment reduced the PCNA labeling index by four folds. The micronuclei analysis in splenocytes also confirms to the chemopreventive activity of NIN. BaP treatment increased the frequency of micronuclei bearing splenocytes (MNBNC) by six folds. NIN treatment during and after BaP administration reduced the frequency of MNBNC in a dose dependent manner up to 10 mg/kg where a highest reduction in MNBNC was observed, thereafter the frequency of MNBNC showed a marginal increase up to a dose of 250 mg/kg NIN however, it was two folds lower than BaP treatment alone. A similar effect on MNBNC decline was observed for pre or post-NIN treated group however,

1 Department of Zoology, Mizoram University, Aizawl – 796 004, India
* *Corresponding author*: E-mail: gc.jagetia@gmail.com

the degree of decline in MNBNC was lesser when compared to pre-post NIN treatment. Our study demonstrates, that the NIN possesses chemopreventive activity and this may be due to reduction in DNA damage as evidenced by lower frequency of MNBNC in the group treated with NIN during and after chemical carcinogenesis.

Keywords: Chemoprevention, Naringin, Micronuclei, Forestomach carcinoma, Mice.

Introduction

Carcinogenesis is a complex interactions between several factors, both exogenous (environmental) and endogenous (genetic, hormonal and/or immunological). Numerous evidences indicate that 50-80 per cent of human cancers can be prevented, because the factors responsible for carcinogenesis are largely exogenous. The several exogenous cancer causing agents or factors identified in humans include: cigarette smoking, occupational and environmental chemicals, radiation, dietary factors, trace metals, metabolic factor, specific viruses, bacteria and parasites (Sporn, 1999; Wogan *et al.*, 2004; Kew, 2009). Environmental pollutants are one of the main risk factors for the induction of cancer and are major public health concern and also a leading cause of death in both developing and developed countries (Wogan *et al.*, 2004). These pollutants include BaP, which is a polycyclic aromatic hydrocarbon (PAH) formed by the pyrolytic process during smoking of cigarettes and other tobacco products as well as in combusted organic matter in automobile exhaust (Wogan *et al.*, 2004). BaP is frequently used as a representative indicator of total PAH levels. It is a complete carcinogen, as it produces initiation and promotion of carcinogenesis (Halliwell and Gutteridge, 1989; Ravindra *et al.*, 2008). BaP, a PAH, is released into the atmosphere from incomplete combustion processes. Humans ingest BaP and other PAHs from charbroiled meat, cigarette smoke, and automobile emissions (Collins *et al.*, 1991; Reinik *et al.*, 2007; Zhang and Tao, 2009; Hoh *et al.*, 2012). CYP-mediated metabolic activation of BaP is necessary for its conversion to form the reactive metabolite, BaP 7,8-diol-9,10-epoxide, which binds to DNA and initiates tumor formation (Levin *et al.*, 1982; Miranda *et al.*, 2006). The cytochrome P450 (CYP)-dependent monooxygenase system consists of CYP, NADPH-CYP reductase, and phospholipids. This monooxygenase plays a major role in the detoxification and bioactivation of xenobiotics including drugs, environmental pollutants, and chemical carcinogens (Guengerich, 1988; Nebert, 1989). The importance of the metabolic activation of BaP has led to the suggestion that inhibitors of BaP hydroxylation (AHH) activity could diminish the mutagenicity and carcinogenicity of BaP (Cassady *et al.*, 1990; Castonguay, 1992). Many studies on rat hepatic CYP enzymes have suggested that CYPs including CYP1A, CYP2C, and CYP3A were involved in the oxidation of BaP (Wood *et al.*, 1976, Shimada, and Fujii-Kuriyama, 2004). CYP1A has the highest AHH activity and CYP3A is the most abundant CYP in mammalian livers (Wood *et al.*, 1976; Bauer *et al.*, 1995; Uppstad *et al.*, 2010). CYP1A1 and CYP1A2 are two major members of the CYP1A subfamily. CYP1A2 is the main hepatic CYP1A member and CYP1A1 is essentially an extrahepatic CYP1A in rodents and humans (Guengerich, 1995).

In spite of great advances made in the clinical management of neoplastic disorders the stated goal of NCI to reduce the cancer related mortality by 50 per cent by the year 2000 has not been met. This has led to the thinking that instead of curing the cancer, its occurrence shall be prevented. This can be achieved by pharmacological intervention with certain chemical compounds. Cancer chemoprevention is recognized as the prevention, inhibition or reversal of carcinogenesis by intervention with chemical substances, which can be administered either as individual drugs or as naturally occurring dietary constituents. Human beings consume several natural products in their daily diet. Many dietary ingredients have been found to alter the development of tumors in experimental animals (Slaga, 1980). Dietary habits have also been linked to various types of cancers (Weisburger, 1991; Reddy *et al.*, 1992).

Fruits and certain vegetables have been found to reduce the risk of cancer (Singletary, 2000). Grapefruit is part of human diet in most countries, where it is usually consumed as a juice. The chemical responsible for the characteristic sour odour of the fruit is NIN, a flavonone that is rapidly transformed into naringenin by the action of enzymes α-rhamnosidase and β-glucosidase (Kim *et al.*, 1998). NIN (glycone of naringenin), a grapefruit bioflavonoid, has been demonstrated as an antioxidant, anti-cancer, radioprotective, free radical scavenging and potent cholesterol-lowering agent (Kroyer, 1986; Francis *et al.*, 1989; Haenen, 1997; Shin *et al.*, 1999; Jagetia and Reddy, 2002; Jagetia *et al.*, 2003). The genotoxicity study of NIN in Ames/Salmonella system (strains TA98 and TA100), showed a 36 per cent reduction in BaP induced DNA damage and it was found to be non-mutagenic (Calomme *et al.*, 1996). It has also been reported to protect rat hepatocytes against the damage induced by 2-amine-1-methyl-6-phenylimidazo (4,5-b) pyridine (Lake *et al.*, 1999). NIN is a potent inhibitor of P450 1A2 protein levels in vivo, which is a major P4501A protein present in the mouse and human liver (Ueng *et al.*, 1999). NIN interferes with BaP induced carcinogenesis because of its BaP (a) pyrene AHH inhibitory activity (Ueng *et al.*, 1999). Our main interest was to know whether NIN, a dietary bioflavonoid would be able to reduce the BaP-induced carcinogenesis and genotoxicity in mice or not? If so what is the optimum dose and best route of administration. Therefore, present study was conceptualized to obtain an insight into the chemopreventive activity of NIN in BaP-induced forestomach carcinoma in mice.

Materials and Methods

Benzo(a)pyrene [BaP purity > 98 per cent Cat no. B 1760] was procured from Sigma Chemical Company, St. Louis, MO, USA. Naringin was procured from Acors Organics Ltd, Geel, Belgium. Proliferating Cell Nuclear Antigen (PCNA) staining kit was obtained from Zymed Laboratories Inc. South San Francisco, CA, USA.

Animal Care and Handling

The animal care and handling were done according to the guidelines issued by the World Health Organization, Geneva, Switzerland and the INSA (Indian National Science Academy, New Delhi, India). Eight to ten weeks old female Swiss albino mice weighing 22 to 24 g were selected from an inbred colony maintained under the controlled conditions of temperature (23 ± 2°C), humidity (50±5 per cent) and light

(10 and 14 h of light and dark, respectively). The animals had free access to the sterile food and water. Four animals were housed in a polypropylene cage containing sterile paddy husk (procured locally) as bedding throughout the experiment. The study was approved by the Institutional Animal Ethical Committee of the Kasturba Medical College, Manipal, India.

Preparation of Drug and Mode of Administration

NIN was freshly dissolved in sterile double distilled water (DDW) immediately before use. The animals were administered with drug either orally *p.o.* or intraperitoneally as the case may be.

Chemopreventive Effect

Induction of BaP Induced Forestomach Tumorigenesis

Forestomach is a dilated lower esophagus (Leininger and Jokinen 1994), and the forestomach carcinoma was induced in the female Swiss albino mice as described by Wattenberg *et al.* (Nguyen *et al.*, 1999) with minor modifications. Briefly, the animals were administered with 100 µl sesame oil or 1 mg of BaP in 100 µl sesame oil *p.o.* twice a week for four weeks (a total of eight administrations). The animals were divided into the following groups:

- ☆ **DDW group**: The animals of this group received sterile double distilled water (DDW) as a sole source of drinking throughout the study period.
- ☆ **Oil group**: The animals of this group received 100 µl of sesame oil by *p.o.* twice a week for four consecutive weeks.
- ☆ **BaP group**: The animals of this group received 1 mg of BaP in 100 µl sesame oil *p.o.* twice a week for four weeks.
- ☆ **NIN group**: The animals of this group received various doses of NIN either orally (1, 2.5, 5, 10, 25, 50, 100 or 250 mg/kg b. wt.) or intraperitoneally (1, 2, 4, 6, 8, 10, 25 or 50 mg/kg b. wt.).
- ☆ **NIN + BaP group (Pre-post treatment):** The animals of this group received various doses of NIN and BaP, depending on the experimental design.

Effect of Oral Administration

The animals were divided into several groups of 10 each. Each group of animals was administered orally with 1, 2.5, 5, 10, 25, 50, 100 or 250 mg/kg b. wt. NIN for five days a week, for 2 weeks before treatment with BaP, followed by the concomitant treatment with NIN and BaP or DDW for 4 weeks during and 2 weeks after the last dose of BaP.

Effect of Intraperitoneal Administration

The animals were divided into several groups of 10 each. Each group of animals was administered intraperitoneally with 1, 2, 4, 6, 8, 10, 25 or 50 mg/kg b. wt. of NIN for five days a weeks for 2 weeks before treatment with BaP, followed by the concomitant treatment with NIN and BaP or DDW for 4 weeks during and 2 weeks after the last dose of BaP.

Effect of Altered Administration Schedule

A separate experiment was conducted to evaluate the effect of alteration in the NIN administration schedule. Since oral administration was most effective further experiments were carried out using this model of treatment. The animals were divided into following two additional groups in addition to the group described above.

- **NIN + BaP group (Pre-treatment):** The animals of this group received 5, 10 and 25 mg/kg b. wt. p.o. of NIN for 5 days a week, for 2 weeks. The last treatment of NIN was given forty-eight hours before the first administration of BaP or sesame oil.
- **BaP + NIN group (Post-treatment):** The animals of this group were provided with normal drinking water and food during the carcinogen treatment for 4 weeks. Forty eight hours after the last administration of BaP or sesame oil the animals were administered with 5, 10 and 25 mg/kg b. wt. NIN *p.o.* for 8 weeks as described above.

The body weights of the animals from each group were recorded at the beginning and at the end of the experiments. The mice were sacrificed 14 weeks after the last dose of BaP and buffered formalin was immediately injected into the stomach of each mouse, so as to distend the stomach and fix the tumors. Thereafter, forestomach was cut open longitudinally and kept in 10 per cent buffered formalin for 24 h for fixation. The stomach papillomas that were 1 mm or larger in diameter were counted under a stereozoom microscope (Leitz, Ernst, Wetzlar, Germany). A total of 440 (220 each for oral and IP administration) animals were used for this experiment. The chemopreventive activity of NIN was assessed on the basis of tumor incidence, mean and multiplicity of tumors (Jagetia *et al.*, 2003). The tumor incidence and multiplicity were compared between the animals fed with BaP or NIN or BaP and NIN.

Histological Examination of Tumors

Tumors found by visual examinations were further confirmed histologically. The stomach samples were excised, fixed in 10 per cent buffered formalin, embedded in paraffin wax and 5 μm thick sections were cut using a rotary microtome. The slides containing sections were stained with hematoxylin and eosin for the histopathological examination. The slides were scored blindly by a pathologist and the tumors were classified according to well-established criteria.

Proliferating Cell Nuclear Antigen (PCNA) Staining

The sections were dewaxed, in xylene, passed through graded alcohol series and rehydrated in distilled water. The hydrated sections were immersed for 30 min in 3 per cent hydrogen peroxidase in methanol to block endogenous peroxidase activity and subsequently washed in PBS. Thereafter, the sections were immersed in citrate buffer and microwaved and allowed to cool for another 20 min, while still being immersed in cirtrate buffer. The PCNA staining was carried out according to the manufacturers instructions. The scorer was unaware of the group to which these specimens belonged.

The PCNA-positive index number (PPIN) was calculated as follows:

$$\text{PPIN} = \frac{\text{Number of PCNA positive nuclei}}{\text{Total number of nuclei scored}} \times 100$$

Splenocyte Culture and Micronuclei Analysis

The splenocytes were cultured as described by Jagetia *et al.* (2001). Briefly, four animals from each group were killed by cervical dislocation at the end of the experiment. They were thoroughly wiped with 70 per cent ethanol and their abdominal cavity was cut open with the help of sterile scissors and forceps in an aseptic environment. The spleens of the animals were removed aseptically and washed with sterile phosphate buffered saline (PBS). The splenocytes were isolated and cultured in RPMI-1640 medium containing 10 per cent fetal calf serum (FCS) and concanavalin-A as mitogen. The splenocytes were incubated at 37°C and allowed to grow for 72 h. Duplicate cultures were set up for each animal for each drug dose. The micronuclei (MN) were prepared according to the method of Fenech and Morley (1985) with minor modifications. Briefly, 40 h after the initiation of splenocyte culture, 3 μg/ml of cytochalasin-B was added to the cultures. The cells were allowed to grow for another 32 h. The splenocytes were centrifuged, subjected to mild hypotonic treatment (0.7 per cent ammonium oxalate) so as to retain the cytoplasm and fixed in Carnoy's fixative (3:1 methanol, acetic acid). The cells were centrifuged again and resuspended in a small volume of fixative and dropped on to precleaned coded slides to avoid observer's bias. Cells were stained with 0.125 per cent acridine orange (BDH, England, Gurr Cat. No. 34001 9704640E) in Sorensen's buffer (pH 6.8). The slides were washed twice in Sorensen's buffer and observed under a fluorescent microscope, equipped with 450-490 nm BP filter set with excitation at 453 nm (Carl Zeiss Photomicroscope III, Germany), using a 40X Neofluar objective. A minimum of 2000 (1000 per culture) binucleate cells (BNC) with well-preserved cytoplasm was scored from each animal for each drug dose for the presence of MN and the frequency of micronucleated binucleate splenocytes (MNBNC) were determined. The MN identification was done according to the criteria of Krisch-Volders *et al.* (2000).

Statistical Analysis

The statistical significance in the alteration in the body weights after various treatments was determined using Student's t-test. The tumor incidence and multiplicity are expressed as the percentage of animals with tumors and the analysis was carried out using ξ^2 –test. The statistical significance for micronuclei test was carried out using one-way analysis of variance ANOVA with the application of Bonferroni's Post-hoc test.

Results

Selection of Optimum Dose and Route of Administration

The optimum drug dose and route of administration was selected by treating the animals with various doses of NIN before or after carcinogen (BaP) treatment. The chemopreventive effect of NIN on BaP induced forestomach papillomas in mice is presented in Table 6.3. The administration of 1 mg BaP by oral gavage twice a week for 4 weeks resulted in 100 per cent incidence of forestomach tumors with a mean of 4.5 tumors per mouse. The administration of BaP alone resulted in 20 per cent mortality during the course of experiment. The mice treated with DDW, oil or NIN without BaP did not show any tumor-induction throughout the study period.

Oral Administration

The treatment of mice with oil or NIN alone did not induce any tumors. Treatment of mice with 1 mg/kg b. wt. NIN *p.o.* caused an approximate 22 per cent reduction in the mean tumor number while the tumor multiplicity was reduced by 48 per cent (Table 6.3). An increase in the dose of NIN reduced the mean number and tumor multiplicity further and a highest reduction of 78 per cent in tumor multiplicity and 77 per cent reduction in tumor mean number was observed in animals that received 10 mg/kg NIN. An increase in NIN dose did not reduce the mean number and tumor multiplicity significantly (Table 6.3). However, these were always lower than the BaP treated group that did not receive NIN. Treatment of mice with 1, 2.5, 5, 10, 25, 50, 100 and 250 mg NIN treatment brought about 1.9, 2.5, 3.2, 4.6, 3.4, 3.2, 2.9 and 2.8 folds reduction in the tumor multiplicity, respectively. The tumor incidence also declined for 10 and 25 mg/kg NIN (Table 6.1). The oral administration was superior to IP administration in reducing the tumor incidence and tumor multiplicity.

Intraperitoneal Administration

The treatment of mice with DDW or NIN alone did not induce any tumors. The intraperitoneal administration of different doses of NIN significantly reduced the mean tumor number when compared with the DDW + BaP group. Treatment of mice with 1 mg/kg b. wt. NIN caused an approximate 22 per cent reduction in the mean number, while the tumor multiplicity was reduced by 36 per cent (Table 2). A further increase in NIN dose reduced the mean number (45 per cent and 33 per cent) and tumor multiplicity and a highest reduction of 60 per cent and 62 per cent in tumor multiplicity was observed in animals that received 6 and 8 mg/kg NIN respectively. An increase in NIN dose further did not reduce the mean tumor number and tumor multiplicity (Table 6.2). However, these were always lower than the BaP treated group that did not receive NIN. Treatment of mice with 1, 2, 4, 6, 8, 10, 25 or 50 mg NIN treatment brought about 1.5, 1.6, 2, 2.5, 2.6, 2.2, 1.9 and 1.6 folds reduction in the tumor multiplicity, respectively. Treatment of mice with various doses of NIN intraperitoneally did not reduce the tumor incidence.

Altered Administration Schedule

The effect of alteration in drug administration was studied for 5, 10 and 25 mg NIN. Treatment of mice with 5, 10 or 25 mg/kg NIN before carcinogen administration resulted in a reduction in tumor mean number and multiplicity when compared with BaP treatment alone. The effect of 5 and 10 mg NIN was similar as both doses caused 22 per cent reduction in mean tumor number, while tumor multiplicity was also reduced by 40 per cent for these doses (Table 6.2). Altered administration schedule did not reduce the incidence of tumors. Similarly mean number and tumor multiplicity also declined when 5, 10 or 25 mg/kg NIN was given to the animals after BaP treatment

Table 6.1: Effect of BaP, Naringin or Naringin and BaP Treatment on the Survival of Mice during Chemical Carcinogenesis

			1	*2*	*3*	*4*	*1*	*2*	*3*	*4*	*5*	*6*	*7*	*8*	*9*	*10*	*11*	*12*	*13*	*14*		
Intraperitoneal administration	Pre and post	Control	–	–	–	–	–	–	–	–	–	–	–	–	–	–	–	–	–	–	10(10)	0(0/10)
		Bap	–	–	–	–	–	–	–	–	–	–	–	–	–	–	–	–	–	1	9(90)	48(9/9)
		NIN1	–	–	–	–	–	–	–	–	–	–	–	–	–	–	–	–	–	–	10(10)	0(0/10)
		NIN2	–	–	–	–	–	–	–	–	–	–	–	–	–	–	–	–	–	–	10(10)	0(0/10)
		NIN4	–	–	–	–	–	–	–	–	–	–	–	–	–	–	–	–	–	–	10(10)	0(0/10)
		NIN6	–	–	–	–	–	–	–	–	–	–	–	–	–	–	–	–	–	–	10(10)	0(0/10)
		NIN8	–	–	–	–	–	–	–	–	–	–	–	–	–	–	–	–	–	–	10(10)	0(0/10)
		NIN10	–	–	–	–	–	–	–	–	–	–	–	–	–	–	–	–	–	–	10(10)	0(0/10)
		NIN25	–	–	–	–	–	–	–	–	–	–	–	–	–	–	–	–	–	–	10(10)	0(0/10)
		NIN50	–	–	–	–	–	–	–	–	–	–	–	–	–	–	–	–	–	–	10(10)	0(0/10)
		BaP+NIN1	–	–	–	–	–	–	–	–	–	–	–	–	–	–	–	–	–	–	10(10)	34(10/10)
		BaP+NIN2	–	–	–	–	–	–	–	–	–	–	–	–	–	–	–	–	–	–	10(10)	33(10/10)
		BaP+NIN4	–	–	–	–	–	–	–	–	–	–	–	–	–	–	–	–	–	–	10(10)	25(10/10)
		BaP+NIN6	–	–	–	–	–	–	–	–	–	–	–	–	–	–	–	–	–	–	10(10)	21(10/10)
		BaP+NIN8	–	–	–	–	–	–	–	–	–	–	–	–	–	–	–	–	–	–	10(10)	20(10/10)
		BaP+NIN10	–	–	–	–	–	–	–	–	–	–	–	–	–	–	–	–	–	–	10(10)	24(10/10)
		BaP+NIN25	–	–	–	–	–	–	–	–	–	–	–	–	–	–	–	–	–	–	10(10)	28(10/10)
		BaP+NIN50	–	–	–	–	–	–	–	–	–	–	–	–	–	–	–	–	–	–	10(10)	32(10/10)

Contd...

Table 6.1–*Contd...*

			1	*2*	*3*	*4*	*1*	*2*	*3*	*4*	*5*	*6*	*7*	*8*	*9*	*10*	*11*	*12*	*13*	*14*		
Oral administration	Pre and post	BaP	–	–	–	–	–	–	–	–	–	–	–	–	–	–	–	–	1	1	8(80)	49(8/8)
		NIN1	–		–	–	–		–	–	–		–	–	–		–	–	–		10(10)	0(0/10)
		NIN2.5	–	–	–	–	–	–	–	–	–	–	–	–	–	–	–	–	–	–	10(10)	0(0/10)
		NIN5	–	–	–	–	–	–	–	–	–	–	–	–	–	–	–	–	–	–	10(10)	0(0/10)
		NIN10	–	–	–	–	–	–	–	–	–	–	–	–	–	–	–	–	–	–	10(10)	0(0/10)
		NIN25	–		–	–	–		–	–	–		–	–	–		–	–	–		10(10)	0(0/10)
		NIN50	–	–	–	–	–	–	–	–	–	–	–	–	–	–	–	–	–	–	10(10)	0(0/10)
		NIN100	–	–	–	–	–	–	–	–	–	–	–	–	–	–	–	–	–	–	10(10)	0(0/10)
		NIN250	–	–	–	–	–	–	–	–	–	–	–	–	–	–	–	–	–	–	10(10)	0(0/10)
		BaP+NIN1	–		–	–	–		–	–	–		–	–	–		–	–	–		10(10)	32(10/10)
		BaP+NIN2.5	–	–	–	–	–	–	–	–	–	–	–	–	–	–	–	–	–	–	10(10)	24(10/10)
		BaP+NIN5	–	–	–	–	–	–	–	–	–	–	–	–	–	–	–	–	–	–	10(10)	19(10/10)
		BaP+NIN10	–	–	–	–	–	–	–	–	–	–	–	–	–	–	–	–	–	–	10(10)	12(9/10)
		BaP+NIN25	–		–	–	–		–	–	–		–	–	–		–	–	–		10(10)	16(9/10)
		BaP+NIN50	–	–	–	–	–	–	–	–	–	–	–	–	–	–	–	–	–	–	10(10)	19(10/10)
		BaP+NIN100	–	–	–	–	–	–	–	–	–	–	–	–	–	–	–	–	–	–	10(10)	21(10/10)
		BaP+NIN250	–	–	–	–	–	–	–	–	–	–	–	–	–	–	–	–	–	–	10(10)	22(10/10)
	Pre or post	BaP	–		–	–	–		–	–	–		–	–	–		–	–	1	1	8(80)	49(8/8)
		NIN+BaP5	–	–	–	–	–	–	–	–	–	–	–	–	–	–	–	–	–	–	10(10)	38(10/10)
		NIN+BaP10	–	–	–	–	–	–	–	–	–	–	–	–	–	–	–	–	–	–	10(10)	37(10/10)
		NIN+BaP25	–	–	–	–	–	–	–	–	–	–	–	–	–	–	–	–	–	–	10(10)	35(10/10)
		Post5	–		–	–	–		–	–	–		–	–	–		–	–	–		10(10)	40(9/10)
		Post10	–	–	–	–	–	–	–	–	–	–	–	–	–	–	–	–	–	–	10(10)	39(9/10)
		Post25	–	–	–	–	–	–	–	–	–	–	–	–	–	–	–	–	–	–	10(10)	36(10/10)

(Post-treatment). The effect was almost similar for 10 and 25 mg, where 33 per cent reduction in mean tumor number was observed, while tumor multiplicity reduced to 36 and 41 per cent respectively for 10 and 25 mg/kg, respectively (Table 6.2).

Micronucleus Assay

Treatment of mice with oil or various doses of NIN did not significantly alter the frequency of micronuclei in the splenocytes of mice (Table 6.3). Treatment of mice with 8 mg/kg b. wt. BaP for the induction of forestomach carcinoma resulted in an approximate six fold increase in MNBNC frequency ($p<0.0001$). Treatment of mice with various doses of NIN before and after carcinogen treatment resulted in a dose dependent but drastic decline in the MNBNCs and the lowest frequency of MNBNC was observed for 10 mg/kg NIN ($p<0.0001$), the dose that gave best chemopreventive

Table 6.2: Effect of Various Doses of Naringin on BaP-induced Carcinogenesis

			Tumor Incidence	*Mean Number*	*Tumor Multiplicity*	*Initial Weight*	*Final Weight*
Oral administration	Pre and post	DDW	0 (0/10)	0	0	22.6±0.26	31.5±0.34
		BaP	100 (8/8)	4.5 (100)	6.125(100)	21.8±0.24	31.7±0.51
		NIN1	0 (0/10)	0	0	21.4±0.22	31.9±0.5
		NIN2.5	0 (0/10)	0	0	21.7±0.3	32.3±0.49
		NIN5	0 (0/10)	0	0	22.0±0.25	32.3±0.21
		NIN10	0 (0/10)	0	0	21.3±0.33	32.0±0.29
		NIN25	0 (0/10)	0	0	21.1±0.34	32.4±0.16
		NIN50	0 (0/10)	0	0	21.3±0.3	32.8±0.53
		NIN100	0 (0/10)	0	0	21.2±0.35	30.8±0.592
		NIN250	0 (0/10)	0	0	21.4±0.49	30.6±0.76
		BaP+NIN1	100 (10/10)	3.5(77.77)	3.2(52.28)	21.6±0.6	30.3±0.63
		BaP+NIN2.5	100 (10/10)	3(66.66)	2.4(39.18	21.1±0.34	30.7±0.80
		BaP+NIN5	100 (10/10)	2(44.44)	1.9(31.02)	21.3±0.3	30.6±0.85
		BaP+NIN10	80 (8/10)	1(22.22)	1.33(21.71)	21.5±0.37	30.2±0.7
		BaP+NIN25	80 (8/10)	1.5(33.33)	1.77(28.89)	21.6±0.3	29.5±0.68
		BaP+NIN50	100 (10/10)	2.5(55.55)	1.9(31.02)	21.5±0.5	31.0±0.64
		BaP+NIN100	100 (10/10)	2(44.44)	2.1(34.08)	21.5±0.34	30.6±0.30
		BaP+NIN250	100 (10/10)	2(44.44)	2.2(35.91)	21.5±0.5	30.3±0.78
	Pre or post	NIN Pre 5	100 (10/10)	3.5(77.77)	3.8(62.04)	22.3±1.22	31.2±0.54
		NIN Pre 10	100 (10/10)	3.5(77.77)	3.7(60.40)	21.4±0.98	32.5±0.55
		NIN Pre 25	100 (10/10)	4(88.88)	3.5(57.14)	23.5±0.54	31.5±0.64
		NIN Post 5	100 (10/10)	3.5(77.77)	4.0(65.30)	22.1±0.34	30.8±0.66
		NIN Post 10	100 (10/10)	3(66.66)	3.9(63.67)	23.4±0.5	34.21±0.3
		NIN Post 25	100 (10/10)	3(66.66)	3.6(58.77)	22.4±0.35	31.7±0.19

Contd...

Table 6.2–*Contd...*

			Tumor Incidence	*Mean Number*	*Tumor Multiplicity*	*Initial Weight*	*Final Weight*
Intraperitoneal administration	Pre and post	NIN1	0 (0/10)	0	0	22.18±2.11	34.56±2.33
		NIN2	0 (0/10)	0	0	20.98±2.04	34.57±3.45
		NIN4	0 (0/10)	0	0	23.14±0.97	35.62±2.51
		NIN6	0 (0/10)	0	0	24.11±1.87	35.78±1.58
		NIN8	0 (0/10)	0	0	22.54±2.11	34.55±2.44
		NIN10	0 (0/10)	0	0	21.04±1.11	33.65±3.14
		NIN25	0 (0/10)	0	0	23.14±2.44	36.14±2.58
		NIN50	0 (0/10)	0	0	22.12±2.21	34.28±2.11
		BaP+NIN1	100 (10/10)	3.5 (77.77)	3.4(63.78)	23.11±1.11	30.56±1.98
		BaP+NIN2	100 (10/10)	3 (66.66)	3.3(61.91)	21.11±2.35	29.88±1.44
		BaP+NIN4	100 (10/10)	3 (66.66)	2.5(46.9)	22.45±3.22	31.25±1.22
		BaP+NIN6	100 (10/10)	2.5 (55.55)	2.1(39.39)	24.11±1.21	31.78±1.48
		BaP+NIN8	100 (10/10)	3 (66.66)	2.0(37.52)	22.55±1.01	29.87±1.45
		BaP+NIN10	100 (10/10)	3.5 (77.77)	2.4(45.02)	21.12±1.54	31.01±1.49
		BaP+NIN25	100 (10/10)	3.5 (77.77)	2.8(52.53)	22.44±1.87	30.11±1.78
		BaP+NIN50	100 (10/10)	3 (66.66)	3.2(60.03)	23.11±1.25	29.87±1.57

effect (Table 6.3). BaP treatment induced not only cells with one MN but also cells bearing two or more than two MN (Figure 6.1). Treatment of mice with various doses of NIN before and after BaP treatment significantly reduced the occurrence of MNBNCs bearing one, two or more than two micronuclei (Figure 6.1) and a greatest reduction was observed for 10 mg/kg NIN (Table 6.3). This reduction was almost 2 fold for 10 and 25 mg/kg NIN, respectively. Similarly, the animals that were treated with different doses of NIN before or after treatment of carcinogen exhibited a dose dependent decline in the frequency of MNBNC when compared with the BaP treated animals (Figure 6.1). NIN treatment before or after BaP administration also reduced the frequency of cells bearing one, two or more than two MN significantly. However, this reduction in MNBNC was not to that extent as was observed for the mice that received NIN before and after (Pre-post) the carcinogen treatment (Table 6.3).

Histopathological Analysis

The majority of papillomas scored in BaP and BaP+NIN group were histologically found to be squamous cell carcinomas (SCC). Forestomach squamous cell carcinomas, often accompanied by inflammation and the presence of abundant PCNA-positive nuclei were observed in BaP treated animals. The PCNA labeling indices in the forestomach tumors are presented in Table 6.4. Histopathological examination of sections from BaP treated group showed an approximate 3.7 fold elevation in the PCNA labeling index, while treatment of mice with different doses of NIN *p.o.* before and after BaP treatment resulted in an almost 4 fold decline in PCNA

Table 6.3: Alteration in the BaP-Induced Micronuclei in the Splenocytes of Mice Treated with different Doses of Naringin Orally during Chemical Carcinogenesis

		One MN		*Two MN*		*Multiple MN*		*Total MN*	
		NIN+oil	*NIN+BaP*	*NIN+oil*	*NIN+BaP*	*NIN+oil*	*NIN+BaP*	*NIN+oil*	*NIN+BaP*
Pre and post treatment	Control	21.9±0.67	134.7±2.4	7.1±0.52	40.8±1.29	0±0	1±0.2582	29.5±1.3	176.5±4.4
	NIN1	21.7±0.7	86.1±0.95[a]	5.5±0.56	30±0.73[b]	0±0	0.7±0.15	26.9 ±1.0	117.2±1.0[a]
	NIN2.5	21.6±0.52	81±1.37[a]	4.9±0.50	30.2±0.5[b]	0±0	0.5±0.16	26.9±0.67	111.9±1.1[a]
	NIN5	21.8±0.59	65.6±1.2[a]	4.9±0.58	22.8±0.7[a]	0±0	0.3±0.15	26.6±1.03	88.3±1.41[a]
	NIN10	23.2±0.67	57.4±1.49[a]	5.7±0.36	19±0.91[a]	0±0	0.3±0.15	29±0.77	76.6±1.6[a]
	NIN25	22.2±0.48	60.5±1.19[a]	5.4±0.22	19±0.93[a]	0±0	0.5±0.16	27.6±0.4	80.4±1.3[a]
	NIN50	22.5±0.40	60.1±1.39[a]	4.8±0.29	21.2±0.6[a]	0±0	0.5±0.16	27.7±0.4	81.7±1.0[a]
	NIN100	21.8±0.59	60.5±1.02[a]	5±0.365	21.5±1.01[a]	0±0	0.5±0.16	26.8±0.7	82.1±1.4[a]
	NIN250	22.4±0.42	61.7±1.23[a]	5.9±0.5	22.2±0.71[a]	0±0	0.6±0.16	29.10±2.4	84±1.67[a]
Pre	NIN5	22.31±1.21	100±4.210[c]	4.19±0.46	25.14±2.8	0±0	0.45±0.02	27.50±1.54	126.2±4.1[b]
	NIN10	23.47±1.95	102.4±5.1[c]	5.87±0.78	20.45±1.5[c]	0±0	0.74±0.09	29.210±2.4	124.0±3.6[b]
	NIN25	21.55±0.98	97.5±3.94[c]	4.45±1.07	21.87±2.1[c]	0±0	0.54±0.08	26.140±2.6	119.1±4.6[b]
Post	NIN5	22.54±1.44	129.5±4.17	5.24±0.97	31.24±3.4	0±0	1.14±0.24	27.90±1.41	162.2±5.68
	NIN10	22.41±1.11	130.9±5.64	4.14±0.87	32.56±2.8	0±0	0.98±0.31	26.540±1.1	163.92±4.1
	NIN25	23.17±2.10	131.2±4.55	5.89±1.01	29.87±3.5	0±0	1.22±0.12	29.510±2.1	162.54±5.8

No symbol – non significant, a-p<0.001, b-p<0.01 and c-p<0.05. n=4.

Figure 6.1: Effect of Naringin on the Benzo-a-pyrene-Induced Genomic Instability in the Spelnocytes during Forestomach Carcinogenesis in Mice.

A: One micronuclei; B: Multiple micronuclei and C: Total micronuclei.

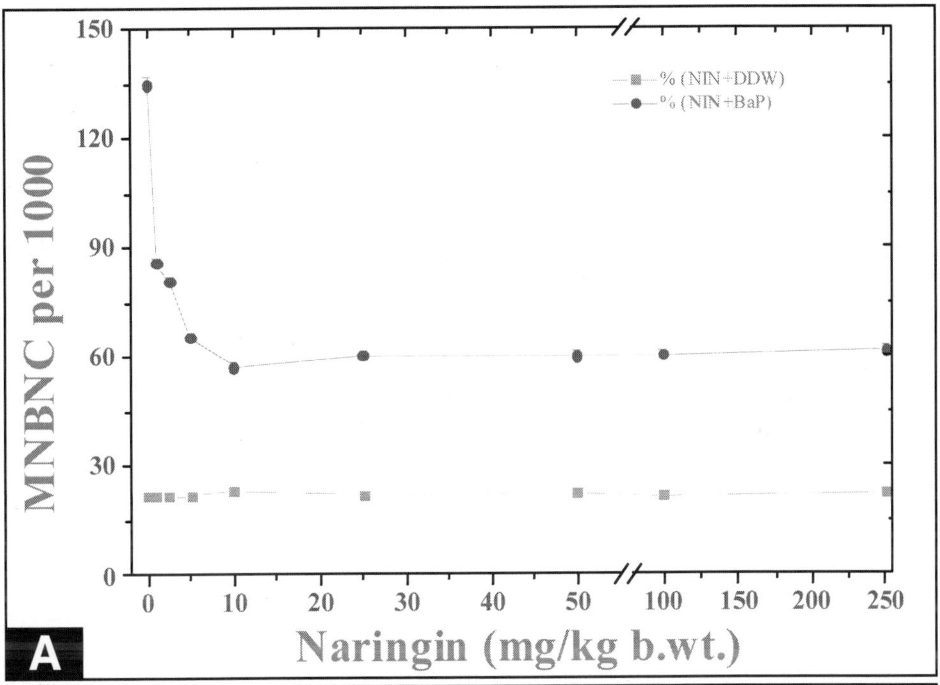

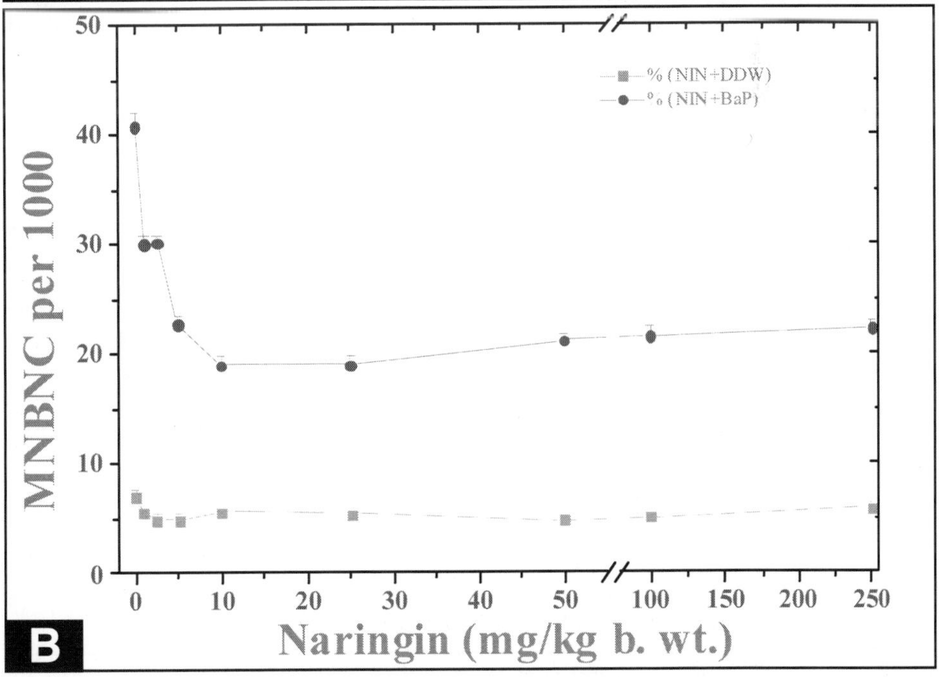

Contd...

Figure 6.1–*Contd...*

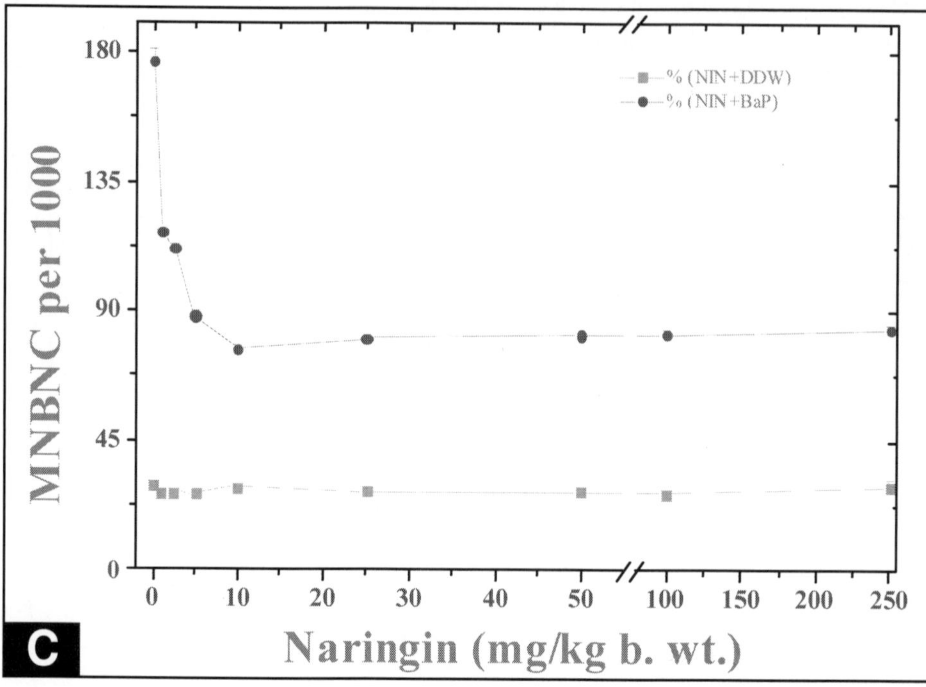

labeling index, when compared to BaP treatment alone (Table 6.4). Similarly, treatment of mice with 5, 10 or 25 mg/kg NIN before or after treatment with BaP also reduced PCNA labeling index. However, this reduction in PCNA labeling index was lesser when compared with the group of animals that received NIN before as well as after the BaP treatment.

Table 6.4: PCNA Labeling Index in the Forestomach Carcinoma of Mice Treated with Various Doses of Naringin during BaP-induced Carcinogenesis

	PCNA Positive Index	
NIN mg/kg b.wt.	*NIN*	*NIN+BaP*
Control	132±2.87	487±4.12
NIN1	120±3.22	272±2.19[a]
NIN2.5	129±3.01	265±3.84[a]
NIN5	135±2.97	269±4.12[a]
NIN10	141±5.11	271±4.22[a]
NIN25	121±3.4	275±5.31[a]
NIN50	129±3.78	274±3.56[a]
NIN100	100±5.11	300±3.55[a]
NIN250	105±3.1	305±3.61[a]

No symbol – non significant, a-p<0.001. n=4.

Discussion

The changes in the environment, life style and dietary habits and increased exposure to mutagenic agents have been responsible for increasing number of cancers worldwide. despite of the great advances being made to cure cancer, the treatment of advanced invasive disease, such as carcinoma of the lung, colon, breast, prostate and pancreas remains elusive, indicating the need for new approaches to control cancer. In general the old adage "prevention is better than cure" may be the best approach to control cancer. The strategies that are capable to control cancer by slowing, blocking, or reversing the process of carcinogenesis due to exposure to various exogenous or endogenous carcinogens by the administration of one or more naturally occurring dietary and or other pharmacological agents will be useful in reducing the cancer worldwide (Kelloff *et al.*, 1994; Stoner and Mukhtar, 1995, Sarkar and Li, 2009). The present study has been undertaken to evaluate the effect of naringin, a grape fruit flavonone on the benzo[*a*]pyrene- induced forestomach carcinoma of mice.

Our results indicate that treatment of mice with BaP caused 100 per cent incidence of forestomach tumors, while the oil treatment did not induce any tumors in the recipient animals. The tumor multiplicity in the BaP group was also high. A similar effect of BaP induced carcinogenesis has been reported earlier (Nagabhushan and Bhide,1987; Azuine and Bhide, 1992; Deshpande *et al.*, 1997; Agha *et al.*, 2001; Jagetia *et al.*, 2003). The oral administration of dietary ingredient, NIN before-during and after BaP treatment reduced the mean tumor number, tumor multiplicity and tumor incidence in mice. Phytochemicals like *Xanthophylls, Astaxanthin* and *Canthaxanthin* have been reported to inhibit chemically induced oral carcinogenesis in rats (Tanaka *et al.*, 1995). Several other synthetic or phytochemicals have been found to inhibit chemical carcinogenesis (Ito and Hirose 1989; Balansky *et al.*, 1996). Several dietary ingredients like β-carotene, ascorbic acid, tochopherols and have been found to be chemopreventive in human studies (Omenn *et al.*, 1996; De Flora *et al.*, 2001; Lee *et al.*, 2003).

NIN treatment also inhibited tumors when it was given either before or after the BaP treatment. However, chemopreventive effect of NIN was lesser when compared with the continuous treatment (pre-post). A similar effect has been observed for turmeric and *Alstonia scholaris* earlier (Deshpande *et al.*, 1997; Jagetia *et al.*, 2003). The intraperitoneal administration of NIN although inhibited BaP-induced carcinogenesis its effect was lesser than that of oral administration. The reason of this difference lies in the conversion of NIN to naringenin by bacterial hydrolysis in the gastrointestinal tract (Fuhr and Kummert, 1995), and also oral administration brings the target tissue into the direct contact of NIN.

The results of present study indicate that BaP treatment increased the frequency of MNBNC by six folds. A similar effect of BaP has been observed earlier in the splenocytes (Benning *et al.*, 1994; Winker *et al.*, 1995; Dertinger *et al.*, 2001; Jagetia *et al.*, 2003). Treatment of mice with various doses of NIN caused a significant decline in the MNBNC and the highest reduction was observed at the dose that gave best-chemopreventive effect. This indicates that the micronucleus assay, which gives an indirect measurement of chromosome damage, may serve as a surrogate marker. Our results support the hypothesis that evaluation of chromosome damage may act as surrogate biomarker in cancer chemoprevention studies (Kelloff *et al.*, 2000). The micronuclei frequencies were higher in mice that received NIN intraperitoneally than those that received it orally. A similar effect was found in mice that received NIN either before or after the BaP treatment in the present study. The reason for the lesser DNA damage in mice receiving NIN orally may be due to the conversion of NIN to naringenin as stated earlier (Kelloff *et al.*, 2000). The reduction in micronuclei in splenocytes of mice receiving extract of *Alostonia scholaris* during chemically induced carcinogenesis has been reported earlier (Jagetia *et al.*, 2003).

Alterations in the native DNA play an important and crucial role in carcinogenesis. The formation of DNA adducts inflicts loss of nuclear functioning that leads to mutations and chromosome aberrations. The mutational events and chromosomal instability are key events in carcinogenesis and many types of cancer have been associated with chromosomal aberrations (Heim and Mitelman, 1987; Heim and Mitelman, 1989). Damage to the chromosomes is expressed as breaks and fragments which appear as MN in the proliferating cells (Heddle and Harris, 1975). The chromatid breaks and exchanges that lead to chromosome anomalies must occur during carcinogenesis to attain the neoplastic property. The tumor cell population is composed of one or few clones of cells with particular chromosome anomalies and this phenomenon is detectible by an increased frequency of micronuclei in the proliferating cells (Heim and Mitelman, 1989; Kelloff *et al.*, 1994). The cell proliferation also allows endogenous adducts to be converted into mutations and makes more sensitive single-stranded DNA target for carcinogenesis. Therefore the evaluation of micronuclei gives an indication on the quantitative aspect on the insult to the cellular DNA. In chronic administration studies it is always desirable to study the MN formation in the spleen, because the irreparable damage to the cellular DNA gets accumulated, which becomes manifest when the splenocytes are stimulated to divide. BaP has been reported to be immunotoxic and has profound inhibitory effect on the spleen (Ginsberg *et al.*, 1989; Zhao, 1990). BaP treatment has been reported to increase the BaP-DNA adducts formation and frequency of mutation in the spleen cells (Benning *et al.*, 1994; Winker *et al.*, 1995; Dertinger *et al.*, 2001; Keshava *et al.*, 2005). The treatment of mice with NIN may have reduced the DNA damage as evident by a significant reduction in the frequency of micronuclei. Therefore, protection against the DNA damage by NIN during tumorigenesis may be one of the reasons for lesser frequency of tumors. In this study we have observed that the chemopreventive effect was best when the NIN is administered before during and after (pre-post BaP treatment).

NIN may have inhibited BaP-induced forestomach carcinogenesis by several putative mechanisms. t BaP requires metabolic activation, mediated by cytochrome P450 (CYP) dependent monooxygenase, for carcinogenesis (Singh *et al.*, 1998; Ueng *et al.*, 1999; Uppstad *et al.*, 2010) and NIN may have inhibited this action. Covalent interaction of carcinogen with nucleophilic sites in DNA is essential for BaP induced tumerogenesis (Singh *et al.*, 1998) and presence of NIN may have suppressed this interaction leading to reduced forestomach carcinoma. BaP-induce carcinogenesis by metabolic activation, mediated by cytochrome-450 (CYP) dependent monooxygenase (Singh *et al.*, 1998; Ueng *et al.*, 1999; Uppstad *et al.*, 2010). NIN has been reported to inhibit benzo[*a*]pyrene hydroxylase (AHH), CYP450 3A4 and expression of CYP4501A2 protein (Guengerich and Shimada, 1991; Ueng *et al.*, 1999; Alvarez-Gonzalez *et al.*, 2001). P4503A4 also appears to play a more dominant role in the conversion of 7,8-dihydroxy-7,8 dihydrobenzo(a)pyrene to 9, 10-epoxide during carcinogenesis (Guengerich and Shimada, 1991; Uppstad *et al.*, 2010). The consumption of grape fruit juice has led to a marked reduction of CYP3A4 activity in the gastrointestinal tract earlier (Ho *et al.*, 2001). The chemopreventive activity of NIN seems to be because of inhibition of AHH and CYP4503A4. The crucial importance of DNA damage in carcinogenesis and inhibition of BaP-induced DNA damage by NIN may also be one of the important mechanisms of chemoprevention in this study. This is evident from the reduction in the frequency of micronuclei in the NIN+BaP treated groups when compared with BaP treatment alone. BaP induce carcinogenesis by induction of DNA adduct and NIN may have reduced the formation of DNA adduct. NIN has been reported to reduce doxorubicin-induced DNA adduct formation earlier (Keshava *et al.*, 2005; Jagetia and Reddy, 2014). The chemopreventive action of NIN may also be due to inhibition of enzyme lipooxygenease and cyclooxygenase. Since these enzymes are known to cause hyperproliferative responses (Frstenberger and Marks, 1980). NIN has been reported to inhibit lipooxygenase and cyclooxygenase (Corvazier and Maclouf, 1985). NIN may have also inhibited cell proliferation thereby reducing the tumor multiplicity. This is supported by PCNA labeling studies, where the PCNA labeling index has been found to be significantly lower in the animals receiving NIN and BaP than those receiving BaP only. Last but not least NIN may have scavenged free radicals and raised the antioxidant status, resulting in the reduction of tumors. NIN has been reported to scavenge free radicals and increase antioxidant status in vitro earlier (Jagetia *et al.*, 2003). NIN has been found to be an antioxidant and anti-inflammatory agent and protect cells from ethanol, ockadic acid, isofamide, aflotoxin B_1 and H_2O_2 induced oxidative stress (Guengerich and Kim, 1990; Martin *et al.*, 1994; Gordon *et al.*, 1995; Wilcox *et al.*, 2001; Alvarez-Gonzalez *et al.*, 2001; Kanno *et al.*, 2003). NIN may have reduced the NF-κB and inflammatory responses induced by BaP thereby reducing the forestomach carcinoma in mice in the present study. Naringin has been reported to inhibit the NF-κB activity earlier (Liu *et al.*, 2011; Ang *et al.*, 2011)

NIN treatment has reduced the BaP induced forestomach carcinoma in recipient mice, which may be due to the inhibition of BaP metabolism, CYPs, BaP-induced DNA damage including DNA adducts, scavenging of free radicals, NF-κB activation and elevation in the antioxidant status.

References

Agha, A.M., El-Fattah, A.A., Al-Zuhair, H.H., and Al-Rikabi, A.C. (2001). Chemopreventive effect of *Ginkgo biloba* extract against benzo[*a*]pyrene -induced forestomach carcinogenesis in mice: amelioration of doxorubicin cardiotoxicity. *Journal of Experimental and Clinical Cancer Research*, **20**: 39-50.

Alvarez-Gonzalez, I., Madrigal-Bujaidar, E., Dorado, V., and Espinosa-Aguirre, J.J. (2001). Inhibitory effect of naringin on the micronuclei induced by ifosfamide in mouse, and evaluation of its modulatory effect on the Cyp3a subfamily. *Mutation Research*, **1**: 480-481.

Ang, E.S., Yang, X., Chen, H., Liu, Q., Zheng, M.H., and Xu, J. (2011). Naringin abrogates osteoclastogenesis and bone resorption via the inhibition of RANKL- induced NF-κB and ERK activation. *FEBS Letters*, **585(17)**: 2755–2762.

Azuine, M.A., and Bhide, S.V. (1992). Chemopreventive effect of turmeric against stomach and skin tumors induced by chemical carcinogens in Swiss mice. *Nutrition and Cancer*, **17**: 77-83.

Balansky, R., Izzotti, A., Scatolini, L., D'Agostini, F., and DeFlora, S. (1996). Induction by carcinogens and chemoprevention by N-acetylcysteine of adducts to mitochondrial DNA in rat organs. *Cancer Research*, **56**: 1642-7.

Bauer, E., Guo, Z., Ueng, Y.F., Bell, L.C., Zeldin, D., and Guengerich, F.P. (1995). Oxidation of benzo[*a*]pyrene by recombinant human cytochrome P450 enzymes. *Chemical Research and Toxicology*, **8**: 136-142.

Benning, V., Brault, D., Duvinage, C., Thybaud, V., and Melcion, C. (1994). Validation of the *in vivo* CD1 mouse splenocyte micronucleus test. *Mutagenesis*, **9**: 199-204.

Calomme, M., Pieters, L., Vlietinck, A., and Vanden Berghe, D. (1996). Inhibition of bacterial mutagenesis by citrus flavonoids, *Planta Medica*, **62**: 222–226.

Cassady, J.M., Baird, W.M., and Chang, C.J. (1990). Natural products as a source of potential cancer chemotherapeutic and chemopreventive agents. *Journal of Natural Products*, **53**: 23-41.

Castonguay, A. (1992). Methods and strategies in lung cancer control. *Cancer Research*, **52**: 2641s-2651s.

Collins, J.F., Brown, J.P., Dawson, S.V., and Marty, M.A. (1991). Risk assessment for benzo[*a*]pyrene. *Regulatory Toxicology and Pharmacology*, **13**: 170-184.

Corvazier, E., and Maclouf, J. (1985). Interference of some flavonoids and non-steroidal anti-inflammatory drugs with oxidative metabolism of arachidonic acid by human platelets and neutrophils. *Biochimica Biophysica Acta*, **9**: 315-21.

De Flora, S., Izzotti, A., D'Agostini, F., Balansky, R.M. Noonan, D., and Albini, A. (2001). Multiple points of intervention in the prevention of cancer and other mutation-related diseases. *Mutation Research*, **1**: 480-481.

Dertinger, S.D., Nazarenko, D.A., Silverstone, A.E., and Gasiewicz, T.A. (2001). Aryl hydrocarbon receptor signaling plays a significant role in mediating benzo[a]pyrene- and cigarette smoke condensate-induced cytogenetic damage *in vivo*. *Carcinogenesis*, **22**: 171-177.

Deshpande, S.S., Ingle, A.D., and Maru, G.B. (1997). Inhibitory effects of curcumin-free aqueous turmeric extract on benzo[a]pyrene-induced forestomach papillomas in mice. *Cancer Letters*, **16**: 79-85.

Fenech, M., and Morley, A.A. (1985). Measurement of micronuclei in lymphocytes. *Mutation Research*, **147**: 29-36.

Francis, A.R., Shetty, T.K., and Bhattacharya, R.K. (1989). Modulating effect of plant flavonoids on the mutagenicity of N-methyl-N9-nitro-N-nitrosoguanidine. *Carcinogenesis,* **10**: 1953–1955.

Frstenberger, G., and Marks, F. (1980). Early prostaglandin E synthesis is an obligatory event in the induction of cell proliferation in mouse epidermis *in vivo* by the phorbol ester TPA. *Biochemical and Biophysical Research Communication,* **92**: 749-756.

Fuhr, U., and Kummert, A.L. (1995). The fate of naringin in humans: a key to grapefruit juice-drug interactions? *Clinical Pharmacology and Therapeutics*, **58**: 365-73.

Ginsberg, G.L., Atherholt, T.B., and Butler, G.H. (1989). Benzo[a]pyrene-induced immunotoxicity: comparison to DNA adduct formation *in vivo*, in cultured splenocytes and in microsomal systems. *Journal of Toxicology and Environmental Health,* **28**: 205-220.

Gordon, F.B., Holen, I., and Seglen P.O. (1995). Protection by naringin and some other flavonoids of hepatocytic autophagy and endocytosis against inhibition by okadaic acid. *Journal of Biological Chemistry,* **270**: 5830 - 5838.

Guengerich, F.P. (1988). Roles of cytochrome P-450 enzymes in chemical carcinogenesis and cancer chemotherapy. *Cancer Research,* **48**: 2946-2954.

Guengerich, F.P., and Kim, D.H. (1990). *In vitro* inhibition of dihydropyridine oxidation and aflotoxin B_1 activation in human liver microsomes by naringenin and other flavonoids. *Carcinogenesis,* **11**: 2275-2279.

Guengerich, F.P., and Shimada, T. (1991). Oxidation of toxic and carcinogenic chemicals by human cytochrome P-450 enzymes. *Chemical Research in Toxicology,* **4**: 391-407.

Haenen, G.R., Paquay, J.B., Korthouwer, R.E., and Bast, A. (1997). Peroxynitrite scavenging by flavonoids. *Biochemical and Biophysical Research Communication*, **236**: 591–593.

Halliwell, B., and Gutteridge, J.M. (1989). Free Radicals in Biology and Medicine. Second Ed. New York Oxford University.

Heddle, J.A., and Harris, J.W. (1975). Letter: rapid screening of radioprotective drugs *in vivo*. *Radiation Research,* **61**: 350-353.

Heim, S., and Mitelman, F. (1987). Ninteen of 26 cellular oncogenes precisely localized in the human genome map to one of the 83 bands involved in primary cancer specific rearrangements. *Human Genetics,* **75**: 70-72.

Heim, S., and Mitelman, F. (1989). Primary chromosome abnormalities in human neoplasia. *Advances in Cancer Research,* **52**: 1-43.

Ho, P.C, Saville, D.J., and Wanwimolruk, S. (2001). Inhibition of human CYP3A4 activity by grapefruit flavonoids, furanocoumarins and related compounds. *Journal of Pharmacy and Pharmaceutical Sciences*, **4**: 217-27.

Ito, N., and Hirose, M. (1989). Antioxidants–carcinogenic and chemopreventive properties. *Adv Cancer Res.*, **53**: 247-302.

Jagetia, G.C., and Reddy, T.K. (2002). The grapefruit flavanone naringin protects against the radiation-induced genomic instability in the mice bone marrow: a micronucleus study. *Mutation Research*, **26**: 37-48.

Jagetia, G.C., and Reddy, T.K. (2014). The grape fruit flavonone naringin protects mice against doxorubicin-induced cardiotoxicity. *Journal of Molecular Biochemistry*, **3**: 34-49

Jagetia, G.C., Baliga, M.S., and Venkatesh, P. (2003). Effect of Sapthaparna (Alstonia scholaris Linn) in modulating the benzo(a)pyrene-induced forestomach carcinogenesis in mice. *Toxicology Letters*, **144**: 183-193.

Jagetia, G.C., Menon, K.S., and Jain, V. (2001). Genotoxic effect of hydroquinone on the cultured mouse spleenocytes. *Toxicology Letters*, **8**: 15-20.

Jagetia, G.C., Venkatesha, V.A., and Reddy, T.K. (2003). Naringin, a citrus flavonone, protects against radiation-induced chromosome damage in mouse bone marrow. *Mutagenesis*, **18**: 337-43.

Kanno, S., Shouji, A., Asou, K., and Ishikawa, M. (2003). Effects of naringin on hydrogen peroxide-induced cytotoxicity and apoptosis in P388 cells. *Journal of Pharmacological Sciences*, **92**: 166-170.

Kelloff, G.J., Boone, C.W., Steele, V.E., Crowell, J.A., Lubet, R., and Sigman, C.C. (1994). Progress in cancer chemoprevention: perspectives on agent selection and short-term clinical intervention trials. *Cancer Res.*, 1: 2015s-2024s.

Kelloff, G.J., Sigman, C.C., Johnson, K.M., Boone, C.W., Greenwald, P., Crowell, J.A., Hawk, E.T., and Doody, L.A. (2000). Perspectives on surrogate end points in the development of drugs that reduce the risk of cancer. *Cancer Epidemiology Biomarkers and Prevention*, **9**: 127-37.

Kew, M.C. (2009). Hepatic iron overload and hepatocellular carcinoma. *Cancer Letters*, **286**: 38–43.

Kim, D.H., Jung, E.A., Shong, I.S., and Han, J.A. (1998). Intestinal bacterial metabolism of flavonoids and its relation to some biological activities. *Archives of Pharmacal Research*, **21**: 17–23.

Krisch-Volders, M., Souni, T., Aardema, M., Albertini, S., Eastmond, D., Fenech, M., Ishidate, M., Lorge, E., Norppa. H., Surralles, J., Von DurHude, W., and Wakata, A. (2000). Report from the *in vitro* micronucleus assay-working group. *Environmental and Molecular Mutagenesis*, **35**: 167-172.

Kroyer, G. (1986). The antioxidant activity of citrus fruit peels. *Zeitschrift fur Ernahrungswissenschaft*, **25**: 63–69.

Lake, B.G., Beamand, J.A., Tredger, J.M., and Barton, P.T. (1999). Inhibition of xenobiotic-induced genotoxicity in cultured precision-cut human and rat liver slices. *Mutation Research*, **440**: 91–100.

Lee, K.W., Lee, H.J., Surh, Y.J., and Lee, C.Y. (2003). Vitamin C and cancer chemoprevention: reappraisal. *American Journal of Clinical Nutrition*,**78**: 1074-1078.

Leininger, J.R., and Jokinen, M.P. (1994). Tumors of the oral cavity, pharynx, oesophagus, and stomach. Tumors of the Mouse. Turusov VS, Mohr U (eds). International Agency for Research on Cancer Lyon, France, pp. 2 167-193.

Levin, W., Wood, A., Chang, R., Ryan, D., and Thomas, P. (1982). Oxidative metabolism of polycyclic aromatic hydrocarbons to ultimate carcinogens. *Drug Metabolism Reviews*, **13**: 555-580.

Liu, Y., Wu, H., Nie, Y.C., Chen, J.L., Su, W.W., and Li, P.B. (2011). Naringin attenuates acute lung injury in LPS-treated mice by inhibiting NF-κB pathway. *International Immunopharmacology*, **11(10)**: 1606-1612.

Martin, M.J., Marhuenda, E., Perez-Guerrero, C., and Franco, J.M. (1994). Antiulcer effect of naringin on gastric lesions induced by ethanol in rats. *Pharmacology*, **49**: 144-150.

Nagabhushan, M., and Bhide, S.V. (1987). Antimutagenicity and anticarcinogenicity of turmeric (*Curcuma longa*). *Journal of Nutrition Growth and Cancer*, **4**: 83-89.

Nebert, D.W. (1989). The Ah locus; genetic differences in toxicity, cancer, mutation, and birth defects. *Critical Reviews in Toxicology*, **20**: 153-174.

Nguyen, C.F., Porter, L., Ren, W.W. Roberts, R.F., Roche, A.B., Subbaramaiah, N.S., and Sporn, M.B. (1999). Inhibitory effects of phenolic compounds on benzo(a)pyrene-induced neoplasia. *Cancer Research*, **40**: 2820-2823.

Omenn, G.S., Goodman, G.E., Thornquist, M.D., Balmes, J., Cullen, M.R., Glass, A., Keogh, J.P., Meyskens, F.L. J., Valanis, B., Williams, J.H. Jr., Barnhart, S., Cherniack, M.G., Brodkin, C.A., and Hammar, S. (1996). Risk factors for lung cancer and for intervention effects in CARET, the β-carotene and Retinol Efficacy Trial. *Journal of National Cancer Institute*, **6**: 1550-1559.

Ravindra, K., Sokhi, R., and Van Grieken, R. (2008a). Atmospheric polycyclic aromatic hydrocarbons: source attribution, emission factors and regulation. *Atmospheric Environment*, **42**: 2895-2921.

Reddy, B.S., Tokumo, K., Kulkarni, N., Aligia, C., and Kelloff, G. (1992). inhibition of colon carcinogenesis by prostaglandin synthesis inhibitors and related compounds. *Carcinogenesis*, **13**: 1019-1023.

Reinik, M., Tamme, T., Roasto, M., Juhkam, K., Tenno, T., and Kiis, A. (2007). Polycyclic aromatic hydrocarbons (PAHs) in meat products and estimated PAH intake by children and the general population in Estonia. *Food Addit Contam.*, **24(4)**: 429-437.

Sarkar, F.H., and Li Y-W. (2007). Targeting multiple signal pathways by chemopreventive agents for cancer prevention and therapy. *Acta Pharmacologica Sinica*, **28 (9)**: 1305-1315.

Shimada, T., and Fujii-Kuriyama, Y. (2004). Metabolic activation of polycyclic aromatic hydrocarbons to carcinogens by cytochromes P450 1A1 and 1B1. *Cancer Science*, **95(1)**: 1-6.

Shin, Y.W., Bok, S.H., Jeong, T.S., Bae, K.H., Jeoung, N.H., Choi, M.S., Lee, S.H., and Park, Y.B. (1999). Hypocholesterolemic effectof naringin associated with hepatic cholesterol regulating enzyme changes in rats. International Journal of Vitamin. *Nutrition Research*, **69**: 341–347.

Singh, S.V., Hu, X., Srivastava, S.K., Singh, M., Xia, H., Orchard, J.L., and Zaren, H.A. (1998). Mechanism of inhibition of benzo[a]pyrene-induced forestomach cancer in mice by dietary curcumin. *Carcinogenesis*, **19**: 1357-1360.

Singletary, K. (2000). Diet, natural products and cancer chemoprevention. *Journal of Nutrition*, **130**: 465S-466S.

Slaga, T.J. (1980). Cancer: etiology, mechanisms, and prevention–a summary. *Carcinog Compr Surv.*, **5**: 243-262.

Sporn, B.M. (1999). Prevention of cancer in the next millennium: Report of the chemoprevention working group to the American association of cancer research. *Cancer research*, **59**: 4743-4758.

Stoner, G.D., and Mukhtar, H. (1995). Polyphenols as cancer chemopreventive agents. *Journal of Cell Biochemistry Suppl.*, **22**: 169-180.

Tanaka, T., Makita, H., Ohnishi, M., Mori, H., Satoh, K., and Hara, A. (1995). Chemoprevention of rat oral carcinogenesis by naturally occurring xanthophylls, astaxanthin and canthaxanthin. *Cancer Research*, **15**: 4059-64.

Ueng, Y.F., Chang, Y.L., Oda, Y., Park, S.S., Liao, J.F., Lin, M.F., and Chen, C.F. (1999). *In vitro* and *in vivo* effects of naringin on cytochrome P450-dependent monooxygenase in mouse liver. *Life Sciences*, **65**: 2591-2602.

Uppstad, H., Øvrebø, S., Haugen, A., and Mollerup, S. (2010). Importance of CYP1A1 and CYP1B1 in bioactivation of benzo[a]pyrene in human lung cell lines. *Toxicology Letters*, **192(2)**: 221-228.

Weisburger, J.H. (1991). Nutritional approach to cancer prevention with emphasis on vitamins, antioxidants, and carotenoids. *American Journal of Clinical Nutrition*, **53**: 226S-237S.

Wilcox, L.J., Borradaile, N.M., deDreu, L.E., and Huff, M.W. (2001). Secretion of hepatocyte apoB is inhibited by the flavonoids, naringenin and hesperetin, via reduced activity and expression of ACAT2 and MTP. *Journal of Lipid Research*, **42**: 725-34.

Winker, N., Weniger, P., Klein, W., Ott, E., Kocsis, F., Schoket, B., and Korpert, K. (1995). Detection of polycyclic aromatic hydrocarbon exposure damage using different methods in laboratory animals. *Journal of Applied Toxicology*, **15**: 59-62.

Wogan, G.N., Hecht, S.S., Felton, J.S., Conney, A.H., and Loeb, L.A. (2004). Environmental and chemical carcinogenesis. *Seminars in Cancer Biology*, **14**: 473–486.

Wood, A.W/, Levin, W., Lu, A.Y.H., Yagi, H., Hernandez, O., Jerina, D.W., and Conney, A.H. (1976). Metabolism of benzo[*a*]pyrene and benzo(a)pyrene derivatives to mutagenic products by highly purified hepatic microsomal enzymes. *Journal of Biological Chemistry,* **251**: 4882- 4890.

Zhang, Y., and Tao, S. (2009). Global atmospheric emission inventory of polycyclic aromatic hydrocarbons (PAHs) for 2004. *Atmospheric Environment,* **43**: 812–819.

Zhao, X.L. (1990). Effects of benzo[a]pyrene on the humoral immunity of mice exposed by single intraperitoneal injection. *Zhonghua,* **24**: 220-222.

Bioactive Phytochemicals: Perspectives for Modern Medicine Vol. 3 (2015)
Editor: **V.K. Gupta**
Published by: **DAYA PUBLISHING HOUSE, NEW DELHI**

Pages **201–209**

7

Capsaicin Prevents Oxidative Stress During D-galactosamine Induced Experimental Hepatitis

P. Anandakumar[1*] and T. Devaki[1]

ABSTRACT

The effect of capsaicin on oxidative stress produced during D-galactosamine induced hepatitis was studied in rats. Administration of D-galactosamine to rats caused a significant increase in oxidative stress indicated by abnormal changes in lipid peroxidation, enzymic antioxidants (superoxide dismutase, catalase, glutathione peroxidase, glutathione reductase and glutathione-S-transferase) and non-enzymic antioxidants (reduced glutathione, vitamin C, vitamin E and vitamin A). Treatment with capsaicin prevented all the above abnormal changes and restored cellular normalcy suggesting the protective role of capsaicin in curbing the oxidative stress produced during D-galactosamine induced hepatitis.

Keywords: Capsaicin, D-galactosamine, Hepatitis, Lipid peroxidation, Antioxidants.

Introduction

Liver is the major metabolic organ which performs varieties of function. Liver injury arises through different primary hepatotoxins including alcohol, aflatoxin, heavy metals and drugs. Among this D-galactosamine (DGalN) is well established as suitable experimental model of liver toxicity (Han *et al.*, 2006). DGalN is an amino sugar normally found *in vivo* only in acetylated form in certain structural polysaccharides. Administration of single dose of this compound to certain species results in dose-dependent hepatic damage resembling viral hepatitis, with focal

1 Department of Biochemistry, University of Madras, Chennai – 25, T.N., India
* *Corresponding author*: E-mail: paksuccess@gmail.com

necrosis and periportal inflammation (Ravikumar *et al.*, 2005a). Free radical mediated oxidant damage can contribute to acute hepatitis (Devaki *et al.*, 2009). High levels and/or inadequate removal of reactive oxygen species may cause severe metabolic imbalance and oxidative damage to biological macromolecules resulting in lipid peroxidation and depletion of cellular antioxidants (Sathivel *et al.*, 2008).

Many epidemiological and animal studies have shown that dietary intake of foods rich in fruits and vegetables decreased the occurrence of hepatitis (Wang *et al.*, 1999; Gyamfi *et al.*, 1999). Pepper fruits (*Capsicum annuum* L.) are important vegetables used as vegetable foods and as spices with well-known antioxidant properties (Materska Malgorzata and Perucka Irena, 2005). Capsaicin (CAP) (trans-8-methyl-N-vannilyl-6-nonemide) is the major pungent principle found in hot red and chilli peppers of the plant genus Capsicum that has long been used as spices, food additives and drugs (Cordell and Araiyo, 1993). Different studies on CAP have also revealed the antioxidant activity of CAP in several dimensions (Rice Evan, 1997; Lugman and Rizvi, 2006; De and Ghosh, 1993, Anandakumar *et al.*, 2008a).

The present study is an attempt to explore the antioxidant potential of CAP in ameliorating the oxidative stress produced during DGalN induced hepatitis in rats.

Materials and Methods

Materials

DGalN and CAP were purchased from M/s. Sigma chemicals, St. Louis, USA. All other chemicals were of analytical grade procured from M/s. SRL Chemicals Pvt. Ltd., Mumbai.

Animals

Adult male albino rats of Wistar strain weighing around 120 to 150 g obtained from Tamil Nadu Veterinary and Animal Sciences University (TANUVAS), Madhavaram, Chennai, India were used in this study. The animals were housed under conditions of controlled temperature (26 ±2°C) with 12-hr day/night cycle. They were fed standard rat/mice pellet diet (M/s. Hindustan Lever Ltd., Mumbai) under the trade name Amrut rat/mice feed and were given access to water *ad libitum*.

Experimental Design

Experimental animals were divided into four groups of six rats each as follows.

- Group I: Control animals received olive oil throughout the course of the experiment.
- Group II: Animals were treated with a single dose of DGalN (500 mg/kg body weight) intraperitoneally (Sathivel *et al.*, 2008).
- Group III: Animals received CAP alone (10 mg/kg body weight dissolved in olive oil) intraperitoneally to assess the cytotoxicity (if any) induced by CAP.
- Group IV: Animals received DGalN (as in Group II) along with CAP (10 mg/kg body weight dissolved in olive oil) intraperitoneally. CAP pre treatment was started 4 weeks prior to the administration of DGalN.

At the end of the experimental period, animals were sacrificed by cervical decapitation under ether anesthesia and liver was excised immediately and washed with ice-cold saline. A 10 per cent homogenate of the washed tissue (liver) was prepared in 0.01 M phosphate buffer (pH 7.4). The homogenate was centrifuged at a speed of 12,000 x g for 30 min in a refrigerated high-speed centrifuge at 4°C. Blood was also collected and the serum was separated for other estimations. The following analysis was carried out in the supernatant.

Biochemical Analysis

Protein estimation was carried out (Lowry *et al.*, 1951). LPO was assayed by the method in which the malondialdehyde (MDA) released served as the index (Ohkawa *et al.*, 1979). Superoxide dismutase (SOD) and catalase (CAT) were assayed (Marklund and Marklund, 1974; Sinha, 1974). The activities of glutathione peroxidase (GPx), glutathione reductase (GR) and glutathione-S-transferase were also was determined. (Rotruck *et al.*, 1973; Beutler, 1968; Habig *et al.*, 1974). Reduced glutathione (GSH), vitamin E, vitamin C and vitamin A were assayed (Moron *et al.*, 1979; Desai,1984; Omaye *et al.*, 1971; Bayfield and Cole, 1980).

Data Analysis

All data were expressed as mean ± S.D for six rats The results were computed statistically (SPSS Software Package) using one-way ANOVA. Post-hoc testing was performed for inter comparisons using the LSD. ($P < 0.05$) was considered significant.

Results

Effect of D-galactosamine and Capsaicin on Lipid Peroxidation in Rat Liver

Figure 7.1 shows the effect of DGalN and CAP on liver lipid peroxides (MDA) levels. DGalN induced group II rats showed significantly ($P < 0.05$) increased levels of MDA in liver compared to control rats (Group I). Pre treatment with CAP (Group IV) markedly ($P < 0.05$) decreased the levels of MDA in liver when compared with Group II animals.

Effect of D-galactosamine and Capsaicin on Enzymic Antioxidants in Rat Liver

Table 7.1 depicts the effect of DGalN and CAP on liver enzymic antioxidant status. Significant ($P < 0.05$) reduction in the activities of enzymic antioxidants SOD, CAT, GPx, GR and GST were observed in the DGalN administered group (Group II). CAP pretreatment resulted in a free radical quenching effect and thereby significantly ($P < 0.05$) reinstated the enzymic antioxidant activities to near normalcy in Group IV animals.

Effect of D-galactosamine and Capsaicin on Non-enzymic Antioxidants in Rat Liver

Table 7.2 shows the levels of non-enzymic antioxidants GSH, vitamin C, vitamin E and vitamin A in control and experimental group of animals. DGalN

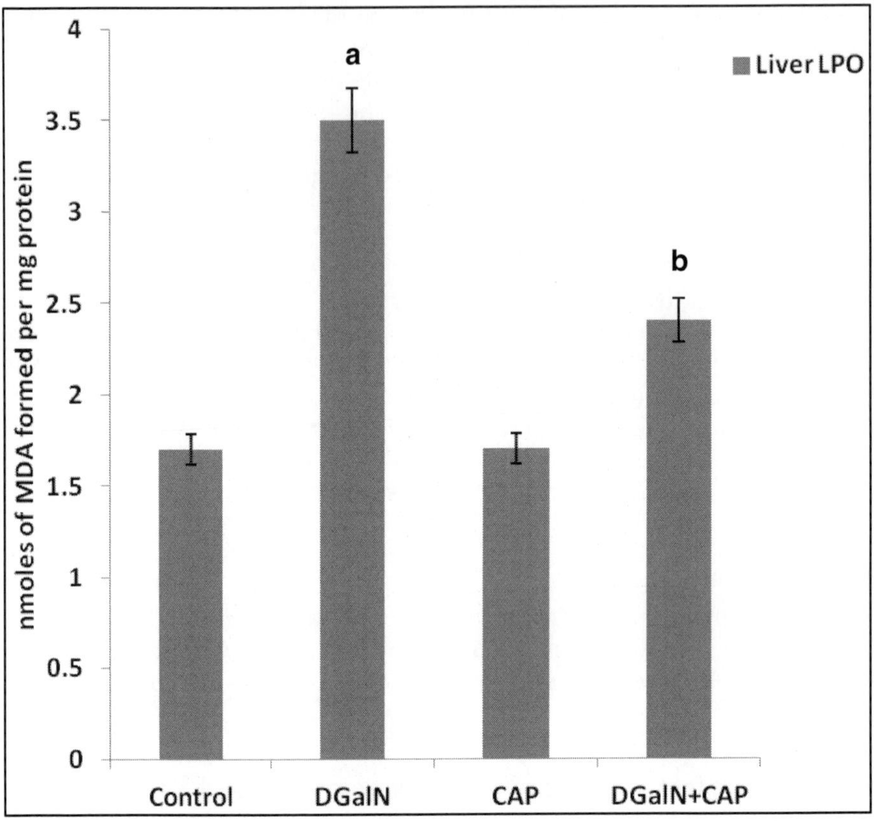

Figure 7.1: Effect of D-galactosamine and Capsaicin on Lipid Peroxidation in Rat Liver. Each value is expressed as mean ± S.D for six rats in each group. Statistical significance at $P<0.05$, as compared with [a]Group I, [b]Group II.

Table 7.1: Effect of D-galactosamine and Capsaicin on Enzymic Antioxidants in Rat Liver

Parameters	*Group I (Control)*	*Group II (DGalN)*	*Group III (CAP)*	*Group IV (DGalN + CAP)*
SOD	6.93 ± 0.06	3.88 ± 0.04[a]	6.96 ± 0.09	5.80 ± 0.04[b]
CAT	72.13 ± 1.30	53.03 ± 1.31[a]	71.59 ± 1.23	63.66 ± 1.27[b]
GPx	104.32 ± 1.85	58.71 ± 1.08[a]	104.06 ± 2.53	86.68 ± 1.77[b]
GR	4.39 ± 0.43	1.28 ± 0.13[a]	4.37 ± 0.43	4.08 ± 0.08[b]
GST	235.27 ± 6.20	149.36 ± 3.81[a]	235.64 ± 7.25	207.51 ± 7.06[b]

Each value is expressed as mean ± S.D for six rats in each group.

SOD: units/mg protein (One unit is equal to the amount of enzyme required to inhibit autoxidation of pyrogallol by 50 per cent); CAT: μg of H_2O_2 consumed/min/mg protein; GPx: μg of reduced GSH utilized/min/mg protein; GR: nmoles of NADPH oxidized/min/mg protein; GST: nmoles of CDNB - GSH conjugate formed/min/mg protein.

Statistical significance at $P<0.05$, as compared with [a]Group I, [b]Group II.

treatment markedly ($P < 0.05$) reduced the levels of GSH, vitamin C, vitamin E and vitamin A in Group II animals that were significantly ($P < 0.05$) restored to near normalcy on CAP pretreatment in Group IV animals.

Table 7.2: Effect of D-galactosamine and Capsaicin on Non-enzymic Antioxidants in Rat Liver

Parameters	*Group I (Control)*	*Group II (DGalN)*	*Group III (CAP)*	*Group IV (DGalN + CAP)*
GSH	6.56 ± 0.37	2.99 ± 0.10[a]	6.55 ± 0.34	5.88 ± 0.32[b]
Vitamin C	4.32 ± 0.23	2.40 ± 0.18[a]	4.31 ± 0.15	3.79 ± 0.5[b]
Vitamin E	1.65 ± 0.25	0.59 ± 0.04[a]	1.62 ± 0.10	1.37 ± 0.19[b]
Vitamin A	0.55 ± 0.05	0.19 ± 0.0[a]	0.54 ± 0.05	0.37 ± 0.04[b]

Each value is expressed as mean ± S.D for six rats in each group.

GSH: μg/mg protein; Vitamin C: μg/mg protein; Vitamin E: μg/mg protein; Vitamin A: μg/mg protein.

Statistical significance at $P<0.05$, as compared with [a]Group I, [b]Group II.

Discussion

LPO is regarded as one of the basic mechanism of cellular damage caused by free radicals (Anandakumar *et al.*, 2008a). An increase in LPO indicates serious damage to cell membranes, inhibition of several enzymes, cellular function and cell death (Ramakrishnan *et al.*, 2006). In recent years, it has been suggested that reactive oxygen species produced by activated hepatic macrophages might be the primary cause of LPO leading to DGalN - induced liver damage (Sathivel *et al.*, 2013). Our results were in consistent with the previous findings as we observed increased liver LPO in group II DGalN induced rats.

The major mechanism accountable for alkaloid substances in combating the ROS induced oxidative damage is due to the antioxidant effect of these compounds (Anandakumar *et al.*, 2008a). CAP is one such alkaloid whose potential antioxidant role has been reported (Surh *et al.*, 1995). Previous reports confirm that the radical scavenging site of CAP is the C7-benzyl carbon (Kogure *et al.*, 2002). The above reports were substantiated by our present study, where pretreatment with CAP reduced liver LPO induced by DGalN in group IV animals suggesting its antioxidant efficacy.

To prevent oxidative damage in the cell, a variety of antioxidants scavenge free radicals. The primary defense against oxidative stress in the tissue rests with antioxidants. SOD, an important antioxidant enzyme protects cells against the toxic effects of superoxide anion (Ravikumar *et al.*, 2005b). CAT catalyses the direct degradation of H_2O_2 to water. It protects the cellular constituents against oxidative damage (Balaji Raghavendran *et al.*, 2005). GPx and the cellular NADPH generating mechanisms together form a system for removing the hydroperoxides from the cell (Balaji Raghavendran *et al.*, 2005). GST is a group of multifunctional proteins that perform tasks ranging from catalyzing the detoxification of electrophilic compounds to protection against peroxidative damage (Anandakumar *et al.*, 2008b). GR plays a major role in regenerating GSH from GSSG, thus maintaining the balance between the redox couple (Kamaraj *et al.*, 2007). The decreased activities of these antiperoxidative enzymes during DGalN administration in the present study are compatible with earlier findings (Sathivel *et al.*, 2008). The decreased activity of these enzymatic antioxidants may be due to the accumulation of H_2O_2 which inturn causes the inhibition of these enzymes. The reduced activities of these enzymes were normalised upon pretreatment with CAP.

GSH, a chief endogenous antioxidant system is found in particularly high concentration in liver and is known to have key functions in protective processes (Pushpavalli *et al.*, 2010). The protective role of GSH against cellular lipid peroxidation has been well recognized (Sheriff and Devaki, 2013). Low concentration of GSH has been implicated in D-GalN-induced hepatitis (Pushpavalli *et al.*, 2008). Vitamin C a major antioxidant acts in tissues, involving ROS in aqueous phase and it has been reported that the tissue concentration of vitamin C is a good indicator of oxidative stress (El-Beshbishy, 2008). Vitamin E is a principal lipid soluble antioxidant in cell membranes that protects critical cellular structures against oxidative damage (El-Beshbishy, 2008). The concentration of vitamin E has been inversely correlated to LPO (Sheriff and Devaki, 2013). Vitamin A as an antioxidant is involved in counteracting free radicals and is known to help in the repair of damaged tissues (Serbecic *et al.*, 2005). Vitamin A at pharmacological doses is reported to ameliorate the oxidative stress mediated membrane lipid peroxidation and membranes enriched with vitamin A are protected against oxidative stress *in vivo* and exhibit resistance to LPO induced *in vitro* (Britton *et al.*, 2000). Vitamin C, E and A levels were found to be reduced in DGalN administered groups (Group II) suggesting an increase in LPO in these animals. The levels of these vitamins in rats challenged with DGalN were almost normalized upon CAP pretreatment. Our results were in consistent with Kempaiah *et al.* (Kempaiah *et al.*, 2004) who reported that CAP was effective against oxidative stress by countering the depleted antioxidant molecules and antioxidant enzymes.

Thus our present findings clearly demonstrate the role of CAP as a potent antioxidant that prevented oxidative stress and in turn paved way for its protective role against DGalN induced hepatitis in rats.

Acknowledgments

First author Anandakumar P wishes to thank Mr. Pandi, Mrs. Padmavathi, Mrs. Kalaivani and Mrs. Prabhavathy for their moral support and encouragement throughout the period of study.

References

Anandakumar, P., Kamaraj S., Jagan S., Ramakrishnan G., Vinodhkumar R., and Devaki T. (2008a). Capsaicin modulates pulmonary antioxidant defense system during benzo(a)pyrene-induced lung cancer in Swiss albino mice. *Phytotherapy Research*, **22**: 529–533.

Anandakumar, P., Kamaraj, S., Jagan, S., Ramakrishnan, G., Vinodhkumar R., and Devaki T. (2008b). Stabilization of pulmonary mitochondrial enzyme system by capsaicin during benzo(a)pyrene induced experimental lung cancer. *Biomedicine and Pharmacotherapy*, **62**: 390–394.

Balaji Raghavendran, H.R., Sathivel, A., and Devaki, T. (2005). Antioxidant effect of Sargassum polycystum (Phaeophyceae) against acetaminophen induced changes in hepatic mitochondrial enzymes during toxic hepatitis. *Chemosphere*, **61(2)**: 276-281.

Bayfield, R.F., and Cole, E.R. (1980). Colorimetric estimation of vitamin A with trichloroacetic acid. *Methods in Enzymology*,**67**: 189.

Beutler, E. (1968). Active transport of glutathione disulfide from erythrocytes. *In:* Larson A, Orrenius S, Holmgren A, Mannerwik B, editors. *Functions of glutathione: Biochemical, physiological, toxicological and clinical aspects.* New York: Raven Press; p. 65.

Cordell, G.A., and Araiyo, O.E. (1993). Capsaicin identification, nomenclature and pharmacotherapy. *Annals of Pharmacotherapy*, **27**: 330.

De, A.K., and Ghosh, J.J. (1993). Capsaicin pretreatment protects free radical induced rat lung damage on exposure to gaseous chemical lung irritants. *Phytotherapy Research*,**7**: 87.

Desai, I.D. (1984). Vitamin E analysis methods for animal tissues. *Methods in Enzymology*, **105**: 138.

Devaki, T., Sathivel, A., and Balaji Raghavendran, H.R. (2009). Stabilization of mitochondrial and microsomal function by polysaccharide of *Ulva lactuca* on D-Galactosamine induced hepatitis in rats. *Chemico Biological Interactions*, **177(2)**: 83-88.

El-Beshbishy, H.A. (2008). Aqueous garlic extract attenuates hepatitis and oxidative stress induced by galactosamine/lipoploysaccharide in rats. *Phytotherapy Research*, **22(10)**: 1372-1379.

Gyamfi, M.A., Yonamine, M., and Aniya, Y. (1999). Free radical scavenging action of medicinal herbs from Ghana thonningia sanguine on experimentally-induced liver injuries. *General Pharmacology*, **32**: 661-667.

Habig, W.H., Pabst, M.J., and Jacob, W.B. (1974). Glutathione-S-transferase. The first enzymatic step in mercapturic acid formation. *Journal of Biological Chemistry*, **249**: 7130.

Han, K.H., Hashimoto, N., Shimada, K., Sekikawa, M., Noda, T., Yamauchi, H., Hashimoto, M., Chiji, H., Topping, D.L., and Fukushima, M. (2006). Hepatoprotective effects of purple potato extract against D-galactosamine-induced liver injury in rats. *Bioscience, Biotechnology and Biochemistry*, **70(6)**: 1432-1437.

Kamaraj, S., Vinodhkumar, R., Anandakumar, P., Jagan, S., and Ramakrishnan, G. (2007). The effects of quercetin on antioxidant status and tumor markers in the lung and serum of mice treated with benzo(a)pyrene. *Biological Pharmaceutical Bulletin*, **30**: 2268–2273.

Kempaiah, P., and Srinivasan, K. (2004). Influence of dietary curcumin, capsaicin and garlic on the antioxidant state of red blood cells and the liver in high-fat fed rats. *Annals of Nutritional Metabolism*,**48**: 314.

Kogure Kentaro., Goto Satoru., Nishimura Miki., Yasumoto Mina., Abe Kazutoyo., and Ohiwa Che. (2002). Mechanism of potent antiperoxidative effect of capsaicin. *Biochima et Biophysics Acta*, **1573**: 84.

Lowry, O.H., Rosenbrough, N.J., Farr, A.L., and Randall R.J. (1951). Protein measurement with the Folin's phenol reagent. *Journal of Biological Chemistry*, **193**: 265.

Lugman, S., and Rizvi, S.I. (2006). Protection of lipid peroxidation and carbonyl formation in proteins by capsaicin in human erythrocytes subjected to oxidative stress. *Phytotherapy Research*, **20**: 303.

Marklund, S., and Marklund, G.(1974). Involvement of superoxide anion radical in the autooxidation of pyrogallol and a convenient assay for superoxide dismutase. *European Journal of Biochemistry*, **47**: 469.

Materska Malgorzata., and Perucka Irena. (2005). Antioxidant activity of the main phenolic compounds isolated from hot pepper fruit (*Capsicum annuum* L.). *Journal of Agricultural Food Chemistry*, **53**: 1750.

Moron, M.S., Despierre, J.W., and Minnervik, B.(1979). Levels of glutathione, glutathione reductase and glutathione-S-transferase activities in rat lung and liver. *Biochima et Biophysics Acta*, **582**: 67.

Ohkawa, H., Ohish, N., and Yagi, K. (1979). Assay of lipid peroxides in animal tissues by thiobarbituric acid reaction. *Analytical Biochemistry*, **95**: 351.

Omaye, A.T., Turnbull, J.D., and Sauberdich, H.E. (1971). Selected method for determination of ascorbic acid in animal cells, tissues and fluids. *Methods in Enzymology*,**62**: 1.

Pushpavalli, G., Kalaiarasi, P., Veeramani, C., and Pugalendi, K.V. (2010). Effect of chrysin on hepatoprotective and antioxidant status in D-galactosamine-induced hepatitis in rats. *European Journal of Pharmacology*, **10**: 36-41.

Pushpavalli, G., Veeramani, C., and Pugalendi, K.V. (2008). Influence of Piper betle on hepatic marker enzymes and tissue antioxidant status in D-galactosamine-induced hepatotoxic rats. *J Basic Clin Physiol Pharmacol.*, 1**9(2)**: 131-50.

Ramakrishnan Gopalakrishnan., Raghavendran Hanumantha Rao Balaji., Vinodh Kumar Radhakrishnan., and Devaki Thiruvengadam. (2006). Suppression of N-nitrosodiethylamine induced hepatocarcinogenesis by silymarin in rats. *Chemico Biological interactions*, **161**: 104.

Ravikumar, V., Shivashangari, K.S., and Devaki, T. (2005a). Hepatoprotective activity of Tridax procumbens against d-galactosamine/lipopolysaccharide-induced hepatitis in rats. *Journal of Ethnopharmacology*, **101(1-3)**: 55-60.

Ravikumar, V., Shivashangari, K.S., and Devaki, T. (2005b). Effect of Tridax procumbens on liver antioxidant defense system during lipopolysaccharide-induced hepatitis in D-galactosamine sensitised rats. *Molecular and Cellular Biochemistry*, **269(1-2)**: 131-136.

Rice Evans, C.A., Miller, J., and Paganga, G. (1997). Antioxidant properties of phenolic compounds. *Trends in Plant Science*, **2**: 152.

Rotruck, J.T., Pope, A.L., Ganther, H.E., Swanson, A.B., Hajeman, D.G., and Hoekstra, W.G. (1973). Selenium-biochemical role as a component of glutathione purification and assay. *Science*,**179**: 588.

Sathivel, A., Balavinayagamani., Hanumantha Rao,B.R., and Devaki, T. (2013). Sulfated polysaccharide isolated from *Ulva lactuca* attenuates d-galactosamine induced DNA fragmentation and necrosis during liver damage in rats. *Pharmaceutical Biology*, (In Press).

Sathivel, A., Raghavendran, H.R., Srinivasan, P., and Devaki, T. (2008). Anti-peroxidative and anti-hyperlipidemic nature of Ulva lactuca crude polysaccharide on D-galactosamine induced hepatitis in rats. *Food and Chemical Toxicology*, **46(10)**: 3262-3267.

Serbecic, N., Ehmann, A.K., and Beutelspacher, S.C. (2005). Reduction of lipid peroxidation and apoptosis in corneal endothelial cells by vitamin A. *Ophthalmologe*, **6**: 607.

Sinha, A.K. (1974). Colorimetric assay of catalase. *Analytical Biochemistry*, **47**: 389.

Sheik Abdulazeez, S., and Thiruvengadam, D. (2013). Effect of lycopene on oxidative stress induced during D-galactosamine/lipopolysaccharide-sensitized liver injury in rats. *Pharmaceutical Biology*, **51(12)**: 1592-1599.

Surh, Y.J., Lee, R.C., Park, K.K., Mayne, S.T., Liem, A., and Miller, J.A. (1995). Chemopreventive effects of capsaicin and diallyl sulfide against mutagenesis or tumorigenesis by vinyl carbamate and N-nitrosodimethylamine. *Carcinogenesis*, **16**: 2467.

Wang, H., Nair, M.G., Strasburg, G.M., Chang, Y.C., Booren, A.M., Gray, J.L., and Dewitt, D.L. (1999). Antioxidant and anti-inflammatory activities of anthocyanins and their aglycon, cyaniding from tart cherries. *Journal of Natural Products*, **62**: 294-296.

Bioactive Phytochemicals: Perspectives for Modern Medicine Vol. 3 (2015) *Pages* **211–234**
Editor: **V.K. Gupta**
Published by: **DAYA PUBLISHING HOUSE, NEW DELHI**

8

A Review on *Rhizophora* Genus: Therapeutically Important Perspective Phytochemical Constituents

V. Balasubramanian[1*], P. Rajesh[2],
R. Rajaram[1] and V. Rajesh Kannan[2]

ABSTRACT

The main objective of the comprehensive review is to present the research carried out with widely spread genus in the world of Rhizophora in order to determine the forcing function that influences their development and architecture. This review has summarized the phytoconstituents; its chemical structure and the corresponding to application of the pharmacological and biological activities in various species of the Rhizophora. The Rhizophora genus is a tropical coastline plant belonging to the family of Rhizophoraceae and distributed in Coastal area of the Asia, Africa, Australia, South Pacific etc., Mangrove plants are rich source of secondary metabolites as phytomedicines as alkaloids, flavonoids, saponins, steroids, tannins and triterpenes. Extracts and various forms of mangrove plants are reported to possess diverse medicinal properties in various ancient and research development such as antibacterial, antioxidant, hepatoprotective and immunological activity. Mangroves are known for their economic and ecological importance throughout the world and they are occupied about one fourth of tropical coastline. There are many challenges in drug development with plants which includes the mangrove plants, in particularly the Rhizophora is having notable functional groups of drug conserving phytoconstituents. In the past decades, the research study of the Mangroves has also been reported to have the plant phytochemicals (secondary

1 Department of Marine Science, Bharathidasan University, Tiruchirappalli – 620 024, Tamil Nadu, India

2 Department of Microbiology, Bharathidasan University, Tiruchirappalli – 620 024, Tamil Nadu, India

* *Corresponding author*: E-mail: vbv82@rediffmail.com, drrajaram69@rediffmail.com

metabolites) have been reported to have flavonoids, phenolic compounds, pigments, steroids as presence as different phytochemicals and its derivatives. The above reviewed details of the Rhizophora genus will be deserved the reference piece for various biological and pharmaceutical applications.

Keywords: Mangroves, Rhizophora, Antimicrobial, Rhizophorine.

Introduction

The *Rhizophora* species are medicinal plants in mangrove system of eastern and southeastern Asia. Mangrove *Rhizophora* species which are the most common representatives are *Rhizophora apiculata, R. conjugata, R. mucronata, R. mangle, R. mucronata* and *R. stylosa*. The Mangrove plants are a group of trees and shrubs growing along seashores in tropical and subtropical areas (Tomlinson, 1994).

The mangrove environment is challenging for tree growth, as shown by the fact that few, albeit taxonomically diverse, tree species have colonized intertidal areas (Tomlinson, 1994). Mangrove species often have anatomical and physiological adaptations to the vagaries of the intertidal, including the 'prop' roots of *Rhizophora* that provide an archetypal tropical mangrove look. These are extensively reviewed and this will not be repeated in depth here (Tomilnson, 1994). The anatomical and physiological adaptations of mangrove species have metabolic costs that are 'the price of survival' in such a difficult environment.

Approximately, 55 species of mangroves from 22 genera are distributed in Indian Ocean region (Kathiresan and Rajendran, 2005). As much as the habitat of mangrove plants takes different names asmangrove swamps, tidal forests, tidal swamp forests or mangals, so they are evidences for its antibacterial (Chandrasekaran *et al.*, 2009), antiviral (Premanathan *et al.*, 1999), Antifungal (Bose and Bose, 2008), mosquito larvicidal (Thangam and Kathiresan, 1989) and antioxidant activity (Babu *et al.*, 2001).

While, the various parts of *Rhizophora mucronata* found its used to treat human ailments like angina, dysentery, hematuria and many more (Joel and Bhimba, 2010). In Malaysia, *Rhizophora apiculata* and *Rhizophora mucronata* or locally known as Bakau Minyak and Bakau Kurapare the famous mangrove plant widely used in charcoal industry and it has been reported to produce high yields of tannins (Jain *et al.*, 2002) which are useful for the immunological disorders.

Extracts of mangrove plants were demonstrated to have biological activity against human animal and plant pathogens, such as human immunodeficiency viruses (Basyuni *et al.*, 2007). *Rhizophora apiculata* is one of the major species of *Rhizophora* genus and the polysaccharide extracted from the leaves of *Rhizophora apiculata* was assessed in cell culture systems, for its activity against human immunodeficiency viruses. The study indicated that a polysaccharide extracted from *Rhizophora apiculata* has anti-HIV activity *in vitro*, apparently due to interference with the adsorption of virus particles to positive human cells (Premanathan *et al.*, 1999). From the above brief of *Rhizophora* genus, the current review is completely discussed on their basic pharmacological and biological properties with their prospective phytochemical constituents and chemicals structures.

Pharmacological and Various activities of Phytochemicals from *Rhizophora* spp.

Rhizophora annamalayana

An endophytic fungus *Fusarium oxysporum* was reported from the *Rhizophora annamalayana* and reported for the taxol **(1)** production (Alaganadham *et al.*, 2012).

Rhizophora apiculata

The study has been reported that the heartwood of *Rhizophora apiculata* was active against fungi, bacteria and boll weevils. Five long chain aliphatic alcohols, 11 long chain aliphatic saturated carboxylic acids **(2)**, three steroids, 2,6-dimethoxy-*p*-benzoquinone **(3)**, syringaldehyde **(4)** and sitosteryl 3-glucoside **(5)** have also been reported from the heartwood of *R. apiculata* (Kokpol *et al.*, 1993).

The *Rhizophora apiculata* was reported as safety assumes of herbivory and not to decrease the productivity estimate of this stand significantly. The particular mangrove plants were reported to possess higher content of the organic matter from the roots. Also, the study was reported that the structure and productivity of a 20 year old stand of *R. apiculata* mangrove forest (Ong Jin-Eong, *et al.*, 1995).

The *Rhizophora apiculata* was reported to possess the phytochemicals such as aliphatic alcohols **(6)**, aldehydes **(7)**, carboxylic acid **(8)**, carotenoids **(9)**, hydrolysable tannins **(10)**, benzoquinones **(11)**, lipids **(12)**, n-alkanes **(13)**, minerals, phenolic compounds **(14)**, polysaccharides **(15)**, steroids **(16)** and triterpenes **(17)**, which are responsible for astringent for diarrhea, nausea, vomiting, typhoid, hepatitis, antiseptic and insecticide (Premanathan *et al.*, 1999).

The growth performance of *Rhizophora apiculata* seedlings enhancement was reported through exogenous gibberellic acid **(18)** in different combinations (Kathiresan and Rajendran, 2002). The plant *R. apiculata* was reported for the efficient and significant inhibition of growth of antibiotic resistant *Staphylococcus* sp. and *Proteus* sp. (Abeysinghe *et al.*, 2004). The hydrolysable tannins **(10)** were reported from the *R. apiculata* extracts and it was reported for the *in vitro* antibacterial and antifungal activity through various pathogenic microbes (Lim *et al.*, 2006).

The *Rhizophora apiculata* barks reported to possess terminal units such as catechin **(19)**, epicatechin **(20)**, epigallocatechin **(21)** and epicatechingallate **(22)** through HPLC analysis and reported as antimicrobial, antioxidative activities (Rahim *et al.*, 2008). The antitermite activity was reported on bark extract of *R. apiculata* and four other species against the subterranean termite *Coptotermes gestroi* and the activity was proved through the phenolic compounds **(14)** (Abdul Khalil *et al.*, 2009).

The accumulative partitioning of Pb and Cu in the *Rhizophora apiculata* was reported on randomly in the mangrove forest, Terengganu. The results were reported on *R. apiculata* shows that the concentration of Pb and Cu were accumulated higher in root tissue compared to bark and leaf tissue but lower than surrounding sediment level. Results of concentration factors (CF) reported that the overall concentration of

Pb and Cu were accumulated much higher in roots system of *R. apiculata* (Kamaruzzaman *et al.*, 2009).

A research was reported that the anticandidal compound of tannins **(23)** extracted from the barks of *R. apiculata*. Tannins **(23)** were reported from the barks of *R. apiculata* was further separated as condensed tannins **(24)** and hydrolysable tannins **(10)**. A strong anticandidal activity was detected and reported in the hydrolysable tannin **(10)** that responsible for the anticandidal activity was also determined using TLC and HPLC. The results were reported that gallic acid **(25)** was the bioactive compound that plays role in inhibiting and killing the *Candida albicans* cells (Lim *et al.*, 2011).

The *Rhizophora apiculata* barks were reported to possess significant antimicrobial properties against 18 bacterial and 12 fungal and 4 yeast species and also reported as significant antioxidant activity through DPPH and H_2O_2 activities on condensed tannins **(24)** (Suraya *et al.*, 2011). The *R. apiculata* has been suggested and reported the compounds phenolic compounds **(14)** and flavonoids **(37)** were producing significant antioxidant activity through DPPH method (Asha *et al.*, 2012).

The *in vitro* antioxidant activity guided phytochemical separation procedures, lyoniresinol-3α-O-β-arabinopyranoside **(26)**, lyoniresinol-3α-O-β-rhamnoside **(27)** and afzelechin-3-O-L-rhamno-pyranoside **(28)** were separated and reported from the butanol fraction of *R. apiculata*. These compounds showed more noticeable antioxidant activity than a BHT standard in the DPPH, ABTS and hydroxyl radical scavenging assays. The HPLC analysis reported that among different plant parts, the highest content of the above compounds was reported in the bark. The results imply that the *R. apiculata* might be a potential source of natural antioxidants and the compounds are antioxidant ingredients (Mingzhe and Hongbin, 2012). The *R. apiculata* reported for the astringent for diarrhoea, treatment of nausea, vomiting, typhoid, hepatitis, an antiseptic, insecticide and amoebiasis (Prabhakaran and Kavitha, 2012).

Rhizophora conjugata

The *Rhizophora conjugata* has been reported for the presence of steroids **(16)**, triterpenes **(17)**, tannins **(23)**, anthocyanins **(29)** and procyanidins **(30)** (Majumdar and Patra, 1976). The *R. conjugata* was reported for the *in vitro* efficiency through antimicrobial properties in various pathogenic bacterial strains (Varahalarao and Chandrshekar, 2009).

Rhizophora gymnorrhiza

The *Rhizophora gymnorrhiza* has been reported for the presence of triterpenes **(17)**, anthocyanins **(29)**, procyanidins **(30)** and anthocyanidins **(31)** (Majumdar and Patra, 1976).

Rhizophora lamarckii

The *Rhizophora lamarckii* has been reported for the antiviral activity (Majumdar and Patra, 1976). The *R. lamarckii* leaves have been reported for the hepatitis treatment (Prabhakaran and Kavitha, 2012).

Rhizophora mangle

The *Rhizophora mangle* was reported to possess sulphur containing nitrogenous compounds **(32)** and having various pharmacological activities against various cancer cells, (carcinomas, melanomas and lymphomas) which are responsible for the diabetes, angina, boils, bruises, fungal infections, diarrhea, dysentery, elephantiasis, fever, malaria, leprosy plaster for fractured bones, tuberculosis and antiseptics (Rollet, 1981). The response of mangrove ecosystems to environmental change has been examined and reported with stable isotopic tracers of carbon and nitrogen. The ^{13}C and ^{15}N of a taphonomic series of *R. mangle* leaves were analyzed from Twin Cays, Belize reported to facilitate reconstruction of past mangrove ecosystems (Matthew *et al.*, 2003).

The report was assessed for herbivory levels on attached fruits of *Rhizophora mangle* in three mangroves with different degrees of structural complexity in Paranagua Bay in South Brazil and also reported that as an important path for organic matter flux in mangroves. The fruits are locally consumed not only by tree-dwelling crabs and insects as previously recognized also by birds, which may play a more significant role in mangrove herbivory (Kalina *et al.*, 2011).

The plant *Rhizophora mangle* has been reported for the significant antiulcer activity through monitoring $PGE_{2,}$ COX-2 inhibitors and histopathological analysis on gastric mucosa and stomach (Felipe *et al.*, 2012). The *R. mangle* was identified and reported to possess a phytochemical such as epicatechin **(20)** through FIA-ESI-IT-MS/MS negative mode (Felipe *et al.*, 2012a).

Rhizophora mucronata

The *Rhizophora mucronata* was reported to possess the phytochemicals such as proteins, minerals, carotenoids **(9)**, hydrolysable tannins **(10)**, lipids **(12)**, polysaccharides **(14)**, steroids **(16)**, triterpenes **(17)**, condensed tannins **(24)**, procyanidins **(30)**, anthocyanidins **(31)**, alkaloids **(33)**, carbohydrates **(34)**, chlorophyll **(35)**, gibberellins **(36)**, flavonoids **(37)**, inositols **(38)**, polyphenols **(39)** and saponins **(40)**, which are responsible for the elephantiasis, hematoma, hepatitis, ulcer and febrifuge (Rollet, 1981).

The alkaloid rhizophorine **(41)** is a major constituent of the leaves of *Rhizophora mucronata* (Bandaranayake, 2002). The growth rings formation and age determination were reported in the mangrove *R. mucronata* through dendrochronological and silvi cultural applications (Anouk *et al.*, 2004).

The variations in the distribution pattern and growth attributes of the two mangrove species *Avicennia marina* and *Rhizophora mucronata* as related to soil factors and tide levels were reported along with the red sea coast, Egypt. The plant height, size index, trunk circumference, number main and lateral branches, leaf number, area and the number of seedlings of *R. mucronata* was high in pure patches than when grow mixed with *A. marina* (El-Khouly *et al.*, 2007).

The plant *Rhizophora mucronata* has been reported for the phytoremediation in highly abundant metals in nature (Pahalawattaarachchi *et al.*, 2009). The *R. mucronata* was reported for the antimicrobial properties against the phytopathogens (Chandrashekar and Varahalarao, 2010).

The mangroves have proven its use worldwide about the specific medicinal properties of *Rhizophora mucronata* depend on the part employed and find its use to treat human ailments like angina, dysentery, hematuria and manymore diseases. The foliar extracts of *R. mucronata* were studied and reported for the bioactivity against *E. coli* and *S. aureus*. A column chromatographic fractionation of the extracts and further UV visible and GC-MS analysis suggested and reported the active principle compound. The GC-MS results of active column fraction reported that the active principles were a mixture of squalene **(42)**, n-hexadecanoic acid **(43)**, phytol **(44)**, 2-cyclohexane-1-one, 4-hydroxy-3,5- **(45)** and oleic acid **(46)**. The leaf extracts was reported to possess antibacterial effects can be clearly reported towards cancer treatment as to inhibiting cancer cell growth (Elsa and Valentin, 2010).

The *Rhizophora mucronata* has been reported for the treatment of elephantiasis, haematoma, hepatitis, ulcers and a febrifuge, bark-powerful astringent useful in diabetes and hemorrhage (Prabhakaran and Kavitha, 2012). The *Neurospora crassa* was isolated and reported *R. mucronata* for the significant antimicrobial and cytotoxic activity (Elsa and Valentin, 2012).

The *Rhizophora mucronata* root extract has been reported for an alternative medicine for the treatment of liver damage through CCl_4 induced hepatic damage and reported their chemical constituents such as alkaloids **(33)**, flavonoids **(37)**, polyphenols **(39)** and coumarins **(47)** (Sundaram Ravikumar, 2012). The most effective concentration of *R. mucronata* leaf extract in decreasing motility of the ileum was reduced motility of the ileum by direct action on smooth muscle cells. It was reported to possess potential gastro intestinal motility such as diarrhea (Yunita *et al.*, 2012).

The antimicrobial potential of endophytic bacteria isolated and reported from the *Rhizophora mucronata* (Anu and Priscilla, 2013). The results were reported on histochemical demonstration for acetyl cholinesterase in supra esophageal ganglion had revealed the inhibition of acetyl cholinesterase by the treatments of plant *R. mucronata* extract and reported significance of bioactive antimosquito larval compound (Meenakshi and Jayaprakash, 2014). Two fractions were reported from the *R. mucronata* and found that the compound as one of the phytochemicals such as hexane-3-ol **(48)** through LC-MS, FT-IR, and ^{1}H NMR techniques (Raut *et al.*, 2014).

Rhizophora racemosa

The *Rhizophora racemosa* was reported to possess the phytochemicals such as polysaccharides **(14)**, triterpenes **(17)**, tannins **(23)**, carbohydrates **(34)**, polyphenols **(39)**, amino acids **(49)**, sugars **(50)** and waxes which are responsible for the bleeding and wound burns (Popp *et al.*, 1984). The corrosion inhibition was reported from the tannins **(23)** produced by *R. racemosa* which was favored because of tannins **(23)** was treated specimens suffered corrosion attack after one week of exposure tests (Makanjuola, 2011).

The *Rhizophora racemosa* plant extracts of bark have been reported antimicrobial properties and the corresponding bioactive compounds are reported to possess saponins **(40)**, quinine **(51)** and terpenoid **(52)** (Ukoima *et al.*, 2013).

Figure 8.1: Chemical Structures through ISIS Chemdraw.

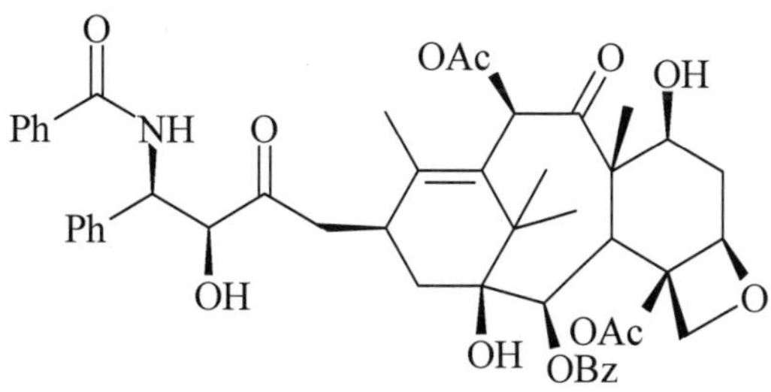

Taxol (1)

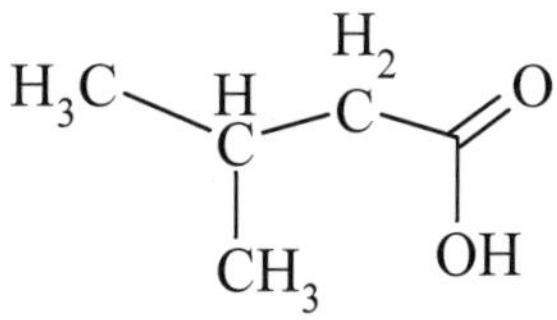

Aliphatic Carboxylic acids (2)

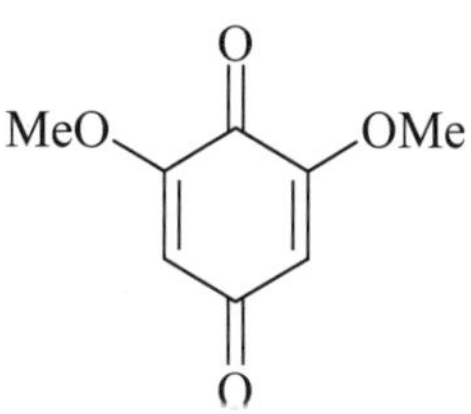

2,6-dimethoxy-*p*-benzoquinone (3)

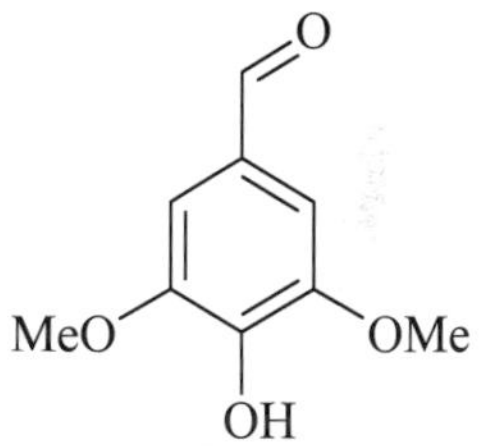

Syringaldehyde (4)

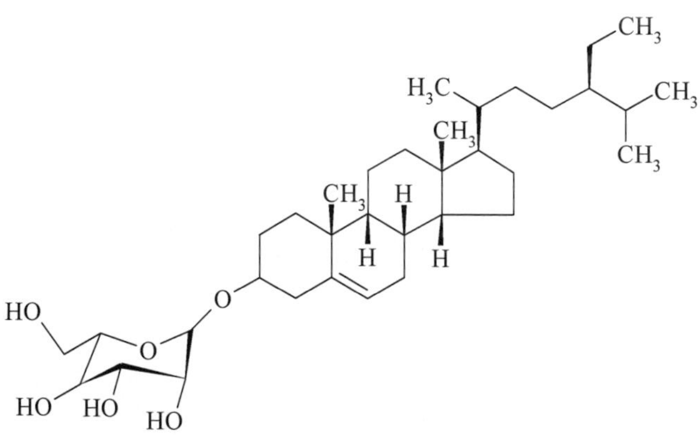

Sitosteryl-3-glucoside (5)

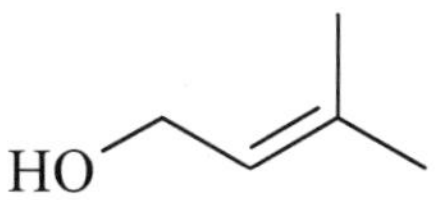

Aliphatic alcohols (6)

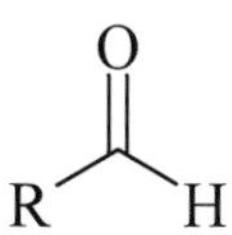

Aldehydes (7)

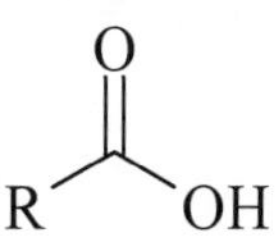

Carboxylic acid (8)

Contd...

Figure 8.1–*Contd...*

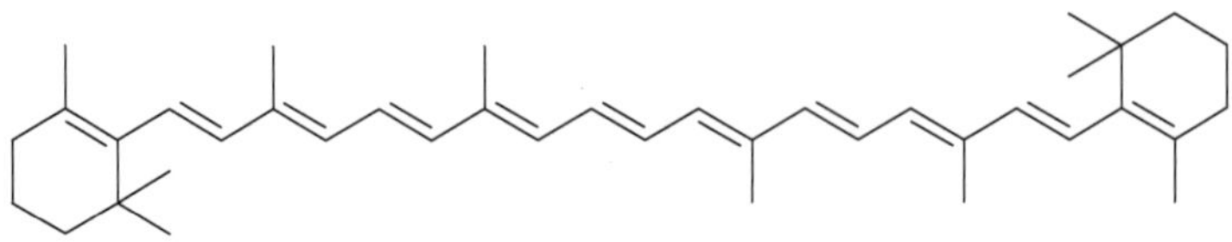

Carotenoids (9)

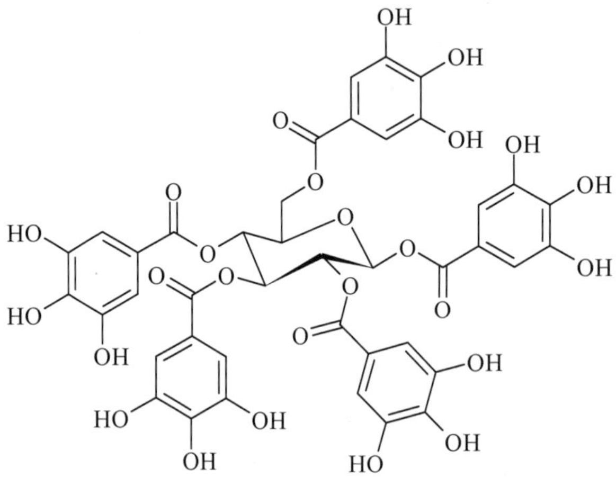

Hydrolysable tannins (10)

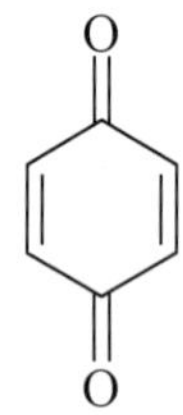

Benzoquinones (11)

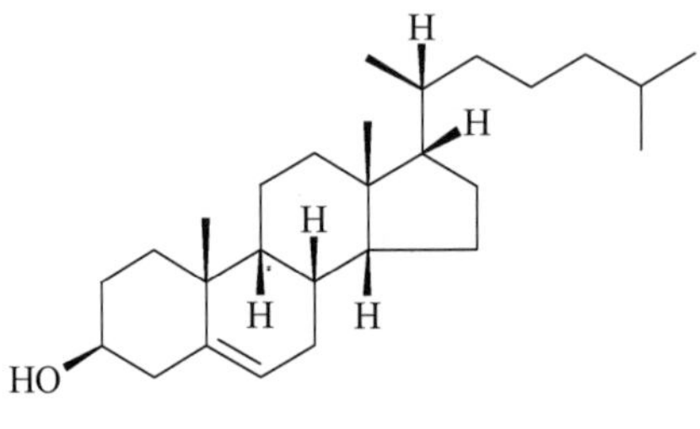

Lipids (12)

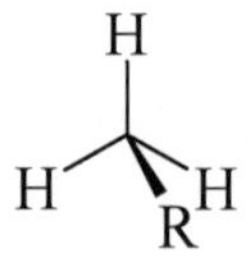

n-Alkanes (13)

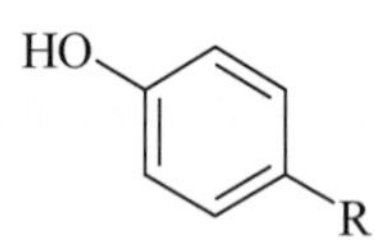

Phenolic compounds (14)

Contd...

Figure 8.1–*Contd...*

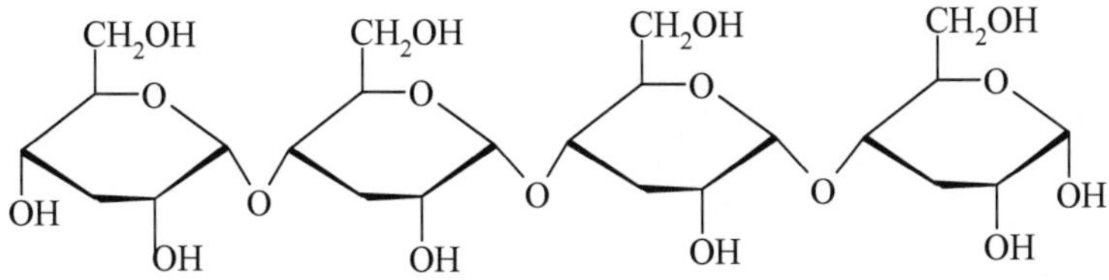

Polysaccharides (15)

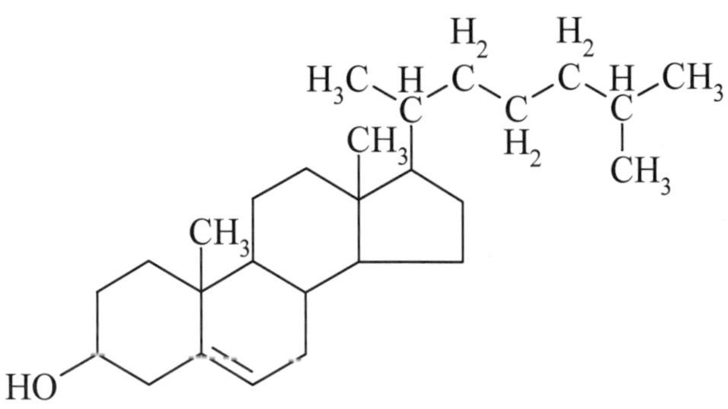

Steroids (16)

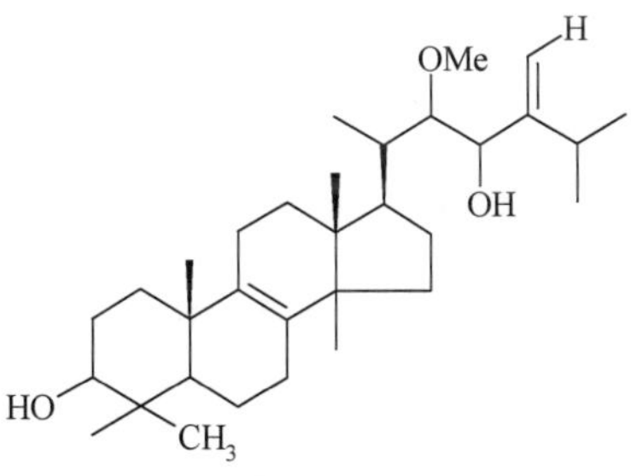

Triterpenes (17)

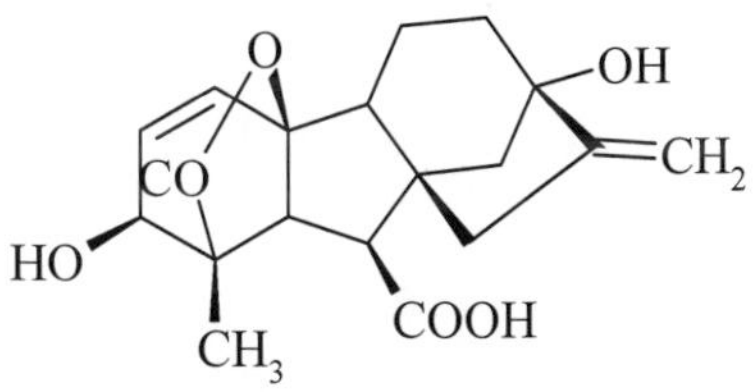

Gibberellic acid (18)

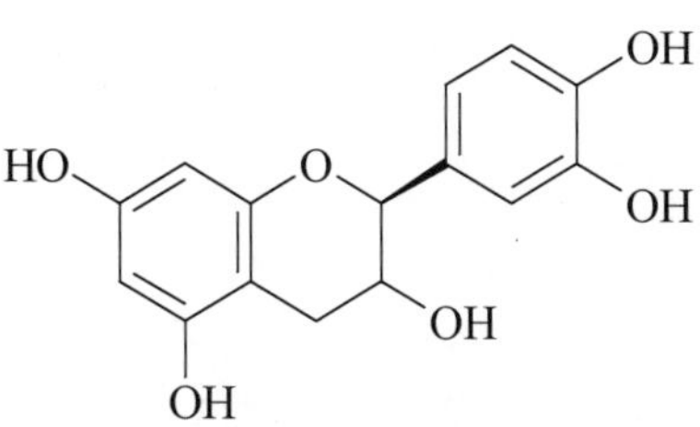

Catechin (19)

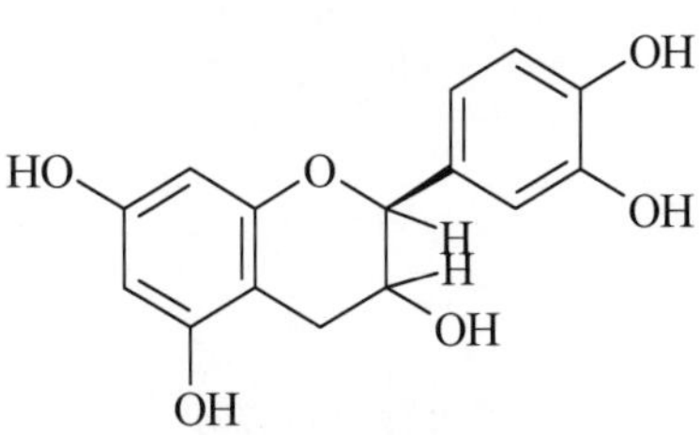

Epicatechin (20)

Contd...

Figure 8.1–*Contd...*

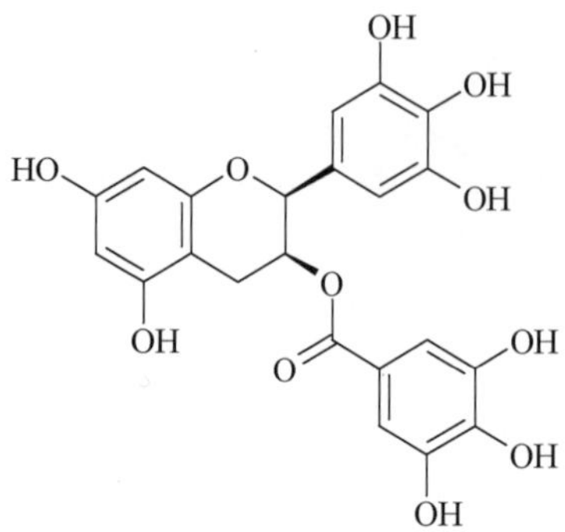

Epigallocatechin (21)

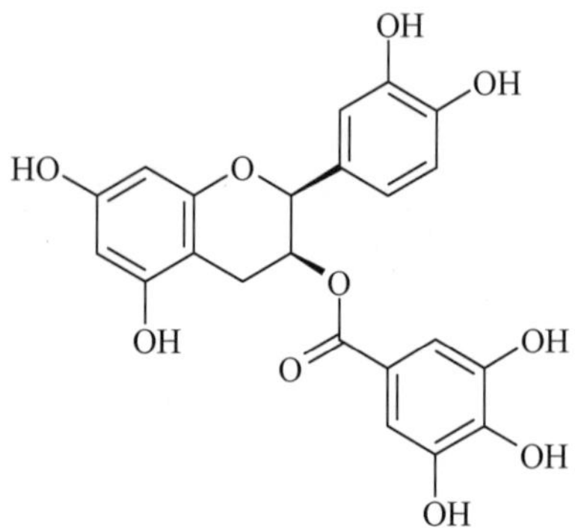

Epicatechingallate (22)

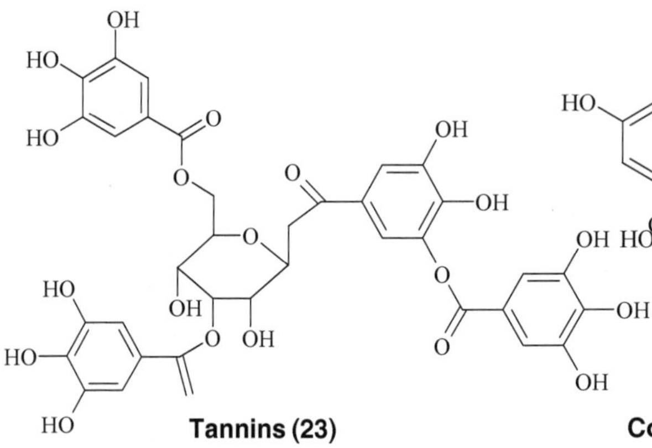

Tannins (23)

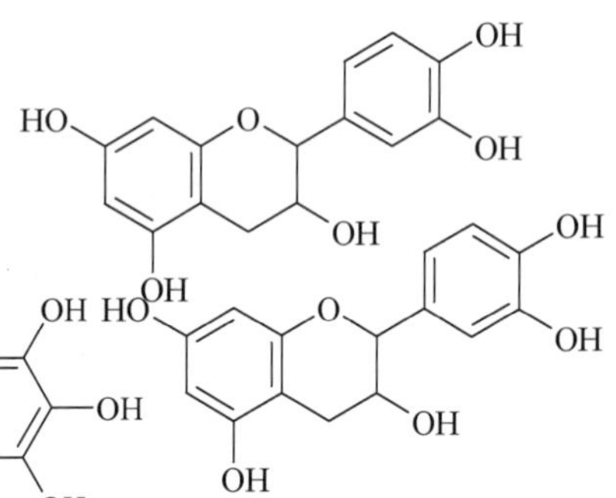

Condensed tannins (24)

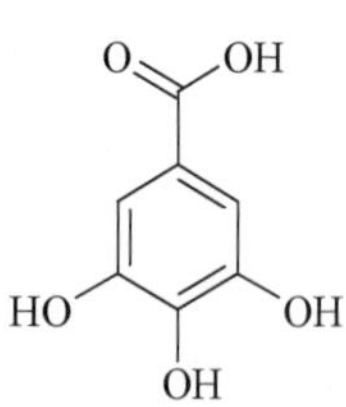

Gallic acid (25)

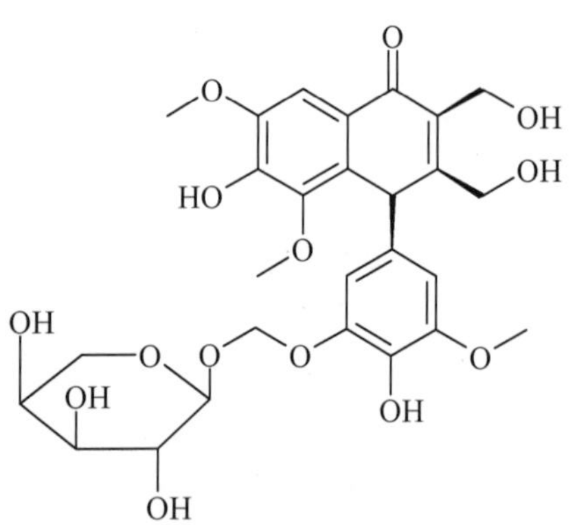

Lyoniresinol-3α-O-β-arabinopyranoside (26)

Contd...

Figure 8.1–*Contd...*

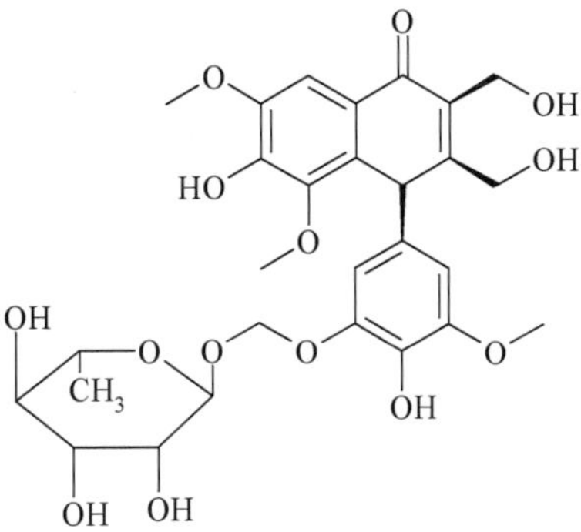

Lyoniresinol-3α-O-α-rhamnoside (27)

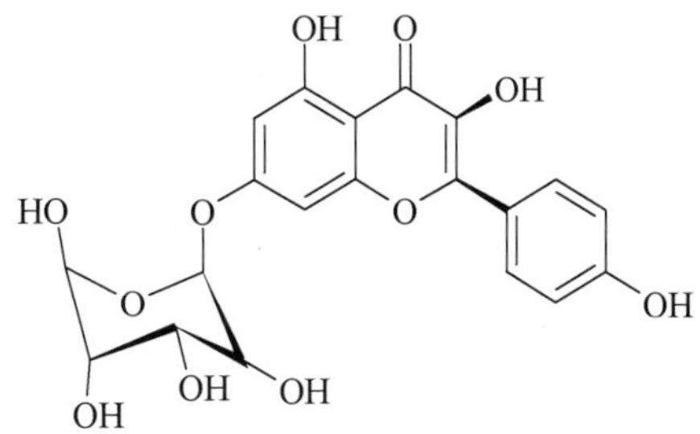

Afzelechin-3-O-L-rhamno-pyranoside (28)

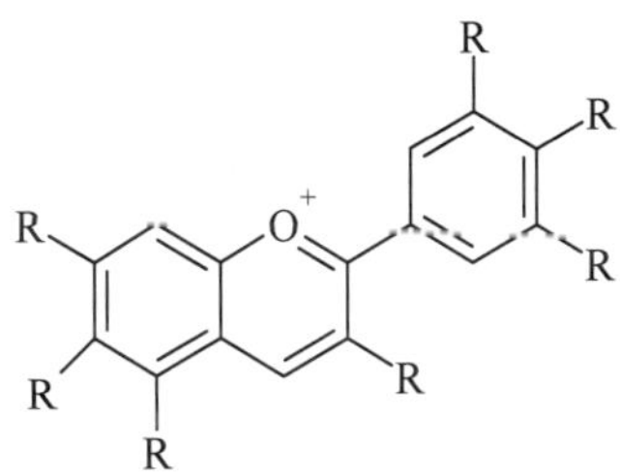

Anthocyanins (29)

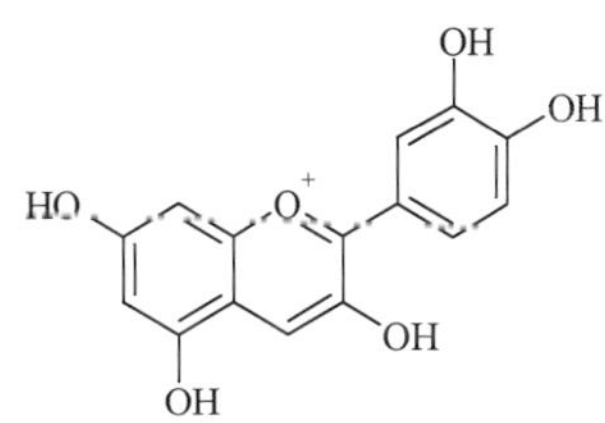

Procyanidins (30)

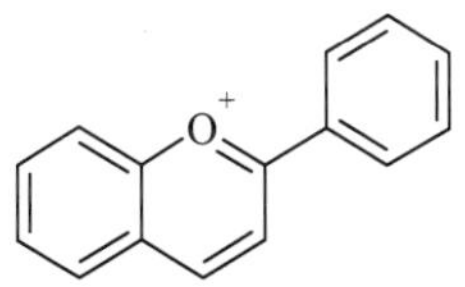

Anthocyanidins (31)

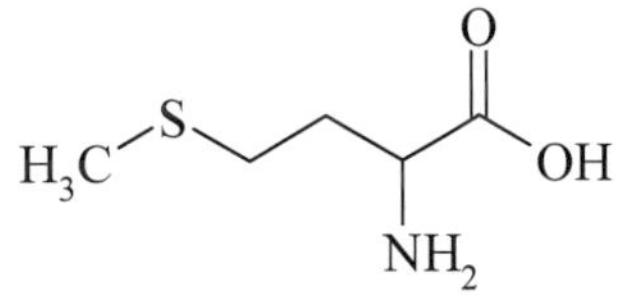

Sulphur contains nitrogenous compound (32)

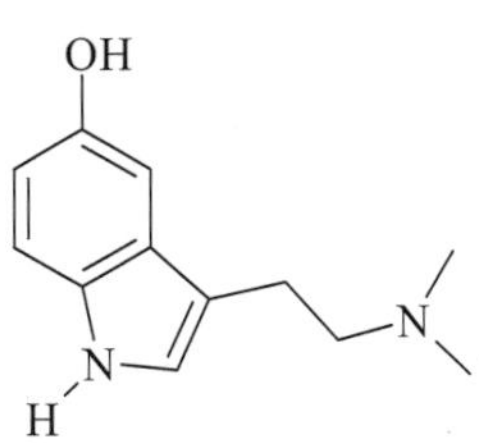

Alkaloids (33)

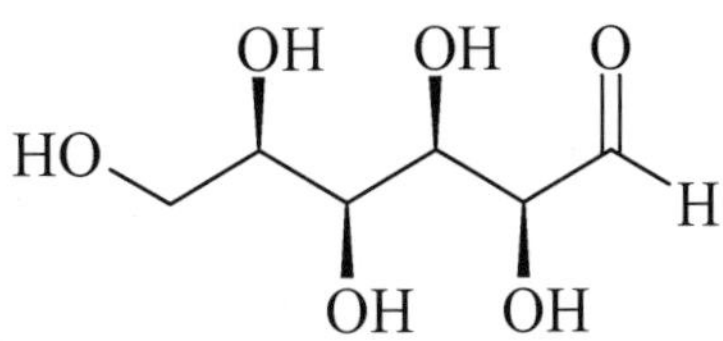

Carbohydrates (34)

Contd...

Figure 8.1–*Contd...*

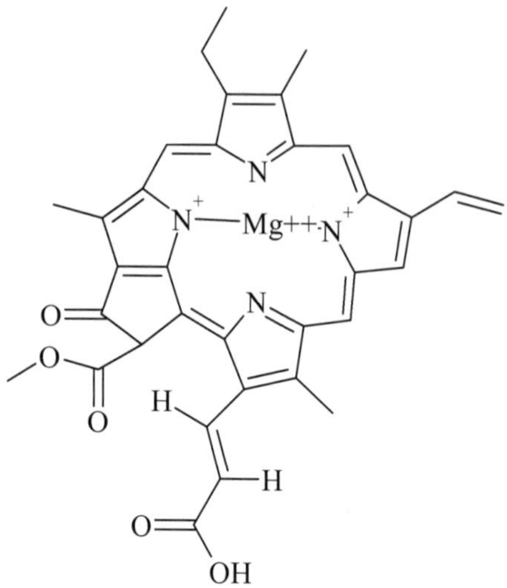

Chlorophyll (35)

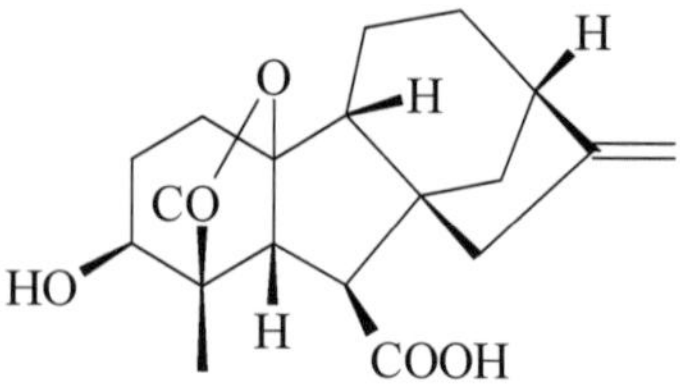

Gibberellins (36)

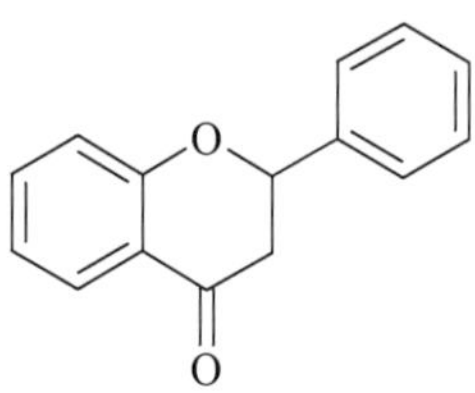

Flavonoids (37)

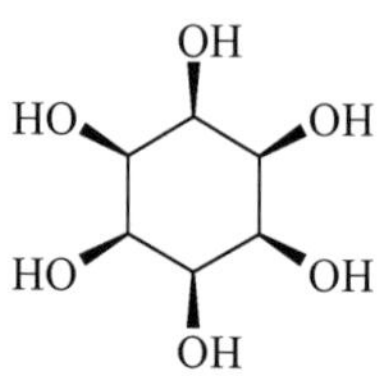

Inositols (38)

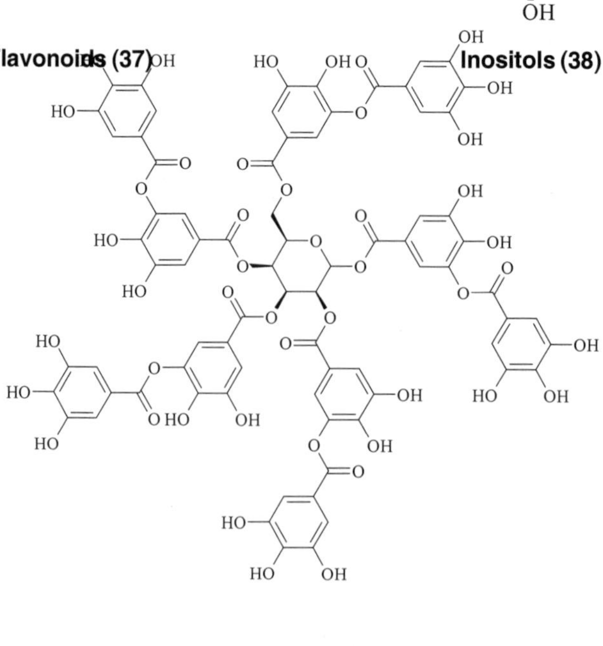

Polyphenols (39)

Contd...

Figure 8.1–*Contd...*

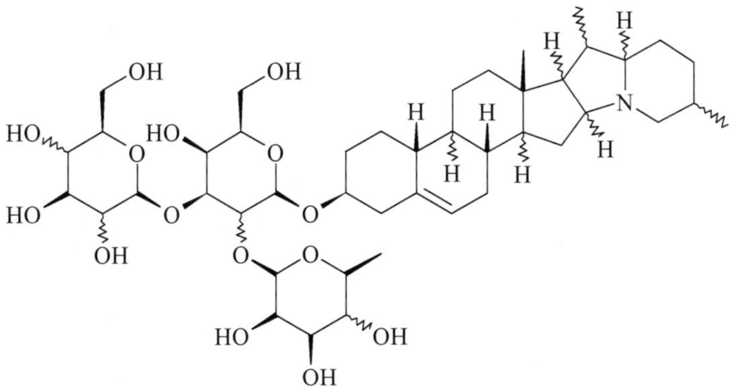

Saponins (40)

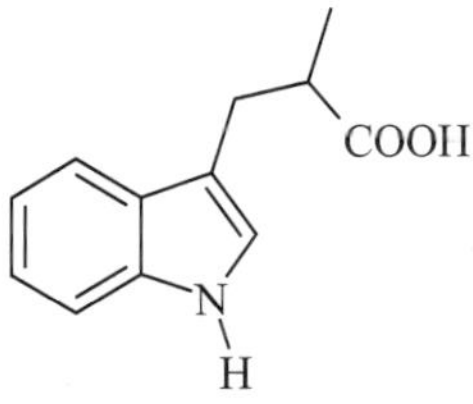

Rhizophorine (41)

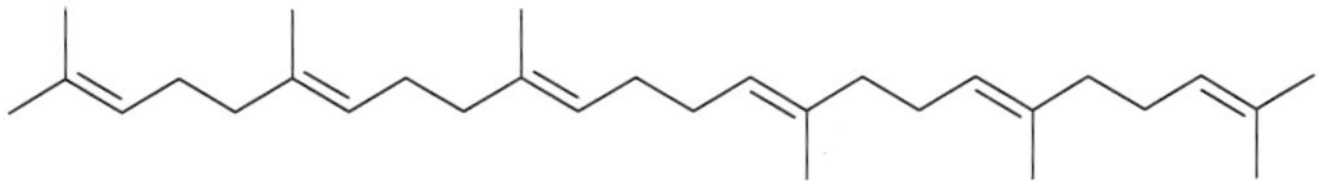

Squalene (42)

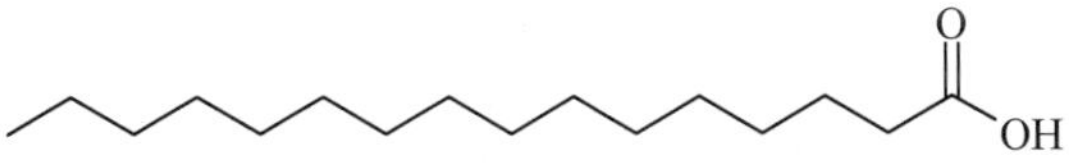

n-Hexadecanoic acid (43)

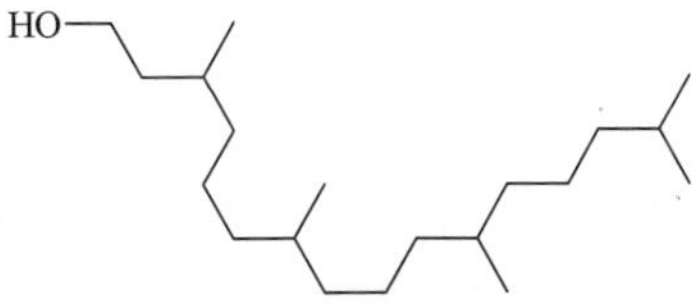

Phytol (44)

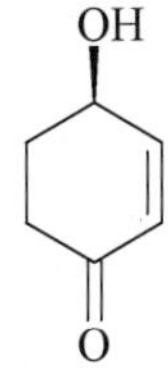

2-Cyclohexane-1-one, 4-hydroxy-3,5- (45)

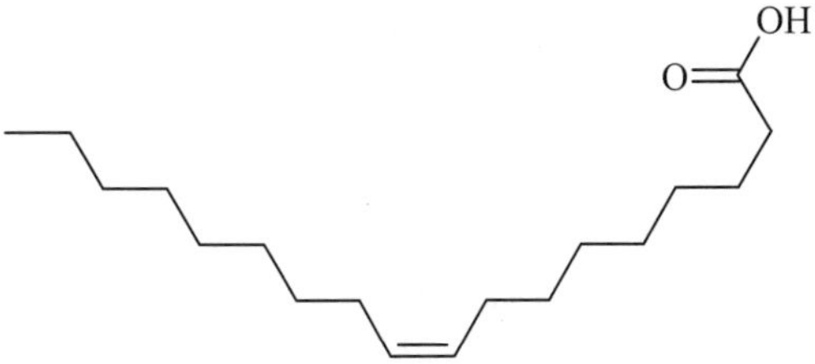

Oleic acid (46)

Contd...

Figure 8.1–*Contd...*

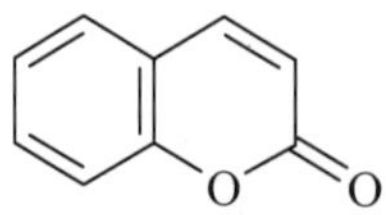

Coumarins (47)

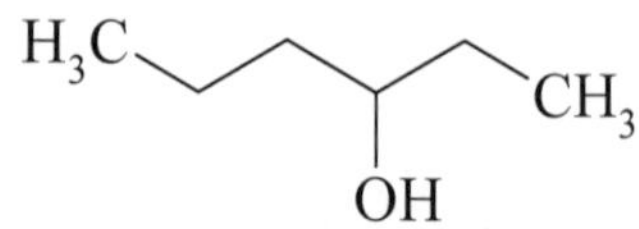

Hexane-3-ol (48)

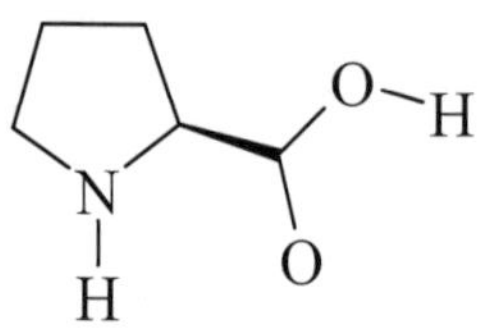

Amino acids (49)

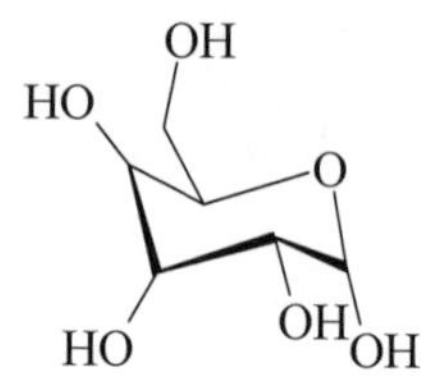

Sugars (50)

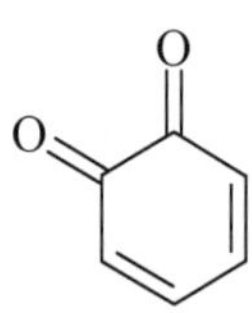

Quinone (51)

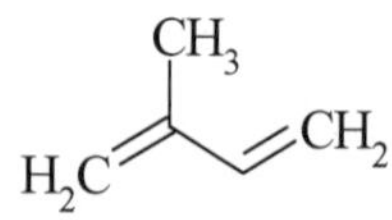

Terpenoid (52)

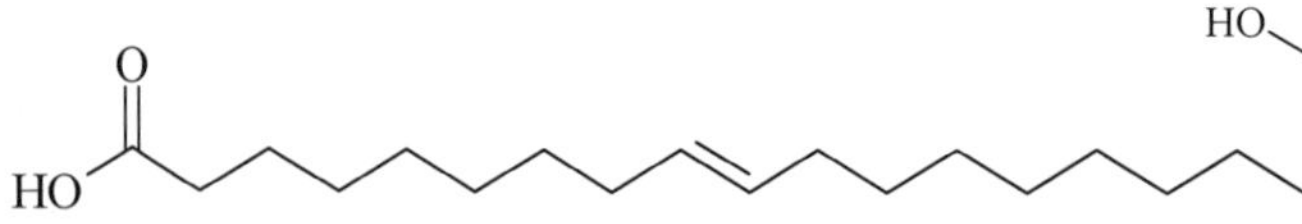

Fatty acid (53)

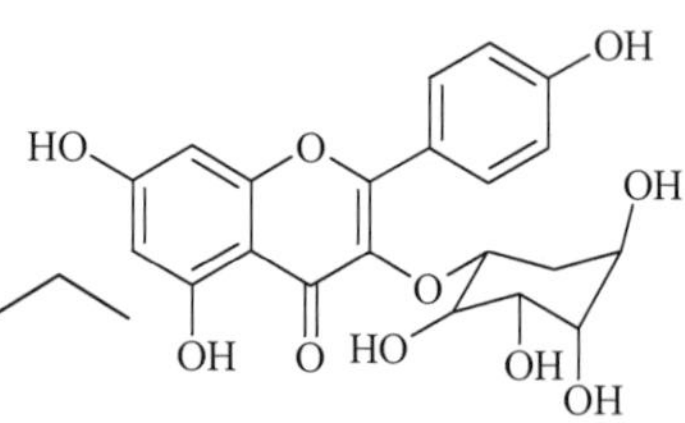

Flavoglycans (54)

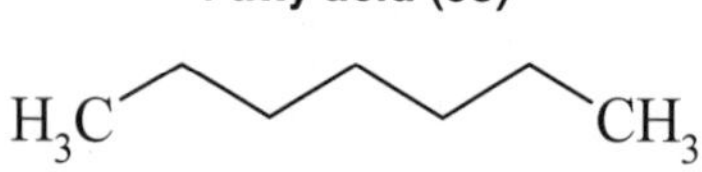

Hydrocarbons (55)

Na—Cl

Inorganic salts (56)

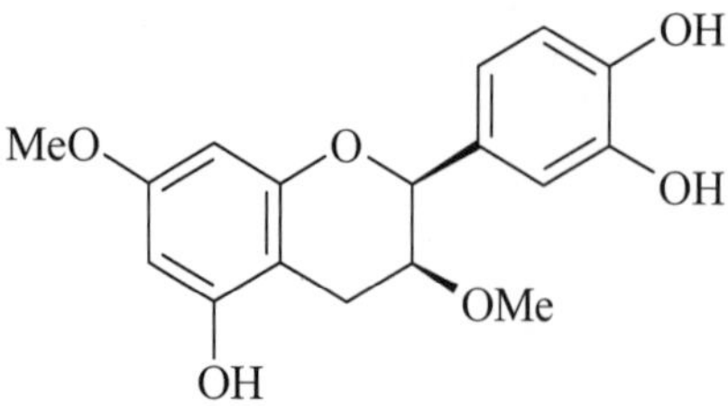

3,7-O-Diacetyl (–)-epicatechin (57)

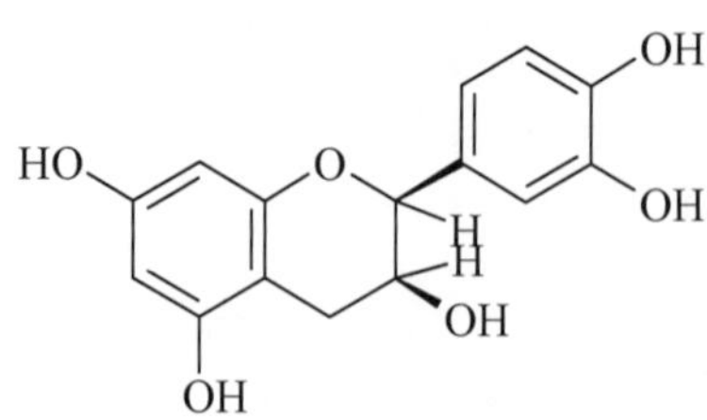

(–)-Epicatechin (58)

Contd...

Figure 8.1–*Contd...*

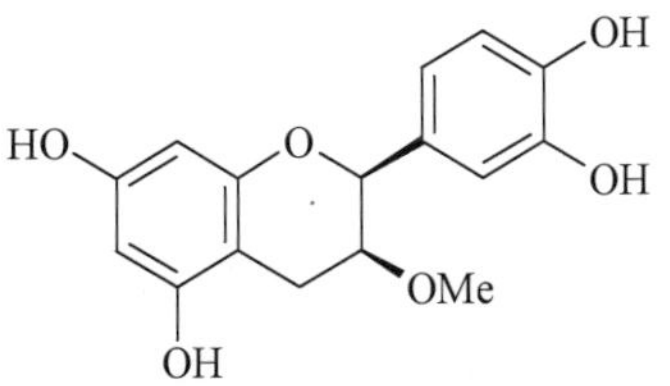

3-O-acetyl (–)-epicatechin (59)

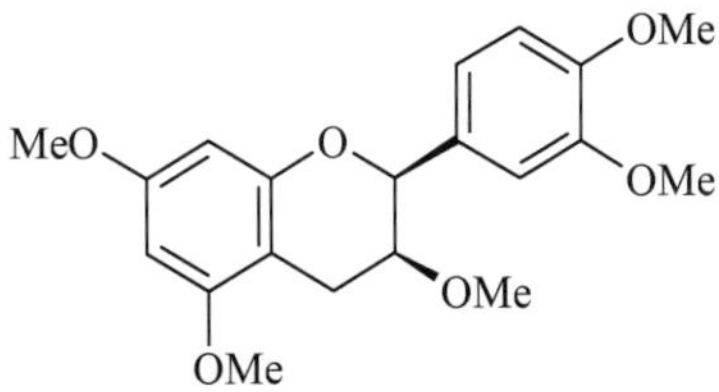

3,32,42,5,7-O-pentaacetyl(–)-epicatechin (60)

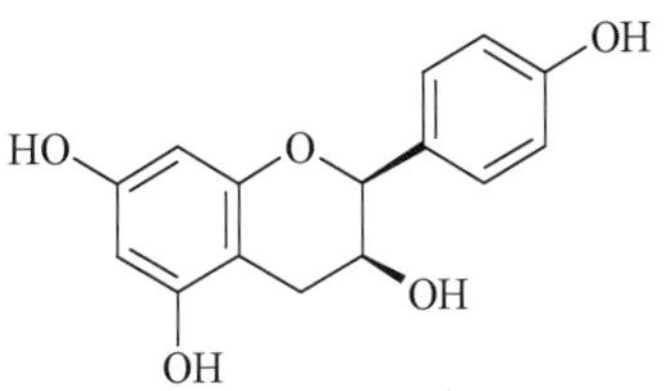

(+)-Afzelechin (61)

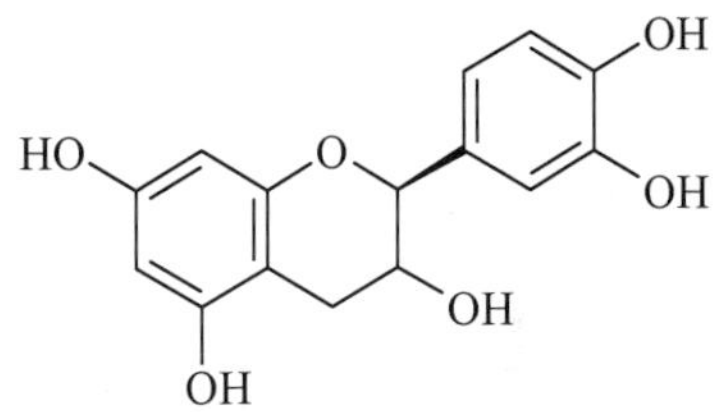

(+)-Catechin (62)

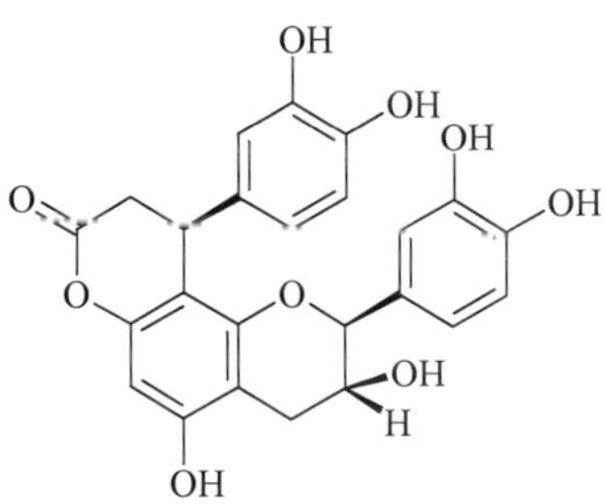

Cinchonain Ib (63)

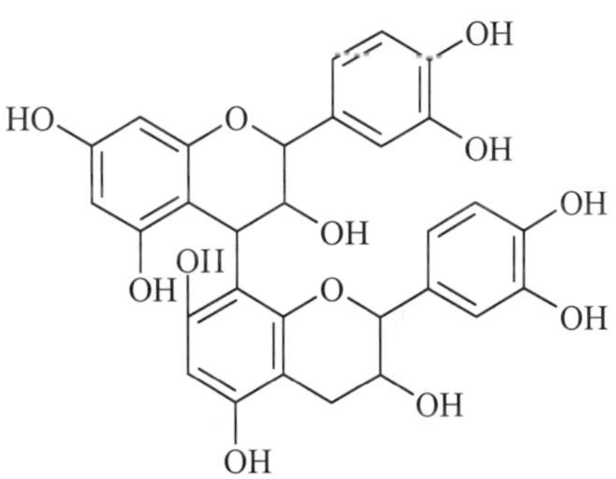

Proanthocyanidin B2 (64)

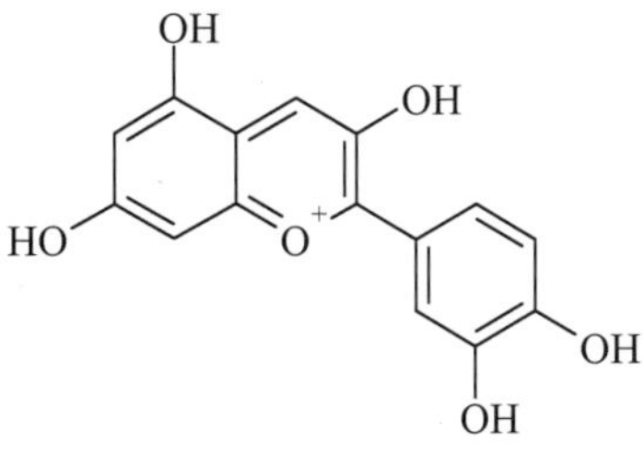

Anthocyanides (65)

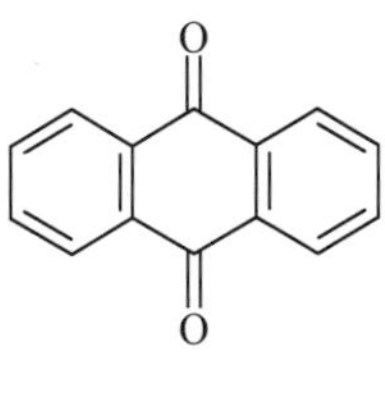

Anthroquinone (66)

Contd...

Figure 8.1–*Contd...*

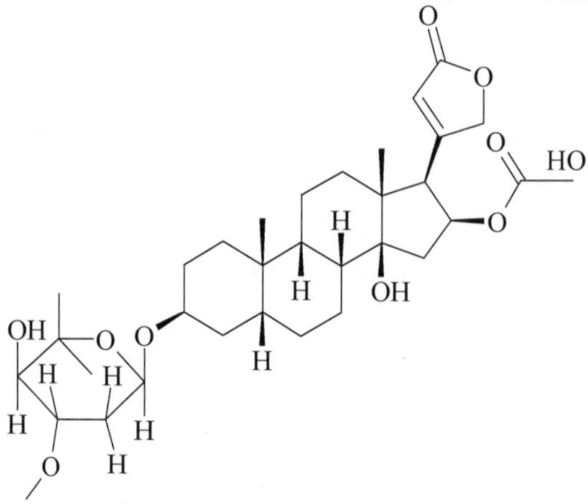

Cardiac glycosides (67)

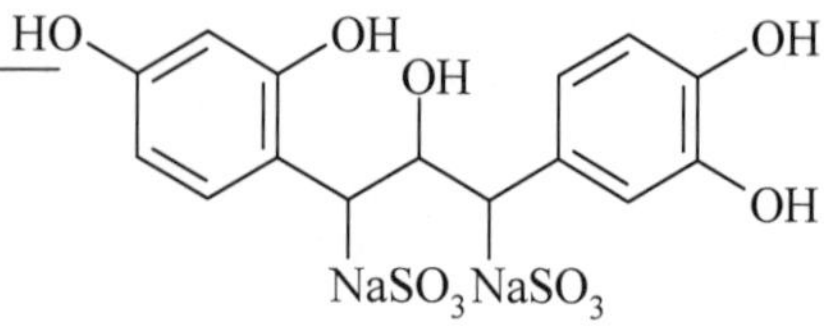

Phlobatanins (68)

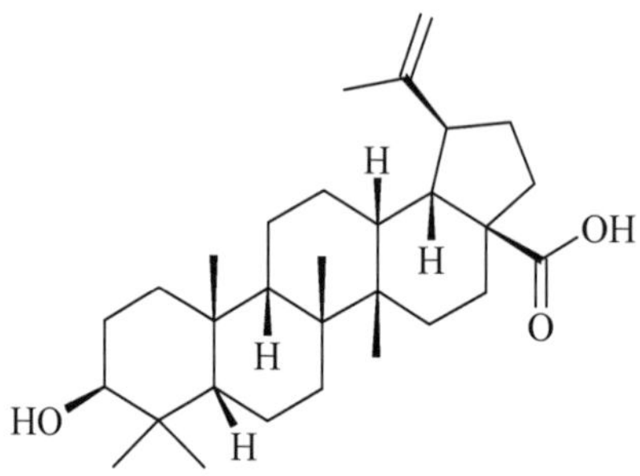

Triterpenoids (69)

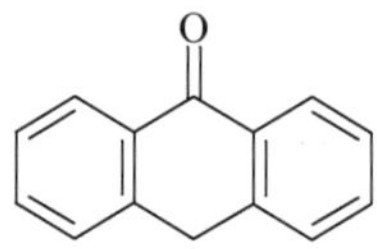

Anthrone (70)

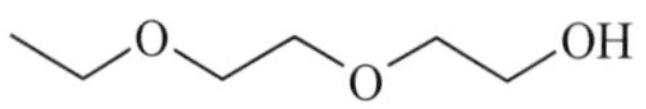

2-(2-ethoxyethoxy)ethanol (71)

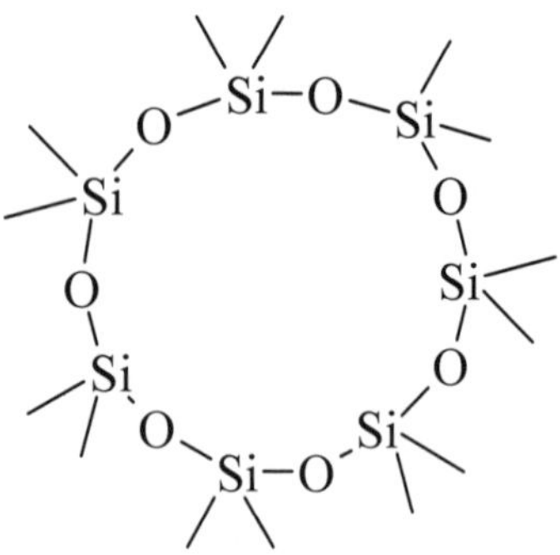

Hexa-decamethylcyclooctasiloxane (72)

Contd...

Figure 8.1–*Contd...*

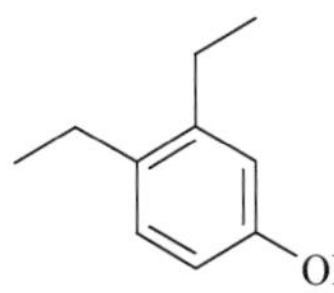

3,4-Diethylphenol (73)

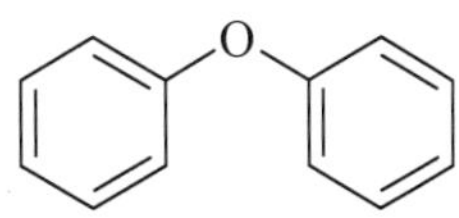

Benzophenone (74)

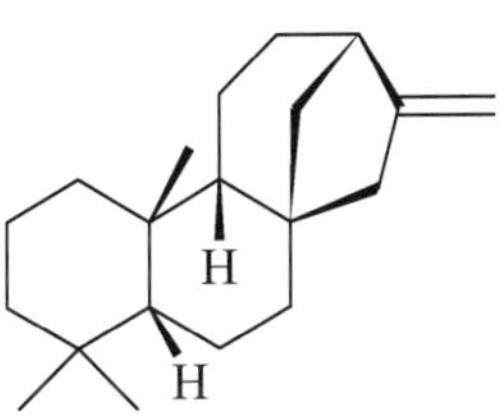

Kaur-16-ene (75)

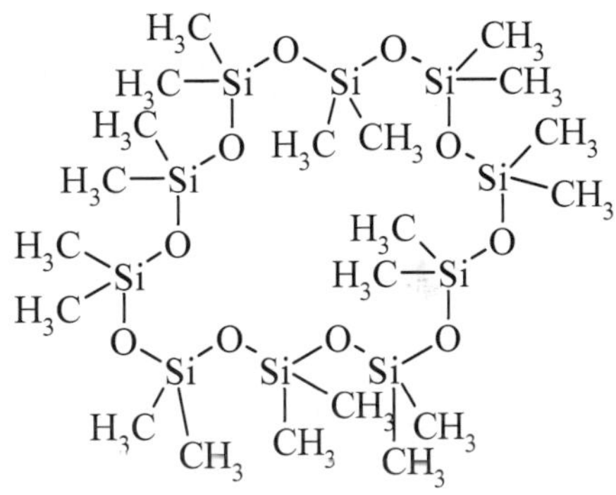

Icosamethylcyclodecasiloxane (76)

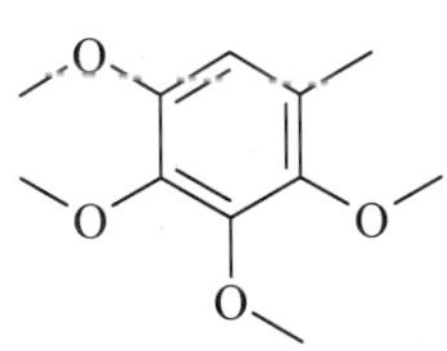

2,3,4,5-Tetramethoxytoluene (77)

Rhizophora stylosa

The *Rhizophora stylosa* has been reported for the phytochemicals such as aliphatic carboxylic acid **(2)**, steroids **(16)**, inositols **(38)**, fatty acids **(53)**, flavoglycans **(54)**, hydrocarbons **(55)** and inorganic salts **(56)** (Richter *et al.*, 1990). A novel type of natural water soluble polymer has been isolated and reported form the *R. stylosa* (Bandaranayake, 2002).

A new acetylated flavanol such as 3,7-O-diacetyl (–)-epicatechin **(57)** and seven known flavanol derivatives *viz.* (–)-epicatechin **(58)**, 3-O-acetyl (–)-epicatechin **(59)**, 3,32,42,5,7-O-pentaacetyl(–)-epicatechin **(60)**, (+)-afzelechin **(61)**, (+)-catechin **(62)**, cinchonain Ib **(63)** and proanthocyanidin B2 **(64)** were isolated and reported from the stems and twigs of the mangrove plant *R. stylosa* and identified and reported from the different fractions and all the purified compounds were evaluated for DPPH radical scavenging activity and reported significant antioxidant activity (Dong Li *et al.*, 2007).

The study has been reported on the phytochemical characterization and antimicrobial efficiency of *Rhizophora stylosa* leaf ethyl acetate extract. The *R. stylosa* has been reported to possess steroids **(16)**, tannins **(23)**, alkaloids **(33)**, flavonoids **(37)**, saponins **(40)**, terpenoids **(52)**, anthocyanides **(65)**, anthroquinone **(66)**, cardiac glycosides **(67)** and phlobatanins **(68)**. The above compounds were reported from the work as antibacterial and antifungal activities (Foukia *et al.*, 2014).

Rhizophora annamalayana and *R. mucronata*

The *Rhizophora annamalayana, R. mucronata* were reported for the phytochemicals constituents and antioxidant properties such as phenolic compounds **(14)** and flavonoids **(37)** contents, DPPH, reducing power, nitric oxides reducing power and the results were reported through flower and leaves of the mangrove plants. The significant antimicrobial activities were reported on pathogenic bacterial strains such as *Escherichia coli, Salmonella typhi, Staphylococcus aereus* and *Proteus valgaris* (Chinnappan *et al.*, 2013).

Rhizophora apiculata and *R. mucronata*

The *Rhizosphora apiculata, R. mucronata* ethanolic extracts were reported on antimicrobial activity against about 150 pathogenic bacterial strains from patients urine samples. Further, the extracts were analyzed for the active compounds presence such as phenolic compounds **(14)**, alkaloid **(33)**, flavonoids **(37)**, anthroquinone **(66)** and triterpenoids **(69)**. The reported results were suggested that potential sources for pathogenic bacterial strains (Ravikumar *et al.*, 2010).

Bioassay guided fractionation of *Rhizophora apiculata* and *R. mucronata* fraction B and C showed inhibitory action. Petroleum ether fractions of both the plants could not show any activity. The HPTLC and IR-spectroscopy study reported the presence of essential oils, tannins **(23)**, coumarins **(47)** and anthrone **(70)** as bioactive compounds (Pimpliskar *et al.*, 2011). The plant *R. apiculata* and *R. mucronata* were reported to possess the significant antimicrobial activity against various pathogenic bacteria (Mukesh *et al.*, 2012).

The *Rhizophora apiculata* and *R. mucronata* are the mangrove plants of the genus *Rhizophora*. The chemical constituents of leaf samples for both species were analyzed by using GC-MS. The analysis of chemical constituents of *R. apiculata* was found to be rich in 2-(2-ethoxyethoxy) ethanol **(71)**, Hexa-decamethylcyclooctasiloxane **(72)**, 3,4-diethylphenol **(73)**, benzophenone **(74)** and kaur-16-ene **(75)**. The phytochemical such as 2-(2-ethoxyethoxy) ethanol **(71)**, benzophenone **(74)**, icosamethylcyclo-decasiloxane **(76)** and 2,3,4,5-tetramethoxytoluene **(77)** were the predominant constituents in *R. mucronata* (Nurul*et al.*, 2013).

Mangrove plants are rich source of secondary metabolites like steroids **(16)**, triterpens **(17)**, tannins **(23)**, alkaloids **(33)**, flavonoids **(37)** and saponins **(40)**. Extracts from different mangrove plants are reported to possess diverse medicinal properties. In view of this *R. apiculata* and *R. mucronata* were selected to study the antimicrobial and antioxidant potential. For this purpose gram negative, gram positive bacteria and fungi were reported for antibacterial and antifungal activity of these plant extracts. The tested extracts showed to varying degrees of antimicrobial potential against the test microorganisms. These promising findings were suggested antibacterial and antifungal activity of plant material indicating presence of bioactive compounds against pathogens. According to HPTLC and IR analysis of potent fractions showed the presence of bioactive principles like tannins **(23)**, coumarin **(47)**, anthrones **(70)** and essential oils. Further, gelatin precipitation test also proves the presence of tannins **(23)**. Similarly biochemical constituents recorded by Pimpliskar (2004) and Cowman (1999) shows the presence of tannins **(23)**, coumarin **(47)**, anthrone **(70)** and essential oils in the mangrove plants (Pimpliskar *et al.*, 2012).

Rhizophora apiculata, R. mucronata, R. mangle and *R. stylosa*

The *Rhizophora apiculata, R. mucronata, R. mangle* and *R. stylosa* were reported for the HPLC analysis of hydrolysable tannins **(10)** (Afidah, 2005).

Rhizophora mangle and *R. harrisonii*

Rhizophora sp., *R. mangle, R. harrisonii* (red mangrove) have been reported to leads by other mangrove such as *Avicennia germinans* (black mangrove), *Laguncularia racemosa* (white mangrove) species. Various species have been found and reported their dominating and leading properties in mangrove plants and their potentiality. The structures and floristics of mangrove forests have been studied and reported in this study (Fernandes, 2000).

Conclusion

The review has been concluded that the *Rhizophora* genus constitutes 55 species constitutes 77 compounds from amino acids, carbohydrates, fatty acids, flavonoids, cardiac glycosides, phenolic compounds, triterpenoids, pigments and intermediate compounds from different species as *Rhizophora annamalayana, R. apiculata, R. conjugata, R. gymnorrhiza, R. harrisonii, R. lamarckii, R. mangle, R. mangle, R. mucronata, R. racemosa* and *R. stylosa.* The secondary metabolites such as lyoniresinol-3α-O-β-rhamnoside, afzelechin-3-O-L-rhamno-pyranoside, hexadecamethylcyclooctasiloxane, kaur-16-ene, icosamethyl cyclodecasiloxane, 2,3,4,5-tetramethoxytoluene *etc.*, compounds were reported from the above mentioned species. Also, the chapter reviewed the pharmacological and biological applications from the reported compounds for various ailments and its useful for the further research on various other endangered species.

Abbreviations

^{1}H NMR: Hydrogen Nuclear Magnetic Resonance

^{13}C NMR: Carbon Nuclear Magnetic Resonance

DPPH: 2,2-diphenyl-1-picrylhydrazyl

FIA-ESI-IT-MS/MS: Flow Injection Analysis - Electro Spectro Ionization - Ion Trap - Mass Spectroscopy/Mass Spectroscopy

FT-IR: Fourier Transform - Infra Red Spectroscopy

GC-MS: Gas Chromatography - Mass Spectroscopy

HPLC: High Performance Liquid Chromatography

HPTLC: High Performance Thin Layer Chromatography
IR: Infra Red Spectroscopy
LC-MS: Liquid Chromatography - Mass Spectroscopy
TLC: Thin Layer Chromatography
UV visible: Ultra Violet Spectroscopy

References

Abdul Khalil, H.P.S., Kong, N.H., Ahmad, M.N., Bhat, A.H., Jawaid, M., and Juma, S. (2009). Selective solvent extraction of the bark of *Rhizophora apiculata* as an anti-termite agent against *Coptotermes gestroi. Journal of Wood Chemistry and Technology.,* **29**: 286-304.

Abeysinghe, P.D., Wijesekara, D., and Pathirana, R.N. (2004). Inhibition of growth of antibiotic resistant *Staphylococcus* sp. and *Proteus* sp. by mangrove plant extracts. *Proceedings of the Second Science Symposium,* **2**: 1-9.

Afidah Abdul Rahim. (2005). Physico-chemical characterization of mangrove tannins as corrosion inhibitors. University of Malaysia.

Alaganadham, E., Gnanaprakash, S.R., and Murugaiyan, K. (2012). Taxol producing mangrove endophytic fungi *Fusarium oxysporum* from *Rhizophora annamalayana*. *Asian Pacific Journal of Tropical Biomedicine,* S1081-S1085.

Anouk, V., James, G.K., Hans, B., and Nico, K. (2004). Growth rings, growth ring formation and age determination in the mangrove *Rhizophora mucronata. Annals of Botany,* **94**: 59-66.

Anu, C.J., and Priscilla, H.C. (2013). Assessment of antimicrobial potential of endophytic bacteria isolated from *Rhizophora mucronata. International Journal of Current Microbiology and Applied Science,* **2(10)**: 188-194.

Asha, K.K., Suseela, M., and Lakshmanan, P.T. (2012). Flavonoids and phenolic compounds in two mangrove species and their antioxidant property. *Indian Journal of Geo-Marine Sciences,* **41(3)**: 259-264.

Babu, B.H., and Shylesh, B.S., and Padikkala, J. (2001). Antioxidant and hepatoprotective effect of *Acanthus ilcifolius*. *Fitoterapia,* **72**: 272-277.

Bandaranayake, W.M. (2002). Bioactivities, bioactive compounds and chemical constituents of mangrove plants. *Wetlands Ecology and Managements,* **10**: 421-452.

Basyuni, M., Oku, H., Tsujimoto, E., Kinjo, K., Baba, S., and Takara, K. (2007). Triterpene synthases from the Okinawan mangrove tribe, Rhizophoraceae. *FEBS J.,* **274(19)**: 5028-5047.

Bose, S., and Bose, A. (2008). Antimicrobial activity of *Acanthus ilcifolius* (L). *Indian Journal of Pharmacy Science,* **70**: 821-3.

Chandrasekaran, M., Kannathasan, K. Venkatesalu V., and Prabhakar, K. (2009). Antibacterial activity of some saltmarsh halophytes and mangrove plants against methicillin resistant *Staphylococcus aureus*. *World Journal Microbiology and Biotechnology*, **25**: 155-160.

Chandrashekar, N.K., and Varahalarao, V. (2010). *In vitro* bioactivity against important phytopathogens of *Rhizophora mucronata* (Lam.) and *Acanthus ilicifolius* Linn. *Der Pharmacia Lettre*, **2(2)**: 107-110.

Chinnappan, R.S., Natarajan, S.B., Kandasamy, K., Sekar, A., Sunil Kumar, S., and Aswin Kumar. (2013). Effect of Bioactive Substances from Mangroves on Anti-Oxidant, Antibacterial Activity and Molecular Docking Study Against Lung and Oral Cancer. *The Journal of Free Radicals and Antioxidants Photon*, **139**: 226-236.

Cowman, M.M. (1999). *Clinical Microbiology Reviews*, **12**: 564-582.

Dong-Li Li., Xiao-Ming Li., Ze-Yu Peng., and Bin-Gui Wang. (2007). Flavanol derivatives from *Rhizophora stylosa* and their DPPH radical scavenging activity. *Molecules*, **12**: 1163-1169.

El-Khouly A. Ahmed Khedr, A., and Abdel-Hamid. (2007). Zonation pattern of *Avicennia marina* and *Rhizophora mucronata* along the Red Sea Coast, Egypt. *World Applied Sciences Journal*, **2(4)**: 283-288.

Elsa Lycias Joel., and Valentin Bhimba, B. (2010). Antibacterial activity and GC-MS analysis of secondary metabolites produced by the mangrove plant *Rhizophora mucronata against* MRSA. *International Journal on Applied Bioengineering*, **4(2)**: 25-28.

Elsa Lycias Joel., and Valentin Bhimba, B. (2012). Biological activity of secondary metabolites isolated from mangrove fungi *Neurospora crassa*. *Journal of Environmental Biology*, **34**: 729-732.

Felipe Meira de Faria, Anderson Luiz-Ferreira, Eduardo Augusto Rabelo Socca, Ana Cristina Alves de Almeida, Ricardo Jose Dunder, Luis Paulo Manzo, Marcelo Aparecido da Silva, Wagner Vi legas, Ariane Leite Rozza, Claudia Helena Pellizzon, Lourdes Campaner dos Santos and Alba Regina Monteiro Souza Brito. (2012). Effects of *Rhizophora mangle* on Experimental Colitis Induced by TNBS in Rats. *Evidence based Complementary and Alternative Medicine*, 1-11.

Felipe Meira de-Faria, Ana Cristina Alves Almeida, Anderson Luiz-Ferreira, Ricardo Jose Dunder, Christiane Takayama, Maria Silene da Silva, Marcelo Aparecido da Silva, Wagner Vilegas, ArianeLeiteRozza, Claudia Helena Pellizzon, Walber Toma, Alba Regina Monteiro Souza-Brito. (2012a). Mechanisms of action underlying the gastric antiulcer activity of the *Rhizophora mangle* L. *Journal of Ethnopharmacology*, **139**: 234-243.

Fernandes, M.E.B. (2000). A Structural Analysis of *Rhizophora*, *Avicennia* and *Lagun cularia* Forests on Maraca Island, Amapa, Brazil. German-Brazilian Workshop on Neotropical Ecosystems-Achievements and Prospects of Cooperative Research Hamburg, September: 3-8.

Foukia E. Mouafi, Shadia M. Abdel Aziz, Awatif A. Bashir and Amal A. Fyiad. (2014). Phytochemical analysis and antimicrobial activity of mangrove leaves (*Avicenna marina* and *Rhizophora stylosa*) against some pathogens. *World Applied Sciences Journal*, **29(4)**: 547-554.

Jain, K., Afidah, A.R., and Azman, I.M. (2002). Proceedings of the Symposium of Malaysian Chemical Engineering, Malaysia. pp. 323-327.

Joel E.L., and Bhimba V. (2010). Antibacterial activity and GC MS analysis of secondary metabolites produced by the mangrove plant *Rhizophora mucronata* against MRSA. *International Journal of Applied Bioengineering*, **4(2)**: 25-28.

Joel, E.L., and Bhimba, V. (2010). Isolation and characterization of secondary metabolites from the mangrove plant *Rhizophora mucronata*. *Asian Pacific Journal of Tropical Medicine*, **3(8)**: 602-604.

Kalina Manabe Brauko, Mauricio Garcia De Camargo and Paulo Da Cunha Lana. (2011). A new method to assess herbivory levels on *Rhizophora mangle* L. fruits in mangroves with different degrees of forest complexity. *Pan-American Journal of Aquatic Sciences*, **6(1)**: 9-15.

Kamaruzzaman, B.Y., Ong, M.C., Jalal, K.C.A., Shahbudin, S. and Mohd Nor, O. (2009). Accumulation of lead and copper in *Rhizophora apiculata* from Setiu mangrove forest, Terengganu, Malaysia. *Journal of Environmental Biology*, **30(5)**: 821-824.

Kathiresan K., and Rajendran, N. (2002). Growth of a mangrove (*Rhizophora apiculata*) seedlings as influenced by Gibberelic acid, light and salinity. *Revista de Biología Tropical.*, **50(2)**: 525-530.

Kathiresan, K., and Rajendran, N. (2005). Mangrove ecosystems of Indian Ocean. *Indian Journal of marine sciences*, **34(1)**: 104-113.

Kokpol, U., Warinthorn, C., Vallapa, C., Bruce, M., Cunningham, G.N., and Miles D.H. (1993). Long chain aliphatic alcohols and saturated carboxylic acids from heartwood of *Rhizophora apiculata*. *Phytochemistry*, **33(5)**: 1129-1131.

Lim, S.H., Darah I., and Jain, K. (2006). Antimicrobial activities of tannins extracted from *Rhizophora apiculata* barks. *Journal of Tropical Forest Science*, **18(1)**: 59-65.

Lim, S.H., Darah, I., Jain, K., and Suraya, S. (2011). Gallic acid: An anticandidal compound in hydrolysable tannin extracted from the barks of *Rhizophora apiculata* Blume. *Journal of Applied Pharmaceutical Science*, **1(6)**: 75-79.

Majumdar, S.G., and Patra, G. (1976). Chemical investigation of some mangrove species. Part II. *Carapaobovata* Bl. *Journal of Indian Chemical Society*, **53**: 947–948.

Makanjuola, O., Ebitei, C., Collins, A., Collins, A., and Tambari, K.O. (2011). Corrosion inhibition of mild steel in Hydrochloric acid by tannins from *Rhizophora racemosa*. **2**: 592-595.

Matthew, W., Barbara, S., Ursula, S., Myrna, J., and Marilyn, F. (2003). A taphonomic study of $\Delta^{13}C$ and $\Delta^{15}N$ values in *Rhizophora mangle* leaves for a multi-proxy approach to mangrove palaeoecology. *Organic Geochemistry*, **34**: 1259-1275.

Meenakshi, S.V., and Jayaprakash, K. (2014). Mosquito larvicidal efficacy of leaf extract from mangrove plant *Rhizophora mucronata* (Family: Rhizophoraceae) against

Anopheles and Aedes species. *Journal of Pharmacognosy and Phytochemistry,* **3(1)**: 78-83.

Mingzhe, G., and Hongbin, X. (2012). Activity guided isolation of antioxidant compounds from *Rhizophora apiculata*. *Molecules,* **17**: 10675-82.

Mukesh, P., Pramod, S., Vijay, S., Vaishali, J., and Jadhav, B.L. (2012). Comparative performance of activity of antimicrobial principles of mangroves *Rhizophora* species along Mumbai coast. *Indo-Global Research Journal of Pharmaceutical Sciences,* **2(4)**: 426-429.

Nurul, A.Z.A., Nurul, H.A.H., and Ropisah, M. (2013). Basic study of chemical constituents in *Rhizophora* species. *The Open Conference Proceedings Journal,* **4(Suppl-2, M7)**: 27-28.

Ong Jin-Eong, Gong Wooi Khoon, and Clough, B.F. (1995). Structure and productivity of a 20-year-old stand of *Rhizophora apiculata* BI. Mangrove forest. *Journal of Biogeography,* **22**: 417-424.

Pahalawattaarachchi, V., Purushothaman, C.S., and Vennila, A. (2009). Metal Phytoremediation potential of *Rhizophora mucronata*. *Indian Journal of Marine Sciences,* **38(2)**: 178-183.

Pimpliskar, M. R., Jadhav, R.N., and Jadhay, B.L. (2011). Study on antimicrobial principles of Rhizophora species along Mumbai coast. *Journal of Aquatic Biology,* **26(1)**: 6-11.

Pimpliskar, M.R. (2004). M.Sc Thesis Mumbai University.

Pimpliskar, M.R, Jadhav, R.N., and Jadhav, B.L. (2012). Evaluation of antimicrobial principles of *Rhizophora* species along Mumbai coast. *Journal of Advanced Scientific Research,* **3(3)**: 30-33.

Popp, M., Larher, F., and Weigel, P. (1984). Chemical composition of Australian mangroves. III. Free amino acids, total methylated onium compounds and total nitrogen. Zeitschr. *Pflanzen.,* 1**14**: 15-25.

Prabhakaran, J., and Kavitha, D. (2012). Ethnomedicinal importance of Mangrove species of Pitchavaram. *International Journal of Research in Pharmaceutical and Biomedical Sciences,* 611-614.

Premanathan, M., Arakaki, R., Izumi, H., Kathiresan, K., Nakano, M., Yamamoto, N., and Nakashima, H. (1999). Antiviral properties of a mangrove plant, *Rhizophora apiculata* Blume. against human immunodeficiency virus. *Antiviral Research,* **44**: 113-122.

Rahim, A.A., Rocca, E., Steinmetz, J., Kassim, M.J., Ibrahim, M.S., and Osman H. (2008). *Food Chemistry,* **10(1)**: 200-207.

Raut, S., Khan, S., and Gaikwad, R. (2014). Isolation and characterization of major phytoconstituents from the leaves of *Rhizophora mucronata* Lamk. and *Acanthusilici folius* Linn. *International Research Journal of Science and Engineering,* **2(2)**: 51-59.

Ravikumar, S., Gnanadesigan, M., Suganthi, P., and Ramalakshmi, A. (2010). Antibacterial potential of chosen mangrove plants against isolated urinary tract infectious bacterial pathogens. *International Journal of Medicine and Medical Sciences,* **2(3)**: 94-99.

Richter, A., Thonke, B., and Popp, M. (1990). 1-D-I-O-Methyl-muco-inositol in Viscumalbum and members of the Rhizophoraceae. *Phytochemistry,* **29**: 1785-1786.

Rollet, B. (1981). Bibliography on mangrove research.1600-1975. UNESCO Paris. Pub. Information Retrieval Ltd., London, pp. 479.

Sundaram Ravikumar and Murugesan Gnanadesigan. (2012). Hepatoprotective and Antioxidant Properties of *Rhizophora mucronata* Mangrove Plant in CCl_4 Intoxicated Rats.*Journal of Experimental and Clinical Medicine,* **4(1)**: 66-72.

Suraya Sulaiman, Darah Ibrahim, Jain Kassim and Lim Sheh-Hong. (2011). Antimicrobial and antioxidant activities of condensed tannin from *Rhizophora apiculata* barks. *Journal of Chemical and Pharmaceutical Research,* **3(4)**: 436-444.

Thangam, T.S., and Kathiresan, K. (1989). Larvicidaleffect of marine plant extracts on mosquito *Culextritaenior hynchus. Journal of the Marine Biological Association of India,* **31**: 306-307.

Tomlinson, P.B. (1994). The Botany of Mangroves. Cambridge University Press: Cambridge.

Ukoima, H.N., Ikata, M., and Pepple, G.A. (2013).Control of *Lasiodiplodia theobromae* on *Rhizophora racemosa* using plants extracts. *American Journal of Biotechnology and Molecular Science,* **3(1)**: 1-7.

Varahalarao, V., and Chandrasekhar, K.N. (2009). *In vitro* bioefficiency of marine mangrove plant activity of *Rhizophora conjugata. International Journal of Pharma Tech Research,* **1(4)**: 1598-1600.

Yunita, E.P., Aniek, M.H., and Eddy, S. (2012). The potency of *Rhizophora mucronata* leaf extract as antidiarrhea. *Journal of Applied Sciences Research,* **8(2)**: 1180-1185.

Bioactive Phytochemicals: Perspectives for Modern Medicine Vol. 3 (2015) *Pages* **235–257**
Editor: **V.K. Gupta**
Published by: **DAYA PUBLISHING HOUSE, NEW DELHI**

9

Rotenoids as Anticancer Agents

Estrella-Parra E.[1], González-Sánchez I.[1,2], Gomez-Verjan J.[1], Vázquez-Martínez E.R.[2], Páez-Franco J.C.[2], Cerbón, M.[2] and Reyes-Chilpa, R.[1*]

ABSTRACT

The rotenoids are secondary metabolites isolated from different plant species of the Fabaceae family, some of them well known due to their insecticide and acaricide properties; in addition, some have shown to possess anticancer activity against several human tumor cell lines. In the present contribution we review 25 rotenoids that have been evaluated in vitro against 48 tumor cell lines, as well as their in vivo antitumor and chemopreventive activity. Two of these rotenoids, rotenone and deguelin, have been thoroughly studied for their anticancer properties. Rotenone has shown high cytotoxic activity against MCF-7 cells (IC_{50}=4.4 nM), as well as chemopreventive and antitumor activity in vivo on mice, by inducing up-regulation of p53, inhibition of proliferation, and down regulation of the C-myc gene. On the other hand, deguelin inhibits 100 per cent of pre-neoplastic injuries on mice at 10 μg/mL. In conclusion, rotenoids are metabolites with high cytotoxic activity against several cell lines, as well as chemopreventive activity in vivo and in vitro. Therefore, rotenoids could be prototypes for the development of new drugs in cancer chemotherapy.

Keywords: Anticancer agents, Cytotoxicity, Deguelin, Rotenoids, Rotenone.

1 Departamento de Productos Naturales, Instituto de Química, Universidad Nacional Autonoma de Mexico, Mexico

2 Departamento de Biología Celular, Facultad de Química, Universidad Nacional Autonoma de México, Mexico

* *Corresponding author*: E-mail: chilpa@unam.mx

Introduction

Cancer

Cancer is defined as a group of diseases characterized by unregulated cell growth, invasion and spread from the original site to other parts of the body (Pecorino, 2012). Any of the 200 or more cell types in the human body can transform to malignant tissue. Tumor cells arise from normal cell by different types of mutations on protooncogenes or tumor suppressor genes. These changes could be result of exposure to physical, chemical or biological carcinogens. Metastasis in cancer is the leading cause of death in patients, and occurs through multiple steps involving the invasion of a primary tumor into the bloodstream, subsequent migration of tumor cells to diverse organs, adhesion to endothelial cells and infiltration into the tissues (Matsuda *et al.*, 2007). Thereby, cancer is classified according to the tissue and cell type where is localized. For example, if cancer arises from epithelial cells it is called "carcinoma"; if it originates from connective tissue or muscle cells is called "sarcoma" if the cancer does not belong to any of these categories is called "leukemia" and so on.

The World Health Organization (WHO) in 2014 estimated that the leading cause of death worldwide in 2012 was cancer, with 8.3 million cases, mainly from lung cancer, stomach, liver, colon and breast (WHO, 2014). These cancer types are different by gender, where in 2012 the most frequents cancers in women are breast, colorectum, cervix uteri, lung and stomach; while in men the most frequents cancers are lung, prostate, colorectum, stomach and liver (Ferlay *et al.*, 2013).

Cancer treatment include several strategies, such as chemotherapy, radiotherapy, immunotherapy and surgery, and it is determined by the cancer type or stage. In the chemotherapy, cytotoxic drugs are administered to induce cell death in tumor cells. However, cancer cells develop resistance to majority of drugs currently used in anticancer therapy. It is also important to note the high costs of these treatments and the harmful side effects for the patient. In this scenario, rotenoids, which are secondary metabolites from plants, could represent an opportunity for development new drugs against cancer.

Rotenoids

Rotenoids (Figure 9.1) are secondary metabolites from plants, that are included in the group of the flavonoids, particularly isoflavonoids. The rotenoids are synthesized by species of the family *Fabaceae*, subfamily *Papilonoideae*. Historically, rotenoids have been known for their insecticidal, acaricidal and pesticidal activity (Estrella-Parra *et al.*, 2014); however, in the last twenty years, rotenoids have acquired pharmacological interest for their antitumor properties (Kardono *et al.*, 1990). Since many rotenoids possess high cytotoxicity against several human tumor cell lines (Lee *et al.*, 2010; Li *et al.*, 1993), they also constitute a source of potential anticancer agents (Ito *et al.*, 2004).

Cytotoxic Properties of Rotenoids

Until 2014, 25 rotenoids have been examined the cytotoxic properties. The comprise 13-α-hydroxytephrosin **(6)**, 1-hydroxytephrosin **(7)**, 4-tephrosin, 5'-dihydro-11, 5'-dihydroxy-4'-metoxitephrosin **(14)**, deguelin, 6a,12a-dehydrodeguelin **(15)**,

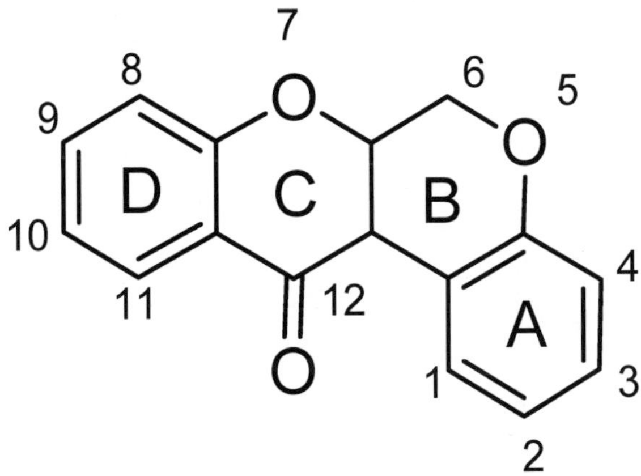

Figure 9.1: General Structure of a Rotenoid.

rotenone **(1)**, 12a hydroxyrotenone **(5)**,12a-hydroxyerosone **(16)**, rotenolone **(11)**, dalpanol **(17)**, 12a,β-hydroxydalpanol **(18)**, 6'-β-O-D-β-glucopyranosildalpanol **(19)**, α-toxicarol **(9)**, 6a,12a-dehydro-α-toxicarol **(4)**, sumatrol **(8)**, 6-deoxyclitoriacetal **(12)**, amorphigenin **(20)**, 12aβ-hydroxyamorphigenine **(21)**, amorphispironone **(10)**, boeravinone G **(22)**, boeravinone H **(23)**, elliptone **(13)**, 6aα,12aα-12a-hydroxyelliptone **(24)** and villosinol **(25)**.

The most studied rotenoids are rotenone **(1)**, deguelin **(2)**, tephrosin **(3)**, 6a,12a-dehydro-α-toxicarol **(4)** and 12a-hydroxyrotenone **(5)**. Most studies were focused on the evaluation of their *in vitro* cytotoxic properties, as well as their *in vivo* antitumor and their chemopreventive properties (preventing the development of cells malignancies). In the current review the cytotoxicity classification of Sangthong *et al.* (2011) was adopted. The cytotoxicity categories are based on average inhibition values (IC_{50}) as follows: very high (< 1 μM), high (1-10 μM), moderate (10-50 μM), low (50-100 μM) and without activity (>100 μM); cytotoxic activity classification depends on the compound and the cancer cell line tested (Sangthong *et al.*, 2011). On the other hand, regarding chemopreventive properties classification (chemopreventive: involves the use of chemicals or dietary compounds to block or inhibit development of cancer in normal or preneoplastic tissue) (Jang *et al.*, 2003), it was assumed chemopreventive effect exists if the inhibition of QR (quinone reductase) is <10μg/mL. To date of the current review, the most potent rotenoids regarding cytotoxic activity are rotenone **(1)** (Table 9.1), deguelin **(2)** (Table 9.3), tephrosin **(3)** (Table 9.5), and 12-hydryxorotenone (Table 9.7). On the other hand, the most effective rotenoids for *in vivo* antitumor and chemopreventive properties are rotenone **(1)** (Table 9.2), deguelin **(2)** (Table 9.4), and tephrosin **(3)** (Table 9.6).

Regarding the *in vitro* cytotoxic activity, rotenoids have been tested against 47 human and mouse origin cancer cells lines. Rotenone **(1)** is the most studied rotenoid, it has been tested against 22 human cancer cells lines (Table 9.1) displaying an IC_{50} of 20-25 nM against MCF-7 and A-549 cells lines, respectively (Sakurai *et al.*, 2006). Other rotenoids with cytotoxic activity at nanomolar concentrations are: deguelin **(2)**

Table 9.1: *In vitro* Cytotoxic Assays and Chemoprevention of Rotenone

Source	*Cell Line*	*Mechanism of Action*	*Reference*
Clitoria macrophylla	P-388 IC_{50}= 0.011 μM KB IC_{50}= 0.9 μM KB-V1 IC_{50}= 6.9 μM	Unknown	(Lin *et al.*, 1992)
Lonchocarpus utilis and *L. urucú*	MCF-7 IC_{50}= 4.4 nM	Inhibits ODC	(Fang and Casida, 1998)
Lonchocarpus aff. fluvialis	LNCaP IC_{50}> 0.4 μM SKNSH IC_{50}= 4.6 μM KB IC_{50}< 0.4 μM Lu 1 IC_{50}< 0.3 μM	Unknown	(Blatt *et al.*, 2002)
Derris trifoliata	Raji cells with EBV-EA Inhibited 100 per cent (32 nM)	Inhibition of EBV-EA	(Ito *et al.*, 2004)
Neurautanenia mitis	MCF-7 IC_{50}= 20 nM A-549 IC_{50}= 25 nM	Unknown	(Sakurai *et al.*, 2006)
	HT-1080: Inhibition of 93.5 per cent -72 h U937 IC_{50}= 13μM (24h), 0.2 μM (48h) and 0.07 μM (72h)	Unknown	(Matsuda *et al.*, 2007)
Derris trifoliata	KB IC_{50}=1.7 μM BC IC_{50}=0.2 μM NCI-H187 IC_{50}=0.05 μM	Unknown	(Cheenpracha *et al.*, 2007)
Lonchocarpus haberi	Molecular computational analysis of prenylated flavonoids, among them rotenone.	Prenylated compounds inhibit PTK, ODC, COX-1 Y2, PKC, the binding site of ATP from topoisomerase II, PI3K	(Cassidy and Setzer, 2010)

Contd...

Table 9.1–*Contd...*

Source	*Cell Line*	*Mechanism of Action*	*Reference*
	MCF-7	ROS induced apoptosis through JNK/p38 and MAPK´s activation	(Deng *et al.*, 2010)
	NIH3T3 IC_{50} =5 μM (48 h)	Unknown	
Leafs of *Antheroporum pierrei*	C-38 IC_{50} = 0.23μg/mL	Unknown	(Gao *et al.*, 2011)
	L1210 IC_{50} =0.045μg/mL	Unknown	
Rotenone (Sigma-Aldrich)	8505-C and CMPBR3 IC_{50} =5μM	Increased activity of *p53* inducing apoptosis.	(Goncalves *et al.*, 2011)
	TPC-1 IC_{50} = 5μM	Nuclear *p53* accumulation, inducing cell death.	
	TPC-1 Rotenone IC_{50} = 500 nM	G2/M induced cell death (15.27 per cent)	
	TPC-1 IC_{50} =500 nM rotenone	Rotenone: Arrest in G2/M phase	

P-388 human leukemia cell. KB: human leukemia cell, KB-V1: Vinblastine-resistant human leukemia cell, MCF-7: human breast adenocarcinoma cell, LNCaP: human prostate adenocarcinoma cell. A549: human lung adenocarcinoma epithelial cell, SKNSH: human neuroblastoma cell, Lu1: lung carcinoma cells, EBV-EA: Epstein Barr virus early antigen, HT1080: human fibrosarcoma cell, BC: breast cáncer cell, NCI-H187: human lung carcinoma cell, Cal27: oral adenosquamous carcinoma cell, Tw2.6: oral adenosquamous carcinoma cell, OMFs: oral mucosa fibroblast, NIH3T3: mouse embryo fibroblast, C38: colon adenocarcinoma cell, L1210: mouse lymphocytic leukemia cells, TPC-1: human thyroid tumor cell.

(Table 9.3), amorphigenine **(20)**, 12-aβ-hydroxyamorphigenine **(21)** (Table 9.8), and 12aβ-hydroxyamorphigenine **(21)** displaying an IC_{50}>1<10 μM in six different cancer cells lines (Table 9.8). Rotenoids that show moderate cytotoxic activity (10 μM <IC_{50}<50 μM) are tephrosin **(3)** (IC_{50}= 86.3 μM against US375-S2 cells; Table 9.5), 12a-hydroxyrotenone **(5)** (IC_{50}= 25 μM against MCF-7 cells, IC_{50}= 15 μM against A-549 cells; Table 9.7) and 6-deoxychlitoriacetal (IC_{50}=30 μM against KB cells; Table 9.8).

Structure/activity relationship also has been examined for rotenoids, Sakurai *et al.* (2006) compared cytotoxic activity between rotenone **(1)** (Table 9.1) and 12a-hydroxyerosone **(16)** (Table 9.7). Rotenone **(1)** is more cytotoxic than 12a-hydroxyerosone **(16)**, which highlight the following structural differences between both compounds (Sakurai *et al.*, 2006). The furan ring (E) of rotenone **(1)** is to C8 and C9, while in 12a-hydroxyerosone **(16)** is lineal to the carbons C9 and C10. This structure/activity relationship was tested *in silico* by Cassidy and Setzer (2010), in which they established that prenilated are more active against several cancer proteins than non prenilated isoflavonoids, for instance 6aα, 12aα-12a-hydroxyelliptone **(24)** shows a high cytotoxic activity against four different cancer cells lines (IC_{50} < 0.3-4.6

Table 9.2: *In vivo* Cytotoxic Assays of Rotenone

Source	*Strain*	*Pharmacological Mechanism*	*Reference*
No source mentioned	75 mg/Kg, 24 months	Tumor inhibition	(Haley, 1978)
No source mentioned	Rats (Fisher 344) with a dietetic exposition during 24 months with different doses (7.5, 37.5, 75.0 mg/Kg)	Did not induced tumors or reproductive problems in rats.	(Marking, 1988)
No source mentioned	Male mouses ((B6C3F1) with hepatic tumors. The treatment with rotenone (75 ppm) inhibits 93 per cent of tumors	No negative effects on hepatocellular β-oxidation and catalase.	(Cunningham *et al.*, 1995)
No source mentioned.	Mouse (B6C3F1). Rotenone (600 ppm) significantly increase in apoptotic hepatocites 90 per cent	Increases *P53* gene activity. H-Ras diminution	(Wang *et al.*, 1999)
No source mentioned.	Rats (F344) Rotenone (500 ppm/266 days)	Inhibitory effect of rotenone on dysplasias lessons (liver and tongue), reducing the size of carcinoma from 53 to 16 per cent. Severe dysplasia size was reduced from 80 to 42 per cent.	(Tanaka *et al.*, 2002)

Table 9.3: *In vitro* Cytotoxic Assays of Deguelin

Source	*Cell Line*	*Mechanism of Action*	*Reference*
Mundulea serícea	308 IC_{50}= 0.0007μM	Inhibits ODC	(Gerhäuser *et al.*, 1995)
Obtained by synthesis from rotenone	BALB/c 3T3 IC_{50}= 0.0005 μg/mL	Inhibits ODC activity	(Gerhauser *et al.*, 1997)
	MCF-7 IC_{50}= 6.9 nM	Unknown	(Fang and Casida, 1998)
Semisynthesis from rotenone (Sigma-Aldrich)	SAS IC_{50}=0.95 μM	Unknown	(Lee *et al.*, 2008)
	Cal27 IC_{50}=0.11 μM		
	Tw2.6 IC_{50}=1.24 μM		
	OMFs IC_{50}=31.43		
	SAS (1 μM)	Release of Cytochrome C	

Contd...

Table 9.3–*Contd...*

Source	*Cell Line*	*Mechanism of Action*	*Reference*
Derris trifoliata	Raji with EBV-EA Inhibits 90.5 per cent (32 nM.)	Inhibition of EBV-EA.	(Ito *et al.*, 2004)
Erycibe expansa	HT 1080 IC_{50}= 30µM-72 h	Unknown	(Matsuda *et al.*, 2007)
	U 937 IC_{50}=42 µM-24 h IC_{50}=16µM-48 h IC_{50}=5.8 µM-72 h		
Amorpha fruticosa	HeLa IC_{50}= 0.22 µM	Inhibition of NF-κB	(Dat *et al.*, 2008)
	RAW2647.7 IC_{50}= 1.75 µM	Unknown	

Hepa 1c1c7: mouse hepatoma cell, HeLa: human cervical carcinoma cell, RAW264.7: Mouse leukemic monocyte-macrophage cell, HL-60: human promyelocytic leukemia cell, HT1080: human fibrosarcoma cell, U937: human histiocytic lymphoma cell, BALB/c-3T3: BALB/c mouse embryos fibroblast cells, Cal27: oral adenosquamous carcinoma cell, Tw2.6: oral adenosquamous carcinoma cell, OMFs: oral mucosa fibroblast.

Table 9.4: *In vivo* Cytotoxic Assays of Deguelin

Species	*Mouse Strain*	*Effect*	*Reference*
Mundulea serícea	CD-1 10µg/mL	Inhibition of proneoplastics injuries (100 per cent) in mammary tissues of mouse.	(Gerhäuser *et al.*, 1995)
Mundulea serícea	CD-1 (female)	33 µg deguelin/0.2 mL acetone reduced 66 per cent of tumor	(Udeani *et al.*, 1997)
		330 µg deguelin/0.2 mL acetone reduced 66 per cent of tumor	
		33 µg deguelin/0.2 mL de acetone reduced (75 per cent) the activity of ODC induced for TPA	
		330 µg deguelin/0.2 mL de acetone reduced (100 per cent) the activity of ODC induced for TPA	
Derris trifoliata	ICR (female, 85 nM)	Inhibited the 100 per cent of mammary tissues of mouse	(Ito *et al.*, 2004)

µM) (Blatt *et al.*, 2002; Table 9.8) (Cassidy and Setzer 2010). In addition, other non-prenilated rotenoids show high and moderate cytotoxic activity against different cancer cells lines (*e.g.* elliptone, boeravinones G and H and 12a-hydroxyerosone), as stated in Table 9.8. On the other hand, boeravinones H **(23)** and G **(22)** (Table 9.8) showed an IC_{50} of 3.0-0.7 µM against HEK-293 cells, respectively (Ahmed-Belkacem *et al.*, 2007). The difference between both rotenoids is a methyl group located at the

Table 9.5: *In vitro* and *In vivo* Cytotoxic Assays of Tephrosin

Source	*Cell Line*	*Mechanism of Action*	*Reference*
		In vitro	
Mundulea sericea	HL-60	PKC not activated	(Gerhäuser *et al.*, 1995)
Lonchocarpus utilis y L. urucú	MCF-7 IC_{50}= 98 nM	Activates ODC	(Fang and Casida, 1998)
Erycibe expansa	HLT1080 IC_{50}= 10 μM	Inhibition of methalo-proteinases 2 and 9	(Matsuda *et al.*, 2007)
	U937 IC_{50}=7.3μM-72 h	Unknown	
Amorpha fruticosa	HeLa IC_{50}= 0.11 μM	Inhibition of NF-κB	(Dat *et al.*, 2008)
	RAW2647.7 IC_{50}=2.0 μM		
Amorpha fruticosa	US375-S2 IC_{50}= 86.3 μM	Unknown	(Jiang *et al.*, 2008)
Derris trifoliata	SNU-484, AGS y MKN-28 1 μM	Induces chromatin condensation and DNA fragmentation. Inhibition of G2/M phase. Apoptosis induction for caspases 3 and 9. Activates Akt	(Lee *et al.*, 2010)
Amorpha fruticosa	HT-29	Inhibits ErB2 and EGFR receptors	(Choi *et al.*, 2010)
Antheroporum pierrei	HCT-116 IC_{50}=0.040 μg/mL	Unknown	(Gao *et al.*, 2011)
		In vivo	

Source	*Strain*	*Mechanism of Action*	*Reference*
Mundulea sericea	CD-1 IC_{50}= 0.005μM 10μg/mL	Inhibits ODC Inhibition of preneo-plastics injuries (89 per cent) in mammary tissues of mouse.	(Gerhäuser *et al.*, 1995)

HL-60: human promyelocytic leukemia cell, HT1080: human fibrosarcoma cell, A549: human alveolar basal epithelial cell, Bel 7402: hepatoma cell line, P388: mouse leukaemia cell, HT 29: human intestinal epithelial cells, HCT-116: colorectal carcinoma cell, HeLa: human cervical carcinoma cell, RAW264.7 mouse leukemic monocyte macrophage cell, US 375-S2: human melanoma cell.

carbon C10 of the ring D in the boeravinone H **(23)**, which is absent in boeravinone G **(22)**. This suggests that the methyl group could be important in the pharmacophore site of this rotenoid.

Table 9.6: *In vitro* and *in vivo* Cytotoxic Assays of 6a, 12a-dehydro-α-toxicarol

Source	*Cell Line*	*Mechanism of Action*	*Reference*
	In vitro		
Tephrosia toxicaria	Hepa 1c1c7 IC_{50} > 47 μM	Unknown	(Jang *et al.*, 2003)
	Hepa 1c1c7 Induction QR (23 μM)	Non activation of QR	
Macaranga triloba	Hepa 1c1c7 IC_{50} > 10 μg/mL	Non activation of QR	(Dae Sik Jang *et al.*, 2004)
Amorpha fruticosa	US375-S2 IC_{50}= 93.5μM	Unknown	(Jiang *et al.*, 2008)
	In vivo		
Source	*Strain*	*Mechanism of Action*	*Reference*
Tephrosia toxicaria	Mouse mammary organ cultura assay	Inhibition of preneoplastic lesions	(D. S. Jang *et al.*, 2003)

QR: Quinone reductase, COX: ciclooxygenase, MMOC: mouse mammary organ culture, Hepa 1c1c7: mouse hepatoma cell, US375-S2: human melanoma cell.

Table 9.7: *In vitro* Cytotoxicity Assays of 12a-hydroxyrotenone

Source	*Cell Line*	*Mechanism of Action*	*Reference*
Neorautanonia mitis	MCF-7: IC_{50}= 25 μM	Unknown	(Sakurai *et al.*, 2006)
	A-549: IC_{50}= 15 μM		
Erycibe expansa	HT 1080 inhibition of 95.0 per cent (72 h)	Unknown	(Matsuda *et al.*, 2007)
	U 937: IC_{50}=3.6 μM-24 h IC_{50}=0.07 μM -48 h IC_{50}=0.09 μM-72 h		
Antheroporum pierrei	L1210 IC_{50}= 0.055 μg/mL	Unknown	(Gao *et al.*, 2011)

HEK-293: Human Embryonic Kidney, MCF-7: human breast adenocarcinoma cell, A549: human lung adenocarcinoma epithelial cell, HT1080: human fibrosarcoma cell, U937: human histiocytic lymphoma cell, L1210: mouse lymphocytic leukemia cell.

Rotenoids may have similar mechanisms of cell death induction on different human cancer cells lines. In particular, rotenone **(1)** (Table 9.1) as well as tephrosin **(3)** (Table 9.5) at 1 μM, induce apoptosis by cytochrome C release, which in turn activates caspases 3 and 9. In addition, rotenone **(1)** also activates the tumor suppressor protein *p53* (Table 9.1) (Goncalves *et al.*, 2011). In contrast, deguelin **(2)** (Table 9.3), tephrosin **(3)**, and 13α-hydroxytephrosin **(6)** (Table 9.8) downregulate the expression of the ornithine decarboxylase gene, a promising target in cancer (Gerhäuser *et al.*,

Table 9.8: *In vitro* cytotoxic and chemoprevention assays of other rotenoids.

Rotenoid	*Source*	*Cell Line*	*Mechanism of Action*	*Reference*
13α-hydroxytephrosin	*Mundulea serícea*	308 IC_{50}= 0.02 μg/mL	Inhibits ODC	(Luyengi *et al.*, 1994)
	Mundulea serícea	308 IC_{50}= 0.05 μM	Inhibits ODC	(Gerhäuser *et al.*, 1995)
		HL-60IC_{50} >10μM	Unknown	
11-hydroxytephrosin	*Tephrosia toxicara*	Hepa 1c1c7 IC_{50}> 23 μM	Unknown	(Jang *et al.*, 2003)
		Hepa 1c1c7 IC_{50}> 47 μM	Activation of QR	
	Amorpha fruticosa	RAW264.7 IC_{50}= 4.21 μM	Inhibits activity of NF-κB	(Dat *et al.*, 2008)
		HeLa IC_{50}= 0.19 μM	Unknown	
Sumatrol	*Lonchocarpus aff. fluvialis*	LNCaP: IC_{50}> 0.4 μM	Unknown	(Blatt *et al.*, 2002)
		SKNSH: IC_{50}= 0.4 μM		
		KB: IC_{50}< 0.3 μM		
		Lu 1 IC_{50}< 0.3 μM		
	Tephrosia toxicaria	Hepa 1c1c71c1c7 IC_{50}> 47 μM	Unknown	(Jang *et al.*, 2003)
		Hepa 1c1c7 1c1c7IC_{50}>23 μM	Unknown	
α-toxicarol	*Derris trifoliata*	Raji with EBV-EA, inhibition of 89.1 per cent at 32 nM	Inhibits EBV-EA	(Ito *et al.*, 2004)
Amorfispironone	*Amorpha fruticosa*	A-549 IC_{50}= 10 μg/mL	Unknown	(Li *et al.*, 1993)
		HCT-8 IC_{50}= 10 μg/mL		
		TE671 IC_{50}= 10 μg/mL		
		P388 IC_{50}= 10 μg/mL		
		RPMI-7951 IC_{50}= 0.61 μg/mL		
		KB IC_{50}= 0.58μg/mL		

Contd...

Table 9.8–*Contd...*

Rotenoid	Source	Cell Line	Mechanism of Action	Reference
Rotenolone	*Lonchocarpus utilis and L. urucú*	MCF-7 IC_{50}= 285 nM	Inhibits ODC	(Fang and Casida, 1998)
	Pongamiopsis pervilleana	BT-549 IC_{50}= 2.6 μM	Unknown	(Harinantenaina *et al.*, 2010)
		DU 145 IC_{50}= 2.7 μM		
		NSCLC NCI-H460 IC_{50}= 2.0 μM		
		HCC-2998 IC_{50}= 2.9 μM		
6-Deoxicloriacetal	*Clitoria macrophylla*	P-388 IC_{50}=0.031 μM	Unknown	(Lin *et al.*, 1992)
		KB IC_{50}=30μM		
		KB-V1 IC_{50}=19μM		
	Stemona collinsae	SW620 IC_{50}> 100 μM	Unknown	(Sangthong *et al.*, 2011)
		KATO IC_{50}> 100 μM		
		BT474 IC_{50}> 100 μM		
		HEP-G2 IC_{50} >100μM		
		KBIC_{50}> 13.28 μM		
		MCF-7 IC_{50}> 23.65 μM		
		NCI-H187 IC_{50}> 3.12 μM		
		CHAGO IC_{50}> 100 μM		
Elliptone	*Derris trifoliata*	Raji with EBV-EA, inhibits 89.1 per cent 32 nM	Inhibits EBV-EA	(Ito *et al.*, 2004)
4′,5′-dihydro-11,5′-dihydroxy-4′-metoxitephrosin	*Tephrosia toxicaria*	Hepa 1c1c7 IC_{50} > 14.9 μM	Unknown	(Jang *et al.*, 2003)
		Hepa 1c1c7 IC_{50} >10.7 μM	Activates the QR	
6a, 12a-dehydrodeguelin	*Amorpha fruticosa*	US375-S2 IC_{50}= 176.2 μM	Unknown	(Jiang *et al.*, 2008)
12a-hydroxyerosone	*Neorautanenia mitis*	MCF-7 IC_{50}= 1.8 μg/mL	Unknown	(Sakurai *et al.*, 2006)
		A-549 IC_{50}= 3.3 μg/mL		

Contd...

Table 9.8–*Contd...*

Rotenoid	*Source*	*Cell Line*	*Mechanism of Action*	*Reference*
Dalpanol	*Amorpha fruticosa*	A-549 IC_{50}= 0.86 μg/mL HCT-8 IC_{50}= 0.48 μg/mL RPMI-7951 IC_{50}=4.83 μg/mL TE671 IC_{50}= 0.49 μg/mL KB IC_{50}= 0.89 μg/mL P388 IC_{50}= 10 μg/mL	Unknown	(Li *et al.*, 1993)
12aβ-hydroxydalpanol	*Amorpha fruticosa*	A-549 IC_{50}=9.28 μg/mL KB IC_{50}=3.67 μg/mL P388 IC_{50}=0.59 μg/mL TE671 IC_{50}= 0.12 μg/mL RPMI-7951 IC_{50}=0.73 μg/mL HCT-8 IC_{50}= 0.56 μg/mL	Unknown	(Li *et al.*, 1993)
6'-O-D-β-gluco-piranosildalpanol	*Amorpha fruticosa*	A-549I C_{50}=10 μg/mL HCT-8 IC_{50}=7.43 μg/mL RPMI-7951 IC_{50}=4.44 μg/mL TE671 IC_{50}=2.94 μg/mL KB IC_{50}=6.32 μg/mL P388 IC_{50}=6.68 μg/mL	Unknown	(Li *et al.*, 1993)
Amorfigenine	*Amorpha fruticosa*	A-549 IC_{50}= 0.05 μg/mL HCT-8 IC_{50}= 0.03 μg/mL RPMI-7951 IC_{50}= 0.05 μg/mL	Unknown	(Li *et al.*, 1993)

Contd...

Table 9.8–*Contd...*

Rotenoid	*Source*	*Cell Line*	*Mechanism of Action*	*Reference*
		KB IC_{50}= 0.04 μg/mL		
		P388 IC_{50}= 0.04 μg/mL		
		TE671 IC_{50} < 0.001 μg/mL		
12aβ-hydroxya-morfigenine	*Amorpha fruticosa*	A-549 IC_{50}<0.001 μg/mL	Unknown	(Li *et al.*, 1993)
		HCT-8 IC_{50}<0.001 μg/mL		
		RPMI-7951 IC_{50}< 0.001 μg/mL		
		TE671 IC_{50}< 0.001 μg/mL		
		KB IC_{50}< 0.001 μg/mL		
		P388 IC_{50}< 0.001 μg/mL		
Boeravinones G and H	*Boerhavia* sp.	HEK-293: Boeravinone G IC_{50}= 0.7 μM	Inhibits BCRP/ ABCG2 activity	(Ahmed-Belkacem *et al.,* 2007)
		HEK-293: Boeravinone H IC_{50}= 3.0 μM		
6aα, 12aα-12a-hydroxyelliptone	*Derris trifoliata*	Raji with EBV-EA, inhibits 89.1 per cent 32 nM	Inhibits EBV-EA	(Ito *et al.,* 2004)
	Lonchocarpus aff. fluvialis	LNCaP IC_{50}> 0.4 μM	Unknown	(Blatt *et al.,* 2002)
		SKNSH IC_{50}= 4.6 μM		
		KB IC_{50}< 0.4 μM		
		Lu 1 IC_{50}< 0.3 μM		
Villosol	*Lonchocarpus aff. fluvialis*	SKNSH IC_{50}= 4.6 μM	Unknown	
		KB IC_{50}< 0.4 μM)		

308: mouse keratinocyte cell, HL-60: human promyelocytic leukemia cell, Hepa 1c1c7: mouse hepatoma cell, HeLa: human cervical carcinoma cell, RAW264.7 mouse leukemic monocyte macrophage cell, LNCaP: human prostate adenocarcinoma cell., SKNSH: human neuroblastoma cell,. KB: human leukemia cell, Lu1: lung carcinoma cells, A549: human alveolar basal epithelial cell, HCT 8: Human ileocecal adenocarcinoma cell, RPMI-7951: Human Skin Malignant Melanoma Cell, TE671: human medulloblastoma cell, P388: human lymphoblastic lymphoma cell, A 2780: human ovarian cancer cell, BT-549: human breast carcinoma cell, DU 145, NSCLC, NCI-H460: human prostate cancer cell, HCC-2998: human colon adenocarcinoma cell, MCF-7: human breast adenocarcinoma cell, KB-V1: Vinblastine-resistant human leukemia cell, SW-620: Human colon adenocarcinoma cell, KATO: Human gastric carcinoma cell, HEP-G2: human liver carcinoma cell, NCI-H187 and CHAGO: Human lung bronchus carcinoma cell, HEK-293: Human Embryonic Kidney cells, US375-S2: human melanoma cell, SKNSH: human neuroblastoma cell, QR: Quinone reductase, EBV-EA: Epstein Barr virus early antigen.

Table 9.9: *In vivo* Antitumor Activity Assays of Three Rotenoids

Rotenoids	*Source*	*Strain*	*Action Mechanism*	*Reference*
13α-hydroxy-tephrosin	*Mundulea serícea*	CD-1 (10 μg/mL)	Inhibition of pre-neoplastics injuries (55 per cent) in mouse mammary tissues	(Gerhäuser *et al.*, 1995)
α-toxicarol	*Derris trifoliata*	ICR (female) Inhibited 73 per cent of pre-neoplastics lesions (85 nM)	Unknown	(Ito *et al.*, 2004)

1995). In addition, the aforementioned rotenoids inhibit NF-kB activation (Dat *et al.*, 2008), an event related with cancer processes and metastasis. Interestingly, until 2014, the tephrosin **(3)** was the only rotenoid that could induce two mechanisms of cell death.

The *in vitro* chemopreventive properties of rotenoids have been evaluated by the quinone reductase (QR) assay. Increased levels of QR *in vitro,* have shown to correlate with induction of other protective phase II enzymes and provides a reasonable biomarker for the potential chemoprotective effect of test agents against cancer initiation. The 6a,12a-dehydro-α-toxicarol **(4)** (Table 9.8) did not induce QR activation in Hepa 1c1c7 cell line at 23 μM (Dae Sik Jang *et al.,* 2004; Jang *et al.,* 2003). Similar results were also observed for 1-hydroxytephrosin **(7)** and sumatrol **(8)** (Table 9.8) (Jang *et al.,* 2003). The *in vitro* chemopreventive properties of rotenoids have been also determined by the ornithine decarboxylase inhibition test, as this enzyme is overexpressed in various human cancer cells lines. In fact, rotenone **(1)** and tephrosin **(3)** (Tables 9.1 and 9.5) inhibited the ornithine decarboxylase (ODC) in the MCF-7 cells line (IC_{50} = 4.4 nM and 98 nM respectively) (Fang and Casida 1998), whereas deguelin **(2)** (Gerhauser *et al.*, 1997; Gerhäuser *et al.*, 1995) inhibit the activation of the ODC at IC_{50} = 0.0007 μM and 0.0005 mg/mL in 308 and BALB/c3T3 cells lines, respectively. Finally, 13α-hydroxytephrosin **(6)** (Gerhäuser *et al.*, 1995; Luyengi *et al.*, 1994) (Table 8) and rotenolone **(11)** (Table 9.8) showed inhibition of ODC at IC_{50}= 0.02 mg/mL and 0.05 μM, against 308 cells line, and 285 nM against MCF-7 cells line, respectively (Fang and Casida 1998). Regarding *in vivo* studies, there are fewer reports on the antitumor properties of rotenoids.

In particular, rotenone **(1)** (Table 9.2), deguelin **(2)** (Table 9.4), tephrosin **(3)** (Table 9.5), 6a,12a-dehydro-α-toxicarol **(4)**, 13-α-hidroxitephrosin **(6)**, and the α-toxicarol

Figure 9.1: Molecular Structures of Rotenoids

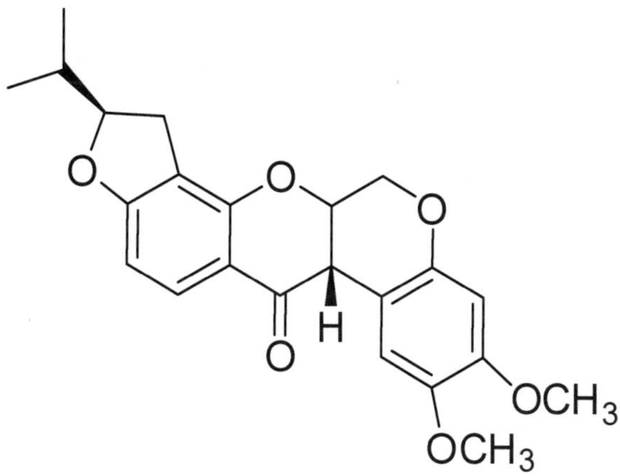

(1) Rotenone

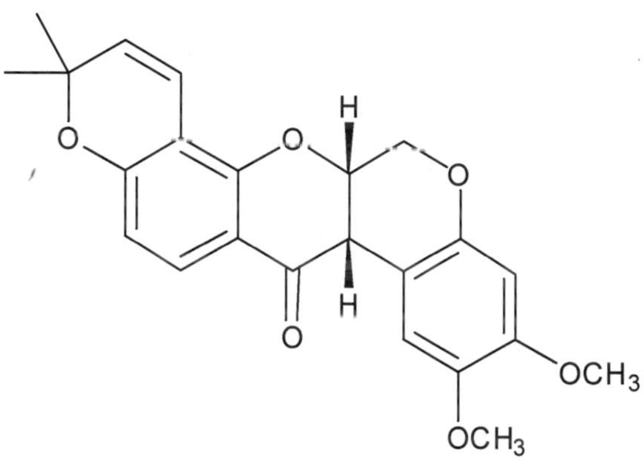

(2) Deguelin

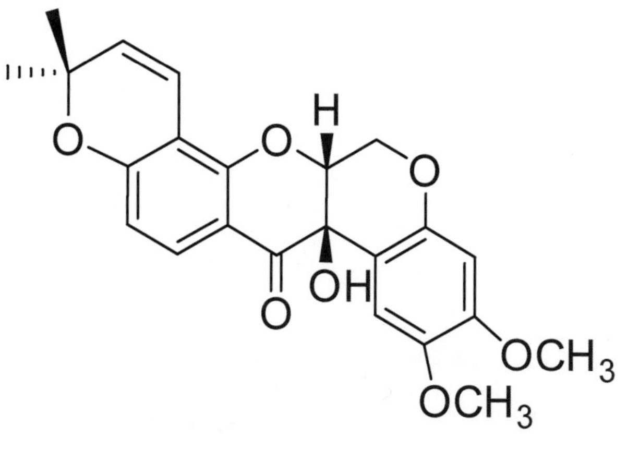

(3) Tephrosin

Contd...

Figure 9.1–*Contd...*

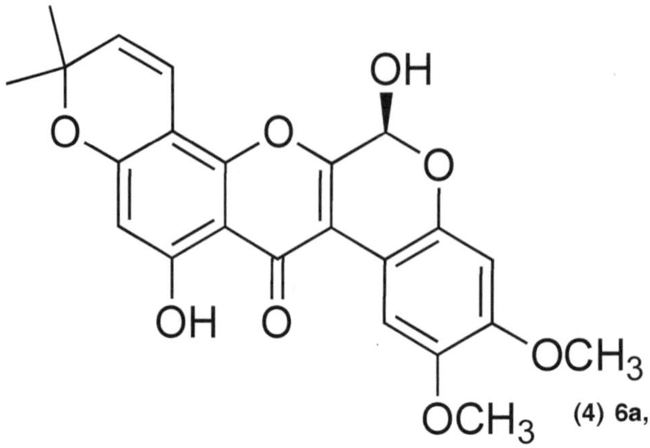

(4) 6a,12a-dehydro-α-toxicarol

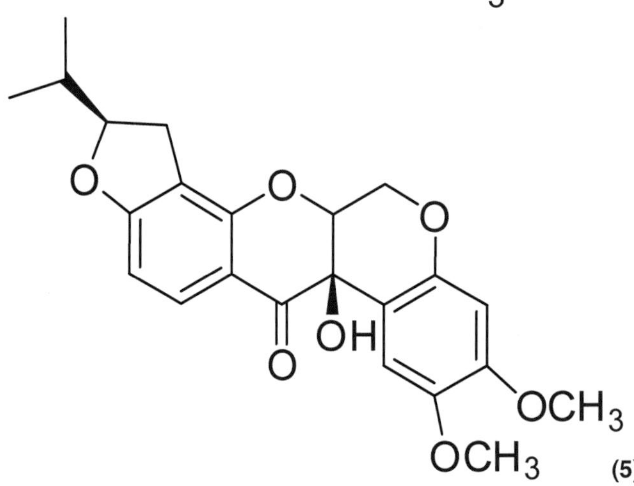

(5) 12a-hydroxyrotenone

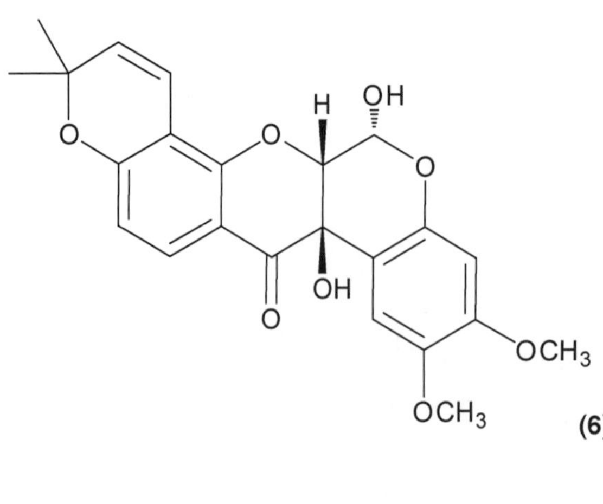

(6) 13α-hydroxytephrosin

Contd...

Figure 9.1–*Contd...*

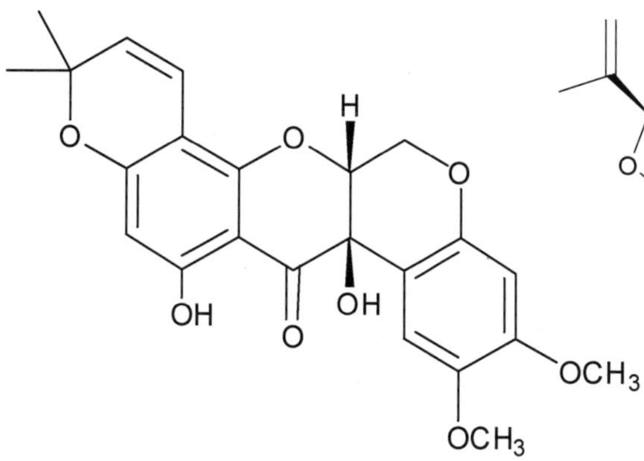

(7) 11-hydroxytephrosin

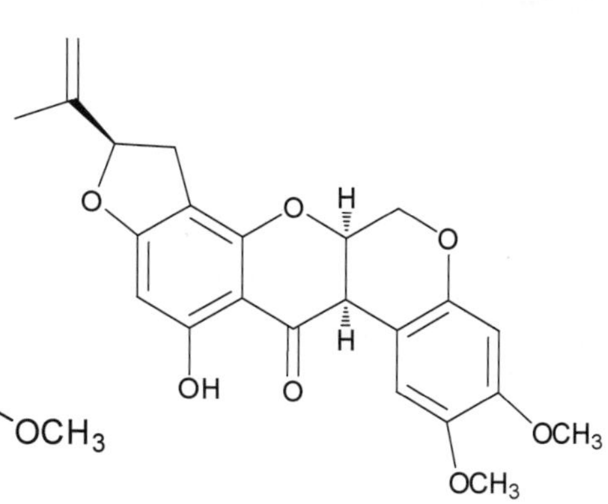

(8) Sumatrol

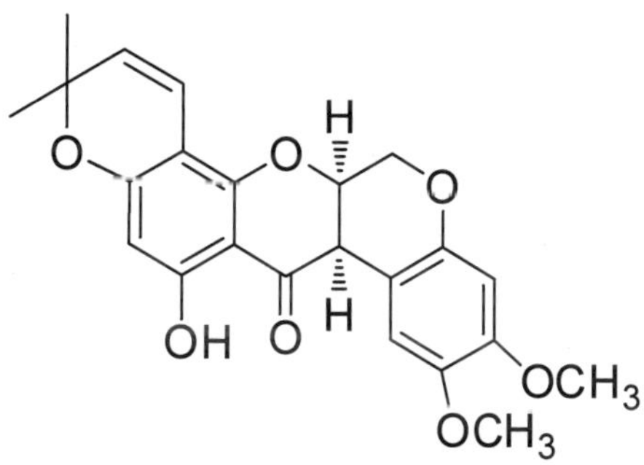

(9) α-toxicarol

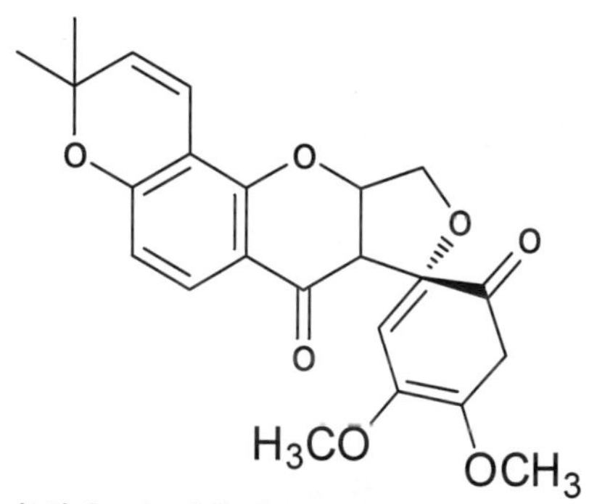

(10) Amorphispironone

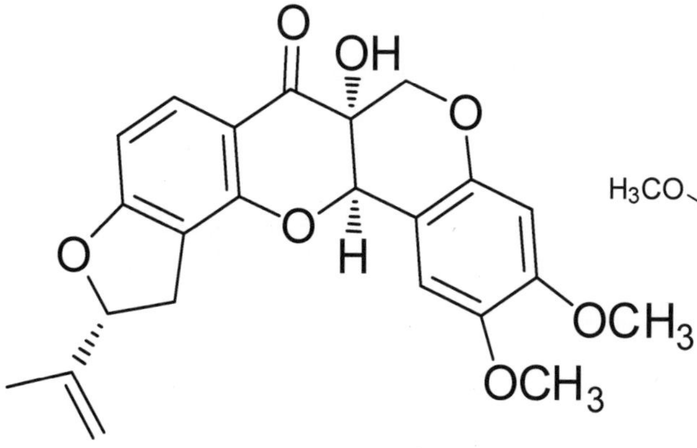

(11) Rotenolone

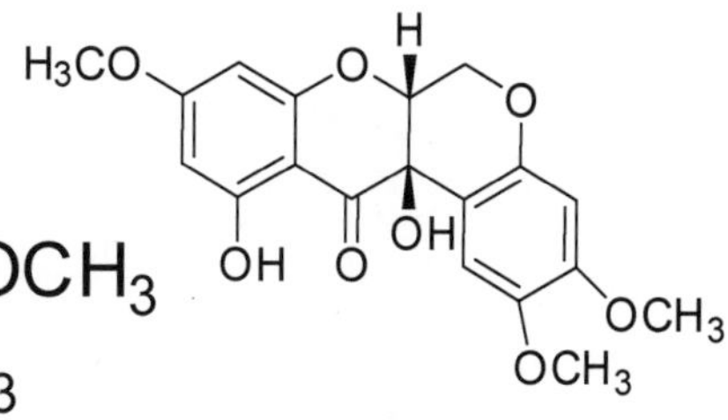

(12) 6-deoxyclitoriacetal

Contd...

Figure 9.1–*Contd...*

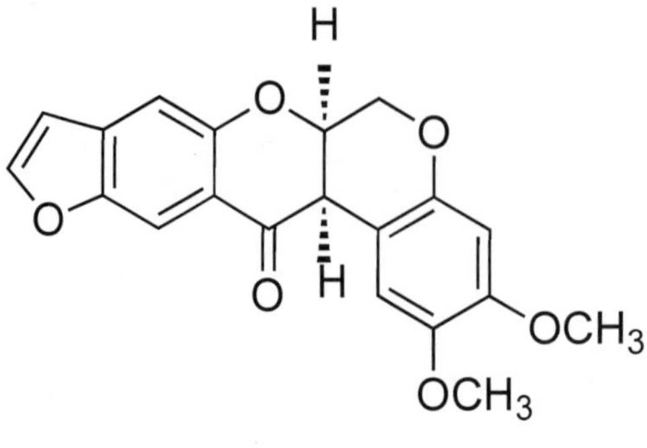

(13) Elliptone

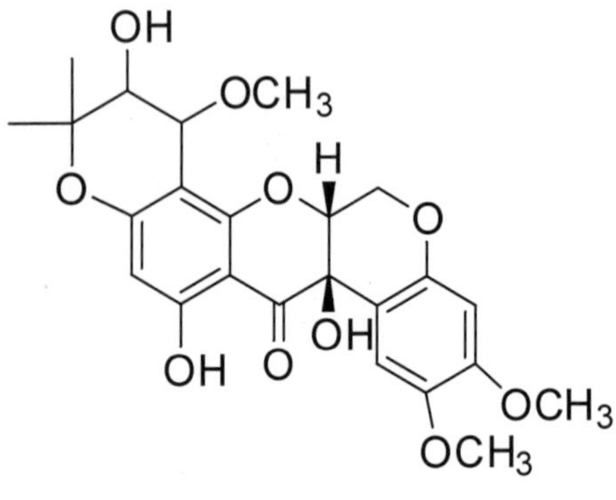

(14) 4′,5′-dihydro-11,5′-dihdroxy-4′-metoxytephrosin

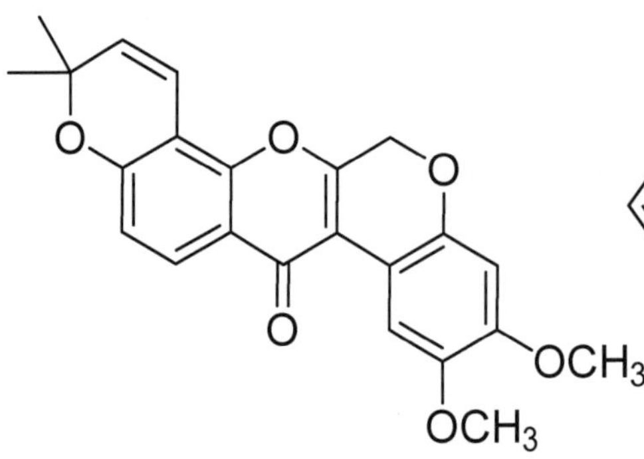

(15) 6a,12a-dehydrodeguelin

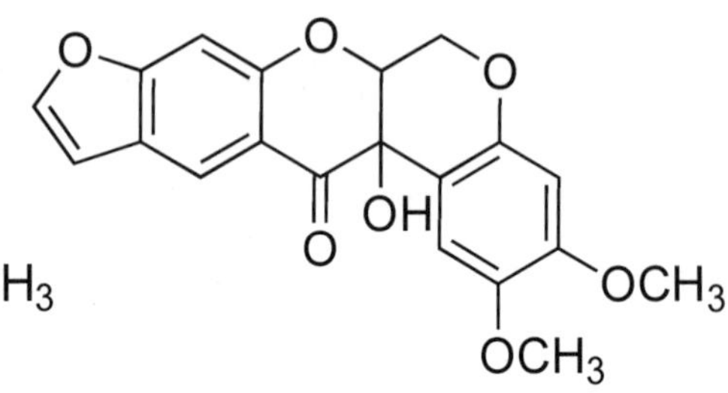

(16) 12a-hydroxyerosone

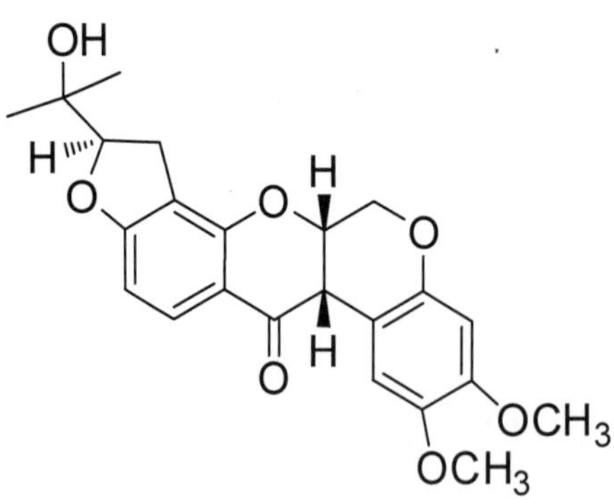

(17) Dalpnol

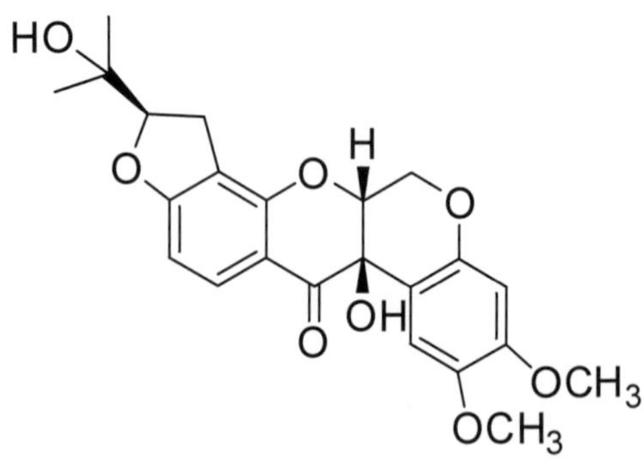

(18) 12a,β-hydroxydalpanol

Contd...

Figure 9.1–*Contd...*

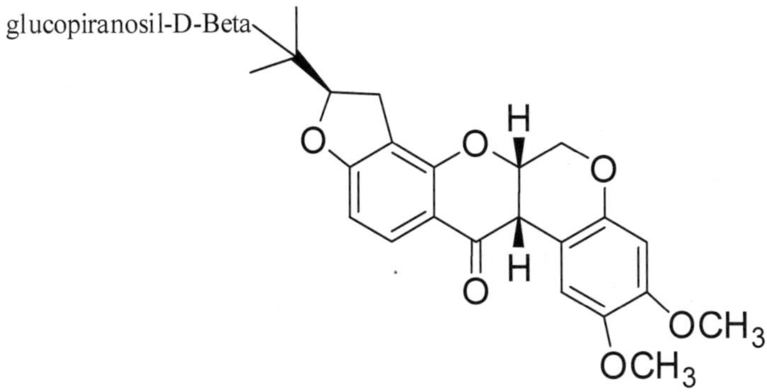

(19) 6'-O-D-β-glucopyranosyldalpanol

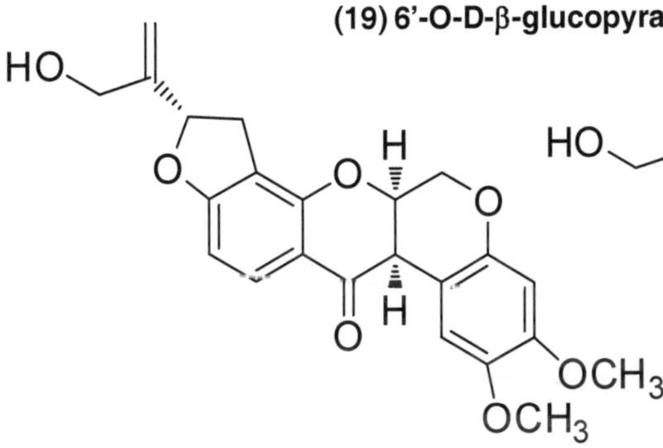

(20) Amorphigenin

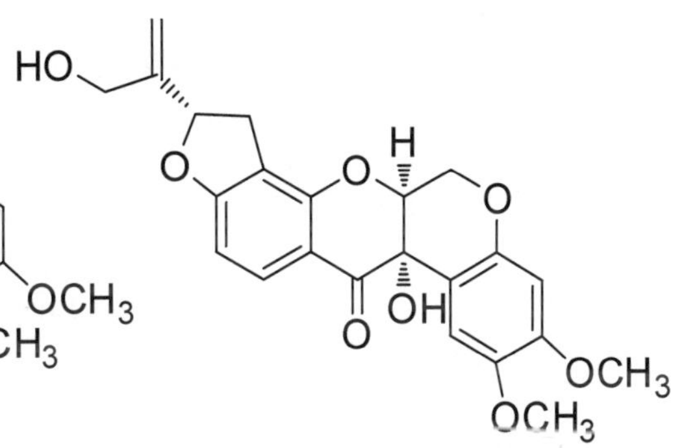

(21) 12a,β-hydroxyamorphigenine

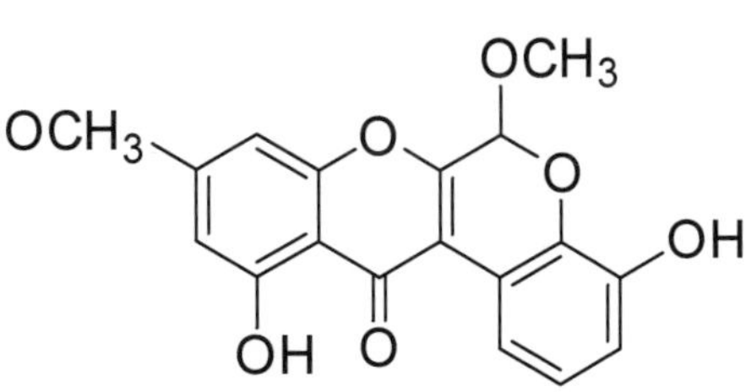

(22) Boeravinone G

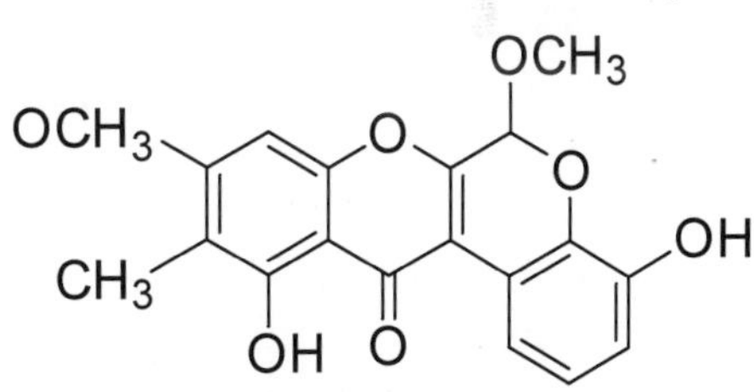

(23) Boeravinone H

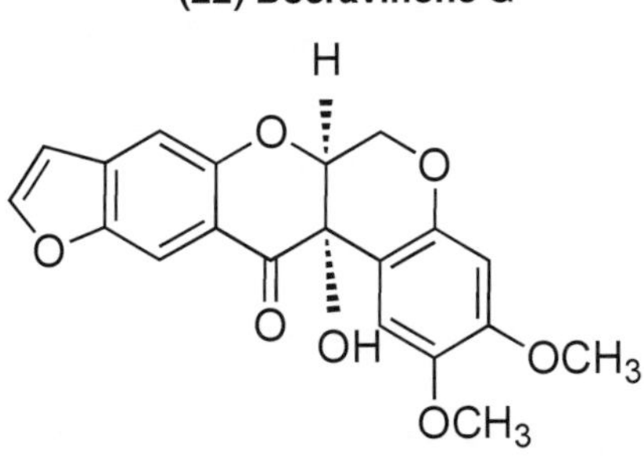

(24) 6aα,12aα-12a-hydroxyelliptone

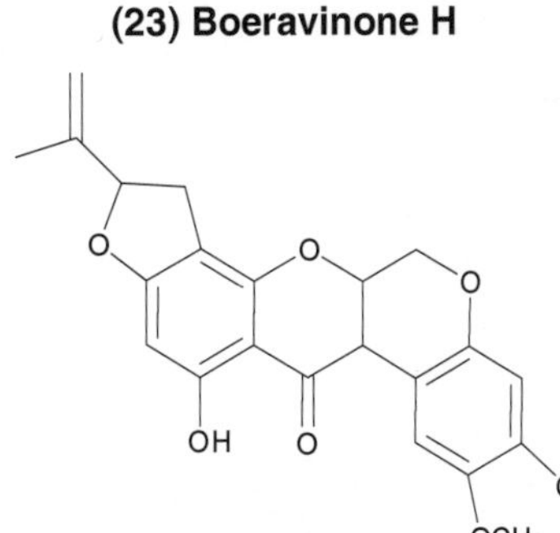

(25) Villosinol

(9) (Table 9.9) inhibits 60 per cent of tumors and lesions in mammary glands on pre-neoplastic mouse at 10 μg/mL. Moreover, rotenone **(1)** inhibits the growth of tumors administered to rats in their diet at 75.0 mg/kg for 2 years, without causing reproductive problems (Haley, 1978). The studies on the mechanism of action of rotenone **(1)** report that it increases expression of *p53* and *c-myc* genes, which are involved in triggering apoptosis (Wang *et al.*, 1999).

Conclusion

Several rotenoids possess potent *in vitro* cytotoxic activity towards several human tumor cell lines, as well as, in *vivo* antiproliferative properties; in addition they can also exhibit high *in vitro* and *in vivo* chemopreventive properties. Therefore, it is of great interest to continue evaluating and exploring these compounds as a potential source of new anticancer and chemopreventive drugs. However, it is important to emphasize that additional toxicological and phamokinetic studies must be performed in order to suggest their use in the clinical practice.

References

Ahmed-Belkacem, A., Macalou, S., Borrelli, F., Capasso, R., Fattorusso, E., Taglialatela-Scafati, O., and Di Pietro, A. (2007). Nonprenylated rotenoids, a new class of potent breast cancer resistance protein inhibitors. *J Med Chem.*, **50**: 1933-1938.

Blatt, C. T. T., Chávez, D., Chai, H., Graham, J. G., Cabieses, F., Farnsworth, N. R., Cordell, G. A., Pezzuto, J. M., and Kinghorn, A. D. (2002). Cytotoxic flavonoids from the stem bark of *Lonchocarpus* aff. *fluvialis*. *Phytotherapy Research*, **16**: 320-325.

Cassidy, C., and Setzer, W. (2010). Cancer-relevant biochemical targets of cytotoxic *Lonchocarpus* flavonoids: A molecular docking analysis. *Journal of Molecular Modeling*, **16**: 311-326.

Cunningham, M. L., Soliman, M. S., Badr, M. Z., and Matthews, H. B. (1995). Rotenone, an anticarcinogen, inhibits cellular proliferation but not peroxisome proliferation in mouse liver. *Cancer Lett.*, **95**: 93-97.

Cheenpracha, S., Karalai, C., Ponglimanont, C., and Chantrapromma, K. (2007). Cytotoxic rotenoloids from the stems of *Derris trifoliata*. *Canadian Journal of Chemistry*, **85**: 1019-1022.

Choi, S., Choi, Y., Dat, N. T., Hwangbo, C., Lee, J. J., and Lee, J. H. (2010). Tephrosin induces internalization and degradation of EGFR and ErbB2 in HT-29 human colon cancer cells. [Research Support, Non-U.S. Gov't]. *Cancer Lett.*, **293**: 23-30.

Dat, N. T., Lee, J. H., Lee, K., Hong, Y. S., Kim, Y. H., and Lee, J. J. (2008). Phenolic constituents of *Amorpha fruticosa* that inhibit NF-κB activation and related gene expression. *J. Nat Prod.*, **71**: 1696-1700.

Deng, Y. T., Huang, H. C., and Lin, J. K. (2010). Rotenone induces apoptosis in MCF-7 human breast cancer cell-mediated ROS through JNK and p38 signaling. [Research Support, Non-U.S. Gov't]. *Mol Carcinog.*, **49**: 141-151.

Fang, N., and Casida, J. E. (1998). Anticancer action of cube insecticide: correlation for rotenoid constituents between inhibition of NADH: ubiquinone oxidoreductase and induced ornithine decarboxylase activities. *Proc Natl Acad Sci U S A*, **95**: 3380-3384.

Ferlay, J., Soerjomataram, I., Ervik, M., Dikshit, R., Eser, S., Mathers, C., Rebelo, M., Parkin, D.M., Forman, D. and Bray, F. Globocan (2012). v1.0, Cancer incidence and mortality worldwide: IARC Cancer Base No. 11 (Internet). Lyon, France: International Agency for Research on Cancer, 2013. Available from: http://globocan.iarc.fr, accessed on 03/10/2014.

Gao, S., Xu, Y. M., Valeriote, F. A., and Gunatilaka, A. A. (2011). Pierreiones A-D, solid tumor selective pyranoisoflavones and other cytotoxic constituents from *Antheroporum pierrei*. *J Nat Prod.*, **74**: 852-856.

Gerhauser, C., Lee, S. K., Kosmeder, J. W., Moriarty, R. M., Hamel, E., Mehta, R. G., Moon, R. C., and Pezzuto, J. M. (1997). Regulation of ornithine decarboxylase induction by deguelin, a natural product cancer chemopreventive agent. *Cancer Res.*, **57**: 3429-3435.

Gerhäuser, C., Mar, W., Lee, S. K., Suh, N., Luo, Y., Kosmeder, J., Luyengi, L., Fong, H. H., Kinghorn, A. D., and Moriarty, R. M. (1995). Rotenoids mediate potent cancer chemopreventive activity through transcriptional regulation of ornithine decarboxylase. *Nat Med.*, 1: 260-266.

Goncalves, A. P., Videira, A., Maximo, V., and Soares, P. (2011). Synergistic growth inhibition of cancer cells harboring the RET/PTC1 oncogene by staurosporine and rotenone involves enhanced cell death. *J Biosci.*, **36**: 639-648.

Haley, T. J. (1978). A review of the literature of rotenone, 1,2,12,12a-tetrahydro-8,9-dimethoxy-2-(1-methylethenyl)-1-benzopyrano[3,5-b]furo[2,3-h][1]benzo-pyran-6(6h)-one. *J Environ Pathol Toxicol.*, 1: 315-337.

Harinantenaina, L., Brodie, P. J., Slebodnick, C., Callmander, M. W., Rakotobe, E., Randrianasolo, S., Randrianaivo, R., Rasamison, V. E., Tendyke, K., Shen, Y., Suh, E. M., and Kingston, D. G. (2010). Antiproliferative compounds from *Pongamiopsis pervilleana* from the Madagascar Dry Forest. *J Nat Prod.*, **73**: 1559-1562.

Ito, C., Itoigawa, M., Kojima, N., Tan, H. T., Takayasu, J., Tokuda, H., Nishino, H., and Furukawa, H. (2004). Cancer chemopreventive activity of rotenoids from *Derris trifoliata*. *Planta Med.*, **70**: 585-588.

Jang, D. S., Cuendet, M., Pawlus, A. D., Kardono, L. B. S., Kawanishi, K., Farnsworth, N. R., Fong, H. H. S., Pezzuto, J. M., and Kinghorn, A. D. (2004). Potential cancer chemopreventive constituents of the leaves of *Macaranga triloba*. *Phytochemistry*, **65**: 345-350.

Jang, D. S., Park, E. J., Kang, Y. H., Hawthorne, M. E., Vigo, J. S., Graham, J. G., Cabieses, F., Fong, H. H., Mehta, R. G., Pezzuto, J. M., and Kinghorn, A. D. (2003). Potential cncer chemopreventive flavonoids from the stems of *Tephrosia toxicaria*. *J Nat Prod.*, **66**: 1166-1170.

Jiang, H., Meng, S., Chen, Z., and Kang, T. (2008). In vitro anticancer activity of flavonoids in *Amorpha fruticosa L. Zhongyaocai.*, **31**: 736-738.

Kardono, L. B. S., Tsauri, S., Padmawinata, K., Pezzuto, J. M., and Kinghorn, A. D. (1990). Cytotoxic Constituents of the Seeds of *Pachyrrhizus erosus. Planta Med.*, **56**: 673-674.

Lee, H., Lee, J. H., Jung, K. H., and Hong, S. S. (2010). Deguelin promotes apoptosis and inhibits angiogenesis of gastric cancer. *Oncol Rep.*, **24**: 957-963.

Lee, J. H., Lee, D. H., Lee, H. S., Choi, J. S., Kim, K. W., and Hong, S. S. (2008). Deguelin inhibits human hepatocellular carcinoma by antiangiogenesis and apoptosis. *Oncol Rep.*, **20**: 129-134.

Li, L., Wang, H. K., Chang, J. J., McPhail, A. T., McPhail, D. R., Terada, H., Konoshima, T., Kokumai, M., Kozuka, M., Estes, J. R., and *et al.* (1993). Antitumor agents, 138. Rotenoids and isoflavones as cytotoxic constitutents from *Amorpha fruticosa. J Nat Prod.*, **56**: 690-698.

Lin, L.-J., Ruangrungsi, N., Cordell, G. A., Shieh, H.-L., You, M., and Pezzuto, J. M. (1992). 6-Deoxyclitoriacetal from *Clitoria macrophylla. Phytochemistry*, **31**: 4329-4331.

Luyengi, L., Lee, I.-S., Mar, W., Fong, H. H. S., Pezzuto, J. M., and Kinghorn, A. D. (1994). Rotenoids and chalcones from *Mundulea sericea* that inhibit phorbol ester-induced ornithine decarboxylase activity. *Phytochemistry*, **36**: 1523-1526.

Marking, L. L. (1988). Oral Toxicity of Rotenone to Mammals. *Federal Government Series: Investigations in Fish Control*, **94**: 1-5.

Matsuda, H., Yoshida, K., Miyagawa, K., Asao, Y., Takayama, S., Nakashima, S., Xu, F., and Yoshikawa, M. (2007). Rotenoids and flavonoids with anti-invasion of HT1080, anti-proliferation of U937, and differentiation-inducing activity in HL-60 from *Erycibe expansa. Bioorg Med Chem.*, **15**: 1539-1546.

Pecorino, L. (2012). *Molecular biology of cancer : mechanisms, targets, and therapeutics* (Third edition. ed.).

Sakurai, Y., Sakurai, N., Taniguchi, M., Nakanishi, Y., Bastow, K. F., Wang, X., Cragg, G. M., and Lee, K. H. (2006). Rautandiols A and B, pterocarpans and cytotoxic constituents from *Neorautanenia mitis. Nat Prod.*, **69**: 397-399.

Sangthong, S., Krusong, K., Ngamrojanavanich, N., Vilaivan, T., Puthong, S., Chandchawan, S., and Muangsin, N. (2011). Synthesis of rotenoid derivatives with cytotoxic and topoisomerase II inhibitory activities. *Bioorg Med Chem Lett.*, **21**: 4813-4818.

Tanaka, T., Kohno, H., Sakata, K., Yamada, Y., Hirose, Y., Sugie, S., and Mori, H. (2002). Modifying effects of dietary capsaicin and rotenone on 4-nitroquinoline 1-oxide-induced rat tongue carcinogenesis. *Carcinogenesis*, **23**: 1361-1367.

Udeani, G. O., Gerhauser, C., Thomas, C. F., Moon, R. C., Kosmeder, J. W., Kinghorn, A. D., Moriarty, R. M., and Pezzuto, J. M. (1997). Cancer chemopreventive activity mediated by deguelin, a naturally occurring rotenoid. *Cancer Res.*, **57**: 3424-3428.

Wang, C., Youssef, J., Saran, B., Rothberg, P. G., Cunningham, M. L., Molteni, A., and Badr, M. (1999). Diminished energy metabolism and enhanced apoptosis in livers of B6C3F1 mice treated with the antihepatocarcinogen rotenone. *Mol Cell Biochem.*, **201**: 25-32.

WHO. (2014). Fact sheet N°297. Cancer Retrieved 03/10/2014, 2012, from http: // www.who.int/mediacentre/factsheets/fs297/en/index.html

Bioactive Phytochemicals: Perspectives for Modern Medicine Vol. 3 (2015) *Pages* **259–281**
Editor: **V.K. Gupta**
Published by: **DAYA PUBLISHING HOUSE, NEW DELHI**

10

Plant Lignans: Potent Anticancer Agents

Deepak M. Kasote[1] and Archana A. Sharbidre[2*]

ABSTRACT

Cancer is a major public health burden in most part the world. Synthetic chemopreventive agents are well practicing as an anticancer drug against treatment of several types of cancer. However, their usage has limitations due to adverse effects. Consequently, these days, the use of botanicals or dietary nutraceuticals for treatment of cancer is becoming more popular. Several phytochemicals mainly lignans found to have anticancer potential. Lignans are the type of polyphenols commonly distributed in higher plants, and is a one of the major classes of phytoestrogens amongst isoflavones and coumestans. Most of these lignan are found to modulate the effect of estrogen by binding competitively with estrogen receptors, and reduce the risk of estrogen-dependent cancers. In addition, they also act as antioxidants and free radical scavengers, which may help to decrease the risk of cancer progression. To date, nearly 65 plant lignans reported to have anticancer potential; however, they are not collectively discussed and documented so far. Hence, the purpose of this chapter is to provide an overview on a source, occurrence, chemistry, metabolism of plant lignans and summarize clinical data regarding their anticancer potential.

Keywords: Anticaner, Lignan, Plant, Dietary nutraceuticals.

Introduction

Plants based medicines have been used for the treatment of various ailments since antiquity, and still around 80 per cent of the world's population primarily depend on herbal medicines for their primary health care. Despite the remarkable

1 Department of Pharmaceutical Sciences, Faculty of Science, Tshwane University of Technology, Private Bag X680, Pretoria, 0001, South Africa

2 Department of Zoology, University of Pune, Pune – 411 007, MS, India

* *Corresponding author*: E-mail: aasharbidre@unipune.ac.in

advancement in the modern pharmaceutical sciences still around 25 per cent of all prescription medicines are of plant origin (Tomlinson and Akerele, 1998; Arroo *et al.*, 2002; Elujoba *et al.*, 2005). Historically, numerous plant species have been used in treatment and prevention of life threatening diseases such as cancer.

Cancer is a large group of diseases characterized by uncontrolled cell growth and spread of abnormal cells. It is a major public health problem and cause of death in almost all parts of the world (Siegel *et al.*, 2013). The causes of cancer are diverse and complex, mainly of environment, genetic and lifestyle origin. Surgery, chemotherapy, radiation therapy, and palliative care are the popular therapies for the control and cure of cancer. However, due to severe side effects of modern cancer therapies, especially the chemo and radiation therapies, the treatment of cancer with botanicals or dietary nutraceuticals has been increasingly accepted. Several accumulating evidences showed that herbal medicines have potential applications in the treatment and control of cancer progression. The search for anti-cancer agents from plant sources were initiated in the 1950s. The *Vinca* alkaloids (vinblastin and vincristine) and podophyllotoxins were the earlier outcomes of these endeavors (Gueritte and Fahy, 2005). Albeit, in last few decades, several important anticancer substances have been investigated from plants, still it is a key area of natural product research. Interestingly, majority of the anticancer agents belong to the phytochemical class, lignan. Plant lignans are the naturally occurring non-steroidal polyphenolic compounds with antioxidant and estrogen like activities. Besides this, they reported to have antiviral, anticancer, cardiovascular, anti-inflammatory and immunosuppressive activities (Saleem *et al.*, 2005). Recent evidences demonstrated that plant lignans have potential application in prevention and treatment of hormone associated-cancers such as breast, prostate and ovary. The anticancer potential of these plant lignans have been found to be linked with their structural similarity with estradiol (17-β-estradiol), and ability to cause estrogenic or/and antiestrogenic effects. There are about 65 plant lignans reported to have anticancer properties (Saleem *et al.*, 2005). However, very few lignan molecules have been well studied regarding their anticancer efficacy and safety. The purpose of this article is to provide an overview on plant lignans in the context of its source, occurrence, chemistry, metabolism and anticancer potential.

Lignans

Sources

Lignans are the type of polyphenols commonly distributed in higher plant predominantly in angiosperms and gymnosperms (Axelson *et al.*, 1982). They occur in roots, rhizomes, stems, leaves, seeds and fruits, usually in the free form. They are also found in the form of glycoside but, in low quantity. Lignans are occurring in most fiber-rich grains such as wheat, barley and oats; legumes such as beans, lentils and soybeans; and vegetables such as garlic, asparagus, broccoli and carrots (Saleem *et al.*, 2005). In plants, lignans are derived from the shikimic acid biosynthetic pathway, and play an important role in plant defense, growth and development (Saleem *et al.*, 2005; Durazzo *et al.*, 2013).

Chemistry

Lignan are 8, 8-coupled dimers of coniferyl alcohol or other cinnamyl alcohols, produced in plants by oxidative dimerization of two phenylpropanoid units (Fuss, 2003; Saleem *et al.*, 2005). They show an enormous structural diversity which originating from different linkage patterns of two phenylpropane (C6–C3) units. Conventionally, lignans are classified into two types, classical lignans and neolignans. Classical lignans are phenylpropane dimers linked in a β–β′ (8–8′) fashion, whereas, neolignans are those dimers whose coupling patterns differ from such a β–β′ (8–8′) linkage. Lignans are optically active compounds and exist in two enantiomeric forms, right and left handed (Durazzo *et al.*, 2013). Besides these classes, other types of lignans such as oligomeric lignans, hybrid lignans and norlignans have also been reported (Pan *et al.*, 2009).

Metabolism

Lignans are one of the major classes of phytoestrogens among isoflavones and coumestans. These phytoestrogens have weak estrogenic activity due to their stereochemical similarity to the hormone 17-b-estradiol (E_2) (Liggins *et al.*, 2000). Besides estrogenic potential, most of the health promoting effects of lignans are linked with their antioxidant activity. Secoisolariciresinol (SECO), lariciresinol (LARI),

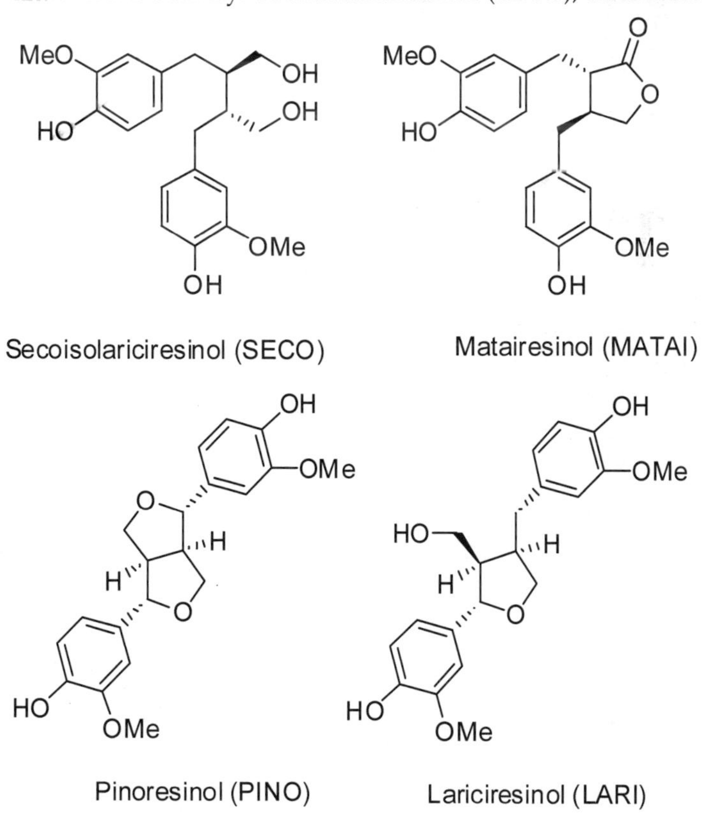

Figure 10.1: Structure of Major Plant Lignans.

matairesinol (MATAI) and pinoresinol (PINO) are the major plant lignans, predominantly occurring in oilseeds and cereals (Mazur, 1998; Gharras, 2009; Durazzo *et al.*, 2013) (Figure 10.1). Among these lignans, SECO is of particular interest because of their wide range of therapeutic activities.

After ingestion, the lignans SECO, MATAI, PINO and LARI are converted by intestinal microorganisms into the enterolignans such as enterodiol and enterolactone (Figure 10.2). It has been found that these phytoestrogens may have an important role in the treatment of estrogen-dependent cancers, as they bind weakly to estrogen receptors, and modulate the response to endogenous estrogens (Adlercreutz, 1995; Fuss, 2003). The extent of lignans conversion depends on the activity of the gut microflora, and varies with individual to individual (Niemeyer *et al.*, 2003).

Anticancer Potential of Lignans

The use of natural, synthetic, or biologic chemical agents to reverse, suppress, or prevent cancer is becoming a rational and appealing strategy in these days (Tsao *et al.*, 2013). It has been found that the cancer chemoprevention effect of natural compounds is linked to their antioxidant, anti-inflammatory, weak estrogenic or/and anti-estrogenic activities, and with their induction of phase II enzymes, apoptosis and cell cycle arrest abilities as well (Pan and Ho, 2008).

The plant lignans are the valuable class of natural compounds with promising anticancer properties. By this time, around 65 different lignan molecules found to have potent anticancer activity, summarized in Table 10.1. However, only few molecules have been well studied in the context of their anticancer efficacy and safety.

Secoisolariciresinol/Secoisolariciresinol Diglucoside (SECO/SDG)

Flaxseed is the richest source of lignan SECO/SDG. Besides this, it is also present in a little amount in sesame seed, pumpkin seed, triticale, wheat, lentils, soyabeans, fruits and certain vegetables such as garlic, asparagus, carrot, etc. (Patel *et al.*, 2012). In flaxseed, SECO is mainly found diglycosylated form so called as SDG, and stored in an ester-linked with 3-hydroxy-3-methylglutaric acid (HMGA) and other phenolic compounds such as *p*-coumaric acid and ferulic acid glycosides to form SDG oligomers of unknown (Ford *et al.*, 2001; Johnsson *et al.*, 2002; Smeds *et al.*, 2007). After ingestion, intestinal bacteria convert SDG into the mammalian lignans ED and EL which has potent antioxidant activity and also act as both anti-estrogens and weak estrogens (Axelson and Setchell, 1981). These properties of SDG proved its importance in the prevention and cure of various types of hormonal associated cancers (Thompson *et al.*, 1996).

The beneficial effect of flaxseed SDG in treatment of breast cancer has been found both animal and human intervention studies (Thompson *et al.*, 1996; Chen *et al.*, 2004; Thompson *et al.*, 2005; Wang *et al.*, 2005). Adlercreutz (2002) showed that a lignan-low diet was related with an increased risk of breast cancer in case-control and prospective studies. It has also been found that feeding with purified lignan at 5 per cent flaxseed diet levels significantly reduced colon and mammary carcinogenesis in animals (Thompson *et al.*, 1996). Later, Hausott *et al.* (2003) showed that SDG

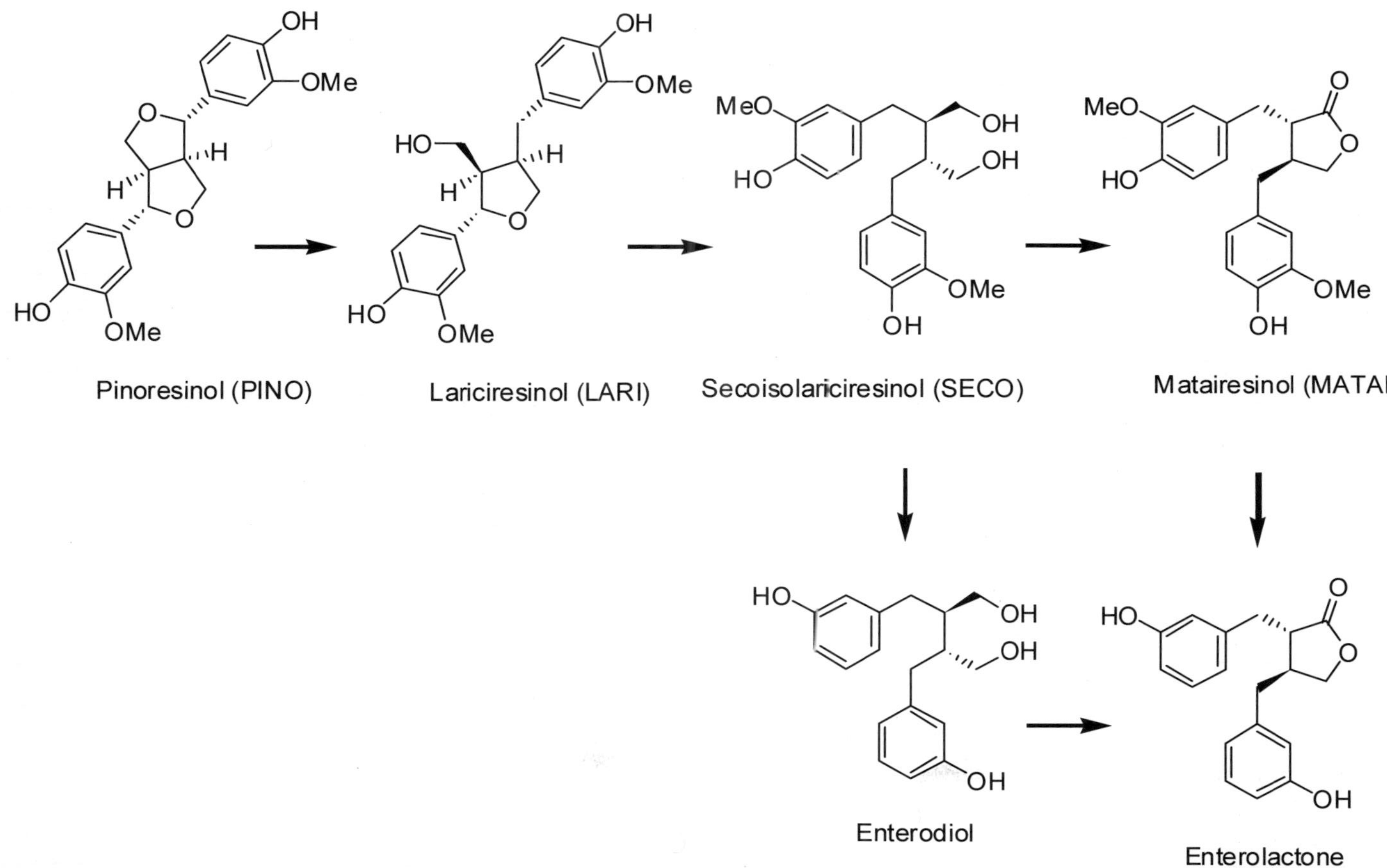

Figure 10.2: The Possible Metabolic Pathway for Conversion of Plant Lignans Secoisolariciresinol (SECO), Lariciresinol (LARI), Matairesinol (MATAI) and Pinoresinol (PINO) to Enterolignans Enterodiol and Enterolactone by Colonic Microflora (Adopted from Patel *et al.*, 2012).

Table 10.1: Plants Lignans with Anticancer Potential

Lignan	*Plant Source*	*Study Model*	*Valuable against Cancer*	*Reference*
(7R,8S,7'R,8'R)-(+)-7'-acetylpicropodophyllin	*Hernandia ovigera* L.	*In vitro*	JB6 cells	Gu *et al.*, 2002
Arctigenin	*Saussurea medusa* Maxim.	*In vitro*	Bladder	Yang *et al.*, 2012
Arctiin	*Saussurea medusa* Maxim.	*In vitro*	Skin	Huang *et al.*, 2004
Arctiin	*Arctium lappa* (burdock) L.	*In vivo*	Mammary, colon and pancreatic	Hirose *et al.*, 2000
Agastinol	*Agastache rugosa* Fisch.	*In vitro*	Not specified	Lee *et al.*, 2002
Austrobailignan-6	*Machilus thunbergii* Forbes.	*In vitro*	Promyeloid leukemic HL-60 cells, HT-29, MCF-7,HT-29, MCF-7 24	Park *et al.*, 2004 Li *et al.*, 2004
Aviculin	*Mallotus furetianus* Mill. Arg.., *Chaenomeles sinensis* Thouin.	*In vitro*	Not specified	Ohashi *et al.*, 2003
Bursehernin	*Hernandia ovigera* L.	*In vitro*	Raji cells	Ito *et al.*, 2001
Cinerins A	*Pleurothyriumcinereum* Henk.	*In vitro*	PC-3, Hep-2, and A549	Coy *et al.*, 2009
Cinerin D	Lauraceae species	*In vitro*	Not Specified	Cuca *et al.*, 2011
Dehydropodophyllotoxin	*Hernandia ovigera* L.	*In vitro*	Raji cells	Ito *et al.*, 2001
4-Demethyl-picropodo-phyllotoxin 7'-O-beta-D-glucopyranoside	*Sinopodophyllum emodi* Wall.	*In vivo*	*Not specified*	Zang *et al.*, 2005
Dibenzyl butyrolactol	*Cedrus deodara* Roxb.	*In vitro*	Leukemia	Shashi *et al.*, 2005
Elenoside	*Justicia hyssopifolia* L.	*In vitro*	Not specified	Navarroet al, 2001
Enterolactone	*Picea abies* L.	*In vivo*	Mammary gland	Saarinen *et al.*, 2002
Enterolactone	*Mammalian lignan* L.	*In vitro*	Human prostate carcinoma LNCaP cells	Chen *et al.*, 2007
Erlangerin (B, C and D)	*Commiphora erlangeriana* Engl.	*In vitro*	Not Specified	Habtemariam,2003
*Erythro-meso-*dihydroguaiaretic acid	*Machilus thunbergii* Forbes.	*In vitro*	Promyeloid leukemic HL-60 cells, HT-29, MCF-7, HT-29, MCF-7 24	Park *et al.*, 2004 Li *et al.*, 2004

Contd...

Table 10.1–*Contd...*

Lignan	*Plant Source*	*Study Model*	*Valuable against Cancer*	*Reference*
Epiashantin	*Hernandia ovigera* L.	*In vitro*	Not specified	Hausott *et al.*, 2003
epi-Magnolin	*Hernandia nymphaeifolia* Presl.	*In vitro*	Not specified	Ito *et al.*, 2001
epi-Yangambin	*Hernandia nymphaeifolia* Presl., *Hernandia ovigera* L.	*In vitro*	JB6 cells	Gu *et al.*, 2002
(+)-Galbacin	*Machilus thunbergii* Forbes.	*In vitro*	Not specified	Lee *et al.*, 2004
(–)-Grandisin	*Piper solmsianum* C.DC.	*In vitro*	LIver	Messiano *et al.*, 2013
Hanultarin	*Berberis amurensis* Rupr.	*In vitro*	Not Specified	Park *et al.*, 2009
2-Hydroxyarctigenin	Seeds of Safflower	*In vitro*	Not specified	Kim *et al.*, 2003
7'-hydroxy-3',4',5,9,9'-pentamethoxy-3,4-methylene dioxy	*Phyllanthus urinaria* L.	*In vitro*	Not specified	Giridharan *et al.*, 2002
7-Hydroxymatairesinol	Food plants	*In vitro*	Prostate	Saarinen *et al.*, 2001
Hydroxymatairesinol	*Picea abies* L.	*In vitro*	Mammary	Kangas *et al.*, 2002
Hypophyllanthin	*Phyllanthus amarus* Schumach	*In vitro*	Human breast cancer cell lines (MCF-7 and MDA-231)	Parvathaneni *et al.*, 2014
Hernanol	*Hernandia peltata* Meisu.	*In vitro*	Leukemia	Pettit *et al.*, 2003
Isochaihulactone	*Bupleurum scorzonerifolium* Wild.	*In vitro*	Lung	Chen *et al.*, 2006
Isolinderanolide E	*Machilus obovatifolia* Hayata	*In vitro*	T47D human breast cancer cells	Kim *et al.*, 2009
Isotaxiresinol	*Taxus wallichiana* Zucc.	*In vivo*	Colon	Chattopadhyay *et al.*, 2003
Kaurenoic acid	Lauraceae species	*In vitro*	Not Specified	Cuca *et al.*, 2011
Licarin A	*Machilus thunbergii* Forbes	*In vitro*	Promyeloid leukemic HL-60 cells, HT-29, MCF-7,HT-29, MCF-7 24	Park *et al.*, 2004 Li *et al.*, 2004
Linderanolide E	*Machilus obovatifolia* Hayata.	*In vitro*	Breast	Kim *et al.*, 2009

Contd...

Table 10.1–*Contd...*

Lignan	*Plant Source*	*Study Model*	*Valuable against Cancer*	*Reference*
Magnolol	*Magnolia* L.	*In vitro*	COLO-205,HCT116	Lin *et al.*, 2001, 2002 Lee *et al.*, 2009
Machilin A	*Machilus thunbergii* Forbes	*In vitro*	Not specified	Lee *et al.*, 2004
Machilin G	*Machilus thunbergii* Forbes.	*In vitro*	Not specified	Lee *et al.*, 2004
Matairesinol 2003	Safflower seeds	*In vitro*	Not specified	Chattopadhyay *et al.*,
Macelignan	*Machilus thunbergii* Forbes.	*In vitro*	Promyeloid leukemic HL-60 cells, HT-29, MCF-7,HT-29, MCF-7 24	Park *et al.*, 2004 Li *et al.*, 2004
5-Methoxyxanthocercin A	*Dipteryx odorata* tonka bean	*In vitro*	Liver	Jang *et al.*, 2003
Nectandrin B	*Machilus thunbergii* Forbes	*In vitro*	Promyeloid leukemic HL-60 cells, HT-29, MCF-7,HT-29, MCF-7 24	Park *et al.*, 2004 Li *et al.*, 2004
Ocophyllal A	Lauraceae species	*In vitro*	Not Specified	Cuca *et al.*, 2011
Oleiferin	*Machilus thunbergii* Forbes	*In vitro*	Promyeloid leukemic HL-60 cells, HT-29, MCF-7,HT-29, MCF-7 24	Park *et al.*, 2004 Li *et al.*, 2004
Perseal F (1)	*Machilus obovatifolia* Hayata	*In vitro*	Breast	Kim *et al.*, 2009
Phyllanthin	*Phyllanthus amarus* Schumuch	*In vitro*	Human breast cancer cell lines (MCF-7 and MDA-231)	Parvathaneni *et al.* (2014)
Pinoresinol	Food plants	*In vitro*	Leukemia	Sepporta *et al.*, 2013
9-OH-pinoresinol	Food plants	*In vitro*	Leukemia	Sepporta *et al.*, 2013
Phillygenol Phillygenoldiglycoside Phillyroside	*Lancea tibetica* Hook.	*In vitro*	Hepatoma cell SMMC-7721, human carcinoma of uterine cervix cell HeLa, hamster lung fibroblast cell V79 and mouse melanoma cell B16	Zhao *et al.*, 2000
Podorhizol	*Hernandia ovigera* L.		Raji cells	Ito *et al.*, 2001
Schizandrin	*Schisandra chinensis* Turcz.	*In vitro*	Breast	Kim *et al.*, 2009

Contd...

Table 10.1–*Contd...*

Lignan	*Plant Source*	*Study Model*	*Valuable against Cancer*	*Reference*
Schinifolisatin A	*Zanthoxylum schinifolium* Zuce	*In vitro*	Leukemia	Li *et al.*, 2013
SECO/SDG	Flaxseed	*In vitro* and *In vivo*	Prostate, breast, thyroid and endometrial	Horn-Ross *et al.*, 2002; Horn-Ross *et al.*, 2003; Lee *et al.*, 2011
Sesamol	Sesame	*In vivo*	Breast	Jacklin *et al.*, 2003
Taiwanin A	*Taiwania cryptomerioides* Hayata	*In vitro*	Lung, breast and colon	Chang *et al.*, 2000
Taiwanin E4	*Taiwania cryptomerioides* Hayata	*In vitro*	Lung, breast and colon	Chang *et al.*, 2000
Taxiresinol	*Taxus wallichiana*	*In vivo*	Colon	Chattopadhyay *et al.*, 2003
Teniposide	Apple	*In vitro*	Lung	Blancy *et al.*, 1989
Vitexin	*Vitex negundo* L.	*In vitro*	breast, prostate and ovarian	Zhou *et al.*, 2009
(–)-Wikstromal	*Cedrus deodara* Roxb.	*In vitro*	Leukemia	Shashi *et al.*, 2005

induced apoptosis in colorectal tumor cells through changing mitochondrial membrane potential and down regulation of the antiapoptotic protein, bcl (xl). In addition to this, lignan-rich flaxseed supplementation to patients with prostate cancer showed beneficial effect on prostate cancer biology and associated biomarkers (Demark-Wahnefried *et al.*, 2001). The dietary intake of SECO also found to reduce the risks of thyroid and endometrial and ovarian cancers in women patients (Horn-Ross *et al.*, 2002; Horn-Ross *et al.*, 2003; McCann *et al.*, 2003). In another study, Hernandez *et al.* (2004) reported a positive association between plasma enterodiol levels and premalignant lesions of the cervix.

Sesamin (SES)

Sesame seed is an oilseed which containing high levels of the oil-soluble lignans – sesamin (SES), episesamin, sesaminol, sesamol and sesamolin (Figure 10.3) (Fukuda *et al.*, 1985; Shimizu *et al.*, 2014). Among these, SES is a major lignan. Similar to SECO, SES is converted to ED and EL, and also possesses weak estrogenic/antiestrogenic activity (Pianjing *et al.*, 2011; Truan *et al.*, 2012). Sesamin found to beneficial in inhibiting the proliferation of a wide variety of tumor cells including leukemia, multiple myeloma, and cancers of the colon, prostate, breast, pancreas and lung. It suppressed NF-κB-regulated cell survival, proliferation, invasion, and angiogenic gene products (Harikumar *et al.*, 2010). SES found to macrophage-enhanced proangiogenic activity of breast cancer cells via inhibition of VEGF and MMP-9 induction (Lee *et al.*, 2011; Truan *et al.*, 2012). Interestingly, it has observed that SES is more effective than SDG in reducing breast tumor growth in mice (Truan *et al.*, 2012). Deng *et al.*(2013) showed that SES induces cell cycle arrest and apoptosis through the inhibition of signal transducer and activator of transcription 3 signaling in human hepatocellular carcinoma cell line HepG2, which confirmed its potential application in treatment for liver cancer. Besides SES, sesaminol derivative sesamol, produced from sesame oil refining or heat treatment, was found to induce growth arrest and apoptosis in MCF-7 and T47D breast cancer cells (Jacklin *et al.*, 2003). Moreover, sesamol was also found to be valuable in the treatment of colon cancer (Shimizu *et al.*, 2014). In epidemiological studies, sesame oil-containing lignans were associated with decreased risk of stomach cancer (Ahn, 1997).

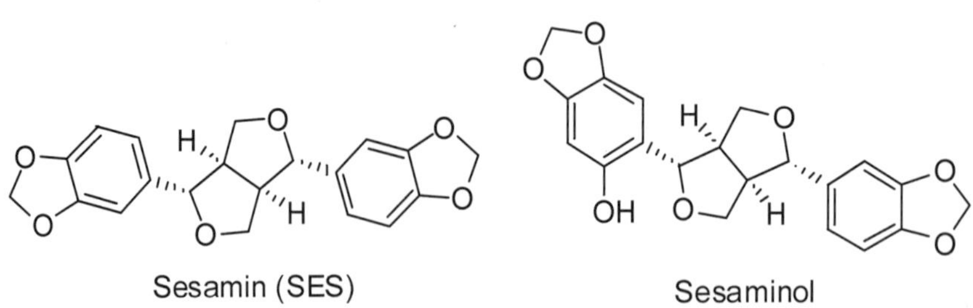

Figure 10.3: Structure of Sesame Lignans: Sesamin and Sesaminol.

Lariciresinol (LARI)

Lignan lariciresinol (LARI) is predominantly found in sesame seeds and *Brassica* vegetables (Milder *et al.*, 2005). On ingestion, LARI is first converted to SECO, and then subsequent to ED and EL (Figure 10.2). Recent investigations showed that the high LARI intake was inversely associated with breast cancer risk. Saarinen *et al.* (2008) showed dietary LARI attenuated mammary tumor growth and reduced blood vessel density in human MCF-7 breast cancer xenografts and carcinogen-induced mammary tumors in rats.

Matairesinol (MATAI)

Matairesinol (MATAI) is also a biologically important plant lignan present in a wide variety of foodstuffs such as seeds, vegetables and fruits (Choi *et al.*, 2014). Similar to other lignan molecules, MATAI is also converted to the mammalian lignans ED and EL by intestinal microbes, which have anti-carcinogenic potential (Pajari *et al.*, 2006). Recent findings confirmed that MATAI has potential application in the treatment of various types of cancers. Peuhu *et al.* (2009) reported that MATAI sensitizes prostate cancer cells to tumor necrosis factor-related apoptosis-inducing ligand induced apoptosis by Inhibition of Akt signaling pathways. In another study, it has been demonstrated that MATAI functions as an anticancer agent by functioning as an angiogenesis inhibitor by suppressing mitochondrial reactive oxygen species signaling (Lee *et al.*, 2012).

Pinoresinol (PINO)

Pinoresinol (PINO) is one of the simplest lignans, present in whole-grain cereals, legumes, fruits and vegetables (Sepporta *et al.*, 2013). Intestinal microbes convert PINO into mammalian lignans which may prevent different types of cancer. However, very little is known about the chemopreventive potential of PINO (*i.e.* antiproliferative and proapoptotic). Sepporta *et al.* (2013) recently demonstrated that PINO inhibits proliferation and induces differentiation on human HL60 leukemia cells by up-regulating of the CDK inhibitor p21 (WAF1/Cip1) both at mRNA and protein levels. Moreover, it has also been found that pinoresinol-rich olive oil induces cell cycle arrest and apoptosis in colon cancer cells by inducing the ATM–p53 cascade (Fini *et al.*, 2008). In addition to PINO, 9-OH-pinoresinol from extracted from *Saussurea salicifolia* was also found to reduced the growth of leukemia mouse lymphoma cells L5178Y to 23.8 per cent.

(–)-Grandisin

(–)-Grandisin is a tetrahydrofuran lignan isolated from plant species *Piperaceae, Lauraceae, Myristicaceae* and *Schisandraceae* (Figure 10.4) (Lopes *et al.*, 1999; Morais *et al.*, 2009; Pu *et al.*, 2008). It reported to have important pharmacological activities such as cytotoxicity and antiangiogenic, antibacterial and trypanocidal (Messiano *et al.*, 2013). Among these, the anticancer potential of, (–)-grandisin and its major metabolite 4-O-demethylgrandisin is well established in both *in vivo* and *in vitro* (Valadares *et al.*, 2011; Vieira Mde *et al.*, 2011). Several *in vitro* studies are available which confirmed cytotoxic and

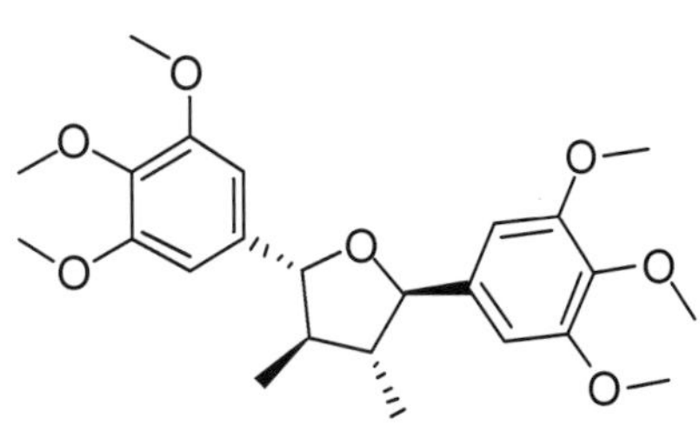

Figure 10.4: Chemical Structure of the Lignan Grandisin.

antitumor activity to (–)-grandisin (Valadares *et al.*, 2009; Valadares, 2011). Valadares *et al.* (2011) recently confirmed of the chemoprotective effect of grandisin within the *in-vivo* rodent micronucleus assay. It has also found that grandisin acted against tumor evolution and prolonged survival in mice (Valadares *et al.*, 2009).

Arylnapthalene Lignans

The majority of natural arylnaphthalene lignans are lactones (Bringmann *et al.*, 1990). These have attracted considerable interest because of their anti-tumor and anti-hyperlipidemic activities (Kimura *et al.*, 1985). Cytotoxicity as well as anti-cancer activities has been reported to arylnapthalene lignan isolated from several genus including *Phyllantus*, *Cleistanthus*, and *Justicia* (Ramesh *et al.*, 2003; Nitiss, 2009; Susplugas *et al.*, 2005) Luo *et al.* (2014) isolated five arylnaphthalene lignans such as 69-hydroxy justicidin A, 69-hydroxy justicidin B, justicidin B, chinensinaphthol methyl ether (CME) and Taiwanin E methyl ether from *Justicia procumbens*, and reported antiproliferative and apoptosis potential to them in human leukemia K562 cell line. Furthermore, structure-activity relationships analysis suggested that hydroxyl substitution at C-1 and C-69 significantly increased the antiproliferative activity of arylnaphthalene lignans while a methoxyl at C-1 significantly decreased this effect.

Arylnaphthalene lignan HJB is a lead compound and may have significant clinical utility in the management of bone cancer and osteoclastogenesis due to its cytotoxic and bone resorption inhibitory properties (Figure 10.5). This compound is the major cytotoxic principle in plant *Linum narbonense* L. (Linaceae) structurally closely related to podophyllotoxin (Mohagheghzadeh *et al.*, 2002). Another arylnaphthalene lignin, elenine is the aglycone of elenoside, obtained from *Justicia hyssopifolia* (family: Acanthaceae) also displayed cytotoxic activity in human tumor cell line (Figure 10.5) (Navarro *et al.*, 2001).

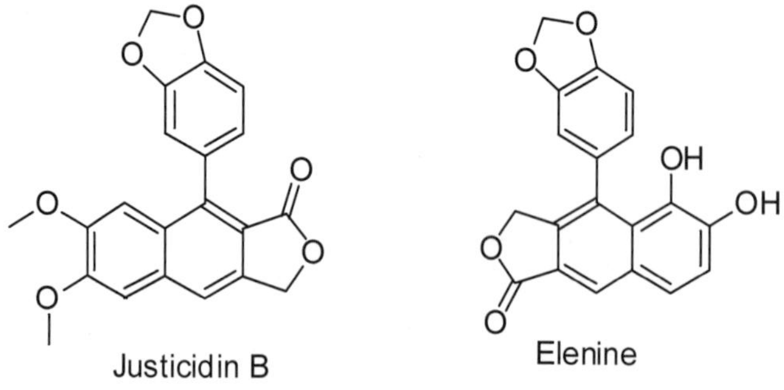

Figure 10.5: Structure of Arylnaphthalene Lignans Justicidin B and Elenine.

Vitexin

Vitexin is a class of nature lignan compounds, mediated its anticancer effect by different mechanisms than the classical lignans. Zhou *et al.* (2009) isolated a series of lignan compounds, named as vitexins, from the seed of Chinese herb *Vitex negundo* and named this lignan extract as EVn-50. Vitexins isolated from EVn-50 have a general structure belong to the class of neolignan (Figure 10.6). Two major lignans namely VB-M1 6-hydroxy-4-(4-hydroxy-3-methoxyphenyl)-3-hydroxymethyl-7-methoxy-3,4-dihydro-2-naphthaldehyde) and VB-M2(6-hydroxy-4-(4-hydroxy-3-methoxyphenyl)-3-hydroxymethyl-5-methoxy-3,4-dihydro-2-naphthaldehyde) were further isolated from EVn-50. In contrary to the classical lignans, Vitexins did not go through metabolic activation to generate mammalian lignans. Vitexin induced antitumor and cytotoxic activity through proapoptotic process, which is mediated by a decreased Bcl-2/Bax ratio and activation of caspases. Vitexin triggered apoptosis in U937 human leukemia cells via a mitochondrial signaling pathway, and also induced autophagy and apoptosis by activating the Jun N-terminal kinase pathway (Lee *et al.*, 2012; Zhou *et al.*, 2013). It has been further found that VB-M1 inhibited choriocarcinoma via inducing cell apoptosis and suppressing the mTOR pathway (Tan *et al.*, 2012)

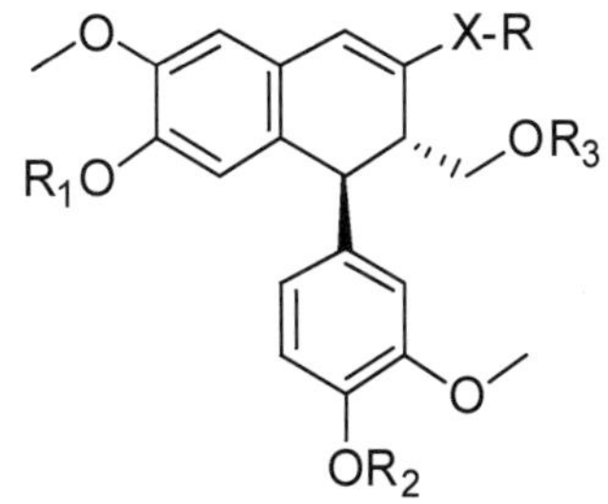

Figure 10.6: General Structure of Lignan Vitexin.

Other Lignans

Chen *et al.* (2006) isolated a novel lignan isochaihulactone from acetone extract of *Bupleurum scorzonerifolium,* which had promising antimitotic and anticancer potential, isochaihulactone showed potent cytotoxic activity in a variety of human tumor cell lines. Within *in vitro* and *in vivo* microtubule assembly assays, it was further found that isochaihulactone inhibited tubulin polymerization in a concentration-dependent manner, and also causes G2/M phase arrest and apoptosis in a time- and concentration-dependent manner. Moreover, isochaihulactone (30 and 50 mg/kg) inhibited the growth of non-small cell lung carcinoma A549 xenograft in nude mice. Park *et al.* (2009) isolated eight phenolic constituents including six lignans from the alcoholic extract from the roots of *Berberis amurensis,* among these lignan hanultarin exhibited moderate cytotoxicity against four human cancer cell lines. Parvathaneni *et al.* (2014) recently isolated two lignans; hypophyllanthin and phyllanthin from *Phyllanthus amarus* (Euphorbiaceae). These lignans showed growth inhibition of human breast cancer cell lines (MCF-7 and MDA-231). Their dietary intake also showed *in vivo* anticancer activity by inhibiting mammary tumor growth in rats at 5mg/kg dose of hypophyllanthin and at 10mg/kg dose of phyllanthin respectively for four weeks.

Toxicity

One of the biggest hurdles in establishing lignans as promising chemopreventive agents is their genotoxic risk and conditional toxicity. It has been reported that pregnant or breastfeeding women should avoid high intake of flaxseed or purified lignans. In one study it has been found that pregnant rats who ate large amounts of flaxseed (5 per cent or 10 per cent of their diet), or a purified lignan present in flaxseed, gave birth to offspring with altered reproductive organs and their functions (Tou *et al.*, 1998). It is noteworthy that eating 25 g of flaxseed per day is equivalent to about 5 per cent lignan of diet (Thompson, 1998). In addition, the high intake of lignans may not be safe for women with a history of estrogen-sensitive cancer, such as breast cancer or uterine cancer. A few test tube studies suggest that certain cancer cells can be stimulated by lignans (Adlercreutz and Mazur, 1997).

Kulling *et al.* (1998) reported genotoxicity to END, ENL, SECO and MAT in cultured Chinese hamster V79 cells. Garcez *et al.* (2005) further showed genotoxic potential to sesamin. However, it is important to note that most of the toxic effect of lignans is linked to their dose concentration, as a result some contradictory reports has been appearing in the literature. Hori *et al.* (2011) recently found that *sesamin* and episesamin had no *genotoxic* activity. Moreover, Resende *et al.* (2010) reported genotoxicity to dibenzylbutyrolactone lignan (-)-hinokinin (HK) isolated from the dry seeds of the *Piper cubeba* and in contrary to this Medola *et al.* (2007) found no genotoxic effect to (-)-hinokinin.

Conclusion and Future Outlook

The findings of several pre-clinical and clinical studies confirmed that lignans are the important herbal origin anticancer agents for the treatment of diverse types of cancer. Most of plants lignans after ingestion converted into mammalian lignans by gut microflora. These mammalian lignans have strong antioxidant activity, and act as both anti-estrogens and weak estrogens, which makes them promising agents in the treatment of hormone-dependent cancers. The positive or negative effects of lignan on cancer cells may depend on dose, type of cancer cell, and levels of hormones present in the body. To date, anticancer potential has been shown to nearly 65 plant lignans, however, among them, very few lignan molecules have been well studied in the context their anticancer efficacy and safety. Hence, there is a need to further explore almost all plant anticancer lignans at efficacy and safety platforms.

References

Adlercreutz, H., and Mazur, W. (1997). Phyto-oestrogens and Western diseases. *Annals of Medicine*, **29(2)**: 95-120.

Adlercreutz, H. (1995). Phytoestrogens: epidemiology and a possible role in cancer protection. *Environmetal Health Perspectives*, **103 (Suppl 7)**: 103-112.

Adlercreutz, H. (2002). Phytoestrogens and breast cancer. *The Journal of Steroid Biochemistry and Molecular Biology*, **83(1-5)**: 113–118.

Ahn, YO (1997). Diet and stomach cancer in Korea. *International Journal of Cancer, Suppl.*, **10**: 7-9.

Arroo, R.R.J, Alfermann, A.W., Medarde, M., Petersen, M., Pras, N., and Woolley J.G. (2002). Plant cell factories as a source for anti-cancer lignans. *Phytochemistry Reviews*, **1**: 27–35.

Axelson, M., Sjövall, J., Gustafsson, B.E., and Setchell, K.D. (1982).Origin of lignans in mammals and identification of a precursor from plants. *Nature*, **12**: 298(5875): 659-660.

Axelson, M., and Setchell, K.D.R. (1981).The excretion of lignans in rats – evidence for an intestinal bacterial source for this new group of compounds, *FEBS letters*, **123**: 337-342.

Blancy, E., Canal, P., Berg, D., and Bugat, R. (1989). Cytotoxic effects of teniposide combined with cis-diammine-dichloroplatinum (II) on the *in vitro* Lewis lung carcinoma model: influence of the treatment schedule. *Fundamental and Clinical Pharmacology*, **3(4)**: 363-370.

Bringmann, G., Walter, R., and Weirich, R. (1990) The Directed Synthesis of Biaryl Compounds: Modern Concepts and Strategies. *Angewandte Chemie,* **29**: 977–991.

Chang, S.T., Wang, D.S., Wu, C.L., Shiah, S.G., Kuo, Y.H., and Chang, C.J. (2000). Cytotoxicity of extractives from *Taiwania cryptomerioides* heartwood. *Phytochemistry*, **55(3)**: 227-232.

Chen, Y-L, Lin, S-Z., Chang, J-Y., Cheng, Y-L., Tsai, N-M., Chen, S-P., Chang, W-L., and Harn, H-J. (2006). *In vitro* and *in vivo* studies of a novel potential anticancer agent of isochaihulactone on human lung cancer A549 cells. *Biochemical pharmacology*, **72**: 308-319.

Chen, J. M., Hui, E., Ip, T., and Thompson, L.U. (2004). Dietary flaxseed enhances the inhibitory effect of tamoxifen on the growth of estrogen-dependent human breast cancer (MCF-7) in nude mice. *Clinical Cancer Research,* **10**: 7703-7711.

Choi, S.W., Park, K.I., Yeon, J.T., Ryu, B.J., Kim, K.J., and Kim, S.H. (2014). Anti-osteoclastogenic activity of matairesinol via suppression of p38/ERK-NFATc1 signaling axis. *BMC Complementary and Alternative Medicine*, **21**: 14-35.

Coy, E.D., Cuca, L.E., and Sefkow, M. (2009). Macrophyllin-type bicyclo[3.2.1]octanoid neolignans from the leaves of *Pleurothyrium cinereum*. *Journal of Natural Products*, **72(7)**: 1245-1248.

Cuca, L.E., Coy, E.D., Alarcón, M.A., Fernández, A., and Aristizábal, F.A. (2011). Cytotoxic effect of some natural compounds isolated from Lauraceae plants and synthetic derivatives. *Biomedica*, **31(3)**: 335-343.

Chen, L-H., Fang, J., Li, H., Demark-Wahnefried, W., and Lin, X. (2007). Enterolactone induces apoptosis in human prostate carcinoma LNCaP cells via a mitochondrial-mediated, caspase-dependent pathway. *Molecular Cancer Therapeutics*, **6(9)**: 2581-2590.

Demark-Wahnefried, W., Price, D.T., Polascik, T.J., Robertson, C.N., Anderson, E.E., Paulson, D.F., Walther, P.J., Gannon, M., and Vollmer, R.T. (2001). Pilot study of dietary fat restriction and flaxseed supplementation in men with prostate cancer before surgery: exploring the effects on hormonal levels, prostate-specific antigen, and histopathologic features. *Urology*, **58**: 47-52.

Deng, P., Wang, C., Chen, L., Wang, C., Du, Y., Yan, X., Chen, M., Yang, G., and He, G. (2013). Sesamin induces cell cycle arrest and apoptosis through the inhibition of signal transducer and activator of transcription 3 signalling in human hepatocellular carcinoma cell line HepG2. *Biological and Pharmaceutical Bulletin*, **36(10)**: 1540-1548.

Durazzo, A., Zaccaria, M., Polito, A., Maiani, G., and Carcea, M. (2013). Lignan Content in Cereals, Buckwheat and Derived Foods. *Foods*, **2(1)**: 53-63.

Elujoba, A. A., Odeleye, O. M., and Ogunyemi, C. M. (2005). Traditional medicine development for medical and dental primary health care delivery system in Africa. *African Journal of Traditional, Complementary and Alternative Medicines*, **2 (1)**: *46-61.*

Fini, L., Hotchkiss, E., Fogliano, V., Graziani, G., Romano, M., De Vol, E.B., Qin, H., Selgrad, M., Boland, C.R., and Ricciardiello, L. (2008). Chemopreventive properties of pinoresinol-rich olive oil involve a selective activation of the ATM-p53 cascade in colon cancer cell lines. *Carcinogenesis*, **29(1)**: 139-146.

Ford, J.D., Huang, K.S., Wang, H.B., Davin, L.B., and Lewis, N.G. (2001). Biosynthetic pathway to the cancer chemopreventive secoisolariciresinol diglucosid hydroxymethyl glutaryl ester- linked lignan oligomers in flax (*Linum usitatissimum*) seed. *Journal of Natural Products*, **64**: 1388-1397.

Fukuda, Y., Osawa, T., Namiki, M., Saki, T. (1985). Studies on antioxidative substances in sesame. *Agricultural and Biological Chemistry*, 49: 301-306.

Fuss, E. (2003). Lignans in plant cell and organ cultures: an overview. *Phytochemistry Reviews*, **2**: 307-320.

Garcez, F.R., Garcez, W.S., Martins, M., Matos, M.F., Guterres, Z.R., Mantovani, M.S., Misu, C.K., and Nakashita, S.T. (2005). Cytotoxic and genotoxic butanolides and lignans from *Aiouea trinervis*. *Planta Medica*, **71(10)**: 923-927.

Gharras, H.E. (2009). Polyphenols: food sources, properties and applications - a review. *International Journal of Food Science and Technology*, **44**: 2512-2518.

Gu, J.Q., Park, E.J., Totura, S., Riswan, S., Fong, H.H., Pezzuto, J.M., and Kinghorn, A.D. (2002). Constituents of the twigs of *Hernandia ovigera* that inhibit the transformation of JB6 murine epidermal cells. *Journal of Natural Products*, **65(7)**: 1065-1068.

Gueritte, F., and Fahy, J. (2005). The vinca alkaloids. *In:* Anticancer Agents from Natural Products, Ed. By Cragg, G.M., Kingston, D.G.I., Newman, D.J., Brunner-Routledge Psychology Press, Taylor and Francis Group, Boca Raton, FL, pp. 123–136 (Chapter 7).

Habtemariam, S. (2003). Cytotoxic and cytostatic activity of erlangerins from *Commiphora erlangeriana*. *Toxicon*, **41(6)**: 723-727

Harikumar, K.B., Sung, B., Tharakan, S.T., Pandey, M.K., Joy, B., Guha, S., Krishnan, S., and Aggarwal, B.B. (2010). Sesamin manifests chemopreventive effects through the suppression of NF-κB-regulated cell survival, proliferation, invasion, and angiogenic gene products. *Molecular Cancer Research*, **8(5)**: 751-761.

Hausott, B., Greger, H., and Marian, B. (2003). Naturally occurring lignans efficiently induce apoptosis in colorectal tumor cells. *Journal of Cancer Research and Clinical Oncology*, **129**: 569-576.

Hernandez,.B.Y., McDuffie, K., Franke, A.A., Killeen, J., and Goodman, M.T. (2004). Plasma and dietary phytoestrogens and risk of premalignant lesions of the cervix. *Nutrition and Cancer*, **49**: 109-124.

Hirose, M., Yamaguchi, T., Lin, C., Kimoto, N., Futakuchi, M., Kono, T., Nishibe, S., and Shirai, T. (2000). Effects of arctiin on PhIP-induced mammary, colon and pancreatic carcinogenesis in female Sprague-Dawley rats and MaIQx-induced hepatocarcinogenesis in male F344 rats. *Cancer Letters*, **155**: 79-88.

Hori, H., Takayanagi, T., Kamada, Y., Shimoyoshi, S., Ono, Y., Kitagawa, Y., Shibata, H., Nagao, M., Fujii, W., and Sakakibara, Y. (2011). Genotoxicity evaluation of sesamin and episesamin. *Mutation Research*, **719(1-2)**: 21-28.

Horn-Ross, P.L., Hoggatt, K.J., and Lee, M. M. (2002). Phytoestrogens and thyroid cancer risk: the San Francisco Bay Area Thyroid Cancer Study. *Cancer Epidemiology, Biomarkers* and *Prevention*, **11**: 43-49.

Horn-Ross, P.L., John, E.M., Canchola, A.J., Stewart, S.L., and Lee, M. M. (2003). Phytoestogen intake and endometrial cancer risk. *Journal of the National Cancer Institute*, **95**: 1158-1164.

Huang, D.M., Guh, J.H., Chueh, S.C., and Teng, C.M. (2004). Modulation of anti-adhesion molecule MUC-1 is associated with arctiin-induced growth inhibition in PC-3 cells. *Prostate*, **59(3)**: 260-267.

Ito, C., Itoigawa, M., Ogata, M., Mou, X. Y., Tokuda, H., Nishino, H., and Furukawa, H. (2001). Lignans as anti tumor-promoter from the seeds of *Hernandia ovigera*. *Planta Medica*, **67(2)**: 166-168.

Jacklin, A., Ratledge, C., Welham, K., Bilko, D., and Newton, C.J. (2003). The sesame seed oil constituent, sesamol, induces growth arrest and apoptosis of cancer and cardiovascular cells. *Annals of the New York Academy of Sciences*, **1010**: 374-380.

Johnsson, P., Peerlkamp, N., Kamal-Eldin, A., Andersson, R.E., Andersson, R., Lundgren, L.N., and Aman, P. (2002). Polymeric fractions containing phenol glucosides in flaxseed. *Food Chemistry*, **76**: 207-212.

Kim, S.J., Min, H.Y., Lee, E.J., Kim, Y.S., Bae, K., Kang, S.S., and Lee, S.K. (2010). Growth inhibition and cell cycle arrest in the G0/G1 by schizandrin, a dibenzocyclooctadiene lignan isolated from *Schisandra chinensis*, on T47D human breast cancer cells. *Phytotherapy Research*, **24(2)**: 193-197.

Kim, J-H., Park, Y-H., Park, S-W., Yang, E-K., and Lee, W-J. (2003). Lignan from Safflower Seeds Induces Apoptosis in Human Promyelocytic Leukemia Cells. *Nutraceuticals and food*, **8(2)**: 113-118.

Kimura, M., Suzuki, J., Yamada, T., Yoshizaki, M., Kikuchi, T., Kadota, S., and Matsuda, S. (1985).Antiinflammatory effect of neolignans newly isolated from the crude drug "Shin-I" (Flos Magnoliae). *Planta Medica*, **51**: 291-293.

Kulling S. E., Rosenberg, B., Jacobs, E., and Metzler, M. (1999).The phytoestrogens coumoestrol and genistein induce structural chromosomal aberrations in cultured human peripheral blood lymphocytes. *Archives of Toxicology*, **73(1)**: 50-54.

Lee, B., Kim, K.H., Jung, H.J., and Kwon, H.J. (2012). Matairesinol inhibits angiogenesis via suppression of mitochondrial reactive oxygen species. *Biochemical and Biophysical Research Communications*, **421(1)**: 76-80.

Lee, C., Kim, H., and Kho, Y. (2002). Agastinol and agastenol, novel lignans from *Agastache rugosa* and their evaluation in an apoptosis inhibition assay. *Journal of Natural Products*, **65(3)**: 414-416.

Lee, C.C., Liu, K.J., Wu, Y.C., Lin, S.J., Chang, C.C., and Huang, T.S. (2011). Sesamin inhibits macrophage-induced vascular endothelial growth factor and matrix metalloproteinase-9 expression and proangiogenic activity in breast cancer cells. *Inflammation*, **34(3)**: 209-221.

Lee, D.H., Szczepanski, M.J., and Lee, Y.J. (2009). Magnolol induces apoptosis via inhibiting the EGFR/PI3K/Akt signaling pathway in human prostate cancer cells. *Journal of Cellular Biochemistry*, **106(6)**: 1113-1122.

Li, G., Lee, C.S., Woo, M.H., Lee, S.H., Chang, H.W., and Son, J.K. (2004). Lignans from the bark of *Machilus thunbergii* and their DNA topoisomerases I and II inhibition and cytotoxicity. *Biological and Pharmaceutical Bulletin*, **27(7)**: 1147-1150.

Li, W., Sun, Y.N., Yan, X.T., Yang, S.Y., Kim, E.J., Kang, H.K., and Kim, Y.H. (2013). Coumarins and lignans from *Zanthoxylum schinifolium* and their anticancer activities. *Journal of Agricultural and Food Chemistry*, **61(45)**: 10730-10740.

Liggins, J., Grimwood, R., and Bingham, SA. (2000). Extraction and quantification of lignan phytoestrogens in food and human samples. *Annals of Biochemistry*, **287(1)**: 102-109.

Lin, S.Y., Chang, Y.T., Liu, J.D., Yu, C.H., Ho, Y.S., Lee, Y.H., and Lee, W.S. (2001). Molecular mechanisms of apoptosis induced by magnolol in colon and liver cancer cells. *Molecular Carcinogenesis*, **32**: 73-83.

Lin, S.Y., Liu, J.D., Chang, H.C., Yeh, S.D., Lin, C.H., and Lee, W.S. (2002). Magnolol suppresses proliferation of cultured human colon and liver cancer cells by inhibiting DNA synthesis and activating apoptosis. *Journal of Cellular Biochemistry*, **84**: 532-544.

Lin, X., Switzer, B.R., and Demark-Wahnefried, W. (2001). Effect of mammalian lignans on the growth of prostate cancer cell lines. *Anticancer Research*, **21(6A)**: 3995-3999.

Lopes, N.P., Kato, M.J., and Yoshida, M. (1999). Antifungal constituents from roots of *Virola surinamensis*, *Phytochemistry*, **51**: 23-33.

Luo, J., Hu, Y., Kong, W., and Yang, M. (2014). Evaluation and Structure-Activity Relationship Analysis of a New Series of Arylnaphthalene lignans as Potential Anti-Tumor Agents. *PLoS ONE*, **9(3)**: e93516.

Mazur, W. (1998). Phytoestrogen content in foods. *Baillieere's Clinical Endocrinology and Metabolism*, **12**: 729-742.

McCann, S.E., Freudenheim, J.L., Marshall, J.R., and Graham, S. (2003). Risk of human ovarian cancer is related to dietary intake of selected nutrients, phytochemicals and food groups. *Journal of Nutrition*, **133**: 1937-1942.

Medola, J,F., Cintra, V.P., Pesqueira, E. Silva, E.P., de Andrade, R. V., da Silva R., Saraiva, J., Albuquerque, S., Bastos, J.K., Andrade, E., Silva, M.L., and Tavares, D.C. (2007). Hinokinin causes antigenotoxicity but not genotoxicity in peripheral blood of Wistar rats. *Food and Chemical Toxicology*, **45(4)**: 638-642.

Messiano, G.B., Santos, R.A., Ferreira Lde S., Simões, R.A., Jabor, V.A., Kato, M.J., Lopes, N.P., Pupo, M.T., and de Oliveira, A.R. (2013). *In vitro* metabolism study of the promising anticancer agent the lignan (-)-grandisin. *Journal of Pharmaceutical and Biomedical Analysis*, **72**: 240-244.

Messiano, G.B., Santos, R.A., Ferreira, Lde S., Simões, R.A., Jabor, V.A., Kato, M.J., Lopes, N.P., Pupo, M.T., and de Oliveira, A.R. (2013). *In vitro* metabolism study of the promising anticancer agent the lignan (-)-grandisin. *Journal of Pharmaceutical and Biomedical Analysis*, **72**: 240-244

Milder, *I.E.*, Feskens, E.J., Arts, I.C., Bueno, de Mesquita, H.B., Hollman, P.C., and Kromhout, D. (2005). Intake of the plant lignans secoisolariciresinol, matairesinol, lariciresinol, and pinoresinol in Dutch men and women. *Journal of Nutrition*, **135(5)**: 1202-1207.

Mohagheghzadeh, A., Schmidt, T.J., and Alfermann, A.W. (2002). Arylnaphthalene lignans from *in vitro* cultures of *Linum austriacum*. *Journal of Natural Products*, **65**: 69-71.

Morais, S.K.R., Teixeira, A.F., Torres, Z.E.S., Nunomura, S.M., Kanashiro, E.H.Y., Lindoso, J.A.L., and Yoshida, M. (2009). Biological activities of lignoids from Amazon Myristicaceae species: *Virola michelii, V. mollissima, V. pavonis* and *Iryanthera juruensis*, *Journal of the Brazilian Chemical Society*, **20**: 1110-1118.

Navarro, E., Alonso, S.J., Alonso, P.J., Trujillo, J., Jorge, E., and Perez, C. (2001). Pharmacological effects of elenoside, an arylnaphthalenelignan. *Biological and Pharmaceutical Bulletin*, **24(3)**: 254-258.

Niemeyer, H.B., Honig, D.M., Kulling, S.E., and Metzler, M. (2003). Studies on the metabolism of the plant lignans secoisolariciresinol and matairesinol. *Journal of Agricultural and Food Chemistry*, **51**: 6317-6325.

Nitiss, J.L. (2009). Targeting DNA topoisomerase II in cancer chemotherapy. *Nature Reviews Cancer*, **9**: 338-350.

Ohashi, K., Winarno, H., Mukai, M., Inoue, M., Prana, M.S., Simanjuntak, P., and Shibuya, H. (2003). Indonesian medicinal plants. XXV. Cancer cell invasion inhibitory effects of chemical constituents in the parasitic plant *Scurrula atropurpurea* (Loranthaceae). *Chemical* and *pharmaceutical bulletin* (Tokyo), **51(3)**: 343-345.

Pajari, A.M., Smeds, A.I., Oikarinen, S.I., Eklund, P.C., Sjöholm, R.E., and Mutanen, M. (2006). The plant lignans matairesinol and secoisolariciresinol administered to Min mice do not protect against intestinal tumor formation. *Cancer Letters*, **233(2)**: 309-314.

Pan, J.Y., Chen, S.L., Yang, M.H., Wu, J., Sinkkonen, J., and Zou, K. (2009). An update on lignans: natural products and synthesis. *Natural Product Reports*, **26**: 1251-1292.

Pan, M.H., and Ho, C.T. (2008). Chemopreventive effects of natural dietary compounds on cancer development. *Chemical Society Reviews*, **37**: 2558-2574.

Park, B.Y., Min, B.S., Kwon, O.K., Oh, S.R., Ahn, K.S., Kim, T.J., Kim, D.Y., Bae, K., and Lee, H.K. (2004). Increase of caspase-3 activity by lignans from *Machilus thunbergii* in HL-60 cells. *Biological and Pharmaceutical Bulletin*, **27(8)**: 1305-1307.

Park, C., Choi, Y.W., Hyun, S.K., Kwon, H.J., Hwang, H.J., Kim, G.Y., Choi, B.T., Kim, B.W., Choi, I.W., Moon, S.K., Kim, W.J., and Choi, Y.H. (2009). Induction of G1 arrest and apoptosis by schisandrin C isolated from *Schizandra chinensis* Baill in human leukemia U937 cells. *International Journal of Molecular Medicine*, **24(4)**: 495-502.

Parvathaneni, M., Battu, G. R., Gray, A.I., and Gummalla, P. (2014). Investigation of anticancer potential of hypophyllanthin and phyllanthin against breast cancer by *in vitro* and *in vivo* methods. *Asian Pacific Journal of Tropical Disease*, **4**: S71-S76.

Patel, D., Vaghasiya, J., Pancholi, S. S., and Paul, A. (2012). Therapeutic Potential of Secoisolariciresinol Diglucoside: A Plant Lignan. *International Journal of Pharmaceutical Sciences and Drug Research*, **4(1)**: 15-18.

Pettit, G.R., Meng, Y., Gearing, R. P., Herald, D. L., Pettit, R.K., Doubek, D.L., Chapuis, J., and Tackett, L. P. (2004). Antineoplastic agents.522. *Hernandia peltata* (Malaysia) and *Hernandia nymphaeifolia* (Republic of Maldives). *Journal of Natural Products*, **67(2)**: 214-220.

Peuhu, E., Rivero-Müller, A., Stykki, H., Torvaldson, E., Holmbom, T., Eklund, P., Unkila, M., Sjöholm, R., and Eriksson, J.E. (2010). Inhibition of Akt signaling by the lignan matairesinol sensitizes prostate cancer cells to TRAIL-induced apoptosis. *Oncogene*, **29(6)**: 898-908.

Pianjing, P., Thiantanawat, A., Rangkadilok, N., Watcharasit, P., Mahidol, C., and Satayavivad, J. (2011). Estrogenic activities of sesame lignans and their metabolites on human breast cancer cells. *Journal of Agricultural and Food Chemistry*, **59(1)**: 212-221.

Jang, D.S., Park, E.J., Hawthorne, M.E., Vigo, J.S., Graham, J.G., Cabieses, F., Santarsiero, B.D., Mesecar, A.D., Fong, H.H., Mehta, R.G., Pezzuto, J.M., and Kinghorn, A.D. (2003). Potential cancer chemopreventive constituents of the seeds of *Dipteryx odorata* (tonka bean). *Journal of Natural Products*, **66(5)**: 583-587.

Pu, J.X., Gao, X.M., Lei, C., Xiao, W.L., Wang, R.R., Yang, L.B., Zhao, Y., Li, L.M., Huang, S.X., Zheng, Y.T., and Sun, H.D. (2008). Three new compounds from *Kadura longipedunculata*. *Chemical* and *pharmaceutical bulletin*, **56**: 1143-1146.

Ramesh, C., Ravindranath, N., Ram, T.S., and Das, B. (2003). Arylnaphthalide lignans from *Cleistanthus collinus*. *Chemical* and *pharmaceutical bulletin* (Tokyo), **51**: 1299-1300.

Resende, F.A., Tomazella, I.M., Barbosa, L.C., Ponce, M., Furtado, R.A., Pereira, A.C., Bastos, J.K., Andrade, E., Silva, M.L., and Tavares, D.C. (2010). Effect of the dibenzylbutyrolactone lignan (-)-hinokinin on doxorubicin and methyl methanesulfonate clastogenicity in V79 Chinese hamster lung fibroblasts. *Mutation Research*, **700(1-2)**: 62-66.

Chattopadhyay, S. K., Kumar, T. R., Maulik, P. R., Srivastava, S., Garg, A., Sharon, A., Negi, A. S., and Khanuja S. P. (2003). Absolute configuration and anticancer activity of taxiresinol and related lignans of *Taxus wallichiana*. *Bioorganic and Medicinal Chemistry*, **11(23)**: 4945-4948.

Saarinen, N.M., Huovinen, R., Wärri, A., Mäkelä, S.I., Valentin-Blasini, L., Needham, L., Eckerman, C., Collan, Y.U., and Santti, R.S. (2001). Uptake and metabolism of hydroxymatairesinol in relation to its anticarcinogenicity in DMBA-induced rat mammary carcinoma model. *Nutrition and Cancer*, **41**: 82-90.

Saarinen, N.M., Huovinen, R., Wärri, A., Mäkelä, S.I., Valentin-Blasini, L., Sjöholm, R., Ämmälä, J., Lehtilä, R., Eckerman, C., Y.U., and Santti, R. S. (2002). Enterolactone inhibits the growth of 7, 12-dimethylbenz (a) anthracene-induced mammary carcinomas in the rat. *Molecular Cancer Therapeutics*, **1**: 869-876.

Saarinen, N.M. (2002). Hydroxymatairesinol from Norway spruce (*Picea abies*), a novel enterolactone precursor with anticarcinogenic properties in experimental mammary carcinoma. Turku University dissertations. ISBN 951-29-2131-4, ISSN 0355-9483, Painosalama Oy, Turku Finland,

Saleem, M., Kim, H.J., Ali, M.S., and Lee, Y.S. (2005). An update on bioactive plant lignans. *Natural Products Reports*, **22**: 696-716.

Sepporta, M.V., Mazza, T., Morozzi, G., and Fabiani, R. (2013). Pinoresinol inhibits proliferation and induces differentiation on human HL60 leukemia cells. *Nutrition and Cancer*, **65(8)**: 1208-1218.

Shashi, B., Jaswant, S., Madhusudana, R.J., Kumar, S.A., and Nabi, Q.G. (2006). A novel lignan composition from *Cedrus deodara* induces apoptosis and early nitric oxide generation in human leukemia Molt-4 and HL-60 cells. *Nitric Oxide*, **14(1)**: 72-88.

Shimizu, S., Fujii, G., Takahashi, M., Nakanishi, R., Komiya, M., Shimura, M., Noma, N., Onuma, W., Terasaki, M., Yano, T., and Mutoh, M. (2014). Sesamol suppresses cyclooxygenase-2 transcriptional activity in colon cancer cells and modifies intestinal polyp development in Apc (Min/+) mice. *Journal of Clinical Biochemistry and Nutrition*, **54(2)**: 95-101.

Siegel, R., Naishadham, D., and Jemal, A. (2013). Cancer statistics. *CA: A Cancer Journal for Clinicians*, **63**: 11-30.

Smeds, A.I., Eklund, P.C., and Sjöholm, R.E. (2007). Quantification of a broad spectrum of lignans in cereals, oilseeds, and nuts. *Journal of Agricultural and Food Chemistry*, **55**: 1337-1346.

Susplugas, S., Hung, N.V., Bignon, J., Thoison, O., Kruczynski, A., Sévenet, T., and Guéritte, F. (2005). Cytotoxic arylnaphthalene lignans from a Vietnamese Acanthaceae, *Justicia patentiflora*. *Journal of Natural Products*, **68(5)**: 734-738.

Tan, Z., Zhang, Y., Deng, J., Zeng, G., and Zhang, Y. (2012). Purified vitexin compound 1 suppresses tumor growth and induces cell apoptosis in a mouse model of human choriocarcinoma. *International Journal of Gynecological Cancer*, **22(3)**: 360-366.

Thompson, L.U. (1998). Experimental studies on lignans and cancer. *Bailliere's Clinical Endocrinology and Metabolism*, **12 (4)**: 691-705.

Thompson, L.U., Chen, J.M., Li, T., Strasser-Weippl, K., and Goss, P.E. (2005). Dietary flaxseed alters tumor biological markers in postmenopausal breast cancer. *Clinical Cancer Research,* **11(10)**: 3828-3835.

Thompson L.U., Li T., Chen J., and Goss P.E. (2000). Biological effects of dietary Flaxseed in patients with Breast Cancer. *Breast Cancer Research and Treatment*, **64**: 50.

Thompson, L.U., Rickard, S.E., and Orcheson, L.J. (1996). Flaxseed and its lignan and oil components reduce mammary tumor growth at a late stage of carcinogenesis. *Carcinogenesis,* **17**: 1373-1376.

Thompson, L.U. Robb, P., Serraino, M. and Cheung, F. (1991). Mammalian lignan production from various foods. *Nutr Cancer,* **16**: 43-52.

Tomlinson, T. R., and Akerele, O. (1998). Medicinal plants: their role in health and biodiversity. University of Pennsylvania Press, Philadelphia. 221 pages.

Tou, J.C., Chen, J., and Thompşon, L.U. (1998). Flaxseed and its lignan precursor, secoisolariciresinol diglycoside, affect pregnancy outcome and reproductive development in rats. *Journal of Nutrition*, **128 (11)**: 1861-1868.

Truan, J.S., Chen, J.M., and Thompson, L.U. (2012). Comparative effects of sesame seed lignan and flaxseed lignan in reducing the growth of human breast tumors (MCF-7) at high levels of circulating estrogen in athymic mice. *Nutrition and Cancer*, **64(1)**: 65-71.

Tsao, A.S., Kim, E.S., and Hong, W.K. (2004). Chemoprevention of cancer. *CA: A Cancer Journal for Clinicians,* **54(3)**: 150-180.

Valadares, M.C., de Carvalho, I.C.T., Junior, L.O., Vieira, M.S., Benfica, P.L., de Carvalho, F.S., Andrade, L.V.S., Lima, E.M., and Kato, M.J. (2009). Cytotoxicity and angiogenic activity of grandisin. *Journal of Pharmacy and Pharmacology*, **61**: 1709-1714.

Valadares, M.C., Júnior, L.M.O., de Carvalho, F.S., Andrade, L.V.S., dos Santos, A.P., de Oliveira, V., Gil, E.S., and Kato, M.J. (2011). Chemoprotective effect of the tetrahydrofuran lignan grandisin in the in vivo rodend micronucleus assay. *Journal of Pharmacy and Pharmacology*, **63**: 447-451.

Vieira Mde S., de Oliveira, V., Lima E.M., Kato, M.J., **and** Valadares, M.C. (2011). *In vitro* basal cytotoxicity assay applied to estimate acute oral systemic toxicity of grandisin and its major metabolite. *Experimental and Toxicologic Pathology*, **63(5)**: 505-510.

Wang, L., Chen, J. M., and Thompson, L. U. (2005). The inhibitory effect of flaxseed on the growth and metastasis of estrogen receptor negative human breast cancer xenografts is attributed to both its lignan and oil components. *International Journal of Cancer*, **116**: 793-798.

Yang, S., Ma, J., Xiao, J., Lv, X., Li, X., Yang, H., Liu, Y., Feng, S., and Zhang, Y. (2012). Arctigenin Anti-Tumor Activity in Bladder Cancer T24 Cell Line through Induction of Cell-Cycle Arrest and Apoptosis. *The Anatomical Record: Advances in Integrative Anatomy and Evolutionary Biology*, **295 (8)**: 1260-1266.

Zhao, C., Qiu, R., and Zheng, R. (2000). *In vitro* Antitumor Activities of Furan Lignans. *Journal-Lanzhou University Natural Sciences*, **36(4)**: 66-68.

Zhang, Q.Y., Jiang, M., Zhao, C.Q., Yu, M., Zhang, H., Ding, Y.J., and Zhai, Y.G. (2005). Apoptosis induced by one new podophyllotoxin glucoside in human carcinoma cells. *Toxicology*, **212(1)**: 46-53.

Zhou, J., Hu, H., Long, J., Wan, F., Li, L., and Zhang, S. (2013). Vitexin 6, a novel lignan, induces autophagy and apoptosis by activating the Jun N-terminal kinase pathway. *Anticancer Drugs*, **24**: 928-936.

Zhou, Y.J., Liu, Y.E., Cao, J.G., Zeng, G.Y., Cui, S., Li, Y.L., Zhou, M.C., Chen, Y., Pu, W., Potters, L., and Shi, E.Y. (2009). Vitexins, nature-derived lignan compounds, induce apoptosis and suppress tumor growth. *Clinical Cancer Research*, **15(16)**: 5161-5169.

Bioactive Phytochemicals: Perspectives for Modern Medicine Vol. 3 (2015) *Pages* **283–310**
Editor: **V.K. Gupta**
Published by: **DAYA PUBLISHING HOUSE, NEW DELHI**

11

Cancer Chemoprevention: Potentials of Dietary Polyphenols to Modulate Wnt/β-catenin Signaling Pathway

T. Rajavel[1] and K. Pandima Devi[1*]

ABSTRACT

Polyphenols are phenolic compounds found throughout plant kingdom. Based on the chemical structure, polyphenols are classified into flavonoids, phenolic acids, phenolic alcohols, stilbenes and lignans. Polyphenols shows anticancer effect by different mechanisms such as removal of carcinogenic agents, modulation of cell signaling, antioxidant enzymatic activities, DNA damage and induction of apoptosis as well as cell cycle arrest. Targeting specific cell signaling pathway to combat cancer is a major focus on chemotherapy. In recent years, large number of studies have attributed that dietary polyphenols prevent cancer by modulating aberrant Wnt/β-catenin signaling pathway. Wnt/β-catenin signaling is the most, conserved intracellular signaling cascade which plays an important role in cell proliferation, differentiation, cell-cell adhesion, and organogenesis. Deregulation of components involved in Wnt/β-catenin signaling has been implicated in a wide spectrum of human cancers, including colorectal, lung, breast, melanoma, prostate and hepatocellular carcinoma. Mutation in extracellular components (Wnt, LRP-5/6 FRZ, DSH), cytoplasmic (APC, Axin, β-catenin, Gsk 3β, CK1), nuclear factors (LEF/Tcf, c-Myc) and Wnt inhibitors (WIF, SFRP1, DKK) leads to tumor development and progression. In this review, we discuss about chemopreventive mechanism of polyphenols (phenolic acids, tannins, flavanoids, stilbenes) in various types of cancer that serve as an antagonist on Wnt/β-catenin signaling pathway.

Keywords: APC, Axin, Chemotherapy, β catenin, ck-1, Dvl, Fzds, Gsk 3β, LEF/Tcf, c-Myc, Polyphenols, Wnt.

1 Department of Biotechnology, Alagappa University, Karaikudi – 630 004, Tamil Nadu, India

* *Corresponding author*: E-mail: devikasi@yahoo.com

Introduction

Cancer is a cluster of disease which involves multiple alterations of genes involved in regulation of cell growth and survival. This results in an imbalance in cell proliferation and cell death that favors growth of a tumor cell population (Lopez *et al.*, 2010). Cancer is one of the most challenging health problems in both developed and developing countries. According to the recent report by GLOBOCON (Global Burden of Cancer Study, 2012), 14.1 million new cancer cases and 8.2 million cancer-related deaths were occurring per year across the world. The most commonly diagnosed cancers worldwide were those of the lung (1.8 million, 13.0 per cent of the total), breast (1.7 million, 11.9 per cent) and colorectum (1.4 million, 9.7 per cent). The highest mortality rate were associated with lung (1.6 million, 19.4 per cent of the total), liver (0.8 million, 9.1 per cent), and stomach (0.7 million, 8.8 per cent). It estimated that nearly 19.3 million new cancer cases will be diagnosed per year by 2025.

Since conventional therapy and surgical approaches have not been able to control cancer due to their side effects and recurrence of cancer. Standard chemotherapy seems to be the attractive strategy in cancer management and treatment (Fan *et al.*, 1998). Cancer chemoprevention refers to the use of synthetic or natural agents to reverse, suppress or prevent the development of cancer. According to ACS (American Cancer Society) chemotherapy offers benefits for certain type of cancer patients by increasing the survival rate and reducing the risk of cancer recurrence. For example, Tamoxifen, the first chemoprevention drug to receive FDA approval, is the most well-known chemopreventive agent for breast cancer. Long-term intake of tamoxifen can reduce the recurrence of breast cancer and also help in preventing breast cancer deaths (Waters *et al.*, 2010). In the last decades, research effort has increased on identifying novel chemopreventive agents against cancer. A large number of dietary phytochemicals has been demonstrated to exhibit anticancer activities by interfering with multiple signaling pathways aberrant in cancer.

Phytochemicals are biologically active compounds in plants which have various health benefit properties. Phytochemicals are categorised into carotenoids, phenolics, alkaloids, and organosulphur compounds are the secondary metabolites that are vital for plant growth and reproduction (Arts *et al.*, 2005). They also serve as defense agents against pathogens and predators that attack plants. They have been found useful in humans for lowering the effect of many chronic diseases including cancer (Scalbert *et al.*, 2005). Recently, prevention of cancer through dietary polyphenols has received much attention in cancer chemotherapy because of their chemical diversity, biological activity, affordability, easy availability, and lack of substantial toxicity. Polyphenols have been reported to interfere at the initiation, promotion and progression of cancer (Margaret *et al.*, 2003). It also has been demonstrated to modulate the signal transduction pathways related to cellular proliferation, differentiation, apoptosis, inflammation, angiogenesis and metastasis. The current review aims to highlight the anticancer properties of polyphenols that target specifically the Wnt/β-catenin signaling pathway in various types of cancers.

Polyphenols and Anticancer Properties

Polyphenols are naturally occurring compounds found largely in vegetables, cereals, beverages and fruits like grapes, apple, pear, cherries and berries. Polyphenols are structurally diverse; approximately more than 8000 different polyphenols were identified from diet. Based on the number of phenol rings, polyphenols were classified into flavonoids, phenolic acids (*e.g.* gallic acid, curcumin), phenolic alcohols (*e.g.* Hydroxytyrosol, oleuropein), stilbenes (*e.g.* resveratrol) and lignans (*e.g.* secoisolariciresinol). Flavanoids is further divided into seven subclasses: flavones (*e.g.* chrysin), flavonols (*e.g.* quercetin, myricetin, and rutin), flavanones (*e.g.* silibilin), anthocyanidins (*e.g.* malvidin), flavan-3-ols (*e.g.* catechin, epicatechin, and EGCG), isoflavones (*e.g.* genistein), and stilbines (*e.g.* resveratrol). Several epidemiological studies indicate that dietary polyphenols from fruits and vegetables reduce cancer risk in humans [Mahmoud *et al.*, 2000].

Defects in programmed cell death (apoptosis), proliferation, differentiation and migration are the major factor for pathogenesis of cancer. Polyphenols affect the pathogenesis of cancer by different mechanisms including antioxidant activities, targeting cell signaling, cell cycle arrest, invasion, angiogenesis, metastasis, transcription factors (NF-κB), protein kinases and apoptosis induction by activation of caspase-9 and caspase-3. For example, EGCG a flavanoid present in green tea acts as an anticancer agent against various types of cancer, such as prostatic cancer, gastric cancer, colon cancer, lung cancer and leukemia [Brusselmans *et al.*, 2003, Chen *et al.*, 2003]. In addition, EGCG inhibits the migration and invasion of mammary cancer cell lines [Punathil *et al.*, 2008]. Phenolic acids like gallic acid induce the oxidative stress and promote apoptotic mode of cell death in human oral cancer cell line [Schuck *et al.*, 2013]. Oleuropein and hydroxytyrosol (3,4-dihydroxyphenylethanol), the main constituent phenolic alcohols present in extra virgin olive oil has been reported to protect against cancer by arresting cell cycle and inducing cytochrome c-dependent apoptosis [Ragione *et al.*, 2000]. Silibinin, a flavanoid found in *Silybum marianum* inhibit the metastasis property in several tumor cell lines and rodent models [Deep *et al.*, 2010]. Catechins are found in fruits such as apricots (250 mg/kg fresh wt) and cherry (250 mg/kg fresh wt) and Green tea (up to 800 mg/L). *In vitro* studies shows that it inhibits the Matrix Metalloproteinase (MMP) in different cancer cell line [Demeule *et al.*, 2000]. Genistein, an isoflavone nutrients derived from soybeans (4.6μg/g) has a chemopreventive effect against breast cancer by targeting estrogen receptors [Fukutake *et al.*, 1996, Shao *et al.*, 2000]. In addition, genistein also has the property of modulating cell cycle, inducing apoptosis and anti-invasive property in various cancers [Shao *et al.*, 2000, Kim *et al.*, 2010, Pavese *et al.*, 2010]. Resveratrol is a stilbenoid, found in more than 70 plant species, including grapes, berries and peanuts. The fresh skin of red grapes is particularly rich in resveratrol (50-100 g/kg net weight) [Baliga *et al.*, 2005]. It has been shown that resveratrol increases hepatic glutathione content, scavenges free radicals and induces enzymes of phase II hepatic metabolism. It also inhibits the transcription factor nuclear factor-κB [Baur *et al.*, 2006 Muriel *et al.*, 2008 Bishayee *et al.*, 2009]. Altogether, these findings underline the fact that polyphenols could be considered as promising anti-cancer agents for cancer treatment and prevention.

Table 11.1: Polyphenols and their Anticancer Mechanisms

Name of the Polyphenol	*Class of the Compound*	*Major Food Source*	*Effective against the Cancer type*	*Mode of Action*	*Reference*
Gallic acid	Phenolic acid	Blueberries, walnuts, apples, flax seed, oak bark and tea	Prostate and Oral cancer	Suppress cycle progression, induce apoptosis and oxidative stress	Komal *et al.*, 2008
Hydroxyl tyrosol	Phenolic alcohol	Olive oil	Breast cancer	Induce apoptosis, and arrest cell cycle	Fabiani *et al.*, 2002
Oleuropein	Phenolic alcohol	Olive oil	Breast cancer	Anti-metastatic effects by inhibiting NF-κB pathway and oncogenic protein	Zeinab *et al.*, 2012
Luteolin	Flavones	Parsley, thyme, celery, oregano, green chilli	Colon cancer	Inhibition of cell survival, invasion, tumor growth and histone deacetylase activity	Cheng *et al.*, 2005, Yang *et al.*, 2006, Bagli *et al.*, 2004
Querctin	Flavonols	Onion, apple, cherry, broccoli, tomato, berries, tea, red wine, leek, lemon	Lung, Colon and Glioma cancer	Cell cycle arrest; Inhibit the angiogenesis; Inhibits cell migration and invasion	Robaszkiewicz *et al.*, 2007, Hosokawa*et al.*,1990 Braganhol *et al.*, 2006
Silibinin	Flavanones	Milk thistle of *Silybum marianum*	Lung, colon, breat	Anti-metastatic effect, Induction of apoptosis, antiinflammatory effects, supression of protein kinases and MAPKs	Mokhtari *et al.*, 2008 Bhatia *et al.*, 1999
Petunidin	Anthocyanidins	Cherry, strawberry, red wine, aubergine, blackberry, black currant, blue berry, black grape.	Hepatoma cells	Anti-invasive effects and inducion of apoptosis	Shin *et al.*, 2009
EGCG	Flavanols	Apple, cacao, tea, apricot, peach, red wine, Apple, cacao, tea, apricot, peach, red wine	Prostatic, gastric, colon, lung cancer and leukemia	Inhibition of cell migration and invasion. Induction of apoptosis	Hibasami *et al.*, 1996, Horie *et al.*, 2005
Genistein	Isoflavones	Soya beans, legumes	Breast	Target estrogen receptor; Inhibit activation of NF-κB and Akt signaling pathways	Li *et al.*, 2012
Resveratol	Stilbines	Grapes, peanuts, Blueberries	Colon	Inhibit the NF-kB pathway	Ren *et al.*, 2013
Sesamol	Lignans	Sesame oil, sunflower oil	Colon	Anti-metastatic effect	Shimizu *et al.*, 2014

Cell Signaling Pathways in Cancer and its Targeting by Anti-cancer Drugs

Cellular signaling pathways play major role in cell proliferation, cell survival, cell death and cell migration. In tumorigenesis, many molecular alterations are associated with cell signaling pathways, especially which regulates cell proliferation and differentiation [Hanahan *et al.,* 2000]. In addition key regulators, activators, repressors, components or even target genes of different pathways are found to be altered (over expressed or under expressed) in various human cancers. Hence, attenuation of cellular signaling pathways has become an attractive target for anticancer therapy and cancer prevention.

In recent years, much progress has been made on understanding wnt/β-catenin signaling in respect to identifying their modulators or antagonists, which can be useful in cancer chemoprevention. In this review we describe the potential effect of polyphenols by targeting Wnt-β-catenin signaling pathway in chemoprevention of cancer.

Overview of Wnt-β Catenin Signaling

Wnt is an intracellular signaling pathway which regulates diverse range of developmental processes such as differentiation, cell migration and embryogenesis. Initially Wnt signaling was identified for its role in tumor development, later it was recognized to function in embryonic development. Wnts are family of secreted glycoprotein that regulates multiple signaling pathways through β-catenin β-dependent (Often referred as canonical) and β-catenin–independent (often refereed as Non-canonical) mechanisms. Wnt proteins are approximately 350 amino acids in length and have conserved pattern of cysteine residues [Clevers *et al.,* 2006]. So far in mammals 19 Wnt genes have been identified [Miller *et al.,* 2001]. Murine WNT3A was the first purified and biochemically characterized Wnt protein [willert *et al.,* 2003]. The term Wnt was derived from combination of two genes such as *Wingless* gene on Drosophila, which controls segment polarity during larval development [Sharma *et al.,* 1976] and mouse proto-oncogene *Int-1* [Nusse *et al.,* 1982]. Based on the intracellular mediators (β-catenin) they are categorized into canonical Wnt pathway (Wnt/β-catenin pathway) and Non-canonical Wnt pathway (planar cell polarity pathway, Wnt/Ca2+ pathway) [Moon *et al.,* 2002, Akiyama *et al.,* 2000, Mlodzik *et al.,* 2002, Kuhl *et al.,* 2000].

Figure 11.1 represents an overview of the wnt/β-catenin signaling pathway. Wnt/β-Catenin signaling is strongly regulated through Wnt dependent and Wnt-independent mechanisms. The key regulator of this pathway is the 88kDa cytoplasmic glycoprotein known as β-catenin which performs dual function including cell-cell adhesion and canonical Wnt signaling pathway [Bullions *et al.,* 1998]. Mutation and over-expression of β-catenin are associated with many cancers. Wnt-β catenin signaling pathway is triggered upon binding of Wnt protein ligand to seven transmembrane frizzled receptors and co-receptors (LRP 5/6) [Pinson *et al.,* 2000]. This complex transduce the signal into cytoplasm of the cell which is further translocated into the nucleus by β-catenin. On other hand, in the absence of Wnt

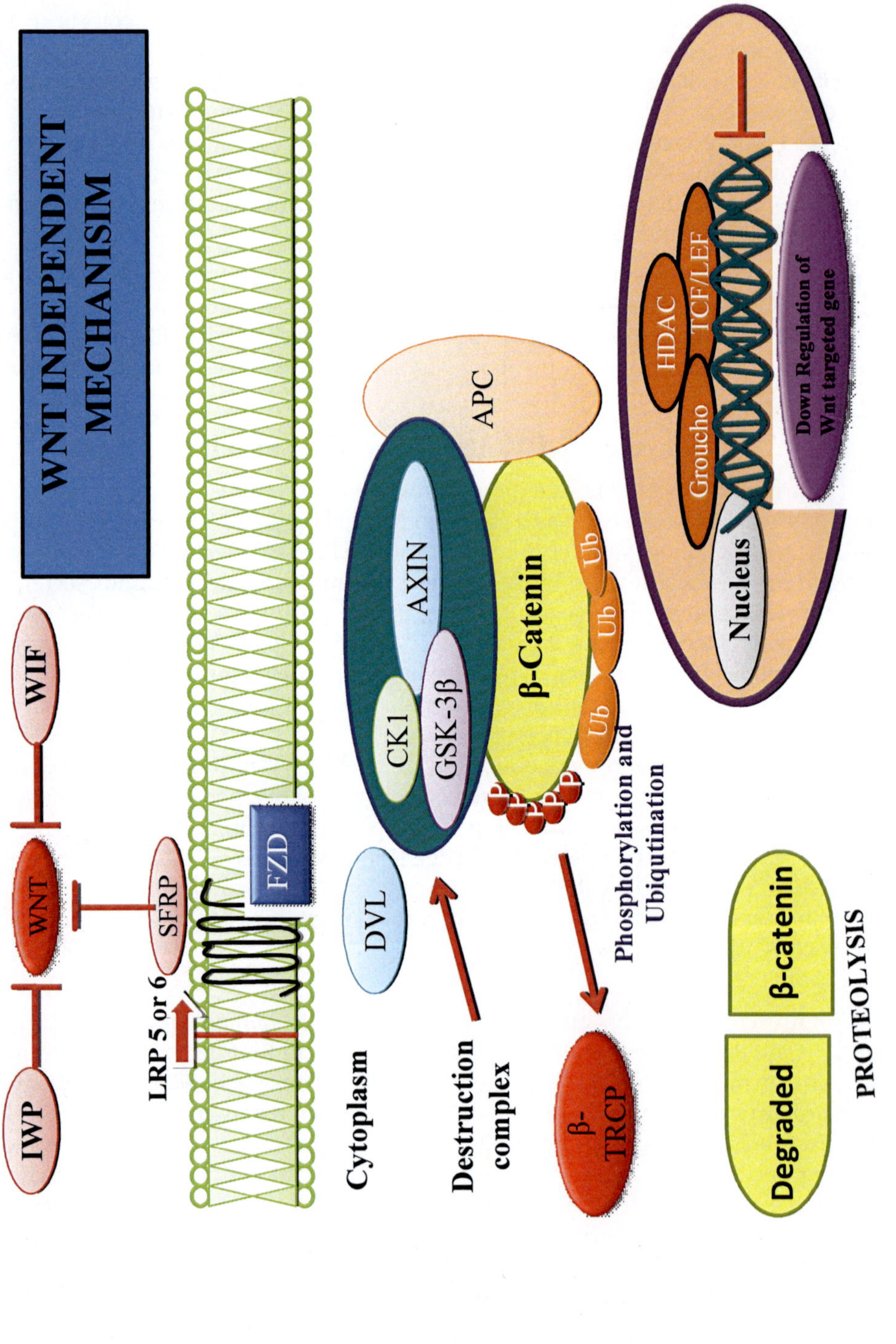
WNT INDEPENDENT MECHANISIM
IWP
WNT
WIF
SFRP
LRP 5 or 6
FZD
Cytoplasm
DVL
CK1
GSK-3β
AXIN
APC
β-Catenin
Ub
Ub
Ub
Ub
P
Phosphorylation and Ubiqutination
Destruction complex
β-TRCP
Degraded
β-catenin
PROTEOLYSIS
Nucleus
Groucho
HDAC
TCF/LEF
Down Regulation of Wnt targeted gene

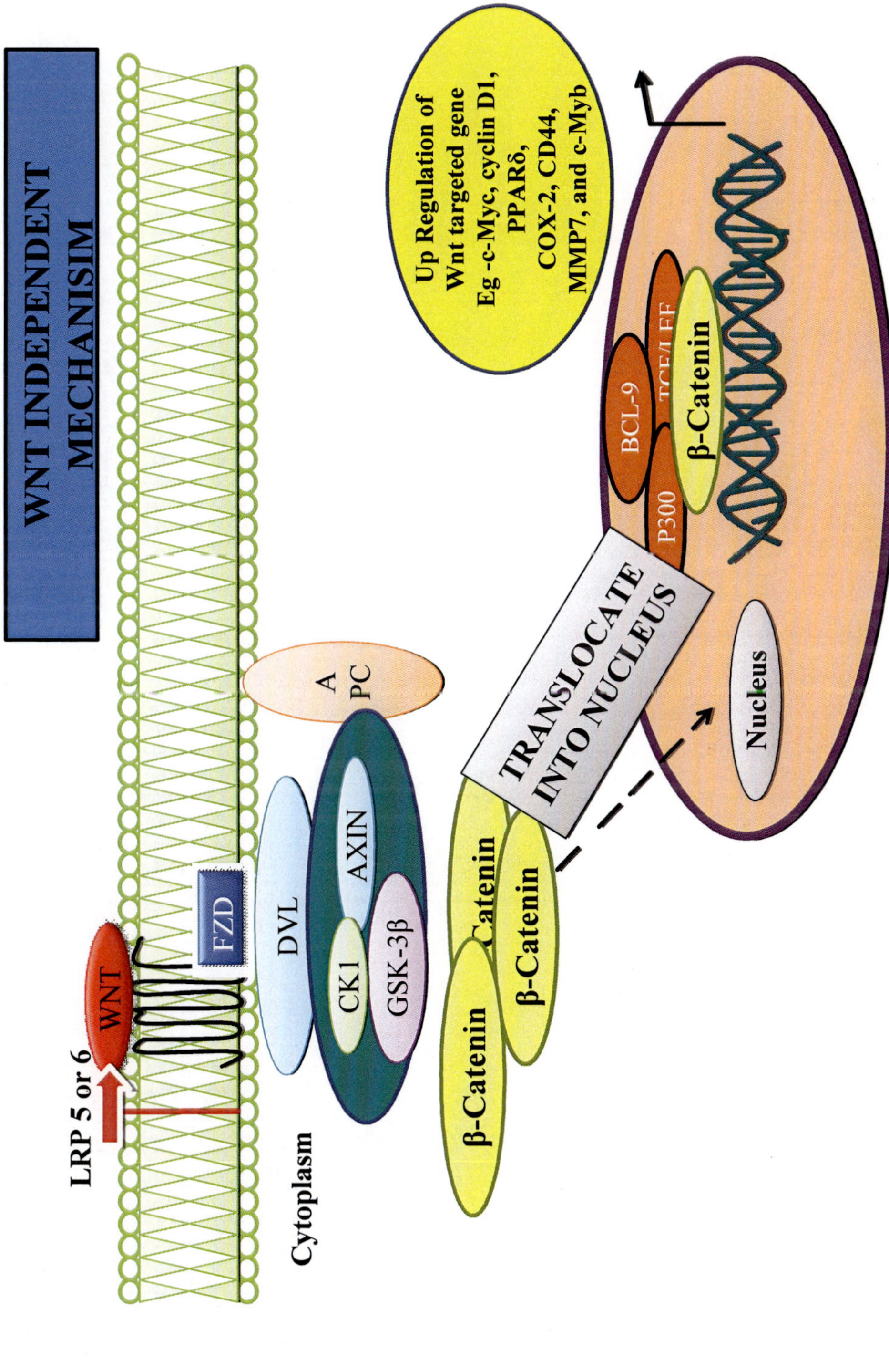
WNT INDEPENDENT MECHANISIM
LRP 5 or 6
WNT
FZD
Cytoplasm
DVL
CK1
GSK-3β
AXIN
A PC
β-Catenin
β-Catenin
β-Catenin
TRANSLOCATE INTO NUCLEUS
Nucleus
P300
BCL-9
β-Catenin
Up Regulation of Wnt targeted gene Eg -c-Myc, cyclin D1, PPARδ, COX-2, CD44, MMP7, and c-Myb

Figure 11.1: Wnt/β-catenin signaling pathway. Wnt/β-catenin signaling pathway mediated by presence and absence of Wnt signals. β-catenin is a cytoplasmic protein perform dual function, it act as a key regulator in Wnt/ β-catenin pathway and play major role in cell-cell adhesion. In the absence of Wnt signals Wnt proteins are inhibited by IWP, SFRP, WIF and cells keep the β-catenin in the cytoplasm at low level. β-catenin was maintained by destruction complex APC, CK, GSK3β and axin. The CK and GSK3β are protein kinase phosphorylate the β-catenin protein. APC and Axin act as a scaffolding protein (localize the β-catenin in cytoplasm). The phosphorylated β-catenin recgoniced by β-TrCP and degraded by proteosomal process. In nucleus Wnt targeted genes are inhibited by Histone De-acetylation (HDAC) process.

Unlike Wnt signals is stimulated it binds to frizilled (Fz) like receptor and co-receptors (LRP5 or 6). This complex recruit Dishevelled protein. The phosphorylated DVL protein inhibit the degradation of β-catenin. The stabilized β-catenin occumulate in cytoplasm and traslocate into nucleus. In nucleus β-catenin binds to transcription factor TCF/LEF and various transcriptional co-factors like BCL-9, P300 and pygopus. As a result various Wnt targeted genes c-Myc, cyclin D1, PPAR Δ, COX-2, CD44, MMP7, and c-Myb are activated.

anticancer property is associated with the induction of apoptosis and inhibition of cell proliferation, metastasis and angiogenesis. Wnt/β-catenin inhibition of luteolin has been reported in human colon cancer. Luteolin decreased the expressions of β-catenin, phosphorylated glycogen synthase kinase-3β, and cyclin D1 expressions at a concentration of 100 μM (IC50) in HCT-15 cells [Pandurangan *et al.*, 2013]. Luteolin inhibit the colon carcinogenesis by decreasing AOM (Azoxymethane)-induced cell proliferation through the involvement of β-catenin, glycogen synthase kinase (GSK)-3β and cyclin D1, the key components in Wnt signaling pathway [Ashokkumar *et al.*, 2011].

Apigenin, also a flavone is abundantly found in common fruits such as grapes, plant-derived beverages and vegetables like parsley, onions, oranges, tea, chamomile and wheat sprouts. Apigenin effectively suppress the prostate carcinogenesis in TRAMP mouse (Transgenic Adenocarcinoma of Mouse) by inhibiting the over accumalation of β-catenin [Shukla *et al.*, 2007]. 3-methoxyapigenin inhibits the β-catenin/LEF transcriptional activity, expression of c-myc and cyclin-D3 in Jurkat leukemic cells [Chuang *et al.*, 2013]. Apigenin reduces the levels of β-catenin and Dsh proteins and accelerates the degradation of β-catenin in the first two hours of treatment, promoting cell cycle arrest in breast cancer cells [Song *et al.*, 2000].

(e) Flavonols - Quercetin and Fisetin

Quercetin is a plant pigment (flavanol) found in red wine, onions, green tea, apples, berries and rich in buckwheat tea. Querecitin has broad spectrum of therapeutic properties which include protection against heart diseases, elevated cholesterol level, blood pressure, diabetes, cataracts, hay fever, peptic ulcer, schizophrenia, inflammation, and asthma. In cancer, quercetin act as apoptosis inducer, block cell cycle and act as anti-metastatic agent [Jakubowicz *et al.*, 2013 Hyeonji *et al.*, 2013 Shan *et al.*, 2009 Bishaye *et al.*, 2013 Shan *et al.*, 2009]. Quercetin directly inhibits the wnt pathway components in cancer cell line. Quercetin reduced β-catenin/Tcf transcriptional activity by about 18-fold. Cyclin D1 and survivin gene were downregulated by quercetin in a dose-dependent manner at both the transcriptional and protein expression levels in colon cancer cell lines. Western blot analysis confirmed that quercetin decreases the nuclear β-catenin and Tcf-4 protein levels in colon cancer cells [Park 2005]. In murine mammary cancer cells, quercetin indirectly inhibit the Wnt/β-catenin pathway by activating the DKK1 (Wnt inhibitor) protein [Park *et al.*, 2005].

Fisetin commonly found in various vegetables and fruits, but abundantly found in strawberries [santi *et al.*, 2002], apples, onions and grapes [Arai *et al.*, 2000]. Treatment of cells with fisetin inhibits the Wnt/β-targeted genes such as cyclin D1 and matrix metalloproteinase 7 (MMP-7) in colon cancer [Suh *et al.*, 2009]. Fisetin-treated melanoma cells showed increased expression level of β-TrCP, Axin and parallelly decreased the expression level of phosphorylated GSK3β and β-catenin [Syed *et al.*, 2011].

(f) Isoflavones, flavonoid - Genistein, Silibinin

Genistein is an isoflavone abundantly found in Soya beans and legumes. It has been reported as Wnt/β-catenin inhibitor in various types of cancer cell lines. Genistein downregulates the Tcf protein and upregulate the Wnt inhibitors like sFRP1, Dkk2, Smad4 in renal cancer cells [Hirata *et al.*, 2013]. Genistein (75μmol/l) decrease the β-catenin level and increase phosphorylated β-catenin in colon cancer cell line. It also increases the Sfrp2 mRNA expression at 4 days treatment [Zhang *et al.*, 2013].

Silibilin, the major active constituents of silymarin possess hepatoprotective property against toxins [Al *et al.*, 2009 Jump *et al.*, 2007]. It also has anticancer property against colon, breast, prostate and lung cancer [Hogan *et al.*, 2007 Sharma *et al.*, 2003]. Silibilin inhibit the migration and invasion property of human melanoma cells by targeting Wnt/β-catenin signaling pathway [Mudit *et al.*, 2011]. In human breast and prostate cancer cells, silibilin inhibits the Wnt/β-catenin signaling pathway by suppressing the Wnt co-receptor LRP6 expression [Lu *et al.*, 2012].

(g) Stilbenoids – Resveratrol

Resveratrol (3, 5, 4′-trihydroxystilbene) is a polyphenolic phytoalexin. It is a stilbenoid, a derivate of stilbene produced by plants with the help of the enzyme stilbene synthase [Hain *et al.*, 1990]. In mouse and rat experiments, anti-cancer, anti-inflammatory and blood-sugar-lowering effects of resveratrol have been reported [Anupam *et al.*, 2009 Lee *et al.*, 2009]. Resveratrol has been shown to inhibit the invasion and metastasis property of colon cancer by inhibiting the expression of c-Myc, MMP-7, as well as MALAT1 [Ji *et al.*, 2013]. Resveratrol inhibit the Wnt/β-catenin signaling pathway in colon cancer by distrupting the binding of β-catenin and TCF4 [Chen *et al.*, 2012]. In SW480 cells, resveratrol decrease the cyclin A, cyclin B1, and β-catenin expression levels within 24 h treatment [Joe *et al.*, 2002]. In colon cancer, at a lowest concentration (10μM), resveratrol inhibit the Wnt/β-catenin signaling pathway [Hope *et al.*, 2008]. In combinational therapy, resveratrol and resveratrol-containing freeze-dried grape powder (GP) effectively inhibit the Wnt pathway in colon cancer [Anthony *et al.*, 2009].

Other Polyphenols

(h) Curcuminoids - Curcumin

Curcumin is a yellow phenolic active ingredient present in turmeric *(Curcuma longa, zingiberaceae)*, and in limited amounts in Ginger. Curcumin is a lipophilic polyphenol and thus is insoluble in water, but is readily soluble in organic solvents such as dimethylsulfoxide, acetone and ethanol. Curcumin has been used extensively in Ayurvedic medicine for centuries, as it is nontoxic and has a variety of therapeutic properties including anti-oxidant, analgesic, anti-inflammatory and antiseptic activities. More recently curcumin has been found to possess anti-cancer activities via its effect on a variety of biological pathways involved in mutagenesis, oncogene expression (Li *et al.*, 2007), cell cycle regulation (Lim *et al.*, 2014), apoptosis (Chang *et al.*, 2013), tumorigenesis and metastasis (Killian *et al.*, 2012).

In Wnt/β-catenin signaling pathway, curcumin inhibits the nuclear translocation of β-catenin protein in HEK293T osteosarcoma cells (Leow *et al.*, 2014). In mouse xenograft model, curcumin inhibit nuclear β-catenin transcription activity and enhance the levels of membrane β-catenin in prostate cancer cells (Vasudha *et al.*, 2012). In colon cancer, curcumin attenuates the Wnt/β-catenin signaling by decreasing the amount of the transcriptional coactivator p300 (Ryu *et al.,* 2008). Curcumin and their derivatives reduce the nuclear β-catenin and Tcf-4 proteins in SW620 cells (park *et al.,* 2005). Treatment of curcumin in breast cancer cells inhibits the Wnt target genes c-myc, c-fos, c-jun and iNOS (Prasad *et al.,* 2009).

(i) Lignans

Lignans are the plant diphenolic compounds found in flaxseed, sesame seed, sunflower, peanut and Cashew. Plant lignans most commonly detected in foods are lariciresinol, matairesinol, pinoresinol and secoisolariciresinol (Milder *et al.,* 2005). Recently lignans were found to be inhibit the Wnt/β-catenin signaling pathway in cancer. The anticancer activity of Hydocarpin, isolated from the aerial parts of *Lonicera japonica* (Caprifoliaceae) (son *et al.,* 1992) is associated with the suppression of Wnt/β-catenin signaling pathway through increasing the stability of axin in cytoplasm (Lee *et al.,* 2013). Arctigenin found in certain plants in the family of asteraceae decreases the transcriptional activity of a TCF binding element (TBE) and reduces β-catenin level by inducing phosphorylation in SW480 cells (Yoo *et al.,* 2010). Magnolol inhibited the nuclear translocation of β-catenin and significantly suppressed the binding of β-catenin/TCF complexes onto their specific DNA-binding sites in the nucleus in colon cancer cells (Kang *et al.,* 2012).

Conclusion

In the last decades, research efforts has increased on preventing cancer by targeting specific signaling pathways related to cell proliferation, apoptosis and cell migration. Identifying modulators or antagonist against cell signaling pathway from natural sources is an attractive approach in chemoprevention of cancer. However, emerging findings suggest that polyphenols has the ability to prevent cancer by modulating cell signaling pathways in cancer. Approximately 8000 different polyphenols are identified from dietary sources. Diversity in their structure is a major factor for anticancer property of polyphenols. Polyphenols are capable of interacting with key regulators in cell signaling pathway. The present review has highlighted that polyphenols are capable of interacting with Wnt/β-catenin signaling pathway. Several components in Wnt/β-catenin signaling pathway are over-expressed or under-expressed in various types of cancers, which offers attractive targets for prevention of cancer.

Wnt/β-catenin signaling pathway cross link with various other pathways like MAP kinase (Ishitani *et al.,* 1999), AKT, Ca++/calmodulin kinase II (Kuhl *et al.,* 2000), TGFβ (Nishita *et al.,* 2000), PKC and retinoid signaling pathways (Easwaran *et al.,* 1999). Targeting Wnt/β-catenin signaling pathway also affects these signaling pathways, which may increase prevention of cancer in a very effective manner. The experimental and clinical results show that single polyphenol is capable of inhibiting various Wnt/β-catenin signaling components in many of cancers. For instance, resveratrol inhibits β-catenin, c-Myc, MMP-7, TCF4 and cyclin A against various cancers, which clearly shows the Structure Activity Relationship (SAR) of polyphenols. These observations also strongly suggest that structure is a key regulator for anticancer mechanism of polyphenols. From this study we conclude that polyphenols are the superior modulators of Wnt/β-catenin signaling pathway and targeting Wnt/β-catenin signaling is an effective approach in treating the cancer.

Acknowledgements

The authors gratefully acknowledge the use of the Bioinformatics Infrastructure Facility, Alagappa University funded by the Department of Biotechnology, Ministry of Science and Technology, Government of India (No. BT/BI/04/055/2001).

Abbreviations

APC: Adenomatous Polyposis Coil

CK1: Casein Kinase 1

DDK: Dickkopf proteins

DSH: Dishevlled Protein

LEF: Lymphoid Enhancer factor

Tcf: T cell specific factor

SFRP1: Secreated Frizzled Related Protein 1.

References

Aberle, H., Bauer A., Stappert, J., Kispert, A., and Kemler, R. (1997). B-catenin is a target for the ubiquitin-proteasome pathway. *Embo J.*, **16**: 3797-804.

Adhami, VM., Siddiqui, IA., Ahmad, N., Gupta, S., and Mukhtar, H. (2004). Oral consumption of green tea polyphenols inhibits insulin-like growth factor-I-induced signaling in an autochthonous mouse model of prostate cancer. *Cancer Res.*, **64**: 8715–8722.

Akiyama, T. (2000). Wnt/β-catenin signaling. *Cytokine Growth Factor Rev.*, **11**: 273–82.

Al-Anati, L., Essid, E., Reinehr, R., and Petzinger, E. (2009). Silibinin protects OTA-mediated TNF-α release from perfused rat livers and isolated rat Kupffer cells. *Mol Nutr Food Res.*, **53**: 460–6.

Alyssa, G. Schuck., Jeffrey, H. Weisburg., Hannah, Esan., Esther, F. Robin., Ayelet, R. Bersson., Jordana, R. Weitschner., Tova Lahasky., Harriet, L. Zuckerbraun., and Harvey Babich. (2013). Cytotoxic and proapoptotic activities of gallic acid to human oral cancer HSC-2 cells. *Oxid Antioxid Med Sci.*, **2**: 265-274.

Andrew, K. Joe., Hui, Liu., Masumi Suzui., Muhammet, E. Vural., Danhua Xiao., and I. Bernard Weinstein. (2002). Resveratrol Induces Growth Inhibition, S-phase Arrest, Apoptosis, and Changes in Biomarker Expression in Several Human Cancer Cell Lines. *Clin Cancer Res.*, **8**: 893-903.

Anupam Bishayee. (2009). Cancer Prevention and Treatment with Resveratrol: From Rodent Studies to Clinical Trials. *Cancer Prev Res.*, **2**: 409-418.

Arai, Y., Watanabe, S., Kimira, M., Shimoi, K., Mochizuki, R., and Kinae, N. (2000). Dietary intakes of flavonols, flavones and isoflavones by Japanese women and the inverse correlation between quercetin intake and plasma LDL cholesterol concentration. *J Nutr.*, 1**30**: 2243–2250.

Arts, I.C., and Hollman P.C. (2005). Polyphenols and disease risk in epidemiologic studies. *Am J Clin Nutr.*, **81**: 317-325.

Ashokkumar, P., and Sudhandiran, G (2011). Luteolin inhibits cell proliferation during Azoxymethane-induced experimental colon carcinogenesis via Wnt/β-catenin pathway. *Invest New Drugs*, **29**: 273-84.

Bagli, E., Stefaniotou, M., Morbidelli, L., Ziche, M., Psillas, K., Murphy, C., and Fotsis, T (2004). Luteolin inhibits vascular endothelial growth factor-induced angiogenesis; inhibition of endothelial cell survival and proliferation by targeting phosphatidylinositol 32-kinase activity. *Cancer Res.*, **64**: 7936–7946.

Bakker, ER., Das, AM., Helvensteijn, W., Franken, PF., Swagemakers, S., van der Valk, MA., Ten Hagen, TL., Kuipers, EJ., van Veelen, W., and Smits, R (2013). Wnt5a promotes human colon cancer cell migration and invasion but does not augment intestinal tumorigenesis in Apc1638N mice. *Carcinogenesis*, **34**: 2629-38.

Baliga, MS., Meleth, S., and Katiyar, SK (2005). Growth inhibitory and antimetastatic effect of green tea polyphenols on metastasisspecific mouse mammary carcinoma 4T1 cells *in vitro* and *in vivo* systems. *Clin Cancer Res.*, **11**: 1918-27.

Baur, JA., and Sinclair, DA. (2006). Therapeutic potential of resveratrol: the *in vivo* evidence. *Nat. Rev. Drug Discov.*, **5**: 493–506.

Bettuzzi, S., Brausi, M., Rizzi, F., Castagnetti, G., Peracchia, G., and Corti, A. (2006). Chemoprevention of human prostate cancer by oral administration of green tea catechins in volunteers with high-grade prostate intraepithelial neoplasia: a preliminary report from a one-year proof-of-principle study. *Cancer Res.*, **66**: 1234–1240.

Bettuzzi, S., Rizzi, F., and Belloni, L. (2007). Clinical relevance of the inhibitory effect of green tea catechins (GtCs) on prostate cancer progression in combination with molecular profiling of catechinresistant tumors: an integrated view. *Pol J Vet Sci.*, 1**0**: 57–60.

Bhatia, N., Zhao, J., Wolf, DM., and Agarwal, R. (1999). Inhibition of human carcinoma cell growth and DNA synthesis by silibinin, an active constituent of milk thistle: comparison with silymarin. *Cancer Lett.*, 1**47**: 77–84.

Bishayee, A. (2009). Cancer prevention and treatment with resveratrol: from rodent studies to clinical trials. *Cancer Prev Res(Phila).*, **2**: 409–418.

Bishayee, K., Ghosh, S., Mukherjee, A., Sadhukhan, R., Mondal, J., and Khuda-Bukhsh, AR. (2013). Quercetin induces cytochrome-c release and ROS accumulation to promote apoptosis and arrest the cell cycle in G2/M, in cervical carcinoma: signal cascade and drug-DNA interaction. *Cell Prolif.*, **46**: 153-63.

Braganhol, E., Zamin, L., Canedo, AD., Horn, F., Tamajusuku, AS., Wink, MR., Salbego, C., and Battastini, AM. (2006). Antiproliferative effect of quercetin in the human U138MG glioma cell line. *Anticancer Drugs*, **17**: 663–71.

Brusselmans, K., de Schrijver, E., Heyns, W., Verhoeven, G., and Swinnen, J. (2003). Epigallocatechin-3- gallate is a potent natural inhibitor of fatty acid synthase in intact cells and selectively induces apoptosis in prostate cancer cells. *Int J Cancer*, **106**: 856–62.

Bryan, T. MacDonald., Keiko Tamai., Xi He. (2009). Wnt/β-catenin signaling: components, mechanisms, and diseases. *Dev. Cell*, **17**: 9–26.

Bullions, LC., and Levine, AJ. (1998). The role of β-catenin in cell adhesion, signal transduction, and cancer. *Curr Opin Oncol.*, **10**: 81– 87.

Cardoso, LC., De Souza, KR., De O Reis, AH., Andrade, RC., Britto AC, Jr., De Lima, MA., Dos Santos, AC., De Faria, PS., Ferman, S., Seuanez, HN., and Vargas, FR. (2013). WT1, WTX and CTNNB1 mutation analysis in 43 patients with sporadic Wilms' tumor. *Oncol Rep.*, **29**: 315-320.

Chang, Z., Xing, J., and Yu, X. (2013). Curcumin induces osteosarcoma MG63 cells apoptosis via ROS/Cyto-C/Caspase-3 pathway. *Tumor Biol.*, **35**: 753-8.

Chen, C., Shen, G., Hebbar, V., Hu, R., Owuor, E., and Kong, A. (2003). Epigallocatechin-3-gallate-inducedstress signals in HT-29 human colon adenocarcinoma cells. *Carcinogenesis*, **24**: 1369–78.

Chen, HJ., Hsu, LS., Shia, YT., Lin, MW., and Lin, CM. (2012). The β-catenin/TCF complex as a novel target of resveratrol in the Wnt/β-catenin signaling pathway. *Biochem Pharmacol.*, 1: 1143-53.

Cheng, A-C., Huang, T-C., Lai, C-S., and Pan, M-H. (2005). Induction of apoptosis by luteolin through cleavage of Bcl-2 family in human leukemia HL-60 cells. *Eur. J. Pharmacol.*, **509**: 1–10.

Che-Pin, Lin., Chien-Ru, Liu., Chun-Nin, Lee., Tze-Sian, Chan., H., and Eugene Liu. (2010). Targeting c-Myc as a novel approach for hepatocellular carcinoma. *World J Hepatol.*, **2**: 16-20.

Chesire, DR., Ewing, CM., Sauvageot, J., Bova, GS., and Isaacs, WB. (2000). Detection and analysis of β-catenin mutations in prostate cancer. *Prostate*, **45**: 323–334.

Chuang, KA., Lieu, CH., Tsai, WJ., Huang, WH., Lee, AR., and Kuo, YC. (2013). 3-Methoxyapigenin modulates β-catenin stability and inhibits Wnt/β-catenin signaling in Jurkat leukemic cells. *Life Sci.*, **92**: 677-86.

Clevers, H. (2006). Wnt/β-catenin signaling in development and disease. *Cell*, **127**: 469–480.

Conney, AH., Lu, Y., Lou, Y., Xie, J., and Huang, M. (1999). Inhibitory effect of green and black tea on tumor growth. *Proc Soc Exp Biol Med.*, **220**: 229–233.

Dang, C. V. (1999). c-Myc target genes involved in cell growth, apoptosis, and metabolism. *Mol. Cell Biol.*, **19**: 1-11.

Dashwood, WM., Orner, GA., and Dashwood, RH. (2002). Inhibition of β-catenin/Tcf activity by white tea, green tea, and epigallocatechin-3-gallate (EGCG): minor contribution of H(2)O(2) at physiologically relevant EGCG concentrations. *Biochem Biophys Res Commun.*, **296**: 584–8.

De Santi, C., Pietrabissa, A., Mosca, F., and Pacifici, G. M. (2002). Methylation of quercetin and fisetin, flavonoids widely distributed in edible vegetables, fruits and wine, by human liver. *Int J Clin Pharmacol Ther.*, **40**: 207–212.

Deep, G., and Agarwal, R. (2010). Antimetastatic efficacy of silibinin: molecular mechanisms and therapeutic potential against cancer. *Cancer Metastasis Rev.*, **29**: 447–63.

Demeule, M., Brossard, M., Page, M., Gingras, D., and Beliveau, R. (2000). Matrix metalloproteinase inhibition by green tea catechins. *Biochim Biophys Acta.*, **1478**: 51–60.

Ding, X., Yang, Y., Han, B., Du, C., Xu, N., H, Huang., T, Cai., A, Zhang., Ze, Han., W, Zhou., and L, Chen. (2014). Transcriptomic Characterization of Hepatocellular Carcinoma with CTNNB1 Mutation. *PLoS ONE*, **9**: e95307.

Dreosti, IE., Wargovich, MJ., and Yang, CS. (1997). Inhibition of carcinogenesis by tea: the evidence from experimental studies. *Crit Rev Food Sci Nutr.*, **37**: 761–770.

Easwaran, V., Pishvaian, M., and Salimuddin, BS (1999). Cross-regulation of β-catenin-LEF/TCF and retinoid signaling pathways. *Curr.Biol.*, **9**: 1415-1418.

Erika A. Waters, Kathleen A. Cronin, Barry I. Graubard, Paul K. Han, and Andrew N.Freedman. (2010). Prevalence of tamoxifen use for breast cancer chemoprevention among U.S. women. *Cancer Epidemiol Biomarkers Prev.*, **19**: 443–446.

Fabiani, R., De Bartolomeo, A., Rosignoli, P., Servili, M., Montedoro, GF., and Morozzi, G. (2002). Cancer chemoprevention by hydroxytyrosol isolated from virgin olive oil through G1 cell cycle arrest and apoptosis. *Eur J Cancer Prev.*, **11**: 351-8.

Facchini, A., Zanella, B., Stefanelli, C., Guarnieri, C., and Flamigni, F. (2003). Effect of green tea extract on the induction of ornithine decarboxylase and the activation of extracellular signal-regulated kinase in bladder carcinoma ECV304 cells. *Nutr Cancer*, **47**: 104–110.

Fan, S., Cherney, B., Reinhold, W., Rucker, K., and Connor, PM. (1998). Disruption of P53 function in immortalized human cells does not affect survival or apoptosis after Taxol or Vincristine treatment. *Clin Cancer Res.*, **4**: 1047-1054.

Fei-jun, Luo., Zhi, Hu., Xi-yun, Deng., Yan, Zhao., Liang, Zeng., Zi-gang, Dong., Wei, Yi., and Ya, Cao. (2001). Effect of tea polyphenols and EGCG on nasopharyngeal carcinoma cell proliferation and the mechanisms involved. *Chin J Cancer Res.*, **13**: 235–242.

Foldynova-Trantirkova, S., Sekyrova, P., Tmejova, K., Brumovsk, E., Bernatik, O., Blankenfeldt, W., Krejci, P., Kozubik, A., Dolezal, T., Trantirek, L., and Bryja, V. (2010). Breast cancer-specific mutations in CK1epsilon inhibit Wnt/β-catenin and activate the Wnt/Rac1/JNK and NFAT pathways to decrease cell adhesion and promote cell migration. *Breast Cancer Res.*, **12**: R30.

Fukutake, M., Takahashi, M., Ishida, K., Kawamura, H., Sugimura, T., and Wakabayashi, K. (1996). Quantification of genistein and genistin in soybeans and soybean products. *Food Chem Toxicol.*, **34**: 457-61.

Gao, Z., Xu, Z., Hung, MS., Lin, YC., Wang, T., Gong, M., Zhi, X., Jablon, DM., and You, L. (2009). Promoter demethylation of WIF-1 by epigallocatechin-3-gallate in lung cancer cells. *Anticancer Res.*, **29**: 2025–30.

Gerstein, AV., Almeida, TA., Zhao, G., Chess, E., Shih, IeM., Buhler, K., Pienta, K., Rubin, MA., Vessella, R., and Papadopoulos, N. (2002). APC/CTNNB1 (β-catenin) pathway alterations in human prostate cancers. *Genes Chromosomes Cancer*, **34**: 9–16.

Granados-Principal, S., Quiles, JL., Ramirez-Tortosa, C., Camacho-Corencia, P., Sanchez-Rovira, P., Vera-Ramirez, L., and Ramirez-Tortosa, MC. (2011). Hydroxytyrosol inhibits growth and cell proliferation and promotes high expression of sfrp4 in rat mammary tumors. *Mol Nutr Food Res.*, **55**: 117-26.

Grunberger, D., Banerjee, R., Eisinger, K., Oltz, E.M., Efros, L., Caldwell, M., Estevez, V., and Nakanishi, K. (1988). Preferential cytotoxicity on tumor cells by caffeic acid phenethyl ester isolated from propolis. *Experientia*, **44**: 230-232.

Hain, R., Bieseler, B., Kindl, H., Schroder, G., and Stocker, R. (1990). Expression of a stilbene synthase gene in Nicotiana tabacum results in synthesis of the phytoalexin resveratrol. *Plant Mol Biol.*, 1**5**: 325-35.

Hanahan, D., and Weinberg, RA. (2000). The hallmarks of cancer. *Cell*, **100**: 57–70.

Hart, MJ., de los Santos, R., Albert, IN., Rubinfeld, B., and Polakis, P. (1998). Downregulation of β-catenin by human Axin and its association with the APC tumor suppressor, β-catenin and GSK3 β. *Curr Biol.*, **8**: 573–81.

Hassan, Z.K., Elamin, M.H., Daghestani, M.H., Omer, S.A., Al-Olayan, E.M., Elobeid, M.A., Virk, P., and Mohammed, OB. (2012). Oleuropein Induces Anti-metastatic Effects in Breast Cancer. *Asian Pacific J Cancer Prev.*, 1**3**: 4555-4559.

He, Y.J., Liu, B.H., Xiang, D.B., Qiao, Z.Y., Fu, T., and He, Y.H. (2006). Inhibitory effect of caffeic acid phenethyl ester on the growth of SW480 colorectal tumor cells involves β-catenin associated signaling pathway down-regulation. *World J Gastroenterol.*, 1**2**: 4981-5.

Hibasami, H., Achiwa, Y., Fujikawa, T., and Komiya, T. (1996). Induction of programmed cell death(apoptosis) in human lymphoid leukemia cells by catechin compounds. *Anticancer Res.*, 1**6**: 1943–6.

Hirata, H., Ueno, K., Nakajima, K., Tabatabai, ZL., Hinoda, Y., Ishii, N., and Dahiya, R. (2013). Genistein downregulates onco-miR-1260b and inhibits Wnt-signalling in renal cancer cells. *Br J Cancer*, **108**: 2070-8.

Hogan, FS., Krishnegowda, NK., Mikhailova, M., and Kahlenberg, MS. (2007). Flavonoid, silibinin, inhibits proliferation and promotes cell-cycle arrest of human colon cancer. *J Surg Res.*, 1**43**: 58–65.

Hope, C., Planutis, K., Planutiene, M., Moyer, MP., Johal, KS., Woo, J., Santoso, C., Hanson, JA., and Holcombe, RF. (2008). Low concentrations of resveratrol inhibit Wnt signal throughput in colon-derived cells: implications for colon cancer prevention. *Mol Nutr Food Res.*, **52**: 52-61.

Horie, N., Hirabayashi, N., Takahashi, Y., Miyauchi, Y., Taguchi, H., and Takeishi, K. (2005). Synergistic effect of green tea catechins on cell growth and apoptosis induction in gastric carcinoma cells. *Biol Pharm Bull.*, **28**: 574–9.

Hosokawa, N., Hosokawa, Y., Sakai, T., Yoshida, M., Marui, N., Nishino, H., Kawai, K., and Aoike, A. (1990). Inhibitory effect of quercetin on the synthesis of a possibly cell-cycle-related 17-kDa protein, in human colon cancer cells. *Int J Cancer*, **45**: 1119–24.

Hyeonji, Kim., Jeong Yong Moon., Kwang Seok Ahn., and Somi Kim Cho. (2013). Quercetin Induces Mitochondrial Mediated Apoptosis and Protective Autophagy in Human Glioblastoma U373MG Cells. *Oxid Med Cell Longev*, Article ID 596496.

Ishitani, T., Ninomiya-Tsuji, J., Nagai, S., Nishita, M., Meneghini, M., Barker, N., Waterman M., Bowerman B., Clevers H., Shibuya H., and Matsumoto K (1999). The TAK1-NLK-MAPK-related pathway antagonizes signalling between β-catenin and transcription factor TCF. *Nature*, **399**: 798-802.

Iwai, S., Katagiri, W., Kong, C., Amekawa, S., Nakazawa, M., and Yura, Y. (2005). Mutations of the APC, β-catenin, and axin 1 genes and cytoplasmic accumulation of β-catenin in oral squamous cell carcinoma. *J Cancer Res Clin Oncol.*, **131**: 773-82.

Jakubowicz-Gil, J., Langner, E., B[1]dziul, D., Wertel, I., and Rzeski, W. (2013). Apoptosis induction in human glioblastoma multiforme T98G cells upon temozolomide and quercetin treatment. *Tumor Biol.*, **34**: 2367-78.

Ji, Q., Liu, X., Fu, X., Zhang, L., Sui, H., L, Zhou., J, Sun., J, Cai., J, Qin., J, Ren., and Q, Li. (2013). Resveratrol Inhibits Invasion and Metastasis of Colorectal Cancer Cells via MALAT1 Mediated Wnt/β-Catenin Signal Pathway.*PLoS ONE*, **8**: e78700.

Johnson, JJ., Bailey, HH., and Mukhtar, H. (2010). Green tea polyphenols for prostate cancer chemo-prevention: a translational perspective. *Phytomedicine*, **17**: 3–13.

Jump up Jayaraj, R., Deb, U., Bhaskar, AS., Prasad, GB., and Rao, PV. (2007). Hepatoprotective efficacy of certain flavonoids against microcystin induced toxicity in mice. *Environ Toxicol.*, **22**: 472–9.

Kane, RC., Farrell, AT., Sridhara, R., and Pazdur, R. (2006). United States Food and Drug Administration approval summary: bortezomib for the treatment of progressive multiple myeloma after one prior therapy. *Clin Cancer Res.*, **12**: 2955–2960.

Kang, YJ., Park, HJ., Chung, HJ., Min, HY., Park, EJ., Lee, MA., Shin, Y., and Lee, SK. (2012). Wnt/β-catenin signaling mediates the antitumor activity of magnolol in colorectal cancer cells. *Mol. Pharmacol.*, **82**: 168-77.

Kidani, T., Nakamura, A., Kamei, S., Norimatsu, Y., Miura, H., and Masuno, H (2014). Overexpression of cytoplasmic β-catenin inhibits the metastasis of the murine osteosarcoma cell line LM8. *Cancer Cell Int.*, **14**: 31.

Killian, PH., Kronski, E., Michalik, KM., Barbieri, O., Astigiano, S., Sommerhoff, CP., Pfeffer U., Nerlich AG., and Bachmeier BE (2102). Curcumin inhibits prostate cancer metastasis in vivo by targeting the inflammatory cytokines CXCL1 and -2. *Carcinogenesis*, **33**: 2507-19.

Kim, H., Lee, MJ., Kim, JE., Park, SD., Moon, HI., and Park, WH (2010). Genistein suppresses tumor necrosis factor-α-induced proliferation via the apoptotic signaling pathway in human aortic smooth muscle cells. *J Agric Food Chem.*, **58**: 2015–9.

Kim, J., Zhang, X., Rieger-Christ, KM., Summerhayes, IC., Wazer, DE., Paulson, KE., and Yee, AS. (2006). Suppression of Wnt signaling by the green tea compound (–)-epigallocatechin 3-gallate (EGCG) in invasive breast cancer cells. Requirement of the transcriptional repressor HBP1. *J Biol Chem.*, **281**: 10865–75.

Kishida, S., Yamamoto, H., Ikeda, S., Kishida, M., Sakamoto, I., Koyama, S., and Kikuchi, A (1998). Axin, a negative regulator of the Wnt signaling pathway, directly interacts with adenomatous polyposis coli and regulates the stabilization of β-catenin. *J Biol Chem.*, **273**: 10823–6.

Koesters, R., Ridder, R., Kopp-Schneider, A., Betts, D., Adams, V., Niggli, F., Briner, J., and von Knebel Doeberitz, M (1999). Mutational activation of the β-catenin protooncogene is a common event in the development of Wilms' tumors. *Cancer Res.*, **59**: 3880–3882

Korinek, V., Barker, N., Morin, PJ., van Wichen, D., de Weger, R., Kinzler, KW., Vogelstein, B., and Clevers H (1997). Constitutive transcriptional activation by a β-catenin-Tcf complex in APC"/" colon carcinoma. *Science*, **275**: 1784–1787.

Kuhl, M., Sheldahl, L.C., Malbon, C.C., and Moon, R.T. (2000). Ca(2+)/calmodulin-dependent protein kinase II is stimulated by Wnt and Frizzled homologs and promotes ventral cell fates inXenopus. *J. Biol. Chem.*, **275**: 12701-12711.

Kuhl, M., Sheldahl, L.C., Park, M., Miller, J.R., and Moon, R.T. (2000). The Wnt/Ca^{2+} pathway: a new vertebrate Wnt signaling pathway takes shape. *Trends Genet.*, **16**: 279–83.

Kusafuka, T., Miao, J., Kuroda, S., Udatsu, Y., and Yoneda, A. (2002). Codon 45 of the β-catenin gene, a specific mutational target site of Wilms' tumor. *Int. J. Mol. Med.*, **10**: 395–399.

Lee, M., Kim, S., Kwon, O.K., Oh, S.R., Lee, H.K., and Ahn, K. (2009). Anti-inflammatory and anti-asthmatic effects of resveratrol, a polyphenolic stilbene, in a mouse model of allergic asthma. *Int Immunopharmacol.*, **9**: 418-24.

Lee, M.A., Kim, W.K., Park, H.J., Kang, S.S., and Lee, S.K. (2013). Anti-proliferative activity of hydnocarpin, a natural lignan, is associated with the suppression of Wnt/b-catenin signaling pathway in colon cancer cells. *Bioorg. Med. Chem. Lett.*, **23**: 5511–5514.

Lee, S.C., Chan, W.K., Lee, T.W., Lam, W.H., Wang, X., Chan, T.H., and Wong, Y.C. (2008). Effect of a prodrug of the green tea polyphenol (–)-epigallocatechin-3-gallate on the growth of androgen-independent prostate. *Nutr Cancer*, **60**: 483-91.

Leow, P.C., Bahety, P., Boon, C.P., Lee, C.Y., Tan, K.L., Yang, T., and Ee, P.L. (2014). Functionalized curcumin analogs as potent modulators of the Wnt/β-catenin signaling pathway. *Eur J Med Chem.*, **71**: 67-80.

Li, H.Q., Luo, Y., and Qiao, C.H. (2012). The mechanisms of anticancer agents by genistein and synthetic derivatives of isoflavone. *Mini Rev Med Chem.*, **12**: 350-62.

Li, M., Zhang, Z., Hill, D.L., Wang, H., and Zhang, R. (2007). Curcumin, a dietary component, has anticancer, chemosensitization, and radiosensitization effects by down-regulating the MDM2 oncogene through the PI3K/mTOR/ETS2 pathway. *Cancer Res.*, **67**: 1988-96.

Li-Hua, Jin., Qiu-Jie, Shao., Wen, Luol., Zhi-Yun, Yel., Qing, Li., and Sheng-Cai, Lin. (2003). Detection of point mutations of the Axin1 gene in colorectal cancers. *Int J Cancer*, **107**: 696–699.

Lim, T.G., Lee, S.Y., Huang, Z., Lim do, Y., Chen, H., Jung, S.K., Bode, A.M., Lee, K.W., and Dong, Z. (2014). Curcumin suppresses proliferation of colon cancer cells by targeting CDK2. *Cancer Prev Res (Phila).*, **7**: 466-74

Lopez-Lazaro, M. (2010). A new view of carcinogenesis and an alternative approach to cancer therapy. *Mol Med.*, **16**: 144-153.

Lu, W., Lin, C., King, T.D., Chen, H., Reynolds, R.C., and Li, Y. (2012). Silibinin inhibits Wnt/β-catenin signaling by suppressing Wnt co-receptor LRP6 expression in human prostate and breast cancer cells. *Cell Signal*, **24**: 2291-6.

Mahmoud, N.N., Carothers, A.M., Grunberger, D., Bilinski, R.T., Churchill, M.R., Martucci, C., Newmark, H.L., and Bertagnolli, M.M. (2000). Plant phenolics decrease intestinal tumors in an animal model of familial adenomatous polyposis. *Carcinogenesis*, **21**: 921–927.

Maiti, S., Alam, R., Amos, C.I., and Huff, V. (2000). Frequent association of β-catenin and WT1 mutations in Wilms tumors. *Cancer Res.*, **60**: 6288–6292.

Margaret, M. (2003). Cancer prevention – the potential for diet to modulate molecular signaling. *Trends Mol Med.*, **9**: 11-8.

Masuda, M., Suzui, M., Lim, J.T., and Weinstein, I.B. (2003). Epigallocatechin-3-gallate inhibits activation of HER-2/neu and downstream signaling pathways in human head and neck and breast carcinomacells. *Clin Cancer Res.*, **9**: 3486–3491.

McDonald, S.L., and Silver, A. (2009). The opposing roles of Wnt-5a in cancer. *Br J Cancer*, **101**: 209–14.

Miean, K.H., and Mohamed, S. (2001). Flavonoid (myricetin, quercetin, kaempferol, luteolin, and apigenin) content of edible tropical plants. *J. Agric. Food Chem.*, **49**: 3106–3112

Milder, I.E., Arts, I.C., van de Putte, B., Venema, D.P., and Hollman, P.C. (2005). Lignan contents of Dutch plant foods: A database including lariciresinol, pinoresinol, secoisolariciresinol and matairesinol. *Br. J. Nutr.*, **93**, 393–402.

Miller, J.R. (2002). The Wnts. *Genome Biol.*, **3**: reviews 3001.

Mitsuyo Noguchi., Masatoshi Yokoyaman., Sumiko Watanabe., Michiko Uchiyama., Yoshifumi Nakao., Kouichi Hara., and Tsuyoshi Iwasaka. (2006). Inhibitory effect of the tea polyphenol, (–)-epigallocatechin gallate, on growth of cervical adenocarcinoma cell lines. *Cancer Lett.*, **234**: 135–142.

Mlodzik, M. (2002). Planar cell polarization: do the same mechanisms regulate Drosophila tissue polarity and vertebrate gastrulation? *Trends Genet.*, **18**: 564–71.

Mokhtari, M.J., Motamed, N., and Shokrgozar, M.A. (2008). Evaluation of silibinin on the viability, migration and adhesion of the human prostate adenocarcinoma (PC-3) cell line. *Cell Biology International*, **32**: 888–92.

Moon, R.T., Bowerman, B., Boutros, M., and Perrimon, N. (2002). The promise and perils of Wnt signaling through β-catenin. *Science*, **296**: 1644–6.

Morin, P.J., Sparks, A.B., Korinek, V., Barker, N., Clevers, H., Vogelstein, B., and Kinzler, K.W. (1997). Activation of β-catenin-Tcf signaling in colon cancer by mutations in β-catenin or APC. *Science*, 275: 1787–1790.

Mudit Vaid., Ram Prasad., Qian Sun., and Santosh K. Katiyar. (2011). Silymarin Targets β-Catenin Signaling in Blocking Migration/Invasion of Human Melanoma Cells. *Plos One*, **6**: e23000.

Muriel, P. (2009) NF-κB in liver diseases: a target for drug therapy. *J. Appl. Toxicol.*, **29**: 91–100.

Nguyen, A.V., Martinez, M., Stamos, M.J., Moyer, M.P., Planutis, K., Hope, C., and Holcombe, R.F. (2009). Results of a phase I pilot clinical trial examining the effect of plant-derived resveratrol and grape powder on Wnt pathway target gene expression in colonic mucosa and colon cancer, **1**: 25 – 37.

Nishita, M., Hashimoto, M.K., Ogata, S., Laurent, M.N., Ueno, N., Shibuya, H., and Cho, K. W. (2000). Interaction between Wnt and TGFβ signalling pathways during formation of Spemann's organizer. *Nature*, **403**: 781-785.

Nusse, R., and Varmus, H. E. (1982). Many tumors induced by the mouse mammary tumor virus contain a provirus integrated in the same region of the host genome. *Cell*, **31**: 99-109.

Pahlke, G., Ngiewih, Y., Kern, M., Jakobs, S., Marko, D., and Eisenbrand, G. (2006). Impact of quercetin and EGCG on key elements of the Wnt pathway in human colon carcinoma cells. *J Agric Food Chem.*, **54**: 7075–82.

Pandurangan, A.K., Dharmalingam, P., Sadagopan, S.K., Ramar, M., Munusamy, A., and Ganapasam, S. (2013). Luteolin induces growth arrest in colon cancer cells through involvement of Wnt/β-catenin/GSK-3β signaling. *J Environ Pathol Toxicol Oncol.*, **32**: 131-9.

Park, C.H., Chang, J.Y., Hahm, E.R., Park, S., Kim, H.K., and Yang, C.H. (2005). Quercetin, a potent inhibitor against β-catenin/Tcf signaling in SW480 colon cancer cells. *Biochem Biophys Res Commun.*, **328**: 227-34.

Park, C.H., Hahm, E.R., Park, S., Kim, H.K., and Yang, C.H. (2005). The inhibitory mechanism of curcumin and its derivative against β-catenin/Tcf signaling. *FEBS Lett.*, **579**: 2965-71.

Pavese, J.M., Farmer, R.L., and Bergan, R.C. (2010). Inhibition of cancer cell invasion and metastasis by genistein. *Cancer Metastasis Rev.*, **29**: 465–82.

Pinson, K. I., Brennan, J., Monkley, S., Avery, B. J., and Skarnes, W. C. (2000). An LDL-receptor-related protein mediates Wnt signalling in mice. *Nature*, **407**: 535–538.

Prasad, C.P, Rath, G., Mathur, S., Bhatnagar, D., and Ralhan, R. (2009). Potent growth suppressive activity of curcumin in human breast cancer cells: modulation of Wnt/β-catenin signaling. *Chem. Biol. Interact.*, **181**: 263–271.

Punathil, T., Tollefsbol, T.O., and Katiyar, S.K. (2008). EGCG inhibits mammary cancer cell migration through inhibition of nitric oxide synthase and guanylate cyclase. *Biochem Biophys Res Commun.*, **375**: 162–7.

Qiao, Y., Cao, J,, Xie, L., and Shi, X. (2009). Cell growth inhibition and gene expression regulation by (–)- epigallocatechin-3-gallate in human cervical cancer cells. *Arch Pharm Res.*, **32**: 1309–1315.

Qin, J., Xie, L.P., Zheng, X.Y., Wang, Y.B., Bai, Y., Shen, H.F., Li, L.C., and Dahiya, R. (2007). A component of green tea, (–)-epigallocatechin-3-gallate, promotes apoptosis in T24 human bladder cancer cells via modulation of the PI3K/Akt pathway and Bcl-2 family proteins. *Biochem Biophys Res Commun.*, **354**: 852–857.

Ragione, F.D., Cucciolla, V., Borriello, A., Pietra, V.D., Pontoni, G., Racioppi, L., Manna, C., Galletti, P., and Zappia, V. (2000). Hydroxytyrosol, a natural molecule occurring in olive oil, induces cytochrome c-dependent apoptosis. *Biochem Biophys Res Commun.*, **278**: 733-9.

Raina, K., Rajamanickam, S., Deep, G., Singh, M., Agarwal, R., and Agarwal, C. (2008). Chemopreventive effects of oral gallic acid feeding on tumor growth and progression in TRAMP mice. *Mol Cancer Ther.*, 7: 1258-1267.

Ren, Z., Wang, L., Cui, J., Huoc, Z., Xue, J., Cui, H., Mao, Q., and Yang, R. (2013). Resveratrol inhibits NF-kB signaling through suppression of p65 and IκB kinase activities. *Pharmazie.*, **68**: 689-94.

Robaszkiewicz, A., Balcerczyk, A., and Bartosz, G. (2007). Antioxidative and prooxidative effects of quercetin on A549 cells. *Cell Biol Int.*, **31**: 1245–50.

Rubinfeld, B., Robbins, P., El-Gamil, M., Albert, I., Porfiri, E., and Polakis, P. (1997). Stabilization of β-catenin by genetic defects in melanoma cell lines. *Science*, **275**: 1790–1792.

Ryu, M.J., Cho, M., Song, J.Y., Yun, Y.S., Choi, I.W., Kim, D.E., Park, B.S., and Oh, S. (2008). Natural derivatives of curcumin attenuate the Wnt/ β-catenin pathway through down-regulation of the transcriptional coactivator p300. *Biochem Biophys Res Commun.*, **377**: 1304-8.

Salic, A., Lee, E., Mayer, L., and Kirschner, M. W. (2000). Control of β catenin stability: reconstitution of the cytoplasmic steps of the wnt pathway in Xenopus egg extracts. *Mol. Cell*, **5**: 523-532.

Scalbert, A., Manach, C., Morand, C., Remesy, C., and Jimenez, L. (2005). Dietary polyphenols and the prevention of diseases. *Crit Rev, Food Sci Nutr.*, **45**: 287-306.

Segditsas, S., and Tomlinson, I. (2006). Colorectal cancer and genetic alterations in the Wnt pathway. *Oncogene*, **25**: 7531–7537.

Sergio Granados., Dong Soon Choil., Anthony M.C. Brown., Jenny Chang (2013). The natural compound hydroxytyrosol inhibits the Wnt/EMT axis and migration of triple-negative breast cancer cells. *Cancer Research*, **73**: 6-10.

Shan, B.E., Wang, M.X., and Li, R.Q. (2009). Effects of quercetin on proliferation, apoptosis, adhesion and migration, and invasion of HeLa cells. *Eur J Gynaecol Oncol.*, **30**: 60-4.

Shan, B.E., Wang, M.X., and Li, R.Q. (2009). Quercetin inhibit human SW480 colon cancer growth in association with inhibition of cyclin D1 and survivin expression through Wnt/β-catenin signaling pathway. *Cancer Invest.*, **27**: 604-12.

Shao, Z.M., Shen, Z.Z., Fontana, J.A., and Barsky, S.H. (2000). Genistein's "ER-dependent and independent" actions are mediated through ER pathways in ER-positive breast carcinoma cell lines. *Anticancer Res.*, **20**: 2409–16.

Sharma, G., Singh, R.P., Chan, D.C., and Agarwal, R. (2003). Silibinin induces growth inhibition and apoptotic cell death in human lung carcinoma cells. *Anticancer Res.*, **23**: 2649–55.

Sharma, R. P., and Chopra, V. L. (1976). Effect of the Wingless (wg1) mutation on wing and haltere development in Drosophila melanogaster. *Dev. Biol.*, **48**: 461-465.

Shimizu, S., Fujii, G., Takahashi, M., Nakanishi, R., Komiya, M., Shimura, M., Noma, N., Onuma, W., Terasaki, M., Yano, T., and Mutoh, M. (2014). Sesamol suppresses cyclooxygenase-2 transcriptional activity in colon cancer cells and modifies intestinal polyp development in ApcMin/+ mice. *J Clin Biochem Nutr.*, **54**.95-101.

Shin, D.Y., Ryu, C.H., Lee, W.S., Kim, D.C., Kim, S.H., Hah, Y.S., Lee, S.J., Shin, S.C., Kang, H.S., and Choi, Y.H. (2009). Induction of apoptosis and inhibition of invasion in human hepatoma cells by anthocyanins from meoru. *Ann N Y Acad Sci.*, 1**171**: 137-48.

Shtutman, M., Zhurinsky, J., Simcha, I., Albanese, C., D' Amico, M., Pestell, R., and Ben-Zeev, A. (1999). The cyclin D1 gene is a target of the β-catenin/LEF-1 pathway. *Proc. Natl. Acad. Sci.*, **96**: 5522-5527.

Shukla, S., MacLennan, G.T., Flask, C.A., Fu, P., Mishra, A., Resnick, M.I., and Gupta, S. (2007). Blockade of β-Catenin Signaling by Plant Flavonoid Apigenin Suppresses Prostate Carcinogenesis in TRAMP Mice. *Cancer Res.*, **67**: 6925-35.

Siddiqui, I.A., Malik, A., Adhami, V.M., Asim, M., Hafeez, B.B., Sarfaraz, S., and Mukhtar, H. (2008). Green tea polyphenols EGCG sensitizes human prostate carcinoma LNCaP cells to TRAIL-mediated apoptosis and synergistically inhibits biomarkers associated with angiogenesis and metastasis. *Oncogene*, **27**: 2055–2063.

Son, K. H., Park, J. O., Chung, K. C., Son, K. H., Park, J. O., Chung, K. C., Chang, H.W., Kim, H. P., Kim, J. S., and Kang, S. S. (1992). Flavonoids from the aerial parts of Lonicera japonica. *Arch. Pharm. Res.*, **15**: 365-370.

Song, D.H., Sussman, D.J., and Seldin, D.C. (2000). Endogenous protein kinase CK2 participates in Wnt signaling in mammary epithelial cells. *J Biol Chem.*, **275**: 23790–7.

Spinella, F., Rosano, L., Di Castro, V., Decandia, S., Albini, A., Nicotra, M.R., Natali, P.G., and Bagnato, A. (2006). Green tea polyphenols epigallocatechin-3-gallate inhibits the endothelin axis and downstream signaling pathways in ovarian carcinoma. *Mol Cancer Ther.*, **5**: 1483–1492.

Stewart, D.J. (2014). Wnt signaling pathway in non-small cell lung cancer. *J Natl Cancer Inst.*, **106**: djt356.

Suh, Y., Afaq, F., Johnson, J.J., and Mukhtar, H. (2009). A plant flavonoid fisetin induces apoptosis in colon cancer cells by inhibition of COX2 and Wnt/EGFR/ NF-κB-signaling pathways. *Carcinogenesis*, **30**: 300-7.

Syed, DN., Afaq, F., Maddodi, N., Johnson, JJ., Sarfaraz, S., Ahmad, A., Setaluri, V., and Mukhtar, H. (2011). Inhibition of human melanoma cell growth by the dietary flavonoid fisetin is associated with disruption of Wnt/β-catenin signaling and decreased Mitf levels. *J Invest Dermatol.*, **131**: 1291-9.

Tetsu, O., and McCormick, F. (1999). B-catenin regulates expression of cyclin D1 in colon carcinoma cells. *Nature*, **398**: 422-426.

Vasudha Sundram., Subhash C. Chauhan., Mara Ebeling., and Meena Jaggi (2102). Curcumin Attenuates β-catenin Signaling in Prostate Cancer Cells through Activation of Protein Kinase D1. *PLoS ONE*, 7: e35368.

Veeck, J., Niederacher, D., An, H., Klopocki, E., Wiesmann, F., Betz, B., Galm, O., Camara, O., Durst, M., Kristiansen, G., Huszka, C., Knuchel, R., and Dahl, E. (2006). Aberrant methylation of the Wnt antagonist SFRP1 in breast cancer is associated with unfavourable prognosis. *Oncogene*, **25**: 3479–3488.

Vo, N., and Goodman, RH. (2001). CREB-binding protein and p300 in transcriptional regulation. *J. Biol. Chem.*, **276**: 13505–8.

Voeller, H.J., Truica, C.I., and Gelmann, E.P. (1998). B-catenin mutations in human prostate cancer.*Cancer Res.*, **58**: 2520–2523.

Waltzer, L., and Bienz, M. (1998). Drosophila CBP represses the transcription factor TCF to antagonize Wingless signalling. *Nature*, **395**: 521-525.

Wang, Z., Desmoulin, S., Banerjee, S., Kong, D., Li, Y., Deraniyagala, R.L., Abbruzzese, J., and Sarkar, F.H. (2008). Synergistic effects of multiple natural products in pancreatic cancer cells. *Life Sci.*, **83**: 293–300.

Watanabe, M., Kakiuchi, H., Kato, H., Shiraishi, T., Yatani, R., Sugimura, T., and Nagao, M. (1996). APC gene mutations in human prostate cancer. *Jpn J Clin Oncol.*, **26**: 77-81.

Wielenga, V. J., Smits, R., Korinek, V., Smit, L., Kielman, M., Fodde, R., Clevers, H., and Pals, S. T (1999). Expression of CD44 in Apc and Tcf mutant mice implies regulation by the WNT pathway. *Am. J.Pathol.*, **154**: 515-523.

Willert, K., Brown, J.D., Danenberg, E., Duncan, A.W., Weissman, I.L., Reya, T., Yates, J.R., and Nusse, R. (2003). Wnt proteins are lipid-modifiedand can act as stem cell growth factors. *Nature*, **423**: 448–452.

Wilson-Simpson, F., Vance, S., and Benghuzzi, H. (2007). Physiological responses of ES-2 ovarian cell line following administration of epigallocatechin-3-gallate (EGCG), thymoquinone (TQ), and selenium (SE). *Biomed Sci Instrum.*, **43**: 378–383.

Xiang, D., Wang, D., He, Y., Xie, J., Zhong, Z., Li, Z., and Xie, J. (2006). Caffeic acid phenethyl ester induces growth arrest and apoptosis of colon cancer cells via the β-catenin/T-cell factor signaling. *Anti-cancer drug*, **17**: 753-62.

Yang, C.S., Kim, S., Yang, G.Y., Lee, M.J., Liao, J., and Chung, J.Y. (1999). Inhibition of carcinogenesis by tea: bioavailability of tea polyphenols and mechanisms of actions. *Proc Soc Exp Biol Med.*, **220**: 213–217.

Yang, J., Mani, S.A., and Weinberg, R.A. (2006). Exploring a new twist on tumor metastasis. *Cancer Res.*, **66**: 4549–4552.

Yokoyama, M., Noguchi, M., Nakao, Y., Pater, A., and Iwasaka, T. (2004). The tea polyphenol, (–)-epigallocatechin gallate effects on growth, apoptosis, and telomerase activity in cervical cell lines. *Gynecol Oncol.*, **92**: 197–204.

Yoo, J.H., Lee, H.J., Kang, K., Jho, E.H., Kim, C.Y., Baturen, D., Tunsag, J., and Nho, C.W. (2010). Lignans inhibit cell growth via regulation of Wnt/β-catenin signaling. *Food Chem Toxicol.*, **48**: 2247-52.

You, X.J., Bryant, P.J., Jurnak, F., and Holcombe, R.F. (2007). Expression of Wnt pathway components frizzled and disheveled in colon cancer arising in patients with inflammatory bowel disease. *Oncol Rep.*, **18**: 691-4.

Zhang, B., Abreu, J.G., Zhou, K., Chen, Y., Hu, Y., Zhou, T., He, X., and Ma, J.X. (2010). Blocking the Wnt pathway, a unifying mechanism for an angiogenic inhibitor in the serine proteinase inhibitor family. *Proc Natl Acad Sci U S A.*, **107**: 6900–5.

Zhang, X., Zhang, H., Tighiouart, M., Lee, J.E., Shin, H.J., Khuri, F.R., Yang, C.S., Chen, Z., and Shin, D.M. (2008). Synergistic inhibition of head and neck tumor growth by green tea (–)-epigallocatechin-3-gallate and EGFR tyrosine kinase inhibitor. *Int J Cancer*, **123**: 1005–1014.

Zhang, Y., Li, Q., and Chen, H. (2013). DNA methylation and histone modifications of Wnt genes by genistein during colon cancer development. *Carcinogenesis*, **34**: 1756-63.

Bioactive Phytochemicals: Perspectives for Modern Medicine Vol. 3 (2015) Pages 311–336
Editor: V.K. Gupta
Published by: DAYA PUBLISHING HOUSE, NEW DELHI

12

Exploitation of Algae as Priceless Source of Potential Commercial High-Value Compounds

G.A. Lutzu[1*] and A. Parsaeimehr[2]

ABSTRACT

Currently, various valuable natural molecules have been identified and isolated from algae. Therefore, it is undoubted that they can represent a brilliant source of several chemical compounds which can find different biological applications, mainly in the field of human health and welfare. These compounds exhibit a wide range of biological actions including anti-viral, antioxidant, anti-allergic, anticancer, and anti-inflammatory. The potential exploitation of both macro- and microalgae as source of valuable components, including carbohydrates, long chain fatty acids, pigments, proteins and vitamins, is encompassed in this review. Applications of these compounds in the pharmaceutical, neutracetical and food market are also discussed.

Keywords: Algae, Antioxidants, Antimicrobials, Astaxanthin, β-carotene, Fatty acids, Lutein, Pigments.

Introduction

Normally the chemical composition of algae can be divided in lipids, carbohydrates and proteins which account for about 5-20 per cent, 10-50 per cent

1 Key Laboratory of Biofuels, Qingdao Institute of Bioenergy and Bioprocess Technology, Chinese Academy of Sciences, Qingdao, 266101, Shandong, People's Republic of China

2 Laboratory of Biosystems Engineering, Institute of Biotechnology, Jiangsu Academy of Agricultural Sciences; Key Laboratory of Agrobiology of Jiangsu Province, Nanjing 210014, Jiangsu, People's Republic of China.

* *Corresponding author:* E-mail: lgiovannian@tiscali.it, giovanni@gibebt.ac.in

and 30-65 per cent, respectively (Becker, 2007). Even though the last two are a major algae biomass component, usually they are undervalued compared to minor components such as pigments or other possible valuable by-products which have a more commercial exploitation.

Lipids are of particular interest mainly because they are considered as the feedstock for biodiesel production. Actually, in the presence of a suitable catalyst and an alcohol, the lipids are converted into biodiesel (fatty acid methyl esters, FAME). However, not all lipids are suitable but only the neutral lipid, including triacylglycerides (TAGs) Kim *et al.*, 2013). Moreover, lipids can also contain essential polyunsaturated fatty acids (PUFAs) which are absent from food crops such as eicosapentaenoic acid (EPA, C20:5ω) and docosahexaenoic acid (DHA, C22:6ω) and some other high-value fatty acids such as omega-3, γ-linolenic acid (GLA) etc. In particular, algae are considered as potential sources of PUFAs of more than 18 carbons, such as GLA, Arachidonic acid (ARA), EPA and DHA (Sajilata *et al.*, 2008).

Carbohydrates are the major products derived from photosynthesis. They can be either accumulated in the plastids as reserve materials such as starch, or become the main component of cell walls such as cellulose, pectin, polysaccharides. In this way microalgae can potentially be used as carbon source for the fermentation process. However, the composition of carbohydrates (mainly starch and cellulose) in algal species strongly depends on different species and their metabolism.

Proteins represent a third main group of compounds produced by algal species. Most algae have high protein content (in some cases more than 50 per cent of the total biomass dry weight in microalgae). The major quality factor for proteins is represented by their amino acid content. In nature 20 different amino acids exist of which 8 are essentials. Most of them can be found in some food such as soya and maize but the main crops contain the complete range of amino acids, although not always in the right ratio. Different algae species can contain different amounts of the essential amino acids and therefore selecting the right species for specific applications can lower the costs in animal production.

A group of high-valued compounds of high commercial interest is represented by carotenoids which are a wide family of isoprenoids with 40-carbon structures. These hydrophobic pigments are essentially classified in xanthophylls and carotenes, respectively, depending on whether their molecules can be oxygenated. The main microalgal carotenoids of commercial interest are astaxanthin, β-carotene and lutein which can be accumulated by many microalgal species. In particular an extensive literature exists on some of these species, such as *Dunaliella salina*, *Haematococcus pluvialis*, *Chlorella zofingiensis* and *Chlorella vulgaris*, due to their capability of commercial production in large scale of cultures (Guedes *et al.*, 2011a; Mulders *et al.*, 2014).

Moreover, scientific evidence has revealed that algal-based compounds exhibit a range of biological actions such as anti-viral, antioxidant, anti-allergic, anticancer, anti-inflammatory and anti-obesity. Furthermore, as mentioned before, algal fast growth rate coupled with simple growth requirements and their valuable compounds makes them attractive enough for industries that are addressed to the production of high value compounds largely demanded by the pharmaceutical market. For instance, seaweeds are rich in bioactive molecules including sulfated polysaccharides, phlorotannins, terpenes and carotenoids (such as fucoxanthin), volatile halogenated organic compounds that could potentially be applied as efficient anti-viral, anti-tumor and anti-cancer agents. In spite of algae being able to produce a wide range of considerable bioactive molecules, there is a scarcity of information about their possible exploitability compared to higher plants or microbes.

The aim of this paper is then to provide a review on the usage of algal species as a priceless source of different metabolites focusing in particular on the role played by fatty acids and antioxidants. The evidence on the presence of antimicrobials and anticancer molecules in some algal species will also be presented.

Algae as a Priceless Source of Metabolites

Some of the chemicals produced by microalgae play an essential role for human nutrition while others can be also utilized in the pharmaceutical and cosmetic market. Potential commercialization of high-value products from microalgae have been recently reviewed in several papers (Borowitzka, 2013; Skjanes *et al.*, 2013). It emerges that these products meet a relevant market demand in which compounds such as β-carotene, astaxanthin, PUFAs (mainly EPA and DHA), and polysaccharides such as β-glucane dominate. However, currently DHA is the only algal PUFA commercially available. Among hundreds of known carotenoids, only very few are used commercially: β-carotene, astaxanthin and to some extent, lutein, xanthophill, zeaxanthin and lycopene. Their primary market is essentially addressed to the food industry mainly as natural food colorants (*e.g.*, orange juice) and as additive for animal feed (poultry, fish). Some of the commercialized carotenoids find also applications in the cosmetics market. β-carotene is indeed highly demanded by the pharma and agro food industry. It is commercialized as dietetic compound, food additive (colorant, antioxidant), animal feed, etc. In particular the microalgae *Dunaliella salina* is the main source of natural β-carotene and several industrial exploitations of *Dunaliella* are operational in Australia, Israel and USA for this purpose (Borowitzka, 1999). Normally the production of these bioactive compounds demands the use of monocultures in order to better control productivity and production efficiency. For these very reasons cultivation systems such as large-scale photobioreactors (PBRs) have been preferred to open ponds.

Fatty Acids

The interest on the cultivation of microalgae is also due to the fact that they are rich in fatty acids (FA). In particular, long-chain polyunsaturated fatty acids (PUFAs) such GLA, ARA, EPA and DHA are considered essential nutrients due to their high physiological and therapeutic significance for humans. For this reason there has been a rising interest over the last years on their potential applications in pharmaceutical, nutraceutical and cosmetic industries. From a nutritional point of view, two of the long chain PUFAs, EPA and DHA, are regarded as the most important bioactive compounds. Actually, these essential FA are necessary in human and animal metabolism even though they are not able to synthesize them themselves and, consequently, they are obliged to obtain them from food sources.

GLA can be used to protect and revitalize the skin and, therefore its market is essentially devoted to therapeutic and cosmetic field. GLA found also applications for the immune system and other processes related to the tissue regeneration, since represents some of the essential nutrients for the synthesis of the cell membrane prostaglandins (Montpoint and Guilhou, 1991). ARA has been proved to be able to act as an aggregative and vasoconstrictive of platelets as well as to act as an antiaggregative and vasodilatative on the endothelium, besides a chemostatic action on the neutrophils (Gordon and Ratliff, 1992). Intensive studies have shown that EPA and DHA have also different effects on leukocyte functions such as phagocytosis, chemotactic response and cytokine production. DHA and EPA modulate differently expression of genes in lymphocytes (Gorjão *et al.*, 2009). For DHA and EPA there are several pharmacological applications since they have been proved to lower hypertension and to reduce problems associated with cardiovascular strokes and with arthritis (Holub, 2009). Furthermore, they also play a fundamental role in lowering lipid content (by decreasing in particular triglycerides and increasing high-density lipoprotein (HDL)) and as anti-inflammatory agents. Amongst the benefits associated with EPA it is possible to list the prevention and treatment of coronary heart disease, tumors, blood platelet aggregation, increased cholesterol levels, inflammatory diseases and even its consumption potentially enhances brain functioning (Sanchez-Lara *et al.*, 2014). At present, PUFAs are almost exclusively obtained from marine fish oil, which is typically obtained from sardine, tuna, anchovy, bass, mackerel or salmon. On the other hand, in the marine food chain these fishes obtain their long chain n3-PUFAs by consumption of marine microalgae indicating that microalgae are considered the primary producers of long chain PUFAs. Precisely, photosynthetic microalgae are considered as primary producers of PUFAs in aquatic environments and their production can be enhanced under stressful conditions. It is well known from some experiments that the respective proportion of EPA and DHA can be altered by changing the cultivation conditions. The development of different cultivation technologies and conditions to improve productivity and yield of EPA has also been recently addressed (Brentner *et al.*, 2011). In particular a marine diatom, *Phaeodactylum tricornutum,* is widely recognized as the best producer of EPA, therefore, it has been extensively investigated in literature (Silva Benavides *et al.*, 2013, Përez-López *et al.*, 2014). According to Ramírez Fajardo *et al.* (2007) this strain is able to accumulate up to 30–45 per cent PUFA amongst which EPA can account for up to 40 per cent of the total FA. Yongmanitchai and Ward (1991) and Sukenik (1991) reported *Phaeodactylum tricornutum* and *Nannochloropsis* sp., respectively, to have an EPA content of up to 39 per cent of total FA under autotrophic conditions. Interestingly, another marine strain, *Pavlova lutheri,* has been found to be particularly rich in EPA as well as also in DHA (Guedes, 2010). As for the DHA content, very few microalgae strains are recognized cotaining high quantity of this FA. Amongst them the genus *Crypthecodinium* (Okuda *et al.*, 2013), *Schizochytrium* (Chang *et al.*, 2013) and *Ulkenia* (Lee Chang *et al.*, 2014). Adarme Vega *et al.* (2012) reported that under heterotrophic fermentative conditions, *Thraustochytrium* and *Schizochytrium limacinum* contained a DHA percentage between 30 and 40 per cent of total FA.

At commercial level oil rich in DHA and EPA is obtained from fish even if, recently some European companies have obtained biomass of omega-3 long chains-PUFA produced by photoautotrophic microalgae. SBAE (Sleidinge, Belgium) commercialize *Thalassiosira pseudonana*, LGem (Voorhout, The Netherlands) *Nannochloropsis gaditana*, Proviron (Hemiksem, Belgium) *Nannochloropsis oculata* and Necton (Olhão, Portugal) *Porphyridium cruentum*, to name a few (Ryckebosch *et al.*, 2014). The marine microalga *Nannochloropsis* too has been reported also by the American company Aurora Algae to produce EPA-rich oils. *Schizochytrium* has been introduced in the market for this purpose. High biomass and commercially acceptable EPA and DHA productivities are achieved with microalgae grown in media with optimized carbon and nitrogen concentrations and controlled pH and temperature conditions (Griffiths *et al.*, 2009). High oil production, including DHA from *Schizochytrium* (50 per cent w/w), can be obtained as a result of high growth rate by controlling some nutrients such as glucose, nitrogen, sodium and some other environmental factors, such as oxygen concentrations as well as temperature and pH, achieving high cell densities and DHA productivities (Ward and Singh, 2005). On the other hand, the fungus *Mortiriella alpina* is commercially cultivated for the production of ARA-rich oil, although the green alga *Parietochloris incise* has be recognized to have a high ARA content (Bigogno *et al.*, 2002).

As for GLA, the best algal source is *Spirulina platensis*, even if its productivity is low, due to the low total lipid content of this cyanobacterium. The main drawback of the commercial production of DHA/EPA-rich oils from microalgae is related to the expensive costs for the phototrophic growth of microalgae, compared to the heterotrophically grown algae and fungi, as well as to other PUFA rich oils such as fish oil. In order to overcome these drawbacks improvements in lipid productivity should be obtained. To reach this goal, and in view of the industrial scaling-up, the current technology should be optimized in terms of isolation of new species (Cohen and Khozin-Goldberg, 2010), selected algal strains (Talebi *et al.*, 2013) as well as design/operating parameters (Tababa *et al.*, 2012). While the creation of new microalgal strains intrinsically characterized by high lipid productivities is an ambitious goal. This can be achieved through genetic manipulation of existing strains (Radakovits *et al.*, 2010; Kilian *et al.*, 2011).

Antioxidants from Algae

The production of reactive oxygen species (ROS) during the cell metabolism generate an oxidative damage on lipids, proteins and nucleic acids that may trigger various chronic diseases, such as coronary heart disease, atherosclerosis, cancer and ageing (Finkel and Holbrook, 2000). Antioxidants contained in fruits and vegetables have been epidemiologically demonstrated to have several positive health effects, including prevention of cardiovascular disorders such as heart disease and atherosclerosis, of certain ageing related diseases such as Alzheimer and of certain types of cancer. Ghiselli *et al.* (1997) supposed that the antioxidants potentialities of carotenoids could be attributed to the prevention of oxidative stress and, in this light, the Mediterranean diet can be regarded as a winning choice, since it is characterized by the consumption of carotenoid and polyphenol-rich vegetables and fruit. For this reason, antioxidants are increasingly being used in food supplements and functional foods. This antioxidant activity is revealed by protecting cells against lipid peroxidation and damage of proteins and DNA, by triggering genes towards the regulation of enzymes like superoxide dismutase, catalase and lipid peroxidase. Furthermore, antioxidants can block lipidic free radicals but also prevent oxidation by chelating metal ions, scavenging oxygen, quenching singlet oxygen or absorbing UV radiation. The antioxidant activity of some unicellular microalgae and cyanobacteria has been studied in the last decade by a growing number of reports, confirming in this way that microalgae are regarded as a promising alternative source of antioxidants (Choochote *et al.*, 2014). Different genera of microalgae have been investigated such as *Botryococcus* (Rao *et al.*, 2013), *Chlorella* (Choochote *et al.*, 2014), *Nannochloropsis* (Goh *et al.*, 2010), *Scenedesmus* sp. (Aremu *et al.*, 2014), *Dunaliella* (Herrero *et al.*, 2006), *Phaeodactylum* (Rodriguez-Garcia and Guil-Guerrero, 2008), *Spirulina* (Rao *et al.*, 2013), *Haematococcus* (Rao *et al.*, 2013), *Chlorococcum* sp. (Choochote *et al.*, 2014), *Porphyridium* (Rodriguez-Garcia and Guil-Guerrero, 2008), *Nostoc* (Ninomiya *et al.*, 2011) and *Chaetoceros* (Goh *et al.*, 2010). The antioxidant capacity and total phenolic content of different fractions of 23 microalgae and 12 soil-isolated strains of microalgae were evaluated by Li *et al.* (2007) and by Hajimahmoodi *et al.* (2010), respectively. The former has found out that the microalgae *Synechococcus* sp. FACHB 283, *Chlamydomonas nivalis* and *Nostoc ellipsosporum* CCAP 1453/17 possessed the highest antioxidant capacities and thus could be potential rich sources of natural antioxidants. The latter demonstrated instead that phenolic compounds were a major contributor to the antioxidant capacities for some of the species investigated, such as *Microchaete tenera*, *Fischerella musicola* and *Fischerella ambigua*. Lee *et al.* (2010b) studied the antioxidant properties of two tidal microalgae, *Halochlorococcum porphyrae* and *Oltamannsiellopsis unicellularis*, isolated from the Korean see. All these studies concluded that several microalgal genera contain potent antioxidants, both from lipophilic and hydrophilic nature that can be regarded as an alternative to higher plants or the production by chemical synthesis. A vast literature on the matter is also available for antioxidants produced by macroalgae. To this regard, compounds such as phlorotannins derived from *Hizikia fusiformis* are regarded as potential radical scavengers and as a valuable natural antioxidative and nutraceuticals source (Siriwardhana *et al.*, 2005). Chkhikvishvili and Ramazanov (2000) reported the antioxidant activity of phenolic substances in 14 species of marine brown algae of the Canary Islands littoral (Spain) while Huang and Wang (2004) screened the lipophilic extracts from 16 species of seaweeds collected along the Qingdao coastline (China).

A well-known class of antioxidants obtained from microalgae is represented by carotenoids, which not only represent secondary pigments in photosynthetic organisms, but also play an important role as antioxidants and provitamin factors for non-photosynthetic organisms that must include them in their diet (Christaki *et al.*, 2013). As for their chemical structure, they are made of eight units of five carbons, having alternate single and double bonds arranged in an alternate manner. If these chains of carbons units end with a cyclic group are named carotenes (such as β-carotene, for which the best producer is the halotolerant microalga *Dunaliella salina* with up to 10 per cent of its dry weight biomass in β-carotene), whereas if they contain an oxygen functional group are called oxycarotenoids or xantophylls (such as astaxanthin for which the best producer is the microalgae *Haematococcus pluvialis* in its encysted status). Several studies have demonstrated that carotenoids contribute significantly to the total antioxidant capacity of microalgae, due to their ability in quenching ROS generated during photosynthesis. Their antioxidant and colorant properties, which are related to the system of conjugated double bonds, are responsible for their therapeutic, dietetic and industrial applications (Abd El-Baky and El-Baroty, 2009). Interestingly, the commercial exploitation of microalgae as a source of carotenoid antioxidants (*e.g.*, *Haematococcus* for astaxanthin, *Dunaliella* for β-carotene) has been recently receiving great attention mainly for being used as additives in food and feed applications, as well as for be used in cosmetics and as food supplements. This rising interest is also confirmed by the work of Guedes *et al.* (2013). They characterized the antioxidant profile of 18 species of cyanobacteria and 23 species of microalgae and found out that the strain *Scenedesmus obliquus* M2-1 exhibited the highest total antioxidant capacity of intracellular extracts. Its scavenger activity correlated well with its protective effects against DNA oxidative damage induced by copper (II)-ascorbic acid.

Astaxanthin

Astaxanthin (3,3'-dihydroxy-b,b-carotene-4,4'-dione; $C_{40}H_{52}O_4$) is a high-value red carotenoid (or pigment) commonly found in marine animals and traditionally used as a pigmentation source for fish aquaculture. It has various biological functions such as species-specific coloration, light-harvesting, photo-protection, antioxidant, and hormone precursor (Zhang *et al.*, 2014). Recently, its importance in medicine sector has been proved since it delays the onset of many diseases such as arteriosclerosis, cataracts, age-related macular degeneration, multiple sclerosis, cardiovascular diseases, and some kinds of cancer. The high antioxidant activity of astaxanthin has been reported to prevent cardiovascular disease and cataract and boost the immune system (Aflalo *et al.*, 2007). Due to its excellent antioxidant properties, astaxanthin has numerous applications; from its use as additive in food and feed industries, nutraceuticals to cosmetics market (Koller *et al.*, 2012). These reasons and many others have led to the drastically increased demand and market growth of astaxanthin. The current astaxanthin world market is dominated by synthetic astaxanthin. The price for synthetic astaxanthin is above \$2,000 kg^{-1}, and its total market value is over \$240 M per year (Misawa, 2009). Because of the high market price and the growing concerns about the safety of using synthetic astaxanthin for aquaculture or direct human consumption, natural astaxanthin represents a preferred and premium choice for human consumption and there are several efforts in using microorganisms (as microalgae and heterobasidiomycete) as a natural source of this product. Astaxanthin can be produced in various amounts by a number of microalgae including *Botryococcus braunii* (up to 0.01 per cent astaxanthin by dry weight [dwt]) (Grung *et al.*, 1994), *Chlamydocapsa* sp. (0.04 per cent astaxanthin/dwt) (Leya *et al.*, 2009), *Chlamydomonas nivalis* (Remias *et al.*, 2005), *Chlorella zofingiensis* (0.7 per cent astaxanthin/dwt) (Orosa *et al.*, 2000), *Chlorococcum* sp. (0.7 per cent astaxanthin/dwt) (Liu and Lee, 2000), *Chloromonas nivalis* (0.004 per cent astaxanthin/

dwt) (Remias *et al.*, 2010), *H. pluvialis* (4 per cent astaxanthin/dwt) (Droop, 1954), *Neochloris wimmeri* (1.9 per cent astaxanthin/dwt) (Orosa *et al.*, 2000), *Coelastrella* sp. (1.8 per cent astaxanthin/dwt) (Hu *et al.*, 2013) *Protosiphon botryoides* (1.4 per cent astaxanthin/dwt) (Orosa *et al.*, 2000), *Scenedesmus* sp. (0.3 per cent astaxanthin/dwt) (Qin *et al.*, 2008), *Scotiellopsis oocystiformis* (1.1 per cent astaxanthin/dwt) (Orosa *et al.*, 2000), and *Trachelomonas volvo-cina* (Green, 1963). Of these species, *H. pluvialis* is recognized as one of the most promising and richest producer of astaxanthin in nature due to its exceptional ability to accumulate large amounts of astaxanthin under stress conditions (Lemoine and Schoefs, 2010). Actually, this microalga stands out for its ability to synthesize astaxanthin in particular high quantities, 1.5-3 per cent of its dry weight (Nonomura, 1989). Compared with other astaxanthin-producing microorganisms, *H. pluvialis* has the highest potential to accumulate large amounts of astaxanthin because it possesses sequestering systems for storing it in lipid bodies. In particular, this pigment starts to be accumulated in the lipid vesicles during the transition between green vegetative cells and red aplanospores after exposure to stress conditions (Aflalo *et al.*, 2007). In the early 1950s Droop (1955) firstly reported *H. pluvialis* as a potential source of astaxanthin. Today it is widely recognized as an astaxanthin-producer commercially yielding 30 g of astaxanthin/kg dry biomass (Olaizola and Huntley, 2000). Starting from 1990s it has been cultivated in large scale by several companies, using different approaches. Commercial production of astaxanthin has been reported by Cynotech Corporation and Aquasearch Inc. both adopting a two step strategy whereby the first stage is done photoautotrophically under controlled culture conditions and consists in growing *Haematococcus* biomass under conditions conducive to fast growth in enclosed systems (either tubular, bubble column or airlift PBRs) followed by a second stage in which carotenogenesis (reddening stage) is induced in open cultivation ponds by changing the cells'environment to stress promoting conditions. Recently, Micro Gaia Inc. has also reported that it is going to start astaxanthin production based on a single step process. However, the cell concentrations obtained with these commercial processes are very low, which in turns leads to the low efficiency of astaxanthin production. Numerous scientific works exist concerning the optimization of astaxanthin production processes by *H. pluvialis*. These papers mainly focus on the assessment of various factors and conditions which affect microalgae growth and induce astaxanthin biosynthesis. Among them, the environmental stress such as increasing light intensity (Kumar Saha *et al.*, 2013), drought (Kobayashi *et al.*, 1997), high temperature (Tjahjono *et al.*, 1994), high salt (Sarada *et al.*, 2002), pH (Lababpour *et al.*, 2004), N and P starvation (Orosa *et al.*, 2001), various carbon sources (Jeon *et al.*, 2006), high carbon to nitrogen ratios (Ip and Chen, 2005).

β-carotene

β-carotene is a hydrocarbon ($C_{40}H_{56}$) having a highly unsaturated chain which forms a chromophore responsible for its yellow-orange colour. Different isomers exist and the all-trans and 9-cis stereoisomers are considered the most important. More than 90 per cent of commercial β-carotene, and more precisely the all-trans isomer, are chemically synthesized, but the 9-cis-β-carotene is produced only from natural sources such as vegetables and microalgae (Leon *et al.*, 2003). The main source of natural β-carotene and, consequently, the most studied microalgae is *Dunaliella* sp. (Raja *et al.*, 2007). In particular the species *Dunaliella salina* can contain typically about 0.5–1 per cent of dry weight in terms of β-carotene, as many as other green microalgae. Its commercialization as dietetic compound (because it physiologically acts as provitamin A and as a radical quencher), food additive (colorant, antioxidant), animal feed has been exploited by several industries which operate mainly in the pharma and agrofood sector in Australia, Israel and USA. In literature many reports are available about strategies to improve β-carotene accumulation. One of the most investigated is the cultivation of microalgae under different stress cultivation conditions. Del Campo *et al.* (2007) have found out that under these conditions microalgae cells are able to accumulate β-carotene up to more than 12 per cent of the algal dry weight inside the chloroplasts. The β-carotene accumulation is related to certain environmental parameters such as nutrients starvation, light, pH, salinity and temperature (Çelekli *et al.*, 2014). Most of the working available on the matter refer to *Dunaliella* sp. or *Duanliella salina*, since it represents the best and well known β-carotene producer. The most evident effect of these stressed culture conditions is the fact that β-carotene accumulation is promoted when cell division rate is either slowed down or arrested (a similar effect is also obtained in the case of astaxanthin accumulation) (Hosseini Tafreshi and Shariati, 2009). For *D. salina* nutrient starvation is well investigated and many reports have demonstrated how β-carotene content can be increased under nitrogen (Lamers *et al.*, 2012), phosphorus (Phadwal and Singh, 2003) and sulfur (Ben-Amotz, 1987) starvation, respectively. Mojaat *et al.* (2008) found out that, by inducing an oxidative stress, Fe^{2+} ions revealed to stimulate β-carotene synthesis in *D. salina*, especially when acting in the presence of the carbon source (acetate and malonate). In mass production the most used technique to promote the production of β-carotene is nitrogen deficiency coupled with a high salinity stress (Ben-Amotz, 1999). *D. salina* is known to be the most halotolerant eukaryotic microorganism, able to tolerate a very wide salinity from 0.5 to as high as 35 per cent v/w NaCl (Hosseini Tafreshi and Shariati, 2009). *Dunaliella* species normally grow well in media containing 1–2 M NaCl while a moderate increase in salt concentration from 4 per cent to 9 per cent results in a 30-fold increase in accumulation of β-carotene (Fazeli *et al.*, 2006). To the contrary, harsher increase in salt concentration resulted in lower β-carotene accumulation. Another method to stimulate β-carotene accumulation is the cultivation under light stress and, in particular, the higher the light intensity the higher the β-carotene content. Aburai *et al.* (2013) enhances carotenogenesis of four aerial microalgae isolated from Japans rocks by increasing the light intensity from 40 to 214 μmol photons $m^{-2} s^{-1}$. Lamers *et al.* (2010) found out that the cultivation of *D. salina* under nitrogen starvation condition combined with light stress resulted in the maximum accumulation of β-carotene (3.1 per cent of dry weight). Also the decrease of culture temperature has been reported to increase the β-carotene (Gómez and González, 2005). Garbayo *et al.* (2008) enhanced production of lutein and β-carotene when *Chlamydomonas acidophila* was grown under standard conditions, but heated at 40 °C. However, recently some other microalgal species have been found to accumulate β-carotene. Guil-Guerrero *et al.* (2008) analyzed the carotenoids content of *Monodus subterraneus* cultivated in an outdoor bubble column photobioreactor and found out that this marine strain exhibited high quantity of neoxanthin and β-carotene. Li *et al.* (2012) screened the profiles of carotenoids and production of β-carotene by six eustigmatophytes, such as *Eustigmatos magnus, Eustigmatos polyphem, Eustigmatos vischeri, Vischeria helvetica, Vischeria punctata* and *Vischeria stellata*. They have found out that β-carotene accounted for over 50 per cent of total carotenoids in all the strains investigated. β-carotene resulted to be one of the most abundant carotenoids found in four new species of microalgae isolated from the surface of rocks in mountainous districts of Japan and identified (based on 18S rDNA analysis) as *Scenedesmus* sp. KGU-Y002, *Scenedesmus* sp. KGU-D002, *Coelastrella* sp. KGU-H001 and *Vischeria helvetica* KGU-Y001, respectively (Aburai *et al.*, 2013). Graziani *et al.* (2013) screened 43 strains of unicellular red microalgae and found out that β-carotene is the main carotenoid of *Galdieria sulphuraria*. They concluded that the low concentration of lipids and the absence of green colour make this microalgae source particularly useful for the addition to many food preparations.

Lutein

Lutein ($C_{40}H_{56}O_2$) is one of the main photosynthetic pigments in the xanthophyllic family, and contains a large conjugated carbon system attached to hydroxyl or carbonyl groups. In addition to acting as the accessory pigment in photo-systems, lutein also prevents or ameliorates cardiovascular diseases, some types of cancer, and age-related diseases (Chiu and Taylor, 2007). Lutein is thus often consumed as a food additive, with sales of related products reaching $150 million in the U.S. (Ceron *et al.*, 2008). At present, marigold petals are the major source for commercial production of lutein, with a lutein content contained in the petals that account for as low as 0.03 per cent per dry weight (Piccaglia *et al.*, 1998). Recently, microalgae have emerged as a promising alternative feedstock to produce lutein. This pigment, depending on operation mode and cultivation conditions, can be produced in various amounts by some microalgae including, *Muriellopsis* sp. (0.55 per cent lutein/dwt) (Blanco *et al.*, 2007), *Chlorella zofingensis* (0.35 per cent lutein/dwt) (Del Campo *et al.*, 2004), *Chlorella protothecoides* (0.46 per cent lutein/dwt) (Shi *et al.*, 2006), *Chlorella citriforme* (0.72 per cent lutein/dwt) (Del Campo *et al.*, 2000), *Chlorella fusca* (0.42 per cent lutein/dwt) (Del Campo *et al.*, 2000), *Chlorella proboscideum* (0.34 per cent lutein/dwt) (Del Campo *et al.*, 2000), *Coccomyxa acidophyla* (0.34 per cent lutein/dwt) (Casal *et al.*, 2011), *Scenedesmus obliquus* (0.45 per cent lutein/dwt) (Ho *et al.*, 2014), *Scenedesmus almeriensis* (0.45 per cent lutein/dwt) (Sanchez *et al.*, 2008), *Muriella aurantica* (0.26 per cent lutein/dwt) (Del Campo *et al.*, 2000), *Muriella decolor* (0.05 per cent lutein/dwt) (Del Campo *et al.*, 2000), *Neospongiococcus gelatinosum* (0.44 per cent lutein/dwt) (Del Campo *et al.*, 2000). There are some strategies reported in literature to promote the productivity of microalgal biomass and the accumulation of lutein. Xie *et al.* (2013) obtained the highest lutein content (0.50 per cent) when *Desmodesmus* sp. F51 was fed-batch cultivated with pulse-feeding of nitrate and the nitrate level was nearly depleted. Ho *et al.* (2014) investigated the effect of light sources and intensity on biomass and lutein productivity of *Scenedesmus obliquus* FSP-3 and found out that the use of white LED resulted in better lutein production efficiency (4.08 mg/L/d) when compared to the other three monochromatic LEDs (red, blue, and green). Similar results were obtained by Sanchez Saavedra and Voltolina (2002) and by Solovchenko *et al.* (2008) indicating that the pigment content of the diatoms investigated (*Chaetoceros* sp.,

Skeletonema costatum, and *Thalassiosira pseudonana*) increased under the illumination of white light. Li *et al.* (2002) have investigated some strategies to isolate and purify lutein from *C. vulgaris* by high-speed counter-current chromatography and by extraction after saponification, respectively. Guedes *et al.* (2011b) found out that temperature plays a more important role on the maximum specific growth rate of *Scenedesmus obliquus* than pH. In terms of antioxidant content, pH and, to a lesser extent temperature have also relevant effects on the production of lutein and β-carotene (203.57 ± 1.41 and 18.20 ± 0.33 mg/mL, respectively). Similar results were also found for *Chlamydomonas acidophila* (Garbayo *et al.*, 2008). The same authors some years later isolated from an acidic river in Huelva, Spain, a heavy-metal-resistant, carotenoid-enriched novel unicellular microalga *Coccomyxa onubensis*. Its pigment profile resulted particularly rich in carotenoids, especially lutein, suggesting that this microalga might have a potential for antioxidant production (Vaquero *et al.*, 2012). Recently, a wastewater chlorophyte isolate, *Kirchneriella* sp. showed an ability to produce several products of commercial value, including lutein as well as β-carotene (Frampton *et al.*, 2013).

Vitamins

Antioxidants activity is reported in literature not only for pigments but also for vitamins, another class of essential compounds that can be produced by microalgae cells. Provitamin A (β-carotene) is one of the well known and it is produced not only by *Dunaliella salina* but also by other microalgae strains such as *Porphidium cruentum* (Sarrobert and Dermoun, 1991). Another vitamin well distributed in microalgae cells is the vitamin E (tocopherols) that can be found in *Navicula ostrearia, D. salina, P. cruentum*. Other vitamins such as vitamins C, vitamin B12 (cobalamin), vitamin B1 (thiamine), vitamin B6 (pyridoxine), vitamin B2 (riboflavin), nicotinic acid and vitamin H (biotin) can be found with different amounts in others microalgae strains such as *Spirulina platensis* (Mendiola *et al.*, 2008), *Pavlova* (Drokova and Popova, 1974), *Euglena gracilis* (Ogbonna *et al.*, 1998), *Dunaliella tertiolecta* (Carballo-Cárdenas *et al.*, 2003), *Tetraselmis suecica* (Carballo-Cárdenas *et al.*, 2003), *Nannochloropsis oculata* (Durmaz, 2007), *Isochrysis galbana* (Bandarra *et al.*, 2003). In literature there is a lack of information about abiotic factors that enhance the accumulation of vitamins in microalgae cells. Durmaz (2007) reported that α-tocopherol content can be increased by decreasing the concentration of nitrogen. Also Herrero *et al.* (1991) demonstrated that variations in the content of vitamin C and E as well as β-carotene in *D. tertiolecta* are strongly influenced by the nature of nitrogen. Abalde *et al.* (1991) found out the accumulation of vitamin C and E is positively enhanced by the presence of urea and nitrate in the culture medium, respectively. In addition, Abd El-Baky *et al.* (2009) succeeded in increasing 4-fold and 8-fold the content of Vitamin C and E, respectively, when *S. platensis* was cultivated under stress condition provoked by the addition of hydrogen peroxide in the culture medium.

Other Bioactive Compounds

The term "bioactive molecule" describes molecules that are "pharmacologically active derived from natural sources and through chemical synthesis". Commonly it refers to secondary metabolites which are organic compounds that are not directly involved in the normal growth, development, or reproduction of an organism. Unlike primary metabolites, absence of secondary metabolites does not result in immediate death, but rather in long-term impairment of the organism's survivability, fecundity, or aesthetics, or perhaps in no significant change at all. The level of production of a definite bioactive molecule is significantly correlated with the presence of its precursors and the activity of particular enzymes, but undoubtedly the action of these enzymes will be managed by gene or multi-gene expression. It is reported that red alga *Rhodomela aculeata* contains antioxidant compounds and its extract was able to scavenge DPPH (2,2-diphenyl-1-picrylhydrazyl) with an IC50 = 90 ìg/mL at a concentration of 20 ìg/mL while also for *Halimeda incrassata* and *Bryothamnion triquetrum* experimental data exposed a significant correlation between phenolic compounds and extracts antioxidant activities (Fallarero *et al.*, 2003). As previously mentioned, currently, different antioxidants have been identified and isolated from algal species algal species among phenolic compounds such as, for example, dieckol and phloroglucinol as well as fucoxanthin which are obtained from edible brown algae *Ecklonia cava* and *Ecklonia stolonifera,* and *Padina tetrastromatica,* respectively. Based on the evidences the majority of purified phenolic compounds from marine algae are responsible for protective actions against oxidative stress which induced the cell damage (Lee *et al.*, 2010a). It is known that nitrogen monoxide (NO) is a cytotoxic, short lived highly diffusible signaling molecule and it causes injury and cell death of oligodendrocytes and neuron. It should be pointed out that also macroalgae such as *Ulva conglobata*, *Ecklonia cava* and *Laminaria japonica* have been shown to possess a considerable anti-neuroinflammatory activity (Pangestuti and Kim, 2011).

Alzheimer is known as a serious, progressive and degenerative disease that destroys brain cells. One of the most realistic approaches to the symptomatic treatment of Alzheimer is the inhibition of acetylcholinesterase (AChE) enzyme, which catalyzes the breakdown of ACh. As mentioned, acetylcholinesterase (AChE) and butyrylcholinesterase (BChE) are cholinesterases that play an important role in cholinergic transmission by hydrolyzing the neurotransmitter acetylcholine, and they play also a significant role on the Alzheimer disease, therefore finding the bioactive molecules with inhibitor activities on AChE and BChE as an approach and rational way for treating Alzheimer's disease. To this end, compounds such as 6, 62-bieckol and diphlorethohydroxycarmalol, derived and identified from brown algae *Ishige okamurae* a brown algae, have been shown to possess an inhibitory influence on AChE and BChE (Heo *et al.*, 2008). Considerably, a number of studies have currently revealed AChE inhibitory activity of several algae species and, in this regard, compounds with acetylcholinesterase (AChE) activities such as eckstolonol, eckol, dieckol, phlorofucofuroeckol, fucoidan have been isolated and purified from different macroalgae species such as *Caulerpa racemosa, Ulva fasciata, Ecklonia stolonifera, Fucus vesiculosus* and *Ishige okamurae* (Pangestuti and Kim, 2011; Cornish *et al.*, 2010).

Antimicrobials are known as agents that kill or inhibit microorganism growth and currently different sources of prokaryotic and eukaryotic algal species are considered to provide novel and useful compounds. To this effect, antimicrobial agents such as phlorotannin, glycerolipids, fisherellin, sulfolipids, cyanovirin, indolocarbazole etc., have been identified and isolated from algal species (Gribble,

1996). Recently, more and more scientific evidence describe the potential of algae species containing antimicrobial agents. Genovese *et al.* (2013) reported red algae *Asparagopsis taxiformis* antifungal activity against *Aspergillus* species with a minimum inhibitory concentration from 0.15 mg ml^{-1} to 5 mg ml^{-1} based on an agar diffusion assay. *Gracilaria cervicornis,* a common species in warm temperate and tropical seas of the Western Atlantic and West Africa, has shown significant inhibitor activities on pathogenic microbes such as *Staphylococcus aureus, Escherichia coli, Bacillus megaterium, Staphylococcus aureus, Streptococcus faecalis* and *Candida albicans* (De Almeida *et al.*, 2011).

Interestingly, the marine alga *Delisea pulchra* has been found to produce a range of metabolites with inhibitory activity on molecules like *N*-acyl-L-homoserine lactones, a class of intercellular signaling molecules known to arrange the expression of particular phenotypes within a population of clones in gram-negative rod-shaped bacterium like *Vibrio fischeri* (Manefield *et al.*, 1999). In sea weeds tannin derivatives like phlorotannins, synthesized through the acetate-malonate pathway with phloroglucinol-based phenolics (1,3,5-trihydroxybenzene) composition, have secondary functions as defensive compounds and primary roles in cell-wall construction. Moreover, volatile halogenated found in *Fucus vesiculosus* and *Leathesia nana* have been reported to act as a natural defense mechanism to prevent biofouling on the surface of *Laminaria digitata* by deactivation of acylated homoserine lactones (Nakai, *et al.*, 2006).

Also oxylipins, compounds which belong to the prostaglandin and leukotriene series, share striking similarities with the products of cyclo-oxygenases and lipo-oxygenases in mammals. They have been shown to play a leading role in chemical attraction and defense mechanisms. The formation of oxylipins in *L. digitata* was up-regulated in sporophytes challenged with lipopolysaccharides which may function as pathogen-associated molecular patterns (Küpper, *et al.*, 2006). Fucoxanthin is the major biofunctional pigment present in brown seaweeds and is one of the most abundant carotenoid found in nature. It has a molecular structure consisting of an unusual allenic bond and a 5,6-monoepoxide. Fucoxanthin has been reported to have anti-oxidant and anti-tumor properties (Thomas *et al.*, 2011). Some studies have revealed the anti-inflammatory effect of fucoxanthin isolated from brown algae via inhibitory effect of nitric oxide production in lipopolysaccharide-induced RAW 264.7 macrophage cells (Heo *et al.*, 2010). In addition, the methyl ester and 3-bromo-4, 5-dihydroxy-benzaldehyde isolated from *Rhodomela confervoides* and *Avrainvillea nigricans* algae have shown anticancer activity with a IC_{50} value ranging from 3.09 to 8.71 μg/mL and 8.9 μg/mL, respectively (Colon *et al.*, 1987). Moreover, other metabolites, such as lanosol, butanone, rhodomelol isolated from *Osmundaria colensoi,* were demonstrated to have cytotoxic activity against human leukemia cells with an IC_{50} value of 8.0 μM. Moreover, researchers have reported how the methanolic extracts from *Jolyna laminarioides* and *Melanothamnus afaqhusainii* have shown antimicrobial activities against a range of bacteria and fungi and, in this regard, compounds such as jolynamine, saringosterol, loliolide, methyl-4-hydroxybenzoate, propyl-4-hydroxybenzoate, 3, 4, 5-trimethylaniline and harmine have been isolated from these algae (Khan *et al.*, 2011). It is also significantly reported that algae can be considered as a valuable source of anti-HIV compounds and currently different classes of compounds such as sesquiterpene, hydroquinones, fucoidan, sulfoglycolipids and carrageenans have been isolated from different algal species (Schaeffer *et al.*, 2000).

Conclusion

This review demonstrates as algae have all the potential to produce a wide range of several high-value compounds. These valuable molecules have already proved their effectiveness in fields of general interest such as human health, food industry, biomedicine and bioengineering. Algae can be easily used to improve food value, they can also be considered a precious source of pharmaceuticals and neutraceticals. Finally, it should be noticed how the production of these compounds by microalgae can be coupled with the production of biodiesel (based on higher lipid content and biomass productivity of microalgae), wastewater treatment, and reduction of carbon dioxide emissions. In this way it would be very appealing for researchers to progress further in order to explore the undoubted potentialities of algae. To reach this goal it could be beneficial to isolate and screen new species, to introduce new technologies and strengthened the cooperation between academic institutions and industrial sector.

Abbreviations

AChE: Acetylcholinesterase
ARA: Arachidonic Acid
BChE: Butyrylcholinesterase
DHA: Docosahexaenoic acid
DNA: Deoxyribonucleic acid
DPPH: 2,2-diphenyl-1-picrylhydrazyl
EPA: Eicosapentaenoic acid
FAME: Fatty acid methyl esters
GLA: γ-linolenic acid
HDL: High-density lipoprotein
IC_{50}: Half maximal inhibitory concentration
LED: Light-emitting diode
NO: Nitrogen monoxide
PBRs: Photobioreactors
PUFAs: Polyunsaturated fatty acids
ROS: Reactive oxygen species
TAGs: Triacylglycerides

References

Abalde, J., Fabregas, J., and Herrero, C. (1991). β-Carotene, vitamin C and vitamin E content of the marine microalga *Dunaliella tertiolecta* cultured with different nitrogen sources. *Bioresource Technology*, **38**: 121–125.

Abd El-Baky, H., El Baz, F.K., and El-Baroty, G. (2009). Enhancement of antioxidant production in *Spirulina platensis* under oxidative stress. *Acta Physiologiae Plantarum*, **31**: 623–31.

Abd El-Baky, H.H., and El-Baroty, G.S. (2013). The potential use of microalgal carotenoids as dietary supplements and natural preservative ingredients. *Journal of Aquatic Food Product Technology*, **22**: 392-406.

Aburai, N., Ohkubo, S., Miyashita, H., and Abe, K. (2013). Composition of carotenoids and identification of aerial microalgae isolated from the surface of rocks in mountainous districts of Japan. *Algal Research*, 2: 237-243.

Adarme-Vega, T.C., Lim, D., Timmins, M., Vernen, F., Li, Y., and Schenk, P.M. (2012). Microalgal biofactories: a promising approach towards sustainable omega-3 fatty acid production. *Microbial Cell Factories*, 11: 96.

Aflalo, C., Meshulam, Y., Zarka, A., and Boussiba, S. (2007). On the relative efficiency of two- vs. one-stage production of astaxanthin by the green alga *Haematococcus pluvialis*. *Biotechnology and Bioengineering*, **98**: 300-305.

Aremu, A.O., Masondo, N.A., Stirk, W, a., Ordog, V., and Van Staden, J. (2014). Influence of culture age on the phytochemical content and pharmacological activities of five *Scenedesmus* strains. *Journal of Applied Phycology*, **26**: 407-415.

Bandarra, N.M., Pereira, P.A., Batista, I., and Vilela, M. (2003). Fatty acids, sterols and α-tocopherol in *Isochrysis galbana*. *Journal of Food Lipids*, **10**: 25–34.

Becker, E.W. (2007). Micro-algae as a source of protein. *Biotechnology Advances*, **25**: 207–210.

Ben-Amotz, A. (1987). Effect of irradiance and nutrient deficiency on the chemical composition of *Dunaliella bardawil* Ben-Amotz and Avron (Volvocales, Chlorophyta). *Journal of Plant Physiology*, **131**: 479–487.

Ben-Amotz, A. (1999) *Dunaliella* β-carotene: From science to commerce. *In*: Enigmatic microorganisms and life in extreme environments. Vol. 1. Ed. By Seckbach, J., Kluwer Academic Publisher, Dordrecht, Netherlands, pp. 401–410.

Bigogno, C., Khozin-Goldberg, I., Boussiba, S., Vonshak, A., and Cohen, Z. (2002). Lipid and fatty acid composition of the green oleaginous alga *Parietochloris incisa*, the richest plant source of arachidonic acid. *Phytochemiatry*, **60**: 497–503

Blanco, A.M., Moreno, J., Del Campo, J.A., Josë, A., Rivas, J., and Guerrero, M.G. (2007). Outdoor cultivation of lutein-rich cells of *Muriellopsis* sp. in open ponds. *Applied Microbiology and Biotechnology*, **73**: 1259-1266.

Borowitzka, M.A. (1993). Products from microalgae. *Infofish International*, **5**: 21–26.

Borowitzka, M.A. (1999). Commercial production of microalgae: ponds, tanks, tubes and fermenters. *Journal of Biotechnology*, **70**: 313–321.

Borowitzka, M.A. (2013). High-value products from microalgae-their development and commercialization. *Journal of Applied Phycology*. **25**: 743-756.

Brentner, L.B., Eckelman, M.J., and Zimmerman, J.B. (2011). Combinatorial life cycle assessment to inform process design of industrial production of algal biodiesel. *Environmental Science and Technology*, **45**: 7060–7067.

Cao, G., and Concas, A. (2010). Process for bio-oil production which makes use of carbon dioxide. Patent EP10158619.6.

Carballo-Cárdenas, E.C., Tuan, P.M., Janssen, M., and Wijffels, R.H. (2003). Vitamin E (α-tocopherol) production by the marine microalgae *Dunaliella tertiolecta* and *Tetraselmis suecica* in batch cultivation. *Biomolecular Engineering*, **20**: 139–147.

Casal, C., Cuaresma, M., Vega, J.M., and Vilchez, C. (2011). Enhanced productivity of a lutein-enriched novel acidophile microalga grown on urea. *Marine Drugs*, **9**: 29–42.

Çelekli, A., Bozkurt, H., and Dönmez, G. (2014). Predictive modeling of β-carotene accumulation by *Dunaliella salina* as a function of pH, NaCI, and irradiance. *Russian Journal of Plant Physiology*, **61**: 215-223.

Ceron, M.C., Campos, I., Sanchez, J.F., Acien, F.G., Molina, E., and Fernandez-Sevilla, J.M. (2008). Recovery of lutein from microalgae biomass: development of a process for *Scenedesmus almeriensis* biomass. *Journal of Agriculture and Food Chemistry*, **56**: 11761–11766.

Chang, G., Gao, N., Tian, G., Wu, Q., Chang, M., and Wang, X. (2013). Improvement of docosahexaenoic acid production on glycerol by *Schizochytrium* sp. S31 with constantly high oxygen transfer coefficient. *Bioresource Technology*, **142**: 400-406.

Chisti, Y. (2007). Biodiesel from microalgae. *Biotechnology Advance*, **25**: 294–306.

Chiu, C.J., and Taylor, A. (2007). Nutritional antioxidants and age-related cataract and maculopathy. *Experimental Eye Research*, **84**: 229–245.

Chkhikvishvili, I.D., and Ramazanov, Z.M. (2000). Phenolic substances of brown algae and their antioxidant activity. *Applied Biochemistry and Microbiology*, **36**: 289–291.

Choochote, W., Suklampoo, L., and Ochaikul, D. (2014). Evaluation of antioxidant capacities of green microalgae. *Journal of Applied Phycology*, **26**: 43-48.

Christaki, E., Bonos, E., Giannenas, I., and Florou-Paneri, P. (2013). Functional properties of carotenoids originating from algae. *Journal of the Science of Food and Agriculture*, **93**: 5-11.

Clarens, A.F., Resurreccion, E.P., White, M.A., and Colosi, L.M. (2010). Environmental life cycle comparison of algae to other bioenergy feedstocks. *Environmental Science and Technology*, **44**: 1813–1819.

Cohen, Z., and Khozin-Goldberg, I. (2010). Searching for polyunsaturated fatty acid-rich microalgae. *In*: Single cell oils: microbial and algal oils. Ed. By Cohen, Z. and Ratledge, C. AOCS Publishing, Urbana, USA, pp. 201–224.

Collet, P., Spinelli, D., Lardon, L., Helias, A., Steyer, J-P., and Bernard, O. (2014). Life-Cycle Assessment of Microalgal-Based Biofuels. In: Biofuels from Algae. Edition:

1st, Ed. By Ashok, P., Lee, D-J., Chisti, Y., Soccol, C. Publisher Elsevier, pp. 287-312.

Colon, M., Guevara, P., Gerwick, W.H., and Ballantine, D. (1987). 5'-Hydroxyisoavrainvilleol, a new diphenylmethane derivative from the tropical green alga *Avrainvillea nigricans*. *Journal of Natural Products,* **50**: 368-374.

Cornish, M.L., and Garbary, D.J. (2010). Antioxidants from macroalgae: potential applications in human health and nutrition. *Algae,* **25**: 155-171.

de Almeida, C.L.F., de S. Falcão, H., de M. Lima, G.R., de A. Montenegro, C., Lira, N.S., de Athayde-Filho, P.F., Rodrigues, L.C., V. de Souza, M.d.F., Barbosa-Filho, J.M., and Batista, L.M. (2011). Bioactivities from marine algae of the genus *Gracilaria*. *International journal of molecular sciences,* **12**: 4550-4573.

Del Campo, J.A., Moreno, J., Rodriguez, H., Vargas, M.A., Rivas, J., and Guerrero, M.G. (2000). Carotenoid content of chlorophycean microalgae: factors determining lutein accumulation in *Muriellopsis* sp. (Chlorophyta). *Journal of Biotechnology,* **76**: 51–59.

Del Campo, J.A., Rodriguez, H., Moreno, J., Vargas, M.A., Rivas, J., and Guerrero, M.G. (2004). Accumulation of astaxanthin and lutein in *Chlorella zofingiensis* (Chlorophyta). *Applied Microbiology and Biotechnology*, **64**: 848–854.

Del Campo, J., García-González, M., and Guerrero, M. (2007). Outdoor cultivation of microalgae for carotenoid production: current state and perspectives. *Applied Microbiology and Biotechnology*, **74**: 1163–1174.

Drokova, T.G., and Popova, R.J. (1974). On the content of tocopherol in the alga *Dunaliella salina* Teod. *Ukrayins'kyi Botanichnyi Zhurnal*, **31**: 229–231.

Droop, M.R. (1954). Conditions governing haematochrome formation and loss in the alga *Haematococcus pluvialis Flotow*. *Archiv fûr Mikrobiologie,* **20**: 391-397.

Droop, M.R. (1955). Carotenogenesis in *Haematococcus pluvialis*. *Nature,* **75**: 42.

Durmaz, Y. (2007). Vitamin E, (α-tocopherol) production by the marine microalgae *Nannochloropsis oculata* (Eustigmatophyceae) in nitrogen limitation. *Aquaculture,* **272**: 717–722.

Fallarero, A., Loikkanen, J.J., Männistö, P.T., Castañeda, O., and Vidal, A. (2003). Effects of aqueous extracts of *Halimeda incrassate* (Ellis) Lamouroux and *Bryothamnion triquetrum* (SG Gmelim) Howe on hydrogen peroxide and methyl mercury-induced oxidative stress in GT1-7 mouse hypothalamic immortalized cells. *Phytomedicine,* **10**: 39-47.

Fazeli, M.R., Tofighi, H., Samadi, N., and Jamalifai, H. (2006). Effects of salinity on β-carotene production by *Dunaliella tertiolecta* DCCBC26 isolated from the Urmia salt lake, north of Iran. *Bioresource Technology,* **97**: 2453-2456.

Finkel, T., Holbrook, N.J. (2000). Oxidants, oxidative stress and the biology of ageing. *Nature,* **408**: 239–247.

Frampton, D.M.F., Gurney, R.H., Dunstan, G.A., Clementson, L.A., Toifil, M.C., Pollard, C.B., Burn, S., Jameson, I.D., and Blackburn, S.I. (2013). Evaluation of growth, nutrient utilization and production of bioproducts by a wastewater-isolated microalga. *Bioresouce Technology*, **130**: 261-268.

Francisco, E.C., Neves, D.B., Jacob-Lopes, E., and Franco, T.T. (2010). Microalgae as feedstock for biodiesel production: carbon dioxide sequestration, lipid production and biofuel quality. *Journal of Chemical Technology and Biotechnology*, **85**: 395–403.

Garbayo, I., Cuaresma, M., Vilchez, C., and Vega, J.M. (2008), Effect of abiotic stress on the production of lutein and β-carotene by *Chlamydomonas acidophila*. *Process Biochemistry*, **43**: 1158-1161.

Genovese, G., Leitner, S., Minicante, S.A., and LassFlörl, C. (2013). The Mediterranean red alga *Asparagopsis taxiformis* has antifungal activity against *Aspergillus* species. *Mycoses*, **56**: 516-519.

Ghiselli, A., D'Amicis, A., and Giacosa, A. (1997). The antioxidant potential of the Mediterranean diet. *European Journal of Cancer Prevention*, **6**: 15–19.

Goh, S-H., Yusoff, F.M., and Loh, S-P. (2010). A comparison of the antioxidant properties and total phenolic content in a diatom, *Chaetoceros* sp. and a green microalga, *Nannochloropsis* sp. *Journal of Agricultural Science*, **2**: 123–130.

Gómez, P., and González, M. (2005). The effect of temperature and irradiance on the growth and carotenogenic capacity of seven strains of *Dunaliella salina* (Chlorophyta) cultivated under laboratory conditions. *Biological Research*, **38**: 151–162.

Gordon, P.T., and Ratliff, V. (1992). The implication of omega"3 fatty acids in human health. *In*: Advances in seafood biochemistry–composition and quality. Ed. By Flick, Jr G.J. and Martin, R.E. Technomic Publishing, Lancaster, USA.

Gorjão, R., Azevedo-Martins, A.K., Gomes Rodrigues, H., Abdulkader, F., Arcisio-Miranda, M., Procopio, J., and Curi, R. (2009). Comparative effects of DHA and EPA on cell function. *Pharmacology and Therapeutics*, 122: 56–64.

Graziani, G., Schiavo, S., Nicolai, M.A., Buono, S., Fogliano, V., Pinto, G., and Pollio, A. (2013). Microalgae as human food: chemical and nutritional characteristics of the thermo-acidophilic microalga *Galdieria sulphuraria*. *Food and Function*, **4**: 144-152.

Green, J. (1963). Occurrence of astaxanthin in euglenoid *Trachelomonas volvocina*. *Comparative Biochemistry and Physiology*, **9**: 313-316.

Gribble, G.W. (1996). The diversity of natural organochlorines in living organisms. *Pure and applied chemistry*, **68**: 1699-1712.

Griffiths, M.J., and Harrison, S.T.L. (2009). Lipid productivity as a key characteristic for choosing algal species for biodiesel production. *Journal of Applied Phycology*, **21**: 493–507.

Grung, M., Metzger, P., and Liaeen-Jensen, S. (1994). Algal carotenoids 53: secondary carotenoids of algae 4. Secondary carotenoids in the green alga *Botryococcus braunii*, race L, new strain. *Biochemical Systematics and Ecology*, **22**: 25-29.

Guedes, A.C., Amaro, H.M., and Malcata, F.X. (2011a). Microalgae as sources of high added-value compounds – A brief review of recent work. *Biotechnology Progress*, **27**: 597–613.

Guedes, A.C., Amaro, H.M., Pereira, R.D., and Malcata, F.X. (2011b). Effect of temperature and pH on growth and antioxidant content of the microalga *Scenedesmus obliquus*. *Biotechnology Progress*, **27**: 1218-1224.

Guedes, A.C., Gião, M.S., Seabra, R., Ferreira, A.C., Tamagnini, P., Moradas-Ferreira, P., and Malcata, F.X. (2013). Evaluation of the antioxidant activity of cell extracts from microalgae. *Marine Drugs*, **11**: 1256-1270.

Guerin, M., Huntley, M.E., and Olaizola, M. (2003). *Haematococcus* astaxanthin: application for human health and nutrition. *Trends in Biotechnology*, **21**: 210–216.

Guil-Guerrero, J.L., and Rebolloso-Fuentes, M.M. (2008). Nutrient composition of *Chlorella* spp. and *Monodus subterraneus* cultured in a bubble column bioreactor. *Food Biotechnology*, **22**: 218-233.

Hajimahmoodi, M., Faramarzi, M.A., Mohammadi, N., Soltani, N., Oveisi, M.R., and Nafissi-Varcheh, N. (2010). Evaluation of antioxidant properties and total phenolic contents of some strains of microalgae. *Journal of Applied Phycology*, **22**: 43-50.

Heo, S.J., Kim, J-P., Jung, W-K., Lee, N-H., Kang, H-S., Jun, E-M., and Park, S-H. (2008). Identification of chemical structure and free radical scavenging activity of diphlorethohydroxycarmalol isolated from a brown alga, *Ishige okamurae*. *Journal of microbiology and biotechnology*, **18**: 676-681.

Herrero, C., Abalde, J., and Fabregas, J. (1991). β-carotene, vitamin C and vitamin E content of the marine microalga *Dunaliella tertiolecta* cultured with different nitrogen sources. *Bioresource Technology*, **38**: 121-125.

Herrero, M., Jaime, L., Martín-Alvarez, P.J., Cifuentes, A., and Ibáñez, E. (2006). Optimization of the extraction of antioxidants from *Dunaliella salina* microalga by pressurized liquids. *Journal of Agriculture and Food Chemistry*, **54**: 5597–5603.

Ho, S-H., Chan, M-C., Liu, C-C., Chen, C-Y., Lee, W-L., Lee, D-J., and Chang, J-S. (2014). Enhancing lutein productivity of an indigenous microalga *Scenedesmus obliquus* FSP-3 using light-related strategies. *Bioresource Technology*, **152**: 275-282.

Holub, B.J. (2009). Docosahexaenoic acid (DHA) and cardiovascular disease risk factors. *Prostaglandins, Leukotrienes and Essential Fatty Acids*, **81**: 199–204.

Hosseini Tafreshi, A., and Shariati, M. (2009). *Dunaliella* biotechnology: methods and applications. *Journal of Applied Microbiology*, **107**: 14–35.

Hu, C-W., Chuang, L-T., Yu, P-C., and Chen, C-N N. (2013). Pigment production by a new thermotolerant microalga *Coelastrella* sp. F50. *Food Chemistry*, **138**: 2071-2078.

Huang, H.L., and Wang, B.G. (2004). Antioxidant capacity and lipophilic content of seaweeds collected from the Qingdao coastline. *Journal of Agricultural and Food Chemistry*, **52**: 4993–4997.

Ip, P.F., and Chen, F. (2005). Production of astaxanthin by the green microalga *Chlorella zofingiensis* in the dark. *Process Biochemistry*, **40**: 733–738.

Jeon, Y-C., Cho, C-W., and Yun, Y-S. (2006). Combined effects of light intensity and acetate concentration on the growth of unicellular microalga *Haematococcus pluvialis*. *Enzyme and Microbial Technology*, **39**: 490–495.

Khan, A.M., Noreen, S., Imran, Z.P., Rahman, A., and Choudhary, M.I. (2011). A new compound, jolynamine, from marine brown alga *Jolyna laminarioides*. *Natural Product Research* **25**: 898-904.

Kilian, O., Benemann, C.S.E., Niyogi, K.K., and Vick, B. (2011). High-efficiency homologous transformation in the oil-producing alga *Nannochloropsis* sp. *Proceedings of the National Academy of Science USA*, **108**: 21265–21269.

Kim, J., Yoo, G., Lee, H., Lim, J., Kim, K., Kim, C.W., Park, S.M., and Jang, J.W. (2013). Methods of downstream processing for the production of biodiesel from microalgae. *Biotechnology Advances*, **31**: 862–876.

Kleinová, A., Cvengrošová, Z., Rimarèík, J., Buzetzki, E., Mikulec, J., and Cvengroš, J. (2012). Biofuels from algae. *Procedia Engineering*, **42**: 231-238.

Kobayashi, M., Kurimura, Y., and Tsuji, Y. (1997). Light-independent, astaxanthin production by the green microalga *Haeamatococcus pluvialis* under salt stress. *Biotechnology Letters*, **19**: 507–509.

Koller, M., Salerno, A., Tuffner, P., Koinigg, M., Böchzelt, H., Schober, S., Pieber, S., Schnitzer, H., Mittelbach, M., and Braunegg, G. (2012). Characteristics and potential of micro algal cultivation strategies: a review. *Journal of Cleaner Production*, **37**: 377-388.

Kumar Saha, S., McHugh, E., Hayes, J., Moane, S, Walsh, D., and Murray, P. (2013). Effect of various stress-regulatory factors on biomass and lipid production in microalga *Haematococcus pluvialis*. *Bioresource Technology*, **128**: 118–124.

Küpper, F. C., Gaquerel, E., Boneberg, E. M., Morath, S., Salaün, J. P., and Potin, P. (2006). Early events in the perception of lipopolysaccharides in the brown alga Laminaria digitata include an oxidative burst and activation of fatty acid oxidation cascades. *Journal of experimental botany*, **57**: 1991-1999.

Lababpour, A., Hada, K., Shimakara, K., Katsuda, T., and Katoh, S. (2004). Effects of nutrient supply methods and illumination with blue light emitting diodes (LEDs) on astaxanthin production by *Haematococcus pluvialis*. *Journal of Bioscience and Bioengineering*; **98**: 452–456.

Lamers, P.P., van de Laak, C.C.W., Kaasenbrood, P.S., Lorier, J., Janssen, M., De Vos. R.C.H., Bino, R.J., and Wijfells, R.H. (2010). Carotenoid and fatty acid metabolism in light-stressed *Dunaliella salina*. *Biotechnology and Bioengineering*, **106**: 638–648.

Lamers, P.P., Janssen, M., De Vos, R.C.H., Bino, R.J., and Wijffels, R.H. (2012). Carotenoid and fatty acid metabolism in nitrogen-starved *Dunaliella salina*, a unicellular green microalga. *Journal of Biotechnology*, **162**: 21–27.

Lee Chang, K.J., Nichols, C.M., Blackburn, S.I., Dunstan, G.A., Koutoulis, A.N., and Peter, D. (2014). Comparison of *Thraustochytrids Aurantiochytrium* sp., *Schizochytrium* sp., *Thraustochytrium* sp., and *Ulkenia* sp. for production of biodiesel, long-chain omega-3 oils, and exopolysaccharide. *Marine Biotechnology*, In Press.

Lee, S.H., Park, M.H., Heo, S.J., Kang, S.M., Ko, S.C., Han, J.S., and Jeon, Y.J. (2010a). Dieckol isolated from *Ecklonia cava* inhibits α-glucosidase and α-amylase in vitro and alleviates postprandial hyperglycemia in streptozotocin-induced diabetic mice. *Food and Chemical Toxicology*, **48**: 2633-2637.

Lee, S-H., Lee, J-B., Lee, K-W., and Jeon, Y-J. (2010b). Antioxidant properties of tidal pool microalgae, *Halochlorococcum porphyrae* and *Oltamannsiellopsis unicellularis* from Jeju Island, Korea. *Algae*, **25**: 45–56.

Lemoine, Y., and Schoefs, B. (2010). Secondary ketocarotenoid astaxanthin biosynthesis in algae: a multifunctional response to stress. *Photosynthesis Research*, **106**: 155–177.

Leon, R., Martin, M., Vigara, J., Vilchez, C., and Vega, J.M. (2003). Microalgae mediated photoproduction of β-carotene in aqueous-organic two phase systems. *Biomolecular Engineering*, **20**: 177–182.

Leya, T., Rahn, A., Lûtz, C., and Remias, D. (2009). Response of arctic snow and permafrost algae to high light and nitro-gen stress by changes in pigment composition and applied aspects for biotechnology. *FEMS Microbiology Ecology*, **67**: 432-443.

Li, H.B., Jiang, Y., and Chen, F. (2002). Isolation and purification of lutein from the microalga *Chlorella vulgaris* by extraction after saponification. *Journal of Agricultural and Food Chemistry*, **50**: 1070–1072.

Li, H., Cheng, K., Wong, C., Fan, K., Chen, F., and Jiang, Y. (2007). Evaluation of antioxidant capacity and total phenolic content of different fractions of selected microalgae. *Food Chemistry*, **102**: 771–776.

Li, Z., Sun, M., Li, Q., Li, A., and Zhang, C. (2012). Profiling of carotenoids in six microalgae (Eustigmatophyceae) and assessment of their β-carotene productions in bubble column photobioreactor. *Biotechnology Letters*, **34**: 2049-2053.

Liu, B-H., and Lee, Y-K. (2000). Secondary carotenoids formation by the green alga *Chlorococcum* sp. *Journal of Applied Phycology*. **12**: 301-307.

Maity J.P, Bundschuh, J., Chen, C-Y., and Bhattacharya, P. (2014). Microalgae for third generation biofuel production, mitigation of greenhouse gas emissions and wastewater treatment: Present and future perspectives - A mini review, Energy, http: //dx.doi.org/10.1016/j.energy.2014.04.003

Manefield, M., de Nys, R., Naresh, K., Roger, R., Givskov, M., Peter, S., and Kjelleberg, S. (1999). Evidence that halogenated furanones from Delisea pulchra inhibit acylated homoserine lactone (AHL)-mediated gene expression by displacing the AHL signal from its receptor protein. *Microbiology*, **145**: 283-291.

Mendiola, J.A., García-Martínez, D., Rupérez, F.J., Martín-Álvarez, P.J., Reglero, G., Cifuentes, A., Barbas, C., Ibaòez, E., and Seòoráns, F.J. (2008). Enrichment of vitamin E from *Spirulina platensis* microalga by SFE. *Journal of Supercritical Fluids*, **43**: 484–489.

Misawa. N. (2009). Pathway engineering of plants toward astaxanthin production. *Plant Biotechnology*. **26**: 93-99.

Mojaat, M., Pruvost, J., Foucault, A., and Legrand, J. (2008) Effect of organic carbon sources and Fe^{2+} ions on growth and β-carotene accumulation by *Dunaliella salina. Biochemical Engineering Journal*, **39**: 177-184.

Montpoint, S., and Guilhou, J.J. (1991). Les microalgues: applications potentielles en dermatologie. Premier Colloque Scientifique Français sur la Biotechnologie des Microalgues et des Cyanobacteries Appliquée au Thermalisme. Amélie-les-bains: Centre d'Études Nucléaires de Cadarache, pp. 93–96. [24et25Octobre].

Mulders, K.J.M., Lamers, P.P., Martens, D.E., and Wijffels, R.H, (2014). Phototrophic pigment production with microalgae: biological constraints and opportunities. *Journal of Phycology*, **50**: 229-242.

Nakai, M., Kageyama, N., Nakahara, K., and Miki, W. (2006). Phlorotannins as radical scavengers from the extract of *Sargassum ringgoldianum*. *Marine Biotechnology*, **8**: 409–414

Ninomiya, M., Satoh, H., Yamaguchi, Y., Takenaka, H., and Koketsu, M. (2011). Antioxidative activity and chemical constituents of edible terrestrial alga *Nostoc commune* Vauch. *Bioscience, Biotechnology and Biochemistry*, **75**: 2175-2177.

Nonomura, A.M. (1989). Industrial biosynthesis of carotenoids. In: Carotenoids, chemistry and biology, Ed. By Krinsky, N.I., Mathews-Roth, M.M. and Taylor, R.F. Plenum Press, New York, pp. 365–375.

Norsker, N-H., Barbosa, M.J., Vermuë, M.H., and Wijffels, R.H. (2011). Microalgal production – a close look at the economics. *Biotechnology Advances*, **29**: 24–27.

Ogbonna, J., Tomiyamal, S., and Tanaka, H. (1998). Heterotrophic cultivation of *Euglena gracilis* Z for efficient production of α-tocopherol. *Journal of Applied Phycology*, **10**: 67–74.

Okuda, T., Ando, A., Sajuradani, E., and Ogawa, J. (2013). Isolation and characterization of a docosahexaenoic acid-phospholipids producing microorganism *Crypthecodinium* sp. D31. *Journal of the American Oil Chemists' Society*, **90**: 1837-1844.

Olaizola, M., and Huntley, M.E. (2000). Recent advances in commercial production of astaxanthin from microalgae. *In*: Biomaterials and bioprocessing. Ed. By Fingerman, M. and Nagabhushanam, R. Science Publishers, Enfield, NH, USA, pp. 143–164.

Orosa, M., Torres, E., Fidalgo, P., and Abalde, J. (2000). Production and analysis of secondary carotenoids in green algae. *Journal of Applied Phycology*, **12**: 553-556.

Orosa, M., Favero, J.F., Herrero, C., and Abalde, J. (2001). Comparison of the accumulation of astaxanthin in *Haematococcus pluvialis* and other green microalgae under N-starvation and high light conditions. *Biotechnology Letters*, **23**: 1079–1085.

Pangestuti, R., and Kim, S. K. (2011). Neuroprotective effects of marine algae. *Marine drugs*, **9**: 803-818.

Patil, V., Källqvist. T., Olsen, E., Vogt. G., and Gislerød, H.R. (2007). Fatty acid composition of 12 microalgae for possible use in aquaculture feed. *Aquaculture International*, **15**: 1–9.

Përez-López, P., González-García, S., Allewaert, C., Verween, A., Murray, P., Feijoo, G., and Teresa Moreira, M. (2014). Environmental evaluation of eicosapentaenoic acid production by *Phaeodactylum tricornutum*. *Science of the Total Environment*, **466-467**: 991-1002.

Phadwal, K., and Singh, P.K. (2003). Effect of nutrient depletion on β-carotene and glycerol accumulation in two strains of *Dunaliella* sp. *Bioresource Technology*, **90**: 55–58.

Piccaglia, R., Marotti, M., and Grandi, S. (1998). Lutein and lutein ester content in different types of *Tagetes patula* and *T-erecta*. *Industrial Crops and Products*, **8**: 45–51.

Qin, S., Liu, G-X., and Hu, Z-Y. (2008). The accumulation and metabolism of astaxanthin in *Scenedesmus obliquus* (Chlorophyceae). *Process Biochemistry*, **43**: 795-802.

Quilodrán, B., Hinzpeter, I., Hormazabal, E., Quiroz, A., and Shene, C. (2010). Docosahexaenoic acid (C22: 6n-3, DHA) and astaxanthin production by *Thraustochytriidae* sp. AS4-A1 a native strain with high similitude to Ulkenia sp.: Evaluation of liquid residues from food industry as nutrient sources. *Enzyme and Microbial Technology*, **47**: 24-30.

Radakovits, R., Jinkerson, R.E., Darzins, A., and Posewitz, M.C. (2010). Genetic engineering of algae for enhanced biofuel production, *Eukaryotic Cell*, **9**: 486–501.

Raja, R., Hemaiswayra, S., and Rengasamy, R. (2007). Exploitation of *Dunaliella* for β-carotene production. *Applied Microbiology and Biotechnology*, **74**: 517-523.

Ramírez Fajardo, A., Cerdán, L.E., Robles Medina, A., Acién Fernández, F.G., González Moreno, P.A., and Molina Grima, E. (2007). Lipid extraction from the microalga *Phaeodactylum tricornutum*. *European Journal of Lipid Science Technology*, **109**: 120–126.

Rao, A.R., Sindhuja, H.N., Dharmesh, S.M., Sankar, K.U., Sarada, R., and Ravishankar, G.A. (2013). Effective inhibition of skin cancer, tyrosinase, and antioxidative properties by astaxanthin and astaxanthin esters from the green alga *Haematococcus pluvialis*. *Journal of Agricultural and Food Chemistry*, **61**: 3842-3851.

Ravi Kumar, S., Bhaskar, N., Divakar, S., and Baskaran, V. (2010). Bioavailability and metabolism of fucoxanthin in rats: structural characterization of metabolites by LC-MS (APCI). *Molecular and cellular biochemistry*. **333**: 299-310.

Rawat, I., Ranjith Kumar, R., Mutanda, T., and Bux, F. (2013), Biodiesel from microalgae: A critical evaluation from laboratory to large scale production. *Applied Energy*, **103**: 444–467.

Razon, L.F., and Tan, R.R. (2011). Net energy analysis of the production of biodiesel and biogas from the microalgae: *Haematococcus pluvialis* and *Nannochloropsis*. *Applied Energy*, **88**: 3507–3514.

Remias, D., Lûtz-Meindl, U., and Lûtz, C. (2005). Photosynthesis, pigments and ultrastructure of the alpine snow alga *Chlamydomonas nivalis*. *European. Journal of Phycology*, **40**: 259-268.

Remias, D., Karsten, U., Lûtz, C., and Leya, T. (2010). Physiological and morphological processes in the alpine snow alga *Chloromonas nivalis* (Chlorophyceae) during cyst for-mation. *Protoplasma*, **243**: 73-86.

Remias, D., Lûtz-Meindl, U., and Lûtz, C. (2005). Photosynthesis, pigments and ultrastructure of the alpine snow alga *Chlamydomonas nivalis*. *European. Journal of Phycology*, **40**: 259-268.

Rodriguez-Garcia, I., and Guil-Guerrero, J. (2008). Evaluation of the antioxidant activity of three microalgal species for use as dietary supplements and in the preservation of foods. *Food Chemistry*, **108**: 1023–1026.

Ryckebosch, E., Brunnel, C., Termote-Verhalle, R., Goiris, K., Muylaert, K., and Foubert, I. (2014). Nutritional evaluation of microalgae oils rich in omega-3 long chain polyunsaturated fatty acids as an alternative for fish oil. *Food Chemistry*, **160**: 393-400.

Sajilata, M.G., Singhai, R.S., and Kamat, M.Y. (2008). Fractionation of lipids and purification of γ-linolenic acid (GLA) from *Spirulina platensis*. *Food Chemistry*, **109**: 580-586.

Sanchez, J.F., Fernandez, J.M., Acien, F.G., Rueda, A., Perez-Parra, J., and Molina Grima, E. (2008). Influence of culture conditions on the productivity and lutein content of the new strain *Scenedesmus almeriensis*. *Process Biochemitry*, **43**: 398–405.

Sánchez-Lara, K., Turcott, J.C., Juárez-Hernández, E., Nuñez-Valencia, C., Villanueva, G., Guevara, P., De la Torre-Vallejo, M., Mohar, A., and Arrieta, O. (2014). Effects of an oral nutritional supplement containing eicosapentaenoic acid on nutritional and clinical outcomes in patients with advanced non-small cell lung cancer: Randomised trial. *Clinical Nutrition*, In Press.

Sanchez-Saavedra, M.P., and Voltolina, D. (2002). Effect of photon fluence rates of white and blue–green light on growth efficiency and pigment content of three diatom species in batch cultures. *Ciencias Marinas*, **28**: 273–279.

Sarada, R., Tripathi, U., and Ravishankar, G.A. (2002). Influence of stress on astaxanthin production in *Haematococcus pluvialis* grown under different culture conditions. *Process Biochemistry*, **37**: 623–627.

Sarrobert, B., and Dermoun, D. (1991). Extraction et valorisation de molecules à haute valeur ajoutée chez la microalgae *Porphyridium cruentum*. Premier Colloque Scientifique Français sur la Biotechnologie des Microalgues et des Cyanobacteries Appliquée au Thermalisme. Amélie-les-Bains, France: Centre d'Études Nucléaires de Cadarache. pp. 109–114. 24-25 Octobre 1991.

Schaeffer, D.J., and Krylov, V.S. (2000) Anti-HIV activity of extracts and compounds from algae and cyanobacteria. *Ecotoxicology and Environmental Safety*, **45**: 208-227.

Shi, X., Wu, Z., and Chen, F. (2006). Kinetic modeling of lutein production by heterotrophic *Chlorella* at various pH and temperatures. *Molecular Nutrition and Food Research*, **50**: 763–8.

Silva Benavides, A.M., Torzillo, G., Kopecký, J., and Masojídek, J. (2013). Productivity and biochemical composition of *Phaeodactylum tricornutum* (Bacillariophyceae) cultures grown outdoors in tubular photobioreactors and open ponds. *Biomass and Bioenergy*, **54**: 115-122.

Singh, A., Olsen, S.I., and Singh Nigam, P. (2011). A viable technology to generate third generation biofuel. *Journal of Chemical Technology and Biotechnology*, **86**: 1349–1353.

Siriwardhana, N., Lee, K.W., and Jeon, Y.J. (2005). Radical scavenging potential of hydrophilic phlorotannins of *Hizikia fusiformis*. *Algae*, **20**: 69-75.

Skjanes, K., Rebours, C., and Lindblad, P. (2013). Potential for green microalgae to produce hydrogen, pharmaceuticals and other high value products in a combined process. *Critical Reviews in Biotechnology*, **33**: 172-215.

Solovchenko, A.E., Khozin-Goldberg, I., Didi-Cohen, S., Cohen, Z., and Merzlyak, M.N. (2008). Effects of light and nitrogen starvation on the content and composition of carotenoids of the green microalga *Parietochloris incisa*. *Russian Journal of Plant Physiology*, **55**: 455–462.

Soratana, K., and Landis, A.E. (2011). Evaluating industrial symbiosis and algae cultivation from a life cycle perspective. *Bioresource Technology*, **102**: 6892–6901.

Suali, E., and Sarbatly, R. (2012). Converstion of microalgae to biofuel. *Renewable and Sustainable Energy Reviews*, **16**: 4316-4342.

Sukenik, A. (1991). Ecophysiological considerations in the optimization of eicosapentaenoic acid production by *Nannochloropsis* sp. (Eustigmatophyceae). *Bioresource Technology*, **35**: 263-269

Tababa, H., Hirabayashi, S., and Inubushi, K. (2012). Media optimization of *Parietochloris incise* for arachidonic acid accumulation in an outdoor vertical tubular photobioreactor. *Journal of Applied Phycology*, **24**: 887–895.

Talebi, A.F., Mohtashami, S.K., Tabatabei, M., Tohidfar, M., Bagheri, A., Zeinalabedini, M., Mirzaei, H.H., Mirzajanzadeh, M., Shafaroudi, S.M., and Bakhtiari, S. (2013). Fatty acids profiling: A selective criterion for screening microalgae strains for biodiesel production. *Algal Research*, **2**: 258-267.

Tannin-Spitz, T., Bergman, M., Van-Moppes, D., Grossman, S., and Arad, S. (2005). Antioxidant activity of the polysaccharide of the red microalga *Porphyridium* sp. *Journal of Applied Phycology*, **17**: 215–222

Thomas, N.V., and Kim, S.-K. (2011). Health Beneficial Aspects of Phloroglucinol Derivatives from Marine Brown Algae. *In*: Handbook of Marine Macroalgae: Biotechnology and Applied Phycology. Ed. By Kim, S-K., John Wiley and Sons, Ltd, Chichester, UK. doi: 10.1002/9781119977087.ch21

Tjahjono, A.E., Hayama, Y., Kakizono, T., Terada, Y., Nishio, N., and Nagai, S. (1994). Hyper-accumulation of astaxanthin in a green alga *Haematococcus pluvialis* at elevated temperatures. *Biotechnology Letters*, **16**: 133–138.

Vaquero, I., Ruiz-Dominguez, M.C., Marquez, M., and Vichez, C. (2012). Cu-mediated biomass productivity enhancement and lutein enrichment of the novel microalga *Coccomyxa onubensis*. *Process Biochemistry*, **47**: 694-700.

Wang, G.Y., Wang, X., and Liu, X.H. (2011). Two-stage hydrolysis of invasive algal feedstock for ethanol fermentation. *Journal of Integrative Plant Biology*, **53**: 246–252.

Ward, O.P., and Singh, A. (2005). Omega-3/6 fatty acids: alternative sources of production. *Process Biochemistry*, **40**: 3627–3652.

Xie, Y., Ho, S-H., Chen, C-N N, Chen, C-F., Ng, I-S., Jing, K-J., Chang, J-S., and Lu, Y. (2013). Phototrophic cultivation of a thermo-tolerant *Desmodesmus* sp. for lutein production: Effects of nitrate concentration, light intensity and fed-batch operation. *Bioresource Technology*, **144**: 435-444.

Yongmanitchai, W., and Ward, O.P. (1991). Growth of and omega-3 fatty acid production by *Phaeodactylum tricornutum* under different culture conditions. *Applied Environmental Microbiology*, **57**: 419-425.

Zhang, J., Sun, Z., Sun, P.P., Chen, T.P., and Chen, F. (2014). Microalgal carotenoids: beneficial effects and potential in human health. *Food and Function*, **5**: 413-425.

Bioactive Phytochemicals: Perspectives for Modern Medicine Vol. 3 (2015)
Editor: **V.K. Gupta**
Published by: **DAYA PUBLISHING HOUSE, NEW DELHI**

Pages **337–353**

13

Hypericum spp.: A Resource from Wild Mediterranean Flora for the Treatment of Mild Depression

Silvia Lazzara[1], Edoordo Napoli[2] and Alessandra Carrubba[3*]

ABSTRACT

The genus Hypericum holds about 480 species (Crockett and Robson, 2011), widely spread throughout the world. A large part of them grows wild in the Mediterranean areas: 30 Hypericum taxa (26 species and 4 sub-species) have been detected in Italy, and about one third of them (11 taxa) are native to Sicily (Castellano and Spadaro, 2010). Actually, traditional and folk medicines in many parts of the world use Hypericum species for a plenty of different purposes. The most important are certainly two: the treatment of wounds and burns (because of the strong effects stimulating the formation of new tissue and lenitive of pain), and the therapy of moderate to mild depression (due to its remarkable hypnotic and tranquilizer effect, with specific antidepressant and anxiolytic effects). Besides these well-known actions, other biological effects of Hypericum extracts have been recognized in time, including antimicrobial, antioxidant, antiproliferative activities. Although many compounds have been identified in Hypericum extracts, however, which compound, or mixture of compounds, is exactly responsible for every specific pharmacological action it is not perfectly clear as far. The available literature agrees in ascribing a great importance to three active compounds, namely hypericin and pseudohypericin (two naphthodianthrones), and hyperforin (a phloroglucinol

1 C.R.A. – S.F.M. (Agricultural Research Council - Research Unit for the recovery and the exploitation of Mediterranean Flower Species), S.S. 113 km 245,500, 90011 Bagheria, Palermo, Italy

2 C.N.R. – I.C.B. (Italian National Research Council – Institue for Biomolecular Chemistry), via P. Gaifami 18, 95126, Catania, Italy

3 D/SAF (Department of Agricultural and Forestry Sciences, Università degli Studi di Palermo), viale delle Scienze ed. 4 ingr. L, 90128 Palermo, Italy

* *Corresponding author*: E-mail: alessandra.carrubba@unipa.it

derivative). The occurrence of these substances in Hypericum extracts is highly variable, as an effect of both genetic factors (species and/or subspecies) and environmental conditions (growing site or cropping techniques). This paper makes a review of the information available in the newest literature about botanical and agronomical concerns, chemical composition and biological activity of Hypericum species, with a special emphasis to the treatment of depressive states. Original data about the content of hypericin, pseudohypericin and hyperforin in several Hypericum species and populations coming from different Italian sites are also exposed and discussed.

Keywords: *Hypericum* spp., Traditional and folk medicines, Hypericin, Pseudohypericin, Hyperforin, Depression.

Hypericum spp.: Taxonomical and Botanical Aspects

Hypericum is one out of the nine genera which form the botanical family Hypericaceae (APG III, 2009). According to Crockett and Robson (2011) the genus contains 484 species, spread worldwide throughout many highly diversified habitats, in so much as in many areas it is claimed to be an invasive weed (Buckley *et al.*, 2003).

Its major diversification center, as arguable by the high number of detected species, may be located in the temperate regions of Northern hemisphere (Crockett and Robson, 2011). Detailed information about the distribution of *Hypericum* taxa is available in Ciccarelli and Garbari (2004). A large part of them grows wild in the Mediterranean areas: 30 *Hypericum* taxa (26 species and 4 subspecies) have been detected in the peninsular part of Italy and in Italian islands (Conti *et al.*, 2005), spanning from coastal areas and low plains to high mountain areas (about 1600 m a.s.l.).

Inside Sicilian flora, the genus *Hypericum* is formed by 11 native taxa (Giardina *et al.*, 2007), homogeneously distributed in the inner part of the isle, from the dry and sunny coastal areas, to the riparian wetlands, to the woody and mountain areas.

Two species (*H. perforatum* and *H. perfoliatum*) are ubiquitous; they may be found in almost every environment, spanning from few to 800 - 1000 meters a.s.l., in arid meadows, grazing lands, wood borders, grasslands and roadsides. *H. calycinum* grows in sunny areas and fits to almost every soil type; it is cultivated rather everywhere as an ornamental plant in gardens and parks, but is considered spontaneous in Sicily as well (from 0 to 1000 m a.s.l.) (Castellano and Spadaro, 2010). *H. triquetrifolium* is typical of arid wildlands, where it may be found from the sea level to 800 m a.s.l. It may be easily encountered in the Eastern part of Sicily. In smaller areas of Sicily other two species are present: *H. pubescens*, typical of humid (sometimes salty) environments, from 0 to 500 m a.s.l., detected in Western Sicily, and *H. tetrapterum*, from 0 to 800 m, typical of humid prairies, marshes, riversides and reeds. *H. androsaemum* may be found sparsely in Sicily from 0 to 1400 m a.s.l., inside woods or in shadowy and fresh slopes, both inside the Madonie and the Nebrodi parks, and *H. hircinum* as well, limited to wet and shadowy areas, from the coast level to 1200 m, in the areas of Messina and Palermo (Pignatti, 1982). *H. aegypticum* is an endemism, retrieved only inside the isle of Lampedusa on cliffs close the sea and in arid garrigue

0 to 200 m a.s.l., although its presence must be confirmed by further investigations. *H. australe* as well, was reported in wet meadows or in wood clearings, but its presence has not been confirmed recently (Giardina *et al.*, 2007). *H. hirsutum* may be found on rather the whole Italian territory, exception made for Val d'Aosta, Sicily and Sardinia; it grows up inside the vegetation with tall woody and herbaceous plants, in coastal areas and clearings, from 0 to 1600 m a.s.l. Similarly, *H. montanum* may be found throughout all Italian territory, although it is missing from the islands. It was retrieved in oaks and beech woods, above all when in degradation phase, 0 to 1800 m a.s.l.

H. perforatum (St. John's Wort) is probably the most studied about all *Hypericum* species. As a morphological typical trait, different types of internal secretory cavity were found in aerial parts of the plant: translucent glands and three different types of secretory canals with different shapes, ontogenesis and localization (Ciccarelli *et al.*, 2001). The frequency and diversity of these secretory structures evidence the intense secretory activity of the species. In *H. perforatum*, the naphthodianthrones hypericin and pseudohypericin are characteristic of the black nodules and they are not present in either glands or canals (Ciccarelli *et al.*, 2001), whereas phloroglucinols, such as hyperforin, seem to be located in translucent glands in leaves, carpellar leaves and sepals (Bruni and Sacchetti, 2009).

Chemical Composition of Extracts

Phytochemical surveys on several *Hypericum* species demonstrated that they contain essential oils, flavonols (catechins), xanthons, cumarins, glycosides, anthraquinones, floroglucynols, flavonoids, flavonolglycosides, lactones, pyrones, lipids, triterpenes, tannins, poliphenolics and phenylpropanes (caffeic, chlorogenic and neochlorogenic acids) (Erken *et al.*, 2001; Poutaraud and Girardin, 2004; Javidnia *et al.*, 2008; Camas *et al.*, 2012; Maltas *et al.*, 2013).

Inside all of these compounds, two groups are identifiable, the first characterized by a fair hydrophily (proantocyanins, flavonoids, biflavonoids, xantones, fenilpropanes and naphtodiantrones) and the second group with a more hydrophobic nature (essential oils and acylfloroglucynols) (Crockett, 2010). From the petroleum ether extract of the aerial parts of *H. calycinum*, a new floroglucynol derivative and five derivatives of cicloesadienone were isolated, only one of which (formerly isolated from *Hypericum chinense* L. and termed chinesin II) was already known in literature (Castellano and Spadaro, 2010).

Some of the identified compounds are responsible for several biological activities, spanning from antioxidant, antibacterial (Maltas *et al.*, 2013), antifungal (Cakir *et al.*, 2004), antiviral (Schmitt *et al.*, 2001), antiproliferative (Donà *et al.*, 2004), and even nematocidal (Guedes *et al.*, 2009). However, plant metabolites that have been subjected to the attention of medicine and phytochemistry are above all naphtodianthrones, such as hypericin and pseudohypericin, many flavonoids, such as hyperoside, quercetin, rutin and quercitrin, xantones, but above all floroglucynols, such as hyperforin and adhyperforin (Castellano and Spadaro, 2010).

Hypericin and pseudohypericin, despite their different chemical structure, often are collectively termed as "hypericins" (Figure 13.1). Their presence in *Hypericum*

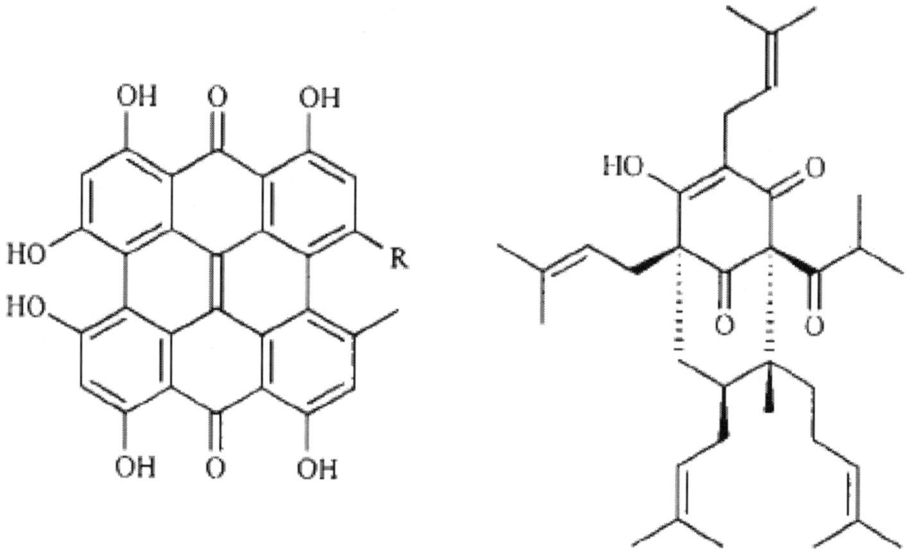

Figure 13.1: Chemical Structures of Hypericin (R = CH_3) and Pseudohypericin (R = CH_2OH) (on the left) and Hyperforin (on the right; Stojanovic *et al.*, 2013, modif.)

plants has an important taxonomic value, since they are specific only for the more phylogenetically advanced taxa, and are completely absent in the primitive sections (Kitanov, 2001). Both of them are contained in aerial flowering parts of plants, in increasing amounts from the bottom to the upper part (Kizil *et al.*, 2013), and tend to decrease as the plant ripening process goes on, being about 10 folds higher in closed buds than in brown capsules (Berger-Büter and Büter, 2002). In *H. perforatum*, pseudohypericin is generally (but not always) detected in higher amounts than hypericin, with a ratio between them that seems mostly depending on the genotype (Poutaraud and Girardin, 2004; Karioti and Bilia, 2010). In *Hypericum* extracts such compounds are the best known and studied, above all because of their activity on the central nervous system. Their occurrence in plant extracts is highly variable, as an effect of both genetic factors (species and/or subspecies) and environmental conditions, such as growing site or cropping techniques (Kizil *et al.*, 2013), harvest and post-harvest management, and extraction techniques (Poutaraud and Girardin, 2005).

In 2012 and 2013 (unpublished data) a survey activity was performed, collecting plant samples (picked up between the stages of full and end of flowering) of various species of *Hypericum* from several Mediterranean environments and at different altitudes. For the measurement of hypericin, pseudohypericin and hyperforin content, about 5 g of air-dried inflorescences were ground and put in ethanol (50 ml) at room temperature for 72 hours, in the dark and under continuous shakering. Each extract was filtered and the filter was washed thrice with 10 ml ethanol, thereafter it was dried with a rotavapor, and extract yield was measured (as percent of d.m.).

Table 13.1: Extract Yield (Per cent) and Average Content in Active Metabolites (mg kg $^{-1}$ d.m.) in the Flowering Tops of Several *Hypericum* Species from Various Provenances

Species	*Provenance*	*Extract Yield (per cent d.m.)*	*Hypericin (mg kg^{-1} d.m.)*	*Pseudo hypericin (mg kg^{-1} d.m.)*	*Hyperforin (mg kg^{-1} d.m.)*
H. aviculariifolium	Turkey (Gümüs)[1]	–	2140	590	–
H. barbatum	Serbia (Suva Planina)[2]	–	300	430	70
H. calabricum	Italy (Calabria)[3]	–	30	–	3450
H. calycinum	Italy (Messina, Sicily)	33,8	–	–	429,5
H. enshiense	China (Badong)[4]	–	3000	4700	–
H. hircinum	Italy(Messina, Sicily)	18,5	–	–	602,2
H. hirsutum	Italy (Siena, Tuscany)[5]	21,4±9,8	38,5±14,5	15,8[6]	103,0±82,6
	Serbia (Suva Planina)[7]	–	40	–	60
H. linarioides	Serbia (Suva Planina)[8]	–	20	–	20
H. lydium	Turkey (Havza)[9]	–	180	340	–
H. maculatum	Serbia (Suva Planina)[10]	–	30	40	50
H. monbretii	Turkey (Çakalli)[11]	–	1390	1170	
H. montanum	Italy (Ancona, Marche)	25,5	417,2	447,8	309,9
	Italy (Arezzo, Tuscany)	23,1	410,3	381,8	135,5
H. orientale	Turkey (Merzifon)[12]	–	–	90	–
H. origanifolium	Turkey (Çakalli)[13]	–	1430	1111	–
H. perfoliatum	Italy (Palermo, Sicily)[14]	23,8± 6,2	304,0± 149,2	878,7± 466,3	6740,7± 5708,9

1. Çirak *et al.,* 2007; data previously expressed in mg g^{-1}
2. Smelcerovic *et al.*, 2006; data previously expressed in mg g^{-1}
3. Statti *et al.,* 2011; data previously expressed in mg g^{-1}
4. Wang *et al.,* 2010; data previously expressed in mg g^{-1}
5. mean value of 2 accessions ± standard deviation
6. value obtained in only one accession over two
7. Smelcerovic *et al.,* 2006; data previously expressed in mg g^{-1}
8. Smelcerovic *et al.,* 2006; data previously expressed in mg g^{-1}
9. Çirak *et al.,* 2007; data previously expressed in mg g^{-1}
10. Smelcerovic *et al.,* 2006; data previously expressed in mg g^{-1}
11. Çirak *et al.,* 2007; data previously expressed in mg g^{-1}
12. Çirak *et al.,* 2007; data previously expressed in mg g^{-1}
13. Çirak *et al.,* 2007; data previously expressed in mg g^{-1}
14. mean value of 10 accessions ± standard deviation

Contd...

Table 13.1–*Contd...*

Species	*Provenance*	*Extract Yield (per cent d.m.)*	*Hypericin (mg kg^{-1} d.m.)*	*Pseudo hypericin (mg kg^{-1} d.m.)*	*Hyperforin (mg kg^{-1} d.m.)*
	Italy (Messina, Sicily)	22,5	252,1	1052,8	12999,5
	Italy (Agrigento, Sicily)[15]	15,3±3,9	322,4± 74,8	756,7± 164,0	1970,0± 1335,1
	Turkey (Çakalli)[16]	–	1060	2110	–
H. perforatum	Italy (Agrigento, Sicily)[17]	20,0± 6,0	357,0± 189,2	358,6± 274,2	8626,5± 5214,8
	Italy (Ancona, Marche)	27,6	291,6	311,3	4855,8
	Italy (Arezzo, Tuscany)[18]	24,0± 6,0	445,6± 206,3	511,3± 302,5	5035,6± 2821,8
	Italy (Firenze, Tuscany)[19]	23,5± 0,1	635,5± 65,6	816,7± 181,2	3412,4± 180,4
	Italy (Isernia, Molise)[20]	22,6± 4,0	238,5± 108,5	481,9± 332,9	6483,7± 853,1
	Italy (Messina, Sicily)	34,5	786,1	1357,2	8906,0
	Italy (Naples, Campania)	25,3	954,2	840,9	3953,3
	Italy (Palermo, Sicily)[21]	25,1± 7,3	515,1± 337,3	555,9± 340,8	8397,7± 7521,2
	Italy (Roma, Latium)[22]	19,5± 10,3	351,7± 79,7	505,3± 288,3	3990,8± 371,7
	Italy (Siena, Tuscany)[23]	20,4± 4,6	261,2± 40,3	542,6± 249,3	6596,3± 1477,3
	Italy (Trento, Trentino)[24]	24,7± 5,0	176,7± 90,5	485,5± 311,1	4060,5± 2521,3
	Italy (various sites, Tuscany)[25]	–	112±38	189±37	4822±1019

15. mean value of 3 accessions ± standard deviation
16. Çirak *et al.,* 2007; data previously expressed in $mg\ g^{-1}$
17. mean value of 11 accessions ± standard deviation
18. mean value of 10 accessions ± standard deviation
19. mean value of 2 accessions ± standard deviation
20. mean value of 2 accessions ± standard deviation
21. mean value of 15 accessions ± standard deviation
22. mean value of 2 accessions ± standard deviation
23. mean value of 4 accessions ± standard deviation
24. mean value of 3 accessions ± standard deviation
25. average ± standard deviation of 14 values from a chemotype without rutin (Mártonfi *et al.,* 2001);

Table 13.1–*Contd...*

Species	*Provenance*	*Extract Yield (per cent d.m.)*	*Hypericin (mg kg⁻¹ d.m.)*	*Pseudo hypericin (mg kg⁻¹ d.m.)*	*Hyperforin (mg kg⁻¹ d.m.)*
	Italy (various sites, Tuscany)[26]	–	115±49	329±151	2764±845
	USA (Montana)[27]	–	97,5±39,6	555,0±125,8	–
	USA (California)[28]	–	230,0±111,7	2105,0±556,9	–
	Turkey (Samsun)[29]	–	2820	1860	–
	Unknown[30]	–	1500	4000	32200
H. pruinatum	Turkey (Gümüs)[31]	–	790	520	–
H. pubescens	Italy (Palermo, Sicily)	29,6± 5,4	228,3± 178,7	799,1± 248,2	1517,7± 1249,7
H. rumeliacum	Serbia (Rudina Planina)[32]	–	180	180	70
H. tetrapterum	Italy (Arezzo, Tuscany)	20,7	844,0	583,0	9384,3
	Italy (Messina, Sicily)	18,5	540,0	431,0	3989,3
	Italy (Roma, Latium)	29,1	252,6	837,4	3298,6
	Serbia (Rudina Planina)[33]	–	90	100	110

26. average ± standard deviation of 12 values from a chemotype without rutin (Mártonfi *et al.*, 2001); data probably expressed in mg g^{-1}

27 mean value of 4 accessions from Montana (Sirvent *et al.*, 2002); data previously expressed in %

28. mean value of 4 accessions from California (Sirvent *et al.*, 2002); data previously expressed in %

29. Çirak *et al.*, 2007; data previously expressed in mg g^{-1}

30. Wang *et al.*, 2010; data previously expressed in mg g^{-1}

31. Çirak *et al.*, 2007; data previously expressed in mg g^{-1}

32. Smelcerovic *et al.*, 2006; data previously expressed in mg g^{-1}

33. Smelcerovic *et al.*, 2006; data previously expressed in mg g^{-1}

The chemical determinations were carried on by means of HPLC diode array analysis, in triplicate, by injecting 20 µL of a 10 mg/mL solution in methanol for each extract. The identification of compounds was performed by comparison of the chromatographic behaviour of the samples with that of standards solutions with a known concentration.

Although it is not easy to ascertain how much of this variability is due to real differences among genotypes and how much is due to differences in analytical methods, experimental management or conditions of the plant material in use, the amounts in hypericin, pseudohypericin and hyperforin show a wide range of variation according to the species and, inside species, according to the genotype. A better understanding of the causes of such variability, however, should imply the elucidation of the reasons why *Hypericum* plants produce such metabolites. One interesting theory, surely deserving of further in-depth examination, suggests that plants synthesize such compounds in response to several stress agents, such as salt and drought (Selmar, 2008) or herbivore attacks (Sirvent *et al.*, 2002).

Hypericum as a Pharmaceutical Item

Traditional and folk medicines in many parts of the world use *Hypericum* species for a plenty of different purposes. They are considered as possessing a range of properties, including antimicrobial, antiviral, antioxidant, antiproliferative, antidepressant, antiepatotoxical, stimulating for blood circulation, beneficial for gastric and duodenal ulcer, intestinal catarrh, cold affections, and visual disturbances (Bruni, 1999; Pistelli *et al.*, 2000; Schmitt *et al.*, 2001; Donà *et al.*, 2004; Sánchez-Mateo *et al.*, 2005; Almeida *et al.*, 2009; Franchi *et al.*, 2011; Guedes *et al.*, 2012; Stojanovic *et al.*, 2013). In Herzegovina, *Hypericum perforatum* is reported to be collected from the wild in large quantities, ranking among the top 5 medicinal plants in the preference of collectors (Radun, 2007). In Portugal, many *Hypericum* species (*H. androsaemum, H. perforatum, H. undulatum*) are used in traditional medicine to treat liver and kidney problems or migraine (Guedes *et al.*, 2012). In Italy, extracts from *H. hircinum* are widely used against cough (Pieroni *et al.*, 2004). In Russia, *Hypericum* is used for wound healing and skin care formulations, but also added in the traditional Russian beverage ("Baikal") to treat winter depression (Kireeva *et al.*, 1999). In Iran, two endemic *Hypericum* species *(H. perforatum* and *H. androsaemum)* are traditionally used as diuretic, wound healing, sedative and antibacterial agents (Mazandarani *et al.*, 2003). Native Americans used the root of several wild *Hypericum* species for internal use in the treatment of severe body impairment and fever, and for external use against the snakebites (Frichsen Brown, 1989). In the Canary Islands, where about 10 *Hypericum* species may be found, some of them are used in folk medicine for the treatment of wounds and also as sedative, diuretic, vermifuge, antihysteric and antidepressant (Rabanal *et al.*, 2005; Sánchez-Mateo *et al.*, 2005). Aerial parts of *Hypericum* plants (mainly *H. perfoliatum*) are largely used to treat contusions, wounds, burns and ulcerations, since they offer a strong lenitive effect of pain and stimulate the formation of new tissue (Frichsen Brown, 1989; Bombardelli and Morazzoni, 1995; Castellano and Spadaro, 2010). In Southern Italy and Sicily, the *Hypericum* extract form that is most used for this purpose is the oil, traditionally obtained by means of a 40-days maceration of the fresh flowers in vegetable oil (olive and sunflower), until the liquid becomes red (Lentini, 2000).

Despite all this variety of traditional uses all over the world, the most important and well-known activities of *Hypericum* extracts are certainly the anti-inflammatory, healing and antidepressant ones. Actually, although many compounds have been identified in *Hypericum* extracts, which active substance, or mixture of substances, is exactly responsible for each specific pharmacological action, it is not perfectly clear as far. For evaluating the quality of the drugs, the *Hypericum* formulations in use for therapy are standardized according to the total content of some selected specific compound; the European Pharmacopoeia, *e.g.*, takes as a reference index the total content in naphthodianthrones, *i.e.*, hypericins (hypericin and pseudohypericin) on total dry extract. The concentration of total hypericins in *Hypericum* sprout and flowers may range among very different values, but for market quality a minimum hypericin amount of 0,04 per cent (400 mg kg^{-1}) is required (Wagner and Bladt, 1994). Hypericin has called the attention of research due to its antiviral and antitumor action associated with a significant photosensitizing activity, that could suggest its utility in some specific antitumor treatments with photodinamic therapy (De Witte, 1998; Miskovsky, 2002; Karioti and Bilia, 2010). As concerns the antidepressant *Hypericum* activity, anyway, several studies seem to conclude that the major responsible for this effect is hyperforin (Chatterjee *et al.*, 1998; Stevinson and Ernst, 1999; Müller *et al.*, 2001; Caccia and Gobbi, 2011). This finding should suggest the opportunity to determine quality standard for hyperforin content, and not only for hypericins, when plant has to be addressed to this kind of therapy. A major problem in such sense is due to the instability of hyperforin in light and air, which requires a special care in handling and storage of extracts (Mennini and Gobbi, 2004).

Antidepressive and Sedative Effects

One of the most concerning aspects of the industrialized western countries lifestyle is the widespread arising of pathologic expressions linked to the emotional and psychological contest, variously expressed as more or less severe anxious-depressive states, sleep disorders and expressions of social maladjustment generically but effectively defined as "stress" (Gabel, 1998). In listing depression among the numerous stress-related problems, WHO claims it as one of the most worrying mental diseases (WHO, 2012 and 2013).

The therapeutic approach toward this pathology takes into consideration the use of a great deal of pharmaceutical items, mostly obtained by chemical synthesis. Following a larger market and production trend, however, this sector of pharmaceutical industry as well is gradually oriented towards the utilization of active compounds of plant origin, in the belief (although under continuous verification) that, besides of causing fewer toxicity phenomena, they do not generate dependence.

Indeed, the utilization of plant extracts in order to cure several widespread pathologic manifestations is rather an ancient practice (Chia, 2005). In several countries, some *Hypericum* species, the most famous being St. John's wort *(Hypericum perforatum* L.), are considered as phytoterapeutic agents and used in many pharmaceutical items of free trading (Larkin, 2000). In the treatment of moderate depression *Hypericum* extracts have been demonstrated more effective than placebo, although less effective than conventional antidepressant (Mennini and Gobbi, 2004; Stevinson and Ernst, 1999). The plant is effectively used against menopause stress syndrome and excitability, above all when they generate depression. It normalizes the sleep both in case of insomnia and hypersomnia. It is effective in the treatment of pain and neuralgic affections. It possesses a sedative effect with specific antidepressant activity, acting in relieving the anxious condition, and is used as a part of therapy for the psychological instability, due to its healthy and regenerating effect on nervous system and on all emotional manifestations.

Hypericum works by means of biochemical mechanisms of action that are similar, although not identical, to those of the elective medicines against mild to moderate depression, *i.e.* the Selective Serotonin Re-uptake Inhibitors (SSRIs), such as fluoxetine

(Prozac), paroxetine (Paxil) and sertraline (Zoloft) (Mennini and Gobbi, 2004). The available studies suggest, in particular, that the extract of *H. perforatum* and *H. perfoliatum* act by means of slowing the re-uptake of neuro transmittants (serotonine, dopamine, noradrenaline) at central nervous system level (Do Rego, 2007). This action, however, seems to exhibit at rather high concentrations. These extracts, moreover, do not show negative effects on the wakefulness state, attention and memory, do not alter the sleep phases and do not generate dependence.

Further experiments allowed to attribute similar effects also to other *Hypericum* species, such as *H. canariense*, *H. glandulosum* and *H. calycinum*. Researches about the effects on the central nervous system of these extracts have shown an effectiveness similar to that of the Tricyclic Antidepressant (TCAs), such as desipramine (Norpramin), trimipramine (Surmontil) and imipramine (Tofranil), that have been compared to these plant extracts in animal models (Sánchez-Mateo *et al.*, 2005; Castellano and Spadaro, 2010).

Although in many controlled trials, no clinically relevant side effects have been reported (Stevinson and Ernst, 1999), some caution is suggested during pregnancy and breastfeeding (Russo *et al.*, 2013). Furthermore, interactions between St John's wort and several drugs have been documented. Among the most relevant interactions, a reduced blood concentration of ciclosporin, indinavir, warfarin, and anticancer drugs has been claimed (Breidenbach *et al.*, 2000; WHO, 2006; Borrelli and Izzo, 2009), as well as serotonine syndrome or lethargy when *Hypericum* is used with SSRIs (Russo *et al.*, 2013), and interferences with hormonal metabolism that could reduce the efficacy of oral contraceptives (Hall *et al.*, 2003).

Wild or Cultivated?

A rich literature takes into consideration many aspects of the researches about *Hypericum*, both agronomical (adaptability, cropping techniques, yields) and chemical-pharmacological (yield in active compounds and their effectiveness, doses and administering ways, clinical effects (Giachetti *et al.*, 1998; Zanoli *et al.*, 1998 a and b; Larkin, 2000; Bruni and Sacchetti, 2009). Unfortunately, most papers referring to the activity of herbal extracts seem to pay little importance to the provenience of the plant material. A deep debate is starting about the opportunity to use only wild plant material, which is sometimes considered more effective than the cultivated one. Actually, many considerations discourage the massive use of plant material taken from the wild (Crockett and Robson, 2011). First, the amounts of active principles in wild plants are subjected to high variations, due to the occurrence of many uncontrollable and unforeseeable environmental factors. Second, picking up from the wild of plant material may be considered an acceptable practice only when the required amounts are low, but becomes unsustainable as the requirements begin to get higher. Many examples all around the world may be done, of plants that after an uncontrolled collection from the natural stations are now at risk of extinction. Hence, the opportunity to achieve sustainable plant collection practices is advocated (Radun, 2007), and cultivation is increasingly recognised as the only real opportunity to obtain high quantities of plant biomass with a known quantity of active principles.

As it is well known, a good management of cropping techniques may put plants in conditions to express their potentialities at maximum level. Of course, much work must still be done, and some crucial aspects of cropping technique, such a fertilization or irrigation, besides post-harvest technology, must be refined.

Some preliminary trials about the suitability of *Hypericum* to the field cultivation have been performed, and the plant has shown a good productivity even under low input conditions (Carrubba *et al.*, 2010). Undoubtedly, as for all other plant secondary metabolites, a proper cropping technique may affect the hypericins content. Experimental activity about this topic is however sparse. A trial performed with different N rates and ways of application allowed to obtain hypericin contents ranging from 0,08 and 0,13 per cent, achieving the maximum values after application of 150 kg N ha^{-1} in two solutions (Berti *et al.*, 2000). Otherwise, Briskin *et al.* (2000) found that N supply in *Hypericum* caused a decrease in hypericin content in leaves, whereas a moderate N stress (although producing a general depression in all growth plant parameters) enhanced the hypericin content. Inoculation of *H. perforatum* with AMF (Arbuscular Mycorrhizal Fungi) significantly enhanced the content in hypericin and pseudohypericin, probably as a consequence of the improved plant nutrient adsorption, whereas no effect on hyperforin concentration was found (Zubek *et al.*, 2012). Other environmental factors, furthermore, are claimed to exert an effect on the content in *Hypericum* active molecules: pseudohypericin content decreased from 2.3 to 1.4 mg g^{-1} in *Hypericum perforatum* plants experiencing a phytoplasma infection, whereas the content in hypericin did not show any significant variation (Bruni *et al.*, 2005).

The amounts of hypericin and hyperforin in plants are not inter-correlated, hence the possibility exists to address plant breeding towards the enhancement of one compound, or both (Poutaraud and Girardin, 2004). Genetic engineering may be therefore a useful tool to obtain highly-yielding genotypes, more suitable to the needs of industry. This goal can be achieved by means of the classical breeding and selection methods: a seven-times increase of the mean content of hypericins was *e.g.* obtained in the fourth generation of fieldgrown *Hypericum perforatum* plants (Koperdáková *et al.*, 2007).

Finally, a strong relevance has to be attributed also to the newest biotechnology techniques, *e.g.*, including *in vitro* cell and tissue cultures (Brutovská *et al.*, 1998). Relevant amounts of hypericin, pseudohypericin and other metabolites (such as flavonoids, procyanidins, and others) have been obtained from cell cultures of *H. perforatum, H. maculatum*, and other *Hypericum* species (Kartnig *et al.*, 1996), also with the help of elicitors such as mannan (Kirakosyan *et al.*, 2000).

References

Almeida, I.F., Fernandes, E., Lima, J.L.F.C., Cardoso Costa, P., and Bahia, M.F. (2009). *In vitro* protective effect of *Hypericum androsaemum* extract against oxygen and nitrogen reactive species. *Basic and Clinical Pharmacology and Toxicology*, **105**: 222–227.

APG III. (2009). An update of the angiosperm phylogeny group classification for the orders and families of flowering plants: APG III. *Botanical Journal of the Linnean Society*, **161**: 105–121.

Berger-Büter, K., and Büter, B. (2002). Ontogenic variation regarding hypericin and hyperforin levels in four accessions of *Hypericum perforatum* L. *J. Herbs, spices and Medicinal Plants*, **9**: 95-100.

Berti, M., Hevia, F., Wilckens, R., Joublan, J.P., Serri, H., and Allende, J. (2000). Fertilizacion nitrogenada del cultivo de Hierba de san Juan (*Hypericum perforatum* L.) en Chillan, provincia de Ñuble, Chile. *Cien. Investig. Agr.*, **27 (2)**: 107-116. (In Spanish, with English abstract).

Bombardelli, E., and Morazzoni, P. (1995). *Hypericum perforatum*. *Fitoterapia*, **66**: 43-68.

Borrelli, F., and Izzo, A.A. (2009). Herb–drug interactions with St John's Wort (*Hypericum perforatum*): an update on clinical observations. *The AAPS Journal*, **11 (4)** : 710-727.

Breidenbach, Th., Hoffmann, M.W., Becker, Th., Schlitt, H., and Klempnauer, J. (2000). Drug interaction of St John's wort with ciclosporin. *The Lancet*, **355**: 1912.

Briskin, D.P., Leroy, A., and Gawienowski, M. (2000). Inuence of nitrogen on the production of hypericins by St. John's wort. *Plant Physiol. Biochem.*, **38 (5)**: 413-420.

Bruni, A. (1999). Farmacognosia generale e applicata. I farmaci naturali. Piccin, Padova: 338 pp. (In Italian).

Bruni, R., Pellati, F., Bellardi, M.G., Benvenuti, S., Paltrinieri, S., Bertaccini, A., and Bianchi, A. (2005). Herbal drug quality and phytochemical composition of *Hypericum perforatum* L. affected by ash yellows phytoplasma infection. *J Agric Food Chem.*, **53 (4)**: 964-968.

Bruni, R., and Sacchetti, G. (2009). Factors affecting polyphenol biosynthesis in wild and field grown St. John's wort (*Hypericum perforatum* L. Hypericacaee/ Guttiferaee). *Molecules*, **14**: 682-725.

Brutovská, R., Cellárová, E., and Doležel, J. (1998). Cytogenetic variability of *in vitro* regenerated *Hypericum perforatum* L. plants and their seed progenies. *Plant Science*, **133**: 221–229.

Buckley, Y.M., Briese, D.T., and Rees, M. (2003). Demography and management of the invasive plant species *Hypericum perforatum*. II. Construction and use of an individual-based model to predict population dynamics and the effects of management strategies. *Journal of Applied Ecology*, **40**: 494–507.

Caccia, S., and Gobbi, M. (2011). Hyperforin in St. John's Wort's central effects: What is the mechanism of action? *Medicinal and Aromatic Plant Science and Biotechnology*, **5 (Special Issue 1)**: 78-85.

Cakir, A., Kordali, S., Zengin, H., Izumi, S., and Hirata, T. (2004). Composition and antifungal activity of essential oils isolated from *Hypericum hyssopifolium* and *Hypericum heterophyllum*. *Flavour and Fragrance Journal*, **19**: 62–68.

Camas, N., Radusiene, J., Stanius, Z., Caliskan, O., and Cirak, C. (2012). Secondary metabolites of *Hypericum leptophyllum* Hochst., an endemic Turkish species. *The Scientific World Journal,* Article ID 501027: 4 pp.

Carrubba, A., Catalano, C., and Militello, M. (2010). Prove di coltivazione di iperico (*Hypericum perforatum* L.) in ambiente semi-arido. Raccolta degli atti - 4° Convegno Nazionale Piante Mediterranee - Le potenzialità del territorio e dell'ambiente: 209-213 (In Italian).

Castellano, G., and Spadaro, V. (2010). *Hypericum calycinum* (Clusiaceae) in Sicilia: aspetti farmacognostici e corologici. *Quaderni di Botanica ambientale e applicata,* **21**: 29-32. (In Italian, with English abstract)

Chatterjee, S.S., Bhattacharya, S.K., Wonnemann, M., Singer, A., and Müller, W.E. (1998). Hyperforin as a possible antidepressant component of *Hypericum* extracts. *Life Sciences,* **63 (6)**: 499-510.

Chia, G. (2005). L'iperico: l'antidepressivo naturale – Macroedizioni- Librisalus (In Italian)

Ciccarelli, D., Andreucci, A.C., and Pagni, A.M. (2001). Translucent glands and secretory canals in *Hypericum perforatum* L. (Hypericaceae): Morphological, anatomical and histochemical studies during the course of ontogenesis. *Annals of Botany,* **88**: 637-644.

Ciccarelli, D., and Garbari F. (2004). Le unità italiane di Hypericum (Clusiaceae), serie Hypericum. *Informatore Botanico Italiano,* **36 (2)**: 413-424. (In Italian)

Çirak, C., Radušiene, J., Janulis, V., Ivanauskas, L. and Arslan, B. (2007). Chemical constituents of some *Hypericum* species growing in Turkey. *Journal of Plant Biology,* **50 (6)**: 632-635.

Conti, F., Abbate, G., Alessandrini, A., and Blasi, C. (Eds.) (2005). An annotated checklist of the Italian vascular flora. *Palombi Editore,* Roma, 420 pp.

Crockett, S.L. (2010). Essential oil and volatile components of the genus *Hypericum (Hypericaceae). Nat. Prod. Commun.,* **5 (9)**: 1493–1506.

Crockett, S.L., and Robson, N.K.B. (2011). Taxonomy and chemotaxonomy of the genus *Hypericum. Medicinal and Aromatic Plant Science and Biotechnology,* **5 (special issue 1)**: 1-13.

De Witte, P. (1998). Hypericin as photosensitizer. *Fitoterapia,* **69 (suppl. 5)**: 26-28.

Donà, M., Dell'Aica, I., Pezzato, E., Sartor, L., Calabrese, F., Della Barbera, M., Donella-Deana, A., Appendino, G., Borsarini, A., Caniato, R., and Garbisa, S. (2004). Hyperforin inhibits cancer invasion and metastasis. *Cancer Res.,* **64 (17)**: 6225-6232.

Do Rego, J.C. (2007). Antidepressant-like effect of hyperfoliatin, a polyisoprenylated phloroglucinol derivative from *Hypericum perfoliatum* (Clusiaceae) is associated with an inhibition of neuronal monoamines uptake. *European Journal of Pharmacology,* **569 (3)**: 197–203.

Erken, S., Malyer, H., Demirci, F., Demirci, B., and Baser, K.H.C. (2002). Chemical investigations on some *Hypericum* species growing in Turkey - I. *Chemistry of Natural Compounds*, **37**: 434–438.

Franchi, G.G., Nencini, C., Collavoli, E., and Massarelli, P. (2011). Composition and antioxidant activity *in vitro* of different St. John's Wort (*Hypericum perforatum* L.) extracts. *Journal of Medicinal Plants Research*, **5 (17)**: 4349-4353.

Frichsen Brown, C. (1989). Medicinal and other uses of North America plants: A historical survey with reference to the Eastern Indian tribes. – Dover Publications, New York: 382 pp.

Gabel, T.L. (1998). Herbal medications, nutraceuticals, and anxiety and depression. Chapt. 11 in: "Herbal Medicinals. A clinician's guide", Miller L.G. and Murray W.J. (Eds.), Haworth Press Inc., New York – London: 205-226.

Giachetti, D., Ghiglieri, O., Tolu, P., Scheggi, S., and Gambarana, C. (1998). Antidepressant activity of *Hypericum perforatum* total extracts on two animal models of depression. *Fitoterapia*, **64 (suppl. 5)**: 29.

Giardina, G., Raimondo, F.M., and Spadaro, V. (2007). A catalogue of plants growing in Sicily. *Bocconea*, **20**: 5-582.

Guedes, A.P., Gregory, F., and Fernandes-Ferreira, M. (2012). *Hypericum* sp.: Essential oil composition and biological activities. *Phytochemistry Reviews*, **11**: 127–152.

Guedes A., Luques R., Ferreira P., Almeida M.T., Fernandes-Ferreira M. (2009). Essential oil components of *Hypericum androsaemum* infusions and their nematotoxic effects against *Meloidogyne javanica* (Treub) Chittwood. 8th Phytochemical Society of Europe (PSE) Meeting on Biopesticides, La Palma, Canary Islands, Spain, 21-25 September 2009. Available at: http: / /repositorium.sdum.uminho. pt/handle/1822/18481 (last accessed July 23rd 2014).

Hall S.D., Wang Z., Huang S.-M., Hamman M.A., Vasavada N., Adigun A.Q., Hilligoss J.K., Miller M. and Gorski J. C. (2003). The interaction between St John's wort and an oral contraceptive. *Clinical Pharmacology and Therapeutics*, **74(6)**: 525-535.

Javidnia K., Miri R., Soltani M., Gholami M. and Khosravi A.R. (2008). Essential oil composition of four *Hypericum* species from Iran. *Chemistry of Natural Compounds*, **44 (3)**: 374-377.

Karioti A. and Bilia A.R. (2010). Hypericins as Potential Leads for New Therapeutics. *International Journal of Molecular Sciences*, **11**: 562-594.

Kartnig T., Göbel I. and Heydel, B. (1996). Production of Hypericin, Pseudohypericin and Flavonoids in cell cultures of various *Hypericum* species and their chemotypes. *Planta Medica*, **62**: 51-53.

Kirakosyan A., Hayashi H., Inoue K., Charchoglyan A. and Vardapetyan H. (2000). Stimulation of the production of hypericins by mannan in *Hypericum perforatum* shoot cultures. *Phytochemistry*, **53**: 345-348.

Kireeva T.B., Sharanov U.L. and Letchamo W. (1999). Biochemical and eco-physiological studies on *Hypericum* spp. In: *Perspectives on new crops and new uses*, Janick J. (Ed.), ASHS Press, Alexandria, VA, pp. 467–468.

Kitanov G.M., 2001. Hypericin and pseudohypericin in some *Hypericum* species. *Biochemical Systematics and Ecology*, **29**: 171–178.

Kizil S., Inan M. and Kirici S. (2013). Determination of the best herbage yield and hypericin content of St. John's wort (*Hypericum perforatum* L.) under semi-arid climatic conditions. *Turkish Journal of Field Crops*, **18(1)**: 95-100.

Koperdáková J., Košuth J. and Èellárová E. (2007). Variation in the content of hypericins in four generations of seed progeny of *Hypericum perforatum* somaclones. *J Plant Res*, **120**: 123–128.

Larkin M. (2000). St John's Wort included in US depression guidelines. *The Lancet*, **355**: 1619.

Lentini F. (2000). The role of ethnobotanics in scientific research. State of ethnobotanical knowledge in Sicily. *Fitoterapia*, **71**: 583 - 588.

Maltas E., Uysal A., Yildiztugay E., Aladag M.O., Yildiz S. and Kucukoduk M. (2013). Investigation of antioxidant and antibacterial activities of some Hypericum species. *Fresenius Environmental Bulletin*, **22(3a)**: 862–869.

Mártonfi P., Repèák M., Ciccarelli D. and Garbari F. (2001). *Hypericum perforatum* L. - chemotype without rutin from Italy. *Biochemical Systematics and Ecology*, **29**: 659 661.

Mazandarani M., Yassaghi S., Rezaei M.B., Mansourian A.R. and Ghaemi E.O. (2003). Ethnobotany and antibacterial activities of two endemic species of *Hypericum* in North-East of Iran. *Asian Journal of Plant Sciences*, **6**: 354-358.

Mennini T. and Gobbi M. (2004). The antidepressant mechanism of *Hypericum perforatum*. *Life Sciences*, **75**: 1021–1027.

Miskovsky P. (2002). *Hypericin* - A New Antiviral and Antitumor Photosensitizer. *Current Drug Targets*, **1(3)**: 55-84.

Müller W.E., Singer A. and Wonnemann M. (2001). *Hyperforin* - Antidepressant Activity by a Novel Mechanism of Action. *Pharmacopsychiatry*, **34 (Suppl1)**: 98-102.

Pieroni A., Quavec C.L. and Santoro R.F. (2004). Folk pharmaceutical knowledge in the territory of the Dolomiti Lucane, inland southern Italy. *Journal of Ethnopharmacology*, **95**: 373–384.

Pignatti S. (1982). Flora d'Italia, 1. Edagricole, Bologna, pp. 343-351.

Pistelli L., Bertoli A., Zucconelli S., Panizzi L and Menichini F. (2000). Antimicrobial activity of crude extracts and pure compounds of *Hypericum hircinum*. *Fitoterapia*, **71 (Suppl. 1)**: 138–140.

Poutaraud A. and Girardin P. (2004). Agronomic and chemical characterization of 39 *Hypericum perforatum* accessions between 1998 and 2000. *Plant Breeding*, **123**: 480-484.

Poutaraud A. and Girardin P. (2005). Improvement of medicinal plant quality: A Hypericum perforatum literature review as an example. *Plant Genetic Resources*, **3(2)**: 178–189.

Rabanal R.M., Bonkanka C.X., Hernández-Pérez M. and Sánchez-Mateo C.C. (2005). Analgesic and topical anti-inflammatory activity of *Hypericum canariense* L. and *Hypericum glandulosum* Ait. *Journal of Ethnopharmacology*, **96**: 591–596.

Radun M. (2007). Conservation and utilisation of St. John's wort *(Hypericum perforatum* L.) in Herzegovina. International Master Programme at the Swedish Biodiversity Centre, *Master Thesis* N. 47, Uppsala Universitet, Sweden: 37 pp.

Russo E., Scicchitano F., Whalley B.J., Mazzitello C., Ciriaco M., Esposito S., Patanè M., Upton R., Pugliese M., Chimirri S., Mammì M., Palleria C. and De Sarro G. (2013). *Hypericum perforatum*: Pharmacokinetic, Mechanism of Action, Tolerability, and Clinical Drug–Drug Interactions. *Phytotherapy Research*, **28(5)**: 643–655.

Sánchez-Mateo C.C., Bonkanka C.X., Prado B. and Rabanal R.M. (2005). Antidepressant properties of some *Hypericum canariense* L. and *Hypericum glandulosum* Ait. extracts in the forced swimming test in mice. *Journal of Ethnopharmacology*, **97**: 541–547.

Schmitt A.C., Ravazzolo A.P. and von Poser G.L. (2001). Investigation of some *Hypericum* species native to Southern of Brazil for antiviral activity. *Journal of Ethnopharmacology*, **77**: 239–245.

Selmar D. (2008). Potential of salt and drought stress to increase pharmaceutical significant secondary compounds in plants. Landbauforschung - vTI. *Agriculture and Forestry Research* **1/2 (58)**: 139-144.

Sirvent T.M., Walker L., Vance N. and Gibson D.M. (2002). Variation in hypericins from wild populations of *Hypericum perforatum* L. in the Pacific Northwest of the U.S.A. *Economic Botany*, **56(1)**: 41–48.

Smelcerovic A., Verma V., Spiteller M., Mudasir A.S., Puri S.C. and Qazi G.N. (2006). Phytochemical analysis and genetic characterization of six *Hypericum* species from Serbia. *Phytochemistry*, **67**: 171–177.

Statti G.A., Conforti F., Menichini F., Marrelli M., Gangale C., Tundis R., Loizzo M.R., Bonesi M. and Menichini F. (2011). Protective effect of *Hypericum calabricum* Sprengel on oxidative damage and its inhibition of nitric oxide in lipopolysaccharide-stimulated RAW 264.7 macrophages. *Biol Res*, **44**: 213-218.

Stevinson C. and Ernst E. (1999). Hypericum for depression. An update of the clinical evidence. *European Neuropsychopharmacology*, **9**: 501–505.

Stojanoviæ G., Đorðeviæ A. and Šmelcerovic A. (2013). Do other Hypericum species have medical potential as St. John's Wort *(Hypericum perforatum)*? *Current Medicinal Chemistry*, **20(18)**: 2273-2295.

Wagner H. and Bladt S. (1994). *Plant drug analysis: a thin layer chromatography atlas*. Springer, Jena: 368 pp.

Wang D., Bai J., Sun F. and Yang D. (2010). Chemical constituents and antidepressant activity of the new species *Hypericum enshiense* occurring in China. *Phytomedicine*, **17**: 410–413.

WHO (2006). The safety of medicines in public health programmes: Pharmacovigilance an essential tool. World Health Organization, Geneva, Switzerland: 60 pp.

WHO (2012). Depression. Fact sheet N° 369, October 2012. World Health Organization, Geneva, Switzerland. Available at: http: //www.who.int/ mediacentre/factsheets/fs369/en/(last accessed: July 1st, 2014)

WHO (2013). Guidelines for the Management of Conditions Specifically Related to Stress. World Health Organization, Geneva, Switzerland. Available at: http: / /apps.who.int/iris/bitstream/10665/85119/1/9789241505406_eng.pdf? ua=1 (last accessed: July 1st, 2014).

Zanoli P., Avallone R., Truzzi C., Vezzalini F. and Baraldi M. (1998a). Pharmacological profile of flavonoids present in medicinal plants with sedative and anxiolytic properties. *Fitoterapia*, **64 (suppl. 5)**: 17.

Zanoli P., Truzzi C., Cannazza G., Vandenbogaerde A., Kamuhabwa A., de Witte P., Merlevede W. and Baraldi M. (1998b). Evidence that *Hypericum perforatum* extracts exert anxiolytic effect in rats. *Fitoterapia*, **64 (suppl. 5)**: 30.

Zubek S., Mielcarek S. and Turnau K. (2012). Hypericin and pseudohypericin concentrations of a valuable medicinal plant *Hypericum perforatum* L. are enhanced by arbuscular mycorrhizal fungi. *Mycorrhyza*, **22**: 149-156.

Bioactive Phytochemicals: Perspectives for Modern Medicine Vol. 3 (2015) *Pages* **355–365**
Editor: **V.K. Gupta**
Published by: **DAYA PUBLISHING HOUSE, NEW DELHI**

14

Herbs and Herbal Products against some Psychiatric Disorders: A Mini Review

Anuradha Mukherjee[1] and Abhijit Dey[2*]

ABSTRACT

The present review reports the use of medicinal plants, plant-derived compounds and herbal formulations against a number of psychiatric disorders such as bipolar disorder (BD), borderline personality disorder (BPD), obsessive-compulsive disorder (OCD), seasonal affective disorder (SAD) etc. Pubmed, Medline, Science direct, Google scholar etc. have yielded a number of references when searched with relevant keywords. Extracts of Hypericum perforatum, Valeriana officinalis, Silybum marianum etc., compound such as gastrodin and herbal formulations such as free and easy wanderer plus (FEWP), yi-gan san (YGS) etc. were reported as psychoactive against the aforesaid psychological disorders in various pharmacological and clinical investigations. The work also describes the safety and efficacy of herbal drugs, need for more clinical trials, use of certain herbal products as adjunctive with synthetic drugs, traditional use of psychoactive herbal preparations alongside a note on future perspectives and directions of herbal psychotherapy.

Keywords: Anxiety, Bipolar disorder, Borderline personality disorder, Herbal, Psychoactive.

Introduction

Herbal psychotherapy has popularly being used in the treatment of a number of psychiatric disorders which include anxiety, depression, OCD, SAD, BPD and so on (Sarris, 2007). Kava and St. John's Wort are reportedly the common medications

1 Assistant Teacher, Biology, MMHS, South 24 Paraganas, West Bengal, India

2 Assistant Professor, UG and PG Department of Biological Sciences, Presidency University (Erstwhile Presidency College), 86/1 College Street, Kolkata – 700 073, W.B., India

* *Corresponding author*: E-mail: abhijitbio25@yahoo.com

against mood and anxiety disorders (Sarris and Kavanagh, 2009). Lack of clinical trials, absence of standardized preparations and chemical complexity of the products are considered as limitations in the development of efficacious treatment of psychiatric disorders using herb based formulations (Beaubrun and Gray, 2000). Safety, adverse effects and probable drug interactions are also considered as other concerns of using herbal drugs in psychiatric practice (Boniel and Dannon, 2000). However, dietary supplements and natural products are considered to prevent and treat psychiatric disorders in a number of literatures (Wong *et al.*, 1998; Fugh-Berman and Cott, 1999). More research is needed to explore the therapeutic efficacies of these botanicals besides considering the safety and effectiveness of such treatments (Wong *et al.*, 1998). The following section describes the characteristics of some unusual psychiatric disorders followed by a brief review on herbs and herbal products against them. Table 14.1 describes the names of herbs, herbal compounds and traditional formulations used against psychiatric disorders performed in various preclinical and clinical investigations with a note on their mode of action. PubMed, Google scholar, Medline etc. were used to generate and tabulate the data. A number of psychiatric disorders such as Borderline personality disorder (BPD), Charles Bonnet Syndrome (CBS), Pervasive developmental disorder (PDD), Asperger's disorder (AD), Restless legs syndrome (RLS): RLS/Willis-Ekbom disease (WED)/Wittmaack-Ekbom syndrome, Treatment-resistant schizophrenia, Bipolar disorder (BD), Tardive dyskinesia (TD), Seasonal affective disorder (SAD), Obsessive-compulsive disorder (OCD), Posttraumatic stress disorder (PTSD) and Nocturnal eating/drinking syndrome with restless legs syndrome (RLS) were found to be treated with various herbs and herbal preparations. Nomenclature of the plants was verified from http://www.tropicos.org. In this present review a total number of 10 plants, herbal compounds and traditional herbal formulations were found to be used against a number of psychiatric disorders.

Characteristics of some Psychiatric Disorders

- ☆ **Borderline personality disorder (BPD):** BPD is a personality disorder, characterized by unstable moods, impulsivity and instability of affects, behaviour, and relationships, the etiology of which includes genetic, constitutional, and environmental factors (Stone, 2014).
- ☆ **Charles Bonnet syndrome (CBS):** CBS is defined by complex visual hallucinations in a partially or severely sighted person, ocular pathology causing visual deterioration, and preserved cognitive status (Miyaoka *et al.*, 2011). It was first described by Charles Bonnet in 1760 and it affects via visual impairments at an old age and the loss of vision was ascribed to macular degeneration and glaucoma.
- ☆ **Pervasive developmental disorder (PDD):** PDDs are neurodevelepmental disorders that are characterized by delays in the development of multiple basic functions such as socialization and communication. More than 60 out of 100,000 children are reported with PDD (Béhérec *et al.*, 2014). PDDs include pervasive developmental disorder not otherwise specified (PDD-NOS), Autism, Asperger syndrome, Rett syndrome and Childhood disintegrative disorder (CDD).

Table 14.1: Herbs and Herbal Products against some Psychiatric Disorders

Herbs and Herbal Products	*Sample*	*Used against*	*Mode of Action*	*Reference*
Yi-gan san (YGS, yokukan-san in Japanese)	20 female BPD outpatients	BPD	↑low mood, ↑impulsivity, ↑aggression	Miyaoka *et al.*, 2008
	22 patients with schizophrenia with neuroleptic-induced TD	neuroleptic-induced TD	↑TD, ↑psychotic symptoms	Miyaoka *et al.*, 2008
		Schizophrenia, BPD, CBS, PDD, AD. neuroleptics induced TD, RLS/WED	↑symptoms	Horiguchi, 2012
		CBS	↓visual hallucination	Miyaoka *et al.*, 2011
		CBS	↓visual hallucination	Miyaoka *et al.*, 2009
	34 patients with schizophrenia	Treatment-resistant schizophrenia	↑symptoms	Miyaoka *et al.*, 2009
	a middle-aged male patient	nocturnal eating/drinking syndrome with RLS	↑symptoms	Kawabe *et al.*, 2012
Yokukansan (TJ-54)		RLS	↑symptoms	Shinno *et al.*, 2010
	20 children and adolescents ages 6-17 years with PDDs	PDD in children and adolescents	↑irritability/agitation, ↑hyperactivity/noncompliance	Wake *et al.*, 2013
	40 subjects, aged 8-40 years	PDD not otherwise specified (PDD-NOS) and AD	↑irritability, ↑lethargy/withdrawal, ↑stereotypic behavior, ↑hyperactivity/noncompliance, ↑inappropriate speech	Miyaoka *et al.*, 2012
	rat	haloperidol-induced TD	↓striatal glutamate level; ↑striatal GLT-1 mRNA level	Sekiguchi *et al.*, 2012
Kamishoyosan	69 schizophrenia patients with/without TD	TD in patients with schizophrenia	↓abnormal involuntary movement	Lee *et al.*, 2007
Saikokeishikankyoto (SKK)	45 participants	PTSD	↑symptoms	Numata *et al.*, 2014

Contd...

Table 14.1–*Contd...*

Herbs and Herbal Products	*Sample*	*Used against*	*Mode of Action*	*Reference*
Xiao-Tan-Jie-Yu-Fang (XTJYF) and placebo separately	Sichuan earthquake survivors with PTSD	PTSD	XTJYF showed better results than placebo; ↑somatization, ↑obsessive-compulsive behavior, ↑depression, ↑anxiety, ↑hostility ↑sleep quality score	Meng *et al.*, 2012
Free and Easy Wanderer Plus (FEWP) as an adjunct to carbamazepine (CBZ)	124 bipolar depressed and 111 manic patients	BPD	↑symptoms, ↑depression	Zhang *et al.*, 2007
FEWP	rats	PTSD	↑PTSD-like behavior ↓cognitive impairments	Wang *et al.*, 2009
St. John's Wort (*Hypericum perforatum* L.)		OCD	↑symptoms	Taylor and Kobak, 2000
	60 subjects	OCD	no efficacy of St John's wort for OCD	Kobak *et al.*, 2005
A concentrated extract of Saint John's Wort	21 RLS patients	RLS/WED	↑symptoms	Pereira *et al.*, 2013
Hypericum (Kira) alone and Kira + light therapy (LT)	168 patients	SAD	↑anxiety, ↑loss of libido, ↑insomnia	Wheatley, 1999
		SAD	↓Hamilton Depression Rating Scale	Kasper, 1997
		SAD	↓Hamilton Depression Rating Scale	Martinez *et al.*, 1994
Silybum marianum (L.) Gaertn. and fluoxetine separately	35 adult outpatients	OCD	No significant difference between extract and fluoxetine treatment	Sayyah *et al.*, 2010
Extract of valerian root (*Valeriana officinalis* L.) and placebo separately	31 adult outpatients	OCD	Antiobsessive and compulsive effects of valerian root; significant difference between the extract and placebo	Pakseresht *et al.*, 2011
Gastrodin	rats	PTSD	↑anxiolytic effect, ↓IL-1β level and p38 MAPK phosphorylation of hippocampus	Peng *et al.*, 2013
Chinese Herbal Drugs and Auricular-Plaster Therapy	50 cases	Child restless syndrome	94 per cent effective	Wang and Fan, 2005

↑ Improved prevented loss of/induced/enhanced/up regulated/elicited/promoted/restored/activated; ↓ Down-regulated/declined/terminated/inhibited.

- **Asperger's disorder (AD):** AD or Asperger syndrome (AS) is an autism spectrum disorder (ASD) characterized by impaired social interaction and communication (Lehnhardt *et al.*, 2013). Five variants of AD were reported such as integrated, inhibitory, peculiar, border-line and hypernormative (Bobrov and Somova, 2013).
- **Restless legs syndrome (RLS)/Willis-Ekbom disease (WED)/Wittmaack-Ekbom syndrome:** RLS is a common sensorimotor neurological disorder characterized by an irresistible urge to move the legs due to uncomfortable and odd sensations and it is divided into two types of etiologies *viz.* primary or idiopathic and secondary (Karroum *et al.*, 2008; Srivanitchapoom *et al.*, 2014).
- **Treatment-resistant schizophrenia:** In treatment-resistant schizophrenia, patients respond unsatisfactorily to antipsychotic treatment and about one third of the schizophrenic patients suffer from this (Mossaheb and Kaufmann, 2012). The patients suffer from prominent negative and cognitive symptoms and severe psychopathology compared to treatment-responsive schizophrenia.
- **Bipolar disorder (BD):** BD is a common, complex genetic disorder reported as both a cyclic and a progressive disorder (Kerner, 2014; Rizzo *et al.*, 2014) and manifested by unusual shifts in mood, energy and activity levels.
- **Tardive dyskinesia (TD):** Hyperkinetic abnormal involuntary movements are noted in TD which is often considered as an incurable form of dyskinesia associated with long term and high dose use of antipsychotic drug (Diefenderfer *et al.*, 2014).
- **Seasonal affective disorder (SAD):** SAD is a subgroup of depression that occurs at the same time every year when symptoms start during autumn, may continue in winter and full remission in spring or early summer (Kasper, 1997). Treatment for SAD includes light therapy, psychotherapy and medications.
- **Obsessive-compulsive disorder (OCD):** OCD is a chronic and potentially disabling disorder characterized by a number of comorbid disorders and outcomes. About 1 to 3 per cent of the general population throughout the world suffers from OCD (Leckman *et al.*, 2010).
- **Posttraumatic stress disorder (PTSD):** Patients with PTSD frequently suffer from sleep disturbances (Khawaja *et al.*, 2014) and possess reduced grey matter (GM) in the left anterior cingulate gyrus (ACC) compared to the normal individuals (Meng *et al.*, 2014).
- **Nocturnal eating/drinking syndrome with restless legs syndrome (RLS):** It is characterized by low level of sleep efficacy, eating huge amount of food rapidly in an uncontrolled way and periodic leg movements (Horiguchi *et al.*, 1999; Kawabe *et al.*, 2012).

Herbs and Herbal Products against some Psychiatric Disorders

Yi-gan san

Yi-gan san (YGS, yokukan-san in Japanese) was developed by Xue Kai in 1555 to treat child restlessness and agitation and later Japanese started using it against dementia in aged people (Horiguchi, 2012). In the treatment of BPD, 20 female outpatients when treated with YGS exhibited improvement in low mood, impulsivity and aggression (Miyaoka *et al.*, 2008). In 22 patients with schizophrenia with neuroleptic-induced TD, YGS improved psychotic symptoms (Miyaoka *et al.*, 2008). Moreover, it also improved symptoms of schizophrenia, BPD, CBS, PDD, AD, neuroleptics induced TD and RLS/WED (Horiguchi, 2012). In addition, it prevented visual hallucination in CBS (Miyaoka *et al.*, 2009, 2011). In another study conducted among 34 patients YGS was found to improve the pathological symptoms of treatment-resistant schizophrenia (Miyaoka *et al.*, 2009). Further, YGS when applied in a middle-aged male patient, it improved the symptoms of nocturnal eating/drinking syndrome with RLS (Kawabe *et al.*, 2012).

Yokukansan (YKS) (TJ-54)

Yokukansan (YKS) is a traditional Japanese medicine made up of seven medicinal herbs used for the treatment of a number of psychiatric and neurological disorders (Nakagawa *et al.*, 2012). In 20 children and adolescents ages 6-17 years with PDDs, the herbal preparation Yokukansan (TJ-54) improved irritability/agitation and hyperactivity/noncompliance in the patients (Wake *et al.*, 2013). In 40 subjects, aged between 8-40 years, suffering from PDD not otherwise specified (PDD-NOS) and AD, the preparation has improved irritability, lethargy/withdrawal, stereotypic behaviour, hyperactivity/noncompliance and inappropriate speech (Miyaoka *et al.*, 2012). Haloperidol-induced TD in rats was also protected by it by decreasing striatal glutamate level and upregulating striatal GLT-1 mRNA level (Sekiguchi *et al.*, 2012).

Kamishoyosan

Kamishoyosan is a traditional Japanese herbal medicine (kampo medicine) (Inoue *et al.*, 2011). In 69 schizophrenia patients with/without TD, kamishoyosan reduced abnormal involuntary movement (Lee *et al.*, 2007).

Free and Easy Wanderer Plus (FEWP)

The Chinese polyherbal preparation FEWP as an adjunct to carbamazepine (CBZ) when applied to 124 bipolar depressed and 111 manic patients, BPD symptoms were found to be improved (Zhang *et al.*, 2007). FEWP was found to reduce PTSD-like behavior and cognitive impairments in rats (Wang *et al.*, 2009).

St. John's Wort (*Hypericum perforatum* L.)

St. John's Wort was found to improve symptoms in OCD patients (Taylor and Kobak, 2000) but contradictory results were noted in another experiment involving 60 subjects suffering from OCD where no efficacy of St John's wort for OCD was found (Kobak *et al.*, 2005). A concentrated extract of Saint John's Wort when applied in 21 RLS patients, symptoms of RLS/WED were found to be improved (Pereira *et al.*, 2013). In another investigation, *Hypericum* (Kira) alone and Kira + light therapy (LT) improved anxiety, loss of libido and insomnia in 168 SAD patients (Wheatley, 1999) which was also found to reduce Hamilton Depression Rating Scale in SAD patients (Martinez *et al.*, 1994; Kasper, 1997).

Silybum marianum (L.) Gaertn.

When *Silybum marianum* (L.) Gaertn. and fluoxetine separately, no significant difference between extract and fluoxetine treatment in 35 adult OCD outpatients (Sayyah *et al.*, 2010).

Valeriana officinalis L.

Extract of valerian root (*Valeriana officinalis* L.) and placebo when applied separately in 31 adult OCD outpatients, antiobsessive and compulsive effects of valerian root was noted alongside significant difference between the extract and placebo (Pakseresht *et al.*, 2011).

Gastrodin

Gastrodin, one of the major constituent of a Chinese herbal medicine alleviated PTSD in rats via anxiolytic effect and reducing IL-1β level and p38 MAPK phosphorylation of hippocampus (Peng *et al.*, 2013).

Saikokeishikankyoto (SKK)

Traditional Japanese herbal formula saikokeishikankyoto (SKK) reduced PTSD symptoms in 45 participants (Numata *et al.*, 2014).

Xiao-Tan-Jie-Yu-Fang (XTJYF)

When the Chinese herbal formula, Xiao-Tan-Jie-Yu-Fang (XTJYF) and placebo were separately applied in Sichuan earthquake survivors with PTSD, XTJYF exhibited better results than placebo by improving obsessive-compulsive behavior, depression, anxiety etc. (Meng *et al.*, 2012).

Discussion

Most of the above mentioned experiments were performed in human samples as it is very difficult to mimic the symptoms of human psychiatric disorders in any *in vitro* and *in vivo* models. However, some of the aforesaid experiments were performed in animal models. The data indicates that yi-gan san (YGS, yokukan-san in Japanese) has been used most prolifically against such disorders followed by *Hypericum perforatum* L. and FEWP. These traditional herbal formulations contain multiple herbs which results into possible synergy among phytochemicals (Dey and De, 2012) leading to increased efficacy against psychiatric disorders. Plants, isolated herbal compounds and traditional formulations are also reported to be used against a number of neurological disorders (Dey and De, 2014) and many of these herbal products have been experimented preclinically and clinically to prepare CNS active drugs. However, the safety, efficacy, side effects and drug interactions are among the possible concerns of using herb based products. Therefore, further research is needed to evaluate the plant based preparations in order to develop therapeutics against human psychiatric and neurological disorders.

References

Beaubrun, G., and Gray, G.E. (2000). A review of herbal medicines for psychiatric disorders. *Psychiatric Services,* **51**: 1130-1134.

Boniel, T., and Dannon, P. (2001). The safety of herbal medicines in the psychiatric practice]. *Harefuah* [Article in Hebrew], **140**: 780-783, 805.

Dey, A., and De, J.N. (2014). Possible anti-Parkinson's disease therapeutics from nature-A review. *Studies in Natural Product Chemistry* **44**: Ed.: Atta-ur-Rahman. Elsevier Science, Amsterdam, The Netherlands. In Press.

Dey, A., and De, J.N. (2012). Ethnobotanical survey of Purulia district, West Bengal, India for medicinal plants used against gastrointestinal disorders. *J Ethnopharmacol.*, **143**: 68-80.

Diefenderfer, L.A., Nelson, L.A., Elliott, E., Liu, Y., Luppa, C., Winans, E., and Sommi, R.W. (2014). Effectiveness evaluation of a pharmacist-driven monitoring database for tardive dyskinesia. *Hosp Pharm.,* **49**: 544-548.

Fugh-Berman, A., and Cott, J.M. (1999). Dietary supplements and natural products as psychotherapeutic agents. *Psychosom Med.,* **61**: 712-728.

Horiguchi, J. (2012). Clinical usage of Yi-gan san-schizophrenia, borderline personality disorder, dyskinesia etc-]. *Seishin Shinkeigaku Zasshi* [Article in Japanese], **114**: 708-718.

Horiguchi, J., Yamashita, H., Mizuno, S., Kuramoto, Y., Kagaya, A., Yamawaki, S., and Inami, Y. (1999). Nocturnal eating/drinking syndrome and neuroleptic-induced restless legs syndrome. *Int Clin Psychopharmacol.*, **14**: 33-36.

Inoue, H., Yamazaki, S., Shimizu, M., Uozaki, H., Goto, T., Ohnishi, S., and Koike, K. (2011). Liver injury induced by the Japanese herbal drug kamishoyosan. *Gastroenterol Hepatol* (N Y)., **7**: 692-695.

Kasper, S. (1997). Treatment of seasonal affective disorder (SAD) with hypericum extract. *Pharmacopsychiatry,* **2**: 89-93.

Kawabe, K., Ueno, S., Hosoda, Y., and Horiguchi, J. (2012). Nocturnal eating/drinking syndrome with restless legs syndrome caused by neuroleptics improved by Yi-Gan San add-on treatment: a case report. *Clin Neuropharmacol.,* **35**: 290-291.

Kobak, K.A., Taylor, L.V., Bystritsky, A., Kohlenberg, C.J., Greist, J.H., Tucker, P., Warner, G., Futterer, R., and Vapnik, T. (2005). St John's wort versus placebo in obsessive-compulsive disorder: results from a double-blind study. *Int Clin Psychopharmacol.,* **20**: 299-304.

Leckman, J.F., Denys, D., Simpson, H.B., Mataix-Cols, D., Hollander, E., Saxena, S., Miguel, E.C., Rauch, S.L., Goodman, W.K., Phillips, K.A., and Stein, D.J. (2010). Obsessive-compulsive disorder: a review of the diagnostic criteria and possible subtypes and dimensional specifiers for DSM-V. *Depress Anxiety,* **27**: 507-527.

Lee, J.G., Shin, B.S., Lee, Y.C., Park, S.W., and Kim, Y.H. (2007). Clinical effectiveness of the Kampo medicine kamishoyosan for adjunctive treatment of tardive dyskinesia in patients with schizophrenia: a 16-week open trial. *Psychiatry Clin Neurosci.,* **61**: 509-514.

Martinez, B., Kasper, S., Ruhrmann, S., and Möller, H.J. (1994). Hypericum in the treatment of seasonal affective disorders. *J Geriatr Psychiatry Neurol.,* **7**: S29-S33.

Meng, X.Z., Wu, F., Wei, P.K., Xiu, L.J., Shi, J., Pang, B., Sun, D.Z., Qin, Z.F., Huang, Y., and Lao, L. (2012). A Chinese herbal formula to improve general psychological status in posttraumatic stress disorder: a randomized placebo-controlled trial on Sichuan earthquake survivors. *Evid Based Complement Alternat Med.,* **2012**: 691258.

Meng, Y., Qiu, C., Zhu, H., Lama, S., Lui, S., Gong, Q., and Zhang, W. (2014). Anatomical deficits in adult posttraumatic stress disorder: A meta-analysis of voxel-based morphometry studies. *Behav Brain Res.,* **270C**: 307-315.

Miyaoka, T., Nagahama, M., Tsuchie, K., Hayashida, M., Nishida, A., Inagaki, T., and Horiguchi, J. (2008). Charles Bonnet syndrome: successful treatment of visual hallucinations due to vision loss with Yi-gan san. *Prog Neuropsychopharmacol Biol Psychiatry,* **33**: 382-383.

Miyaoka, T., Furuya, M., Kristian, L., Wake, R., Kawakami, K., Nagahama, M., Kawano, K., Ieda, M., Tsuchie, K., and Horiguchi, J. (2011). Yi-gan san for treatment of charles bonnet syndrome (visual hallucination due to vision loss): an open-label study. *Clin Neuropharmacol.,* **34**: 24-27.

Miyaoka, T., Furuya, M., Yasuda, H., Hayashia, M., Inagaki, T., and Horiguchi, J. (2008). Yi-gan san for the treatment of borderline personality disorder: an open-label study. *Prog Neuropsychopharmacol Biol Psychiatry,* **32**: 150-154.

Miyaoka, T., Furuya, M., Yasuda, H., Hayashia, M., Nishida, A., Inagaki, T., and Horiguchi, J. (2009). Yi-gan san as adjunctive therapy for treatment-resistant schizophrenia: an open-label study. *Clin Neuropharmacol.,* **32**: 6-9.

Miyaoka, T., Furuya, M., Yasuda, H., Hayashia, M., Nishida, A,. Inagaki, T., and Horiguchi, J. (2008). Yi-gan san for the treatment of neuroleptic-induced tardive dyskinesia: an open-label study. *Prog Neuropsychopharmacol Biol Psychiatry,* **32**: 761-764.

Miyaoka, T., Wake, R., Furuya, M., Liaury, K., Ieda, M., Kawakami, K., Tsuchie, K., Inagaki, T., and Horiguchi, J. (2012). Yokukansan (TJ-54) for treatment of pervasive developmental disorder not otherwise specified and Asperger's disorder: a 12-week prospective, open-label study. *BMC Psychiatry,* **29**: 215.

Mossaheb, N., and Kaufmann. R.M. (2012). Role of aripiprazole in treatment-resistant schizophrenia. *Neuropsychiatr Dis Treat,* **8**: 235-244.

Numata, T., Nagayasu, K., Nishitani, N., Shirakawa, H., Sekiguchi, K., Ikarashi, Y., Kase, Y., and Kaneko, S. (2012). Yokukansan inhibits morphine tolerance and physical dependence in mice: the role of α©üA-adrenoceptor. *Neuroscience,* **227**: 336-349.

Numata, T., Gunfan, S., Takayama, S., Takahashi, S., Monma, Y., Kaneko, S., Kuroda, H., Tanaka, J., Kanemura, S., Nara, M., Kagaya, Y., Ishii, T., Yaegashi, N., Kohzuki, M., and Iwasaki, K. (2014). Treatment of posttraumatic stress disorder using the traditional Japanese herbal medicine saikokeishikankyoto: a randomized, observer-blinded, controlled trial in survivors of the great East Japan earthquake and tsunami. *Evid Based Complement Alternat Med.,* **2014**: 683293.

Pakseresht, S., Boostani, H., and Sayyah, M. (2011). Extract of valerian root (Valeriana officinalis L.) vs. placebo in treatment of obsessive-compulsive disorder: a randomized double-blind study. *J Complement Integr Med.,* **8**: pii: /j/jcim.2011.8.issue-1/1553-3840.1465/1553-3840.1465.xml.

Peng, Z., Wang, H., Zhang, R., Chen, Y., Xue, F., Nie, H., Chen, Y., Wu, D., Wang, Y., Wang, H., and Tan, Q. (2013). Gastrodin ameliorates anxiety-like behaviors and inhibits IL-1β level and p38 MAPK phosphorylation of hippocampus in the rat model of posttraumatic stress disorder. *Physiol Res.,* **62**: 537-545.

Pereira, J.C. Jr., Pradella-Hallinan, M., and Alves, R.C. (2013). Saint John's wort, an herbal inducer of the cytochrome P4503A4 isoform, may alleviate symptoms of Willis-Ekbom's disease. *Clinics (Sao Paulo),* **68**: 469-474.

Khawaja, I., Hashmi, A., Aftab, M., Westermeyer, J., and Hurwitz, T. (2014). Actigraphy in post traumatic stress disorder. *Pak J Med Sci.,* **30**: 438-442.

Sarris, J. (2007). Herbal medicines in the treatment of psychiatric disorders: a systematic review. *Phytother Res.,* **21**: 703-716.

Sarris, J., and Kavanagh, D.J. (2009). Kava and St. John's Wort: current evidence for use in mood and anxiety disorders. *J Altern Complement Med.,* **15**: 827-836.

Sayyah, M., Boostani, H., Pakseresht, S., and Malayeri, A. (2010). Comparison of Silybum marianum (L.) Gaertn. with fluoxetine in the treatment of Obsessive-Compulsive Disorder. *Prog Neuropsychopharmacol Biol Psychiatry,* **34**: 362-365.

Sekiguchi, K., Kanno, H., Yamaguchi, T., Ikarashi, Y., and Kase, Y. (2012). Ameliorative effect of yokukansan on vacuous chewing movement in haloperidol-induced rat tardive dyskinesia model and involvement of glutamatergic system. *Brain Res Bull.,* **89**: 151-158.

Shinno, H., Yamanaka, M., Ishikawa, I., Danjo, S., Nakamura, Y., Inami, Y., and Horiguchi, J. (2010). Successful treatment of restless legs syndrome with the herbal prescription Yokukansan. *Prog Neuropsychopharmacol Biol Psychiatry,* **34**: 252-253.

Taylor, L.H., and Kobak, K.A. (2000). An open-label trial of St. John's Wort (Hypericum perforatum) in obsessive-compulsive disorder. *J Clin Psychiatry,* **61**: 575-578.

Wake, R., Miyaoka, T., Inagaki, T., Furuya, M., Ieda, M., Liaury, K., Kishi, K., and Horiguchi, J. (2013). Yokukansan (TJ-54) for irritability associated with pervasive developmental disorder in children and adolescents: a 12-week prospective, open-label study. *J Child Adolesc Psychopharmacol.,* **23**: 329-336.

Wang, H.N., Peng, Y., Tan, Q.R., Wang, H.H., Chen, Y.C., Zhang, R.G., Wang, Z.Z., Guo, L., Liu, Y., and Zhang, Z.J. (2009). Free and Easy Wanderer Plus (FEWP), a polyherbal preparation, ameliorates PTSD-like behavior and cognitive impairments in stressed rats. *Prog Neuropsychopharmacol Biol Psychiatry,* **33**: 1458-1463.

Wang, W., and Fan. H. (2005). Fifty cases of child restless syndrome treated with the integrated method of Chinese herbal drugs and auricular-plaster therapy. *J Tradit Chin Med.,* **25**: 276-277.

Wheatley, D. (1999). Hypericum in seasonal affective disorder (SAD). *Curr Med Res Opin.,* **15**: 33-7.

Wong, A.H., Smith, M., and Boon, H.S. (1998). Herbal remedies in psychiatric practice. *Arch Gen Psychiatry,* **55**: 1033-1044.

Zhang, Z.J., Kang, W.H.,Tan, Q.R., Li, Q., Gao, C.G., Zhang, F.G., Wang, H.H., Ma, X.C., Chen, C., Wang, W., Guo, L., Zhang, Y.H., Yang, X.B., and Yang, G.D. (2007). Adjunctive herbal medicine with carbamazepine for bipolar disorders: A double-blind, randomized, placebo-controlled study. *J Psychiatr Res.,* **41**: 360-369.

Bioactive Phytochemicals: Perspectives for Modern Medicine Vol. 3 (2015) *Pages* **367–409**
Editor: **V.K. Gupta**
Published by: **DAYA PUBLISHING HOUSE, NEW DELHI**

15

The Current Status of Bioactive Metabolites from the Genus *Juniperus*

Ana M. L. Seca,[1,2] Diana C.G.A. Pinto[2] and Artur M.S. Silva[2*]

ABSTRACT

The genus Juniperus (family Cupressaceae) is one of the most numerous genera of the conifers (there are 102 accepted Latin binominal names). The plants are evergreen shrubs or trees, widely distributed throughout the northern hemisphere from the sea level to above timberline. Some Juniperus species are frequently used in medicinal purposes, for example Juniperus communis L. is used traditionally to cure tuberculosis while Juniperus oxycedrus L. is used in Turkey as a folk remedy in the treatment of diabetes. The richness of Juniperus species in essential oils and secondary metabolites type diterpenes, flavonoids and lignans contributes to its use in the folk medicine. Details on the most recent and relevant pharmacological studies on the bioactive secondary metabolites isolated from Juniperus species will be summarized and thoroughly discussed.

Keywords: Anti-inflammatory, Antimicobacterial, Antimicrobial, Antibiabetic, Cytotoxicity, Diterpenes, *Juniperus*.

Introduction

For centuries, nature has been a source of medicinal products, the plant itself or their secondary metabolites are the source of useful drugs. Currently the scientific community renewed its interest in pharmacologically active natural compounds,

1 DCTD, University of Azores, Rua Mãe de Deus, 9501-801 Ponta Delgada, Azores, Portugal

2 Chemistry Department and QOPNA, University of Aveiro, Campus de Santiago, 3810-193 Aveiro, Portugal

* *Corresponding author*: E-mail: artur.silva@ua.pt

obtained from plants but also from microorganisms or small animals, so that new drugs are obtained, particularly for diseases which cure has not been found yet and/ or for diseases states where our present range of drugs is less effective than we would wish (Cragg and Newman, 2013). Herbal remedies are also enjoying a revival with many sufferers turn away from modern drugs and embraces traditional medicine. In this context *Juniperus* species are of huge importance due their applications on folk medicine.

Depending on the taxonomic viewpoint, there are 67 species of *Juniperus*, 28 varieties and 7 formae (Adams, 2014) or 74 species, 24 varieties and 4 formae ("The Plant List" database). In fact, it consensual that the genus *Juniperus* (Cupressaceae family) is the second most numerous genus of conifers. On the other hand, more than 730 plants are reported as belonging to the *Juniperus* genus but only 102 corresponds to accepted names on "The Plant List" database, being the others synonyms and/or unresolved names. Although understandable, the changes in the species taxonomy may lead to several confusions in the literature and consequently increase difficulties to the phytochemical researchers, usually chemists.

All the botanic names referred herein were confirmed in the "The Plant List" database and the full accepted binominal Latin scientific name will be displayed in the first citation while in subsequent citations *Juniperus* will be indicated by the first capital letter and the authors' names will be omitted.

The genus *Juniperus* is widely distributed throughout the northern hemisphere, from near the equator in Africa and Central America to the Arctic Circle in Alaska, Canada, Greenland, Norway, and Russia (Van Auken and Smeins, 2008). Only one species, *Juniperus procera* Hochst. ex Endl., grows in the southern hemisphere along the rift mountains in east Africa (Adams *et al.*, 2002). The genus *Juniperus* is monophyletic, being recognized three monophyletic sections: sect. *Caryocedrus* with one species in the Mediterranean, sect. *Juniperus* with ten species in East Asia and in the Mediterranean area plus the circumboreal *Juniperus communis* L., and sect. *Sabina* with 56 species mainly in southwestern North America, Asia and Mediterranean region (Mao *et al.*, 2010). The *Juniperus* species are distributed from sea level as for example the *Juniperus procumbens* (Siebold ex Endl.) Miq. to above timberline as *Juniperus zanonii* R.P.Adams (Adams, 2014). The genus *Juniperus* is a major component of arid and semi-arid tree D shrub ecosystems that occur on limestone shallow rocky soils but can also grow on sand dunes of desert [*Juniperus osteosperma* (Torr.) Little] or on the *laurisilva* forest, also known as cloud-zone forest (Figure 15.1) [*Juniperus brevifolia* (Seub.) Antoine (Figure 15.2)] (Adams, 2014; Elias and Dias, 2009).

The species from genus *Juniperus* are evergreen plants with needle-like and/or scale-like leaves. They have a large variation in size, from tall trees (20-40 m) (Adams, 2014) to small trees with pyramidal or columnar forms until low, prostrate forms that are popular for borders, edging and ground cover (Ciesla, 1998). Many of them are popular landscape materials and are especially popular for bonsai because they are relatively easy to care and very popular with beginners.

Applications of *Juniperus* species include the production of dyes in India, whereas the roots of *J. communis* are used to produce a purple-coloured dye and the strips of

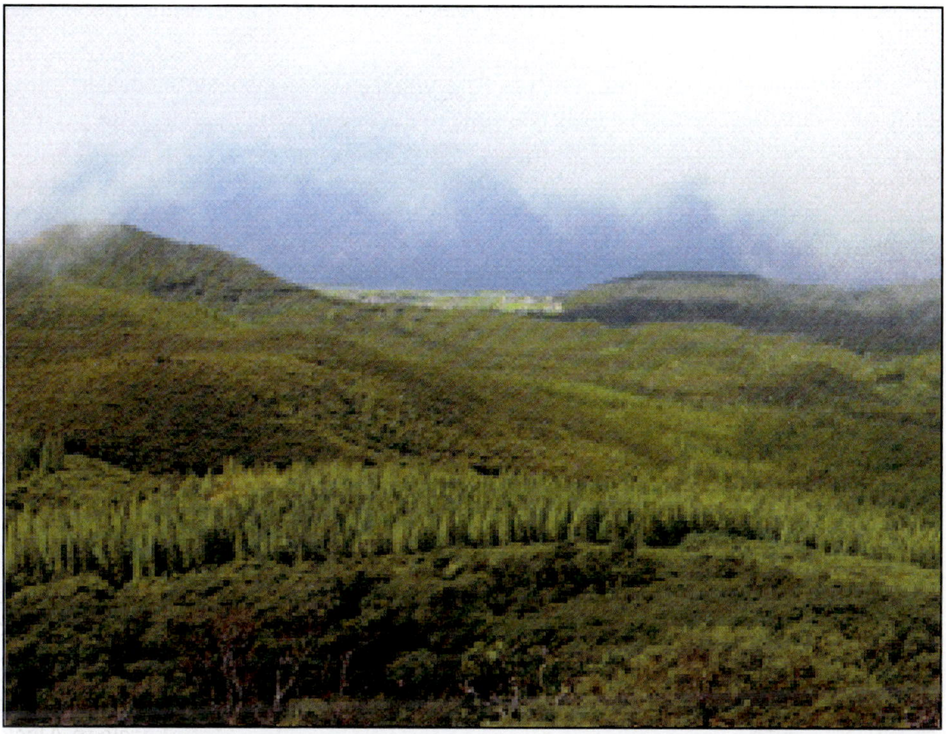

Figure 15.1: *Laurisilva* Forest known as Cloud-Zone Forest in Azores Islands.

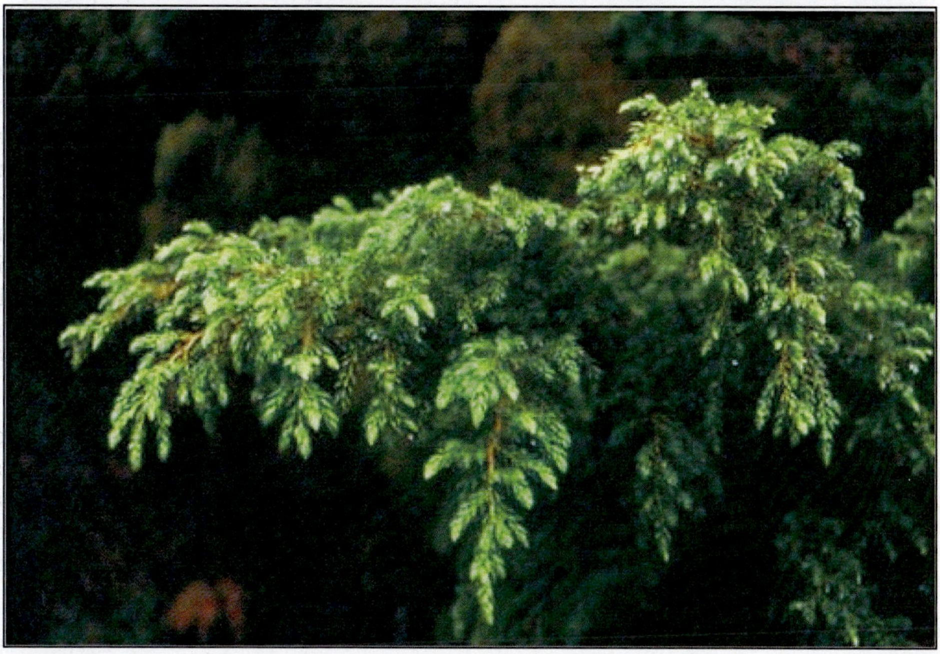

Figure 15.2: *Juniperus brevifolia* (Seub.) Antoine Specimen.

the outer bark of *Juniperus excelsa* M.Bieb is used as roofing material in southwestern Pakistan (Ciesla, 1998).

The *Juniperus* berries, mainly from *J. communis*, are an important spice in many European cuisines, being the only example of a spice coming from a conifer. These berries are used as flavour and spice in a wide variety of culinary dishes and as the primary flavour in the liquor Jenever and sahti-style of beers (Buglass *et al.*, 2010). In Portugal, the traditional homemade alcoholic drink called "aguardente de zimbro" ("zimbro" firewater) is a juniper-flavoured spirit drink, made from the maceration of *J. communis* berries in different distillates like arbutus spirit, marc spirit and wine spirit (Anjos *et al.*, 2013). The berries of *Juniperus oxycedrus* L. are used in northern European and particularly Scandinavian cuisine to impart a sharp, clear flavour to meat dishes (Loizzo *et al.*, 2007).

The seed cones of *Juniperus drupacea* Labill. are used in Turkey for making traditional jam *Pekmez*, a high-energy fruit, mainly consumed in the winter months (Semiz *et al.*, 2007).

There are also reports of toxic effects, for example, cade oil (juniper tar), obtained by distillation from the branches and wood of *J. oxycedrus*, has a dark colour, a strong smoky smell and has toxic effects apparently due to its content in phenols (Koruk *et al.*, 2005). The poisoning of healthy new born treated with a topical application of cade oil for atopic dermatitis was observed (Achour *et al.*, 2011). The ingestion of a spoonful of cade oil cause, within an hour, fever, headache, myalgia, nausea, vomiting, dyspnea, and a productive cough to an adult (Koruk *et al.*, 2005). These and other cases were the incentive to a study on the safety and possible side effects of cade oil (Skalli *et al.*, 2014).

Savin oil (*Juniperus sabina* L. oil), when taken orally in large doses, produced abortions followed by serious poisoning; analysis of the aborted fetus showed the presence of the oil, which proves the permeability of the placenta to the poison (Madari and Jacobs, 2004).

Juniperus species are also used as medicinal plants and secondary metabolites that have proved to be promising therapeutic agents or source of inspiration for the synthesis of new drugs. These topics, until 2004, were reviewed by Seca and Silva (2006). After, several new and known secondary metabolites were isolated from *Juniperus* species, their biological activities evaluated and their mechanisms of action elucidated. Thus, herein we reported the information on traditional medicine applications, bioactive natural compounds isolated from *Juniperus* species since 2005 and their more relevant bioactivities.

Juniperus Genus: Traditional and Pharmacological Applications

The most recent reports on the medicinal uses of *Juniperus* species include *J. communis* (known as juniper) berries and aerial parts used extensively by the indigenous peoples of North America for a variety of medicinal purposes, from respiratory ailments to gynaecological disorders, as a tonic or analgesic (Moerman, 2009; Carpenter *et al.*, 2012). American Indians, such as the Navajo, use this plant to treat coughs, fever, diabetes and as an emetic (Carpenter *et al.*, 2012). In India, the berries of *Juniperus communis* var. *saxatilis* Pall. are used for acute and chronic cystitis, catarrh of the bladder, albuminuria, leucorrhoea as diuretic, carminative, antiseptic, digestive, sudorific, anti-inflammatory and emmenagogue, while aerial parts showed abortive effect (Khare, 2007). The Yurvedic Pharmacopeia of India recommends the dried fruits in malabsorption syndrome (Khare, 2007). The dried ripe berries of *J. communis* are also cited in the European Pharmacopoeia (European Pharmacopoeia, 2008), suggestingtheir significance for medicinal purposes.

Less referred species are *Juniperus virginiana* L. and *J. procera*. The first one is used in India; the berries apparently possess diaphoretic, emmenagogue proprieties while leaves are diuretic and the essential oil is used in the preparation of insecticides (Khare, 2007). The second is used in the Southern part of Saudi Arabia as a traditional remedy for tuberculosis and jaundice (Samoylenko *et al.*, 2008).

The traditional medicine in Turkey includes several *Juniperus* species (Orhan *et al.*, 2011a). Orhan *et al.* (2011b) reported that *J. oxycedrus* fruits and leaves are used in Turkey as a folk remedy for the treatment of diabetes. Later on these authors (Orhan *et al.*, 2012a) reported that the used species was *Juniperus oxycedrus* ssp. *oxycedrus*. Interesting is the fact that this last botanic name does not appear in database "The Plant List" being one of the subspecies for which there is no consensus among taxonomists. Additionally, in Turkey berry decoctions of *J. excelsa* are used to treat common cold and bronchitis, and shoot decoctions of *Juniperus foetidissima* Willd. are used for coughs and common colds, while the fresh berries are used to treat joint calcification (Orhan *et al.*, 2012b). For stomach disorders, eczema and wounds they use *J. sabina* fresh berries (Orhan *et al.*, 2012b). Öztürk *et al.* (2011) showed that the herbal of *J. sabina* is also used as diuretic, emmenagogue, abortive and in the treatment of diabetes mellitus. Fruits of this species are used in Iran, as antifertility, antioxidant and anti-inflammatory agents (Jazayeri *et al.*, 2014).

In Tunisian traditional medicine the decoction of aerial parts of *Juniperus phoenicea* L. is used to treat some skin diseases, pharyngitis, rheumatism, diabetes and diarrhoea (Sassi *et al.*, 2008).

Nepal folk medicine is very popular and for many Nepalese population this traditional medicine are their primary health care. In this context several *Juniperus* species are used; *Juniperus indica* Bertol. seeds are eaten to get relief from kidney problems in the Dolpa district whereas its leaf juice is taken for cough, cold and paralysis in Humla district (Kunwar *et al.*, 2006). In Dolpa and Mustang districts the paste of young leaf shoot from *Juniperus squamata* Buch.-Ham. ex D.Don is used in the fever control and skin disease and its fruits are used as digestive (Kunwar *et al.*, 2006). In the Rasuwa district, fresh fruits and leafs from *Juniperus recurva* Buch.-Ham. ex D.Don are used to treat fever, headache, cough, cold and kidney problems (Uprety *et al.*, 2010). The decoction of *J. drupacea* berries is used as anthelmintic, to treat stomach ache and haemorrhoids and of fresh shoots is used for urinary inflammations, gout and to treat abdominal pain (Miceli *et al.*, 2011). Khan *et al.* (2012), states that *J. excelsa* is used in folk medicine to treat diarrhoea, abdominal spasm, asthma, fever, gonorrhoea, headache and leucorrhoea and also useful as antihypertensive, diuretic, appetizer, carminative, stimulant, anticonvulsant and flavouring agent. These recently cited ethnopharmacology applications confirm the great pharmacological potential of the *Juniperus* species.

Structural Pattern of Bioactive Compounds Isolated from *Juniperus* Species

Isolation of secondary metabolites from *Juniperus* species and the evaluation of their biological activities including the study of their mechanisms of action are important to validate (or not) the traditional medicine based in this species and, ultimately, to find new drugs.

Since phytochemical studies of *Juniperus* are vast, we choose to present in Table 15.1 the most frequent and/or active secondary metabolites isolated from *Juniperus* species published after last review in this subject in 2004 (Seca and Silva, 2006).

Table 15.1: Bioactive Compounds Isolated from *Juniperus* Species (Structures illustrated in Figures 15.3 to 15.18)

Compound	*Juniperus Species**	*Part of Plant*	*Reference*
Totarol	*J. procera*	Bark	Mossa *et al.*, 2004
	J. procera	Berries	Samoylenko *et al.*, 2008
	J. excelsa	Berries	Samoylenko *et al.*, 2008
	J. phoenicea	Berries	Samoylenko *et al.*, 2008
	J. brevifolia	Bark	Seca and Silva, 2008
	J. communis	Roots	Gordien *et al.*, 2009
Ferruginol	*J. procera*	Bark	Mossa *et al.*, 2004
	J. procera	Berries	Samoylenko *et al.*, 2008
	J. brevifolia	Bark	Seca and Silva, 2008
	J. excelsa	Berries	Samoylenko *et al.*, 2008
	J. phoenicea	Berries	Samoylenko *et al.*, 2008
	J. procera	Aerial parts	Alqasoumi and Abdel-Kader, 2012
Hinokiol	*J. brevifolia*	Bark	Seca and Silva, 2008
	J. brevifolia	Leaves	Seca *et al.*, 2008
	J. excelsa	Berries	Samoylenko *et al.*, 2008
	J. phoenicea	Berries	Samoylenko *et al.*, 2008
	J. procera	Berries	Samoylenko *et al.*, 2008
	J. procera	Aerial parts	Alqasoumi and Abdel-Kader, 2012
Sugiol	*Juniperus polycarpos* var. *seravschanica* (Kom.) Kitam.[1]	Fruits	Okasaka *et al.*, 2006
	J. procera		
	Juniperus chinensis L.[2]	Berries	Samoylenko *et al.*, 2008
	J. brevifolia	Bark	Chang *et al.*, 2008

Contd...

Table 15.1–*Contd...*

Compound	*Juniperus Species**	*Part of Plant*	*Reference*
	J. brevifolia	Bark	Seca and Silva, 2008
		Leaves	Seca *et al.*, 2008
	J. procera		Seca and Silva., 2010
		Aerial parts	Alqasoumi and Abdel-Kader, 2012
Dehydroabietinol	*J. brevifolia*	Leaves	Seca *et al.*, 2008
(18-hydroxy-dehydroabietane)			Seca and Silva, 2010
Dehydroabietic acid	*J. brevifolia*	Bark	Seca and Silva, 2008
Abieta-7,13-diene	*J. procera*	Berries	Samoylenko *et al.*, 2008
Abietic acid	*J. phoenicea*	Leaves	Barrero *et al.*, 2004
	Juniperus thurifera Maire var. *africana*	Leaves	Barrero *et al.*, 2004
4-*epi*-Abietinol	*J. procera*	Aerial parts	Alqasoumi and Abdel-Kader, 2012
Communic acid	*J. procera*	Berries	Samoylenko *et al.*, 2008
	J. virginiana	Resinous exudate	Samoylenko *et al.*, 2008
	J. chinensis	Bark	Chang *et al.*, 2008
	J. brevifolia	Leaves	Seca *et al.*, 2008
	Juniperus taxifolia Hook. & Arn.	Leaves	Muto *et al.*, 2008
	J. chinensis	Bark	Chang *et al.*, 2008
	J. communis	Aerial parts	Gordien *et al.*, 2009
	Juniperus rigida Siebold & Zucc.	Aerial parts	Woo *et al.*, 2011
	J. communis	Aerial parts	Carpenter *et al.*, 2012
	J. procera	Aerial parts	Alqasoumi and Abdel-Kader, 2012
(*Z*)-8α-Hydroxylabda-13(16), 14-dien-19-yl coumarate	*J. brevifolia*	Leaves	Moujir *et al.*, 2008
Shikimic acid	*J. phoenicea*	Berries	Aboul-Ela *et al.*, 2005
	J. oxycedrus subsp. *oxycedrus*[3]	Berries	Orhan *et al.*, 2012a
	J. communis	Berries	Falasca *et al.*, 2014
Umbelliferone	*J. communis* subsp. *nana*[4]	Leaves and ripe fruits	Orhan *et al.*, 2011a
		Leaves	
	J. foetidissima	Leaves and ripe fruits	Orhan *et al.*, 2011a

Contd...

Table 15.1–*Contd...*

Compound	*Juniperus Species**	*Part of Plant*	*Reference*
	J. oxycedrus subsp. *oxycedrus*[3]	Leaves	Orhan *et al.*, 2011a
	J. excelsa	Leaves	Orhan *et al.*, 2011a
	J. sabina	Berries	Orhan *et al.*, 2011a
	J. drupacea	Leaves and seed cones	Miceli *et al.*, 2011
	J. foetidissima	Leaves and seed cones	Lesjak *et al.*, 2013
	Juniperus macrocarpa Sm.		Lesjak *et al.*, 2014
Deoxypodo-phyllotoxin	*J. taxifolia*	Leaves	Muto *et al.*, 2008
	J. communis	Aerial parts	Kusari *et al.*, 2009
	J. recurva	twings	Kusari *et al.*, 2009
	J. squamata	twings	Kusari *et al.*, 2009
	J. x media[5]	twings	Kusari *et al.*, 2009
	J. recurva	Aerial parts	Kusari *et al.*, 2011
	J. communis	Aerial parts	Kusari *et al.*, 2011
	J. procumbens	Aerial parts	Kusari *et al.*, 2011
	J. x media[5]	Aerial parts	Kusari *et al.*, 2011
	J. squamata	Aerial parts	Kusari *et al.*, 2011
	Juniperus bermudiana L.	Leaves	Renouard *et al.*, 2011
	J. x media[5]	Leaves	Renouard *et al.*, 2011
	J. procumbens	Leaves	Renouard *et al.*, 2011
	J. squamata	Leaves	Renouard *et al.*, 2011
	J. verginiana	Leaves	Renouard *et al.*, 2011
	J. sabina	Leaves	Renouard *et al.*, 2011
	J. communis	Leaves	Renouard *et al.*, 2011
	J. rigida	Aerial parts	Woo *et al.*, 2011
	J. communis	Aerial parts	Carpenter *et al.*, 2012
	Juniperus thurifera L.	Leaves	Guerrero *et al.*, 2013
	J. communis	Branches and needles	Benzina *et al.*, 2014
Amentoflavone	*J. communis*	Berries	Innocenti *et al.*, 2007
	J. phoenicea	Leaves	Ali *et al.*, 2010
	J drupacea	Berries	Miceli *et al.*, 2011
	J. rigida	Leaves	Jeong *et al.*, 2012

Contd...

Table 15.1–*Contd...*

Compound	*Juniperus Species**	*Part of Plant*	*Reference*
	J. foetidissima	Leaves and seed cones	Lesjak *et al.*, 2013
		Leaves and seed cones	
	J. macrocarpa		Lesjak *et al.*, 2014
Hinokiflavone	*J. polycarpos* var. *seravschanica*[1]	Fruits	Okasaka *et al.*, 2006
	J. phoenicea	Aerial parts	Alqasoumi *et al.*, 2013

* The indicated secondary metabolites were found in several other *Juniperus* species, herein were just mentioned the ones reported after 2004.

1 The botanical name cited in the original work (Okasaka *et al.*, 2006) was *J. polycarpus* var. *seravschanica* however in "The Plant List" database it is named as indicate.

2 The botanical name referred in the original work is *Juniperus chinensis* Linn. However in "The Plant List" database the author's name is as we indicate.

3 This botanical name is not in the "The plant list" database.

4 This name is a synonym of *Juniperus communis* var. *saxatilis* Pall.

5 This plant name is cited as *J. x media* (Pfitzeriana) and authors are not given. This botanical name cannot be found in "The Plant List" database.

Biological Properties of the Isolated Compounds

The aim of this review is not to compile all the literature data on *Juniperus* secondary metabolites and/or their biological potential. However, the most studied activities, such as antimicrobial, anti-inflammatory, antioxidant, cytotoxic and antidiabetic are the main subject of this manuscript, although other more recent studies which were pioneers in the biological activity evaluated are also cited. Studies on nematicidal, antifouling, anticonvulsant, allergenic, antiulcer, gastroprotective, anti-obesity antinociceptive and hepatoprotective activities can be found in the recent literature. The importance of the last one as a topic of research is mainly due to the liver causes of death, such as viral hepatitis and liver cancer, while fortunately, the liver cirrhosis mortality has decreased in recent years (Fedeli *et al.*, 2014). Another original study was the search for testosterone 5α-redutase inhibitors. Apparently the over production of 5α-dehydrotestosterone is associated with acne, benign prostatic hyperplasia and male pattern baldness diseases. Therefore, the inhibition of the enzymatic reductive conversion of testosterone to 5α-dehydrotestosterone represents an important therapeutic target to the selective treatment of these androgen-dependent diseases (Aggarwal *et al.*, 2014).

Within the recent years the infectious diseases have increase to a great extent and antibiotic resistance is a therapeutic problem. The evaluation of antibacterial activity is still of particularly relevance to the drug discovery, even more if we have in mind that 8.6 million cases of *Mycobacterium tuberculosis* infection, the causative agent of tuberculosis, were estimated in 2012, and 1.3 million people died from the disease

(WHO, 2013). New antimycobacterial agents are needed to improve the treatment of several forms of pulmonary, skeletal and soft tissue infections and opportunistic diseases caused by non-tuberculosis mycobacteria which are also increasing (Zheng and Fanta, 2013; Atkins and Gottlieb, 2014).

Conversely, a wide range of new antiviral drugs is needed to tackle virus, such as HIV and HCV, HSV, VZV, pox, influenza, flavi, bunya and filo (Ebola), especially in view of the various strains that emerge each year (Luetkemeyer *et al.*, 2013), but also diseases caused by parasites, such as antileishmanial and antimalarial, which need more effective drugs. Also *Candida albicans*, notorious for causing candidiasis, colonizes the mucosal surfaces of the respiratory tract and the vaginal cavity and is able to cause serious infection depending on the defects of the host immune system (Sharanappa and Vidyasagar, 2013), still needs efficient drugs to be eliminated. Due to the increasing development of drug resistance of the human pathogens as well as the appearance of undesirable side effects, the search of new antimicrobial agents is still a hot topic.

Non-steroidal anti-inflammatory drugs (NSAIDs), steroidal drugs, and immunosuppressant drugs, which have been used usually in the relief of inflammatory diseases, were often associated with severe adverse side effects, such as gastrointestinal bleeding and peptic ulcers. Natural products play a significant role in human health in relation to the prevention and treatment of inflammatory conditions (Lourenço *et al.*, 2012).

Cancer treatment has been moving away from conventional chemotherapy towards targeted therapeutics that has sparked further explorations for novel pathways to inhibit or to better control the cancer. The monoclonal antibodies and kinase inhibitors are the two most successful categories of targeted therapeutics agents (Bailly, 2014). However, conventional cytotoxic agents, some of them natural compounds, continue to be used in daily practice in oncology, mainly when there is no other treatment modality available, in particular for late stage or metastatic diseases.

Diabetes mellitus is a metabolic disorder of multiple aetiologies and is characterised by chronic hyperglycaemia. It is the commonest endocrine disorder that, according to the World Health Organization (WHO, 2014), affects more than 347 million people worldwide. So the search for antidiabetic compounds is vital.

Reactive oxygen species (ROS) and reactive nitrogen species (RNS) such as nitric oxide radical, superoxide radical, hydroxyl radical, hydrogen peroxide and singlet oxygen are by-products of cellular metabolism and also produced by a number of exogenous sources [ionizing radiations (ultraviolet and γ-rays), tobacco, smoke, pesticides, pollutants]. Such species are considered to be the cause of aging-diseases, DNA mutations and degenerative human diseases (cancer, cardio- and cerebral-vascular diseases) (Brieger *et al.*, 2012). Thus antioxidant substances play an important role in health care.

In view of the above mention needs it is expectable that scientists not only isolate the metabolites from medicinal plants but also evaluate their activities. Herein we are going to highlight the most interesting active metabolites isolated from *Juniperus* species and the most interesting synthetic derivatives.

Totarol

Totarol (Figure 15.3a) is a tricyclic phenolic diterpene with a totarane skeleton, which is structurally different from the abieta-8,11,13-trien skeleton (Figure 15.3b) by the isopropyl migration from C-13 to C-14 position. This compound seems to be a good synthon towards new interesting active drugs. It is found in many *Juniperus* species (Seca and Silva, 2006) and is the most abundant compound in the hexane extract of *J. brevifolia* bark (11 per cent) (Seca and Silva, 2008), but it is also found in species from other genus. Since the first biological evaluation in 1977 (Enomoto *et al.*, 1977), several other evaluations demonstrate that totarol displays a range of interesting bioactivities.

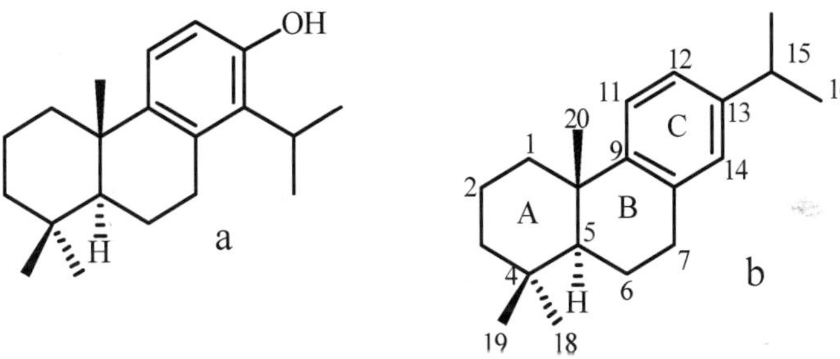

Figure 15.3: Totarol Structure (a) and Abieta-8,11,13-trien Skeleton (b).

More recent studies include the antistaphylococcal activity and the efflux inhibitory activity of totarol. It is worthy to mention that the multidrug-resistant staphylococci have become a major health risk and the need for new antibacterial agents is becoming increasingly urgent. Efflux is a common resistance mechanism employed by bacteria. For example, the *NorA* multidrug resistance (*NorA* MDR) pump of *Staphylococcus aureus* effluxes a broad spectrum of compounds. Some compounds named EPI (efflux pump inhibitors) may inhibit bacterial efflux pumps. The MICs of totarol for NCTC 8325-4 (commonly used laboratory strain), SA-K1758 (*norA* null), SAK3090 (SA-K1758 resistant to totarol) and SA-K3092 (SA-K3090 plasmid-based *norA* over-expresser) strains are 2.5, 1.25, 16 and 16 μg/mL, respectively, indicating that totarol is not a substrate for the *NorA* MDR pump (Smith *et al.*, 2007a). The concentration at which totarol inhibited ethidium bromide (EtBr) efflux by 50 per cent (IC_{50} 4.29 μg/mL) is approximately one-fourth of the MIC for SAK3092 strain (Smith *et al.*, 2007a). The totarol reduces *NorA*-mediated EtBr efflux, but not as effective as the reference compound reserpine [an efficient tetracyclines (TetK) efflux agent and a *NorA* EPI with significant toxicity at the required concentrations]. However, totarol can be a good lead candidate for further development of effective drugs against resistant *S. aureus*.

The FtsZ, prokaryotic homologue of tubulin, is a central protein of bacterial cell division, which is a selective antibacterial target for the development of new antibiotics to fight infections that are resistant to current therapies. In this context the totarol inhibition of *Bacillus subtilis* proliferation, with a MIC of 2 μM, (0.57 μg/mL) (Jaiswal *et al.*, 2007), was evaluated and was found that it presents an antibacterial activity comparable to that of other known FtsZ inhibitors (dichamanetin MIC 1.7 µM). At 1.5 µM the antibacterial activity of totarol is not likely to be associated with a major perturbation in the membrane structure of the bacteria but it is related with a strong inhibition of the cytokinesis by perturbing the formation and functioning of the Z-ring through its binding to FtsZ (Jaiswal *et al.*, 2007), a central protein of bacterial cell division. On the other hand, totarol did not perturb microtubule and chromosome organization in the HeLa cells suggesting that totarol exerted differential activity toward eukaryotic and prokaryotic cells (Jaiswal *et al.*, 2007). A subsequent study, with *B. subtilis* strain 168, showed that totarol decreased the transmembrane potential or perturbed membrane permeability, and influenced the localization of the membrane-associated division protein MinD (Foss *et al.*, 2013). Recently, Kim *et al.* (2012) suggested that totarol is not a specific FtsZ inhibitor, being its antibacterial activity caused by the molecules aggregation.

Totarol exhibit antimycobacterial activity against *Mycobacterium intracellulare*, *M. smegmatis*, *M. xenopei* and *M. chelonei*, with a more potent effect (MIC 1.25-2.5 µg/mL) than the two positive controls, INH and streptomycin (MIC 10 and 20 µg/mL, respectively) (Mossa *et al.*, 2004). Noticeable is the synergetic effect detected when totarol was mixed with INH, the MIC was lowered from 2.5 to 0.3 µg/mL. When tested against the resistant strain of *M. tuberculosis* H37Rv, this diterpene showed to be inactive at lower concentrations (MIC 12.5 µg/mL) (Mossa *et al.*, 2004).

In another study was proposed that the use of *J. communis* in folk medicine to treat tuberculosis is related to its content in totarol. In fact, totarol was found to be the most active and selective compound against *M. tuberculosis* H37Rv (MIC 21.1 µg/mL) and also against the rifampicin-resistant and isoniazid-resistant variants, MIC 5.8 µg/mL and 11.0 respectively (Gordien *et al.*, 2009). However, totarol showed toxicity against Vero cell lines (IC_{50} 7.5 µg/mL). The low selectivity index obtained (IC_{50}/MIC lower than 10) indicated that the isolated diterpene was relatively toxic towards mammalian cells, especially when compared to the high selectivity of the antibiotic rifampicin (IC_{50}/MIC > 90) used as control (Gordier *et al.*, 2009). From these independent studies we can conclude that most likely totarol could be used as activity enhancer of some conventional drug.

The totarol showed interesting activity against *Leishmania donovani* promastigotes (IC_{50} 3.5 µg/mL *vs* 1.3 µg/mL for reference drug) but it has no antimalarial activity (IC_{50} > 4.76 µg/mL) against the two *Plasmodium falciparum* strains (chloroquine-sensitive, D6 and chloroquine-resistant, W2) (Samoylenko *et al.*, 2008).

Later, Tacon *et al.* (2012) showed that totarol exhibit activity against *Plasmodium falciparum* strains D10 (IC_{50} 11.78 µM) and K1 (IC_{50} 11.69 µM), (values more or less equivalents to ~ 3.3 µg/mL). It means that totarol is more active against these strains, but considerably less active than the reference mefloquine (IC_{50} 0.018 and 0.008 µM respectively against D10 and K1 strains) (Tacon *et al.*, 2012). The authors also showed that its cytotoxicity against the CHO mammalian cell lines is lower (IC_{50} 170 µM). The authors synthetized several β-amino alcohol and found that the addition of a 13-*O*-β-amino alcohol side chain to totarol notably improved the antiplasmodial activity (IC_{50} 0.17-6.47 µM), but also increase the cytotoxicity against the CHO mammalian cell lines (Tacon *et al.*, 2012). This was not the first study evaluating the activity of β-amino alcohol totarol derivatives as antimalarial activity. In fact, Clarkson *et al.* (2003) synthetized several derivatives, from which *N,N*-diethyl β-amino alcohol totarol derivative (**1**) (Figure 15.19) was the most active (IC_{50} values of 0.61 and 0.63 µM against the D10 and K1 strains respectively) (Clarkson *et al.*, 2003).

A screening test revealed that, among the several metabolites isolated from *J. procera* berries, totarol is the active one against *Caenorhabditis elegans* (at a concentration of 80 µg/mL) and *Artemia salina*, a model organism for crustaceous foulers like barnacles (at 1 µg/mL), being these activity level identical to the Jansen Pharmaceutica reference compounds (Samoylenko *et al.*, 2008). These results indicate that totarol can be a good candidate to develop new nematicidal and antifouling agents.

Ferruginol

Ferruginol is also a tricyclic phenolic diterpene like totarol but with an abieta-8,11,13-trien skeleton. It is a widely distributed natural product occurring in plants belonging to the Podocarpaceae, Cupressaceae, Lamiaceae, and Verbenaceae families being particularly abundant in the hexane extract of *J. excelsa* berries (32.9 per cent) (Samoylenko *et al.*, 2008). This diterpene has attracted much attention since it exhibits promising bioactivities and is the starting material for the synthesis of several very active compounds.

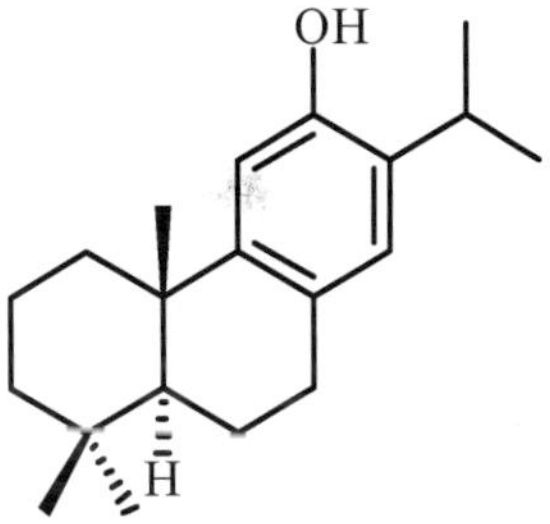

Figure 15.4: Ferruginol Structure.

Ferruginol was evaluated for its antistaphylococcal and modulatory activities against a standard *Staphylococcus aureus* ATCC strain and a clinically isolated methicillin-resistant *S. aureus* (MRSA) (Smith *et al.*, 2007b) and also against five clinically relevant multidrug resistance (MDR) pathogens. Ferruginol was active against all the tested strains, exhibiting MIC values of 4-16 µg/mL, although is less active than tetracycline, norfloxacin, erythromycin and oxacillin, antibiotics used against *S. aureus* ATCC strain. On the other hand, ferruginol proved to be more active than some antibiotics used against MDR and MRSA strains (Smith *et al.*, 2007b). Ferruginol also exhibit modulatory activity. It use at a sub-inhibitory concentration results in a 80-fold potentiation of oxacillin activity against the epidemic MRSA-15 (EMRSA-15) (MIC from 32 to 0.40 µg/mL), demonstrating good modulatory activity in restoring oxacillin sensitivity (Smith *et al.*, 2007b). Ferruginol also potentiate the activity of erythromycin against a strain possessing the MsrA efflux pump. The efflux inhibition experiments using ferruginol (2.86 µg/mL) showed 40 per cent inhibition of the EtBr efflux in SA1199B, a strain which overexpresses the *NorA* pump, (Smith *et al.*, 2007b).

Ferruginol was assayed against *Propionibacterium acnes*, one of the major agents in the skin condition acne, and showed interesting activity (MIC 4 µg/mL) nevertheless was less active than the reference antibiotic clindamycin (MIC 0.125 µg/mL) (Smith *et al.*, 2008).

Ferruginol also have some synergetic effect in INH action, the MIC against nontuberculous agents *Mycobacterium intracellulare, M. smegmatis, M. xenopei* and *M. chelonei* was lowered from 5 to 0.3 µg/mL when applied with ½ MIC of INH (5 µg/mL) (Mossa *et al.*, 2004).

Ferruginol exhibits good antileishmanial activity against *Leishmania donovani* promastigotes (IC_{50} 3.5 µg/mL *vs* 1.3 µg/mL for pentamidine, a reference compound) (Samoylenko *et al.*, 2008). Ferruginol is also active against two strains of the malaria agent *Plasmodium falciparum* (chloroquine-sensitive D6 and chloroquine-resistant W2 strains) (IC_{50} 3.5-4.2 µg/mL), but much less than the positive control ($IC_{50} < 0.264$ µg/mL for chloroquine) (Samoylenko *et al.*, 2008).

Severe acute respiratory syndrome (SARS) is a highly contagious and a life-threatening form of atypical pneumonia caused by infection with a novel human coronavirus (SARS-CoV), whose replication depends of a chymotrypsin-like cysteine proteinase 3CLpro recognized as a key target for anti-SARS drug design (Thanigaimalai *et al.*, 2013). Ferruginol has proved to be a potent inhibitor of SARS-CoV 3CLpro (IC_{50} 49.6 µM), exhibiting nearly a fourfold more potent inhibitor effect on SARS-CoV 3CLpro than the diterpenoid abietic acid (Figure 15.10) used as positive control (IC_{50} 189.1 µM) (Ryu *et al.*, 2010).

Hinokiol

Hinokiol is a 3β,12-dihydroxy-abieta-8,11,13-triene [also known as (3β)-abieta-8,11,13-triene-3,12-diol] and like ferruginol belongs to the abieta-8,11,13-trien diterpene type. It was first isolated from *Chamaecyparis obtusa* (Siebold and Zucc.) Endl. in 1913 but its correct structure (Figure 15.5) was only assigned in 1962 (Chow and Erdtman, 1962). It is not as abundant as ferruginol but it has also attracted great interest in the scientific community as a starting material for synthetic purposes and due to its pharmacological potential.

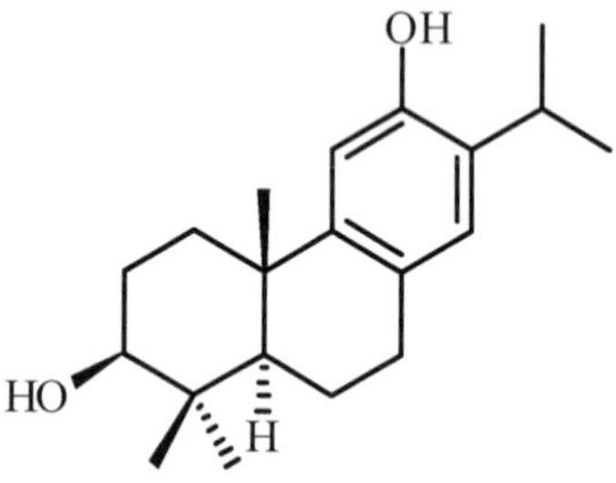

Figure 15.5: Hinokinol Structure.

5-LOX inhibitors are important compounds due to their potential used to treat asthma and in their effort to find anti-inflammatory agents. Fan *et al.* (2012) demonstrate the 5-LOX inhibitory effect of hinokiol (~50 per cent of inhibition at 100 µM). Hinokiol inhibits LTB4 (at 100 µM) and 5-HETE (at 25 µM), however less active than the positive control used (nordihydroguaiaretic acid causes identical inhibition but at 12.5 µM). Hinokiol also showed beneficial effects on COX pathway exhibiting inhibitory effects on TNF-α and NO production (Fan *et al.*, 2012). In *in vitro* assays showed that hinokiol significantly inhibit the NO production in LPS stimulated RAW264.7 macrophages (IC_{50} 26 µM) (Chen *et al.*, 2013). Unfortunately, the authors did not use a positive control in their work so conclusions are not possible.

Another activity assayed was the hinokiol ability to scavenge DPPH radicals and the results showed that its scavenging effect (IC_{50} 201.98 µM) is lower than that of BHT and quercetin (IC_{50} 101.68 µM and 10.96 µM respectively) (Gaspar-Marques *et al.*, 2008).

Sugiol

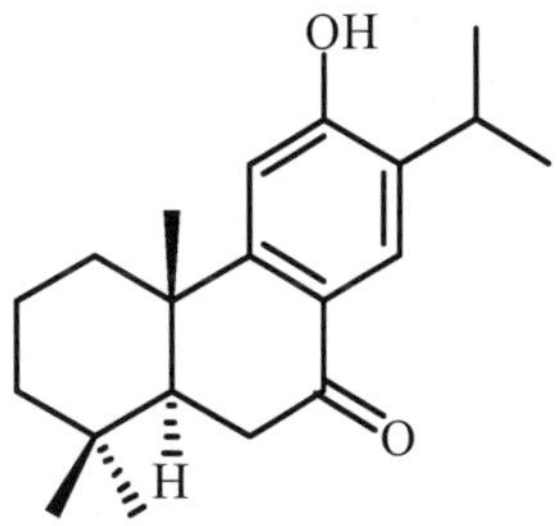

Figure 15.6: Sugiol Structure.

Sugiol is a 12-hydroxy-7-oxo-abieta-8,11,13-triene and like ferruginol is widely distributed in the Taxodiaceae, Lamiaceae and Cupressaceae families. Since oxygen functionality in B and C rings might be responsible for the biological profile of abietatriene derivatives, the carbonyl group at C-7 makes the sugiol an excellent and versatile synthon for new derivatives.

In the search for new hepatoprotective compounds, sugiol was administrated to rats prior to CCl_4 administration and showed significant reductions on the liver levels in the SGOT enzyme and bilirubin (~32-36 per cent), about half the effect produced by the reference drug silymarin. In the levels of SGPT and ALP (37 and 60 per cent respectively) the sugiol effect is similar to the silymarin effect (Alqasoumi and Abdel-Kader, 2012). These results indicated that sugiol can reduce the elevated liver enzymes level and contributes to liver protection. It is noteworthy that, in the same study, ferruginol (identical structure without C-7 carbonyl group) and hinokiol (without C-7 carbonyl group but with an extra C-3 hydroxyl group) do not show significant hepatoprotective effects (Alqasoumi and Abdel-Kader, 2012).

Recently the antioxidant activity of sugiol was evaluated by different methods and its scavenging effect (25-250 µg/mL) against active oxygen and nitrogen species (NO, superoxide and hydroxyl radicals), the lipid peroxidation inhibitory action (25-250 µg/mL) and the ability to reduce ferric ions (Fe^{3+}) (5-25 µg/mL) were demonstrated. The results indicate that sugiol seems to be better than ascorbic acid, BHA and α-tocopherol, antioxidants usually used in food industry (Bajpai *et al.*, 2014). These results reveal that sugiol antioxidant ability is higher than hinokiol (Figure 15.5) when the only structural difference is a 7-C=O group instead a 3-OH group. On the other hand, sugiol showed an IC_{50} > 66 µM in the inhibitory evaluation of NO production (Chen *et al.*, 2013), highlighting in this case the negative effect that the replacement of a 3-OH group by a 7-C=O has in the ability to inhibit NO production.

Dehydroabietinol

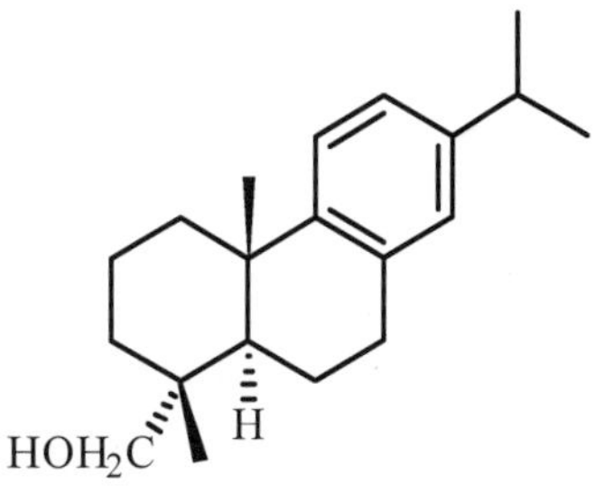

Figure 15.7: Dehydroabietinol Structure.

The dehydroabietinol, also known as pomiferin A and 18-hydroxydehydroabietane, is an isomer of ferruginol but is not a phenolic diterpene. In fact, it is possible to deduce from the last name and analysis of the structures (Figures 15.4 and 15.7) that the hydroxyl group is at C-18 instead of at C-12 (aromatic ring C). Dehydroabietinol has a more restricted distribution in nature than any of the compounds described above. It is known as natural product since 1985 (Kaneko *et al.*, 1985), although in 1992, when it was isolated from *Salvia pomifera*, the authors claimed the isolation of a new natural product and named it as pomiferin A (Ulubelen and Topcu, 1992). Until now it was reported in more than ten species mainly from Pinaceae family.

The antibacterial and antifungal activity of dehydroabietinol was evaluated and the results showed that against *Staphylococcus aureus, Enterococcus faecalis, Escherichia coli, Pseudomonas aeruginosa* and *Candida albicans* is inactive (MIC up to 40 µg/mL), although exhibited activity against two of the Gram-(+) bacteria used *Bacillus cereus, Staphylococcus epidermidis* (Moujir *et al.*, 2011). Furthermore, dehydroabietinol exhibited the highest activity (MIC 2.5–5 µg/mL) against *B. cereus,* higher than cephotaxime used as positive control (MIC 10 µg/mL) (Moujir *et al.*, 2011). The SAR analysis based on the MIC of several dehydroabietane derivatives showed that the 18-hydroxyl group is important for the antimicrobial activity while the presence of a second hydrophilic group reduce the compounds activity (Moujir *et al.*, 2011).

The dehydroabietinol exhibit moderate cytotoxic activity against A549 and MCF-7 human tumor cell lines and it is more active against HeLa when applied in lag phase (IC_{50} 15.7 µM), although less active than the positive control 6-mercaptopurine (IC_{50} 2.9 µM). Dehydroabietinol cytotoxic activity against non-tumor mammalian Vero cells (IC_{50} 28.0 µM) indicate that it is selective towards the tumor cell lines HeLa (Moujir *et al.*, 2011). The same authors evaluated several other dehydroabietane diterpenes and the SAR analysis suggested that one hydrogen-bond-donor group strategically positioned is an important requirement for activity while the presence of one extra hydroxyl group or a carbonyl group at C-7 lower their cytotoxic activity (Moujir *et al.*, 2008, Moujir *et al.*, 2011). The unfavourable position of the hydroxyl group can also be confirmed by the fact that hinokiol (3,12-dihydroxydehydroabietane) (Figure 15.5) is not active against HL-60, A549, and MCF-7 tumor cell lines at 40 µM (Zhao *et al.*, 2011).

Several dehydroabietinol derivatives bearing a triazole moiety were synthetized and their cytotoxic activity against AGS, SK-MES-1, J82 tumor cell lines and MRC-5 normal lung fibroblasts was evaluated (Pertino *et al.*, 2014). The best antiproliferative effect was against SK-MES-1 cells and obtained with compound **(2)** (Figure 15.19). The IC_{50} value is higher (6.1 µM) than the reference drug value etoposide (IC_{50} 1.83 µM) but the derivative is also selective towards tumor cell lines (IC_{50} 17.1 µM against MRC-5) (Pertino *et al.*, 2014).

Dehydroabietic Acid

The dehydroabietic acid has a lipophilic abietan-8,11,13-trien structure with only an equatorial carboxylic group at C-4. It is a component of the mixture known as resin acids very abundant for example in pine resin. This acid is widely distributed in nature, known as natural product at least since the beginning of last century, and has been considered as an interesting starting material for the synthesis of new compounds with interesting biological properties as will be further referred.

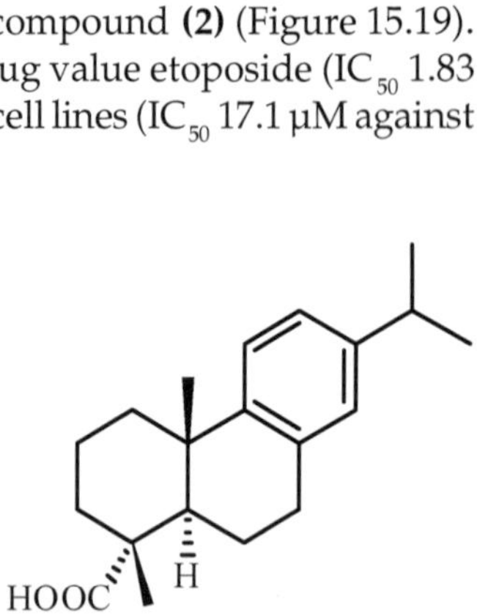

Figure 15.8: Dehydroabietic Acid Structure.

The dehydroabietic acid and some derivatives showed moderate activity against HHV-2 and were not active against HHV-1 (Agudelo-Gómez *et al.*, 2012). The antiviral activity of dehydroabietic acid does not lead to its clinical application but its derivatives can be a powerful tool in the synthesis of new antiviral drugs, since they have some key structural points that influence its antiviral activity, although the inhibition mechanisms remain unclear.

Certain pancreatic cancer cell lines exhibit extraordinary tolerance against extreme nutrient starvation. The elimination of this tolerance could be a novel approach to pancreatic cancer therapy (Awale *et al.*, 2006). The cytotoxicity of dehydroabietic acid derivatives was assayed against PANC-1 cancer cells under nutrient-deprived conditions. The dehydroabietic acid showed moderate cytotoxicity at 50 µg/mL while its methyl ester derivative (methyl abieta-8,11,13-trien-18-oate) at 10 µg/mL showed potent preferential activity. The 12-hydroxyl and the 7-oxo derivatives showed low preferential cytotoxicity at 200 µg/mL (Zaidi *et al.*, 2006). These results suggest that increasing the lipophilicity increases the preferential cytotoxicity. It is a pity that the authors of this study have not evaluated the compounds cytotoxicity towards a non-tumor cell line under the same conditions and did not use an approved clinical drug as positive control. If they had, they would have increased the impact of their work and its contribution to the field.

Dehydroabietic acid and several derivatives were involved in an *in vivo* study of gastroprotective activity on gastric lesions induced by the HCl/EtOH. Dehydroabietic acid and the 18-CH_2OH, 18-CHO and 18-$COOCH_3$ derivatives, at 100 mg/kg, showed slightly greater percentage of lesion reduction (81-85 per cent) compared with the reference drug, lansoprozole at 20 mg/kg (70 per cent) (Sepúlveda *et al.*, 2005). However, these dehydroabietic derivatives are cytotoxic products (IC_{50} of 25-95 µM and 49-297 µM towards AGS cells and fibroblasts, while the reference drug exhibit an IC_{50} of 162 and 306 µM towards AGS cells and fibroblasts, respectively). The exception goes to the 18-CHO derivatives which are less cytotoxic than the reference against AGS cells (Sepúlveda *et al.*, 2005). In the same study, the best gastroprotective activity with lower cytotoxicity was exhibit by the synthetic *N*-(*o*-chlorophenyl)abieta-8,11,13-trien-18-amide (**3**) (87 per cent of lesion reduction) and IC_{50} > 1000 µM towards AGS cells and fibroblasts (Sepúlveda *et al.*, 2005).

Abieta-7,13-diene

The abieta-7,13-diene is the only example of a tricyclic diterpene with a no-oxygenated and non-aromatic abietane skeleton given in this work. It is much less frequent than the above mentioned compounds.

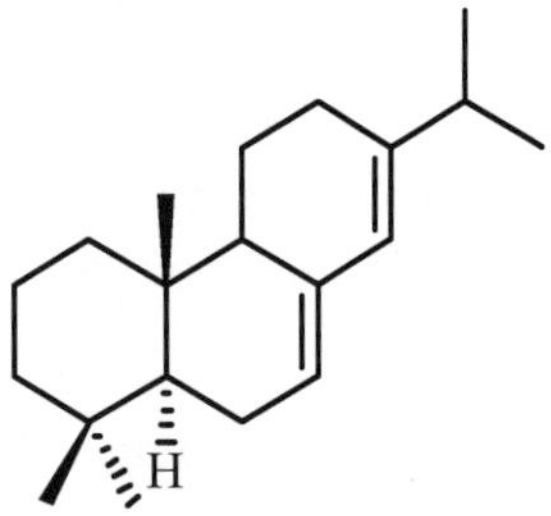

Figure 15.9: Abieta-7,13-diene Structure.

The abieta-7,13-diene was the most active antimalarial agent isolated from berries of *J. procera* against *P. falciparum* D6 and W2 clones (IC_{50} values of 1.9 and 2.0 µg/mL respectively) and it was also selective [selectivity index (SI) of ~2.5. SI values can be therapeutically relevant for designing and synthesizing new drugs since it refers to the ability of a compound to recognize its target without interacting with other targets]. Furthermore, it exhibits no cytotoxicity against Vero cell line at 4.76 µg/mL. However, when compared with reference compound (IC_{50} < 0.264 µg/mL for chloroquine) its activity is much lower (Samoylenko *et al.*, 2008).

Abietic Acid

Abietic acid is an abietan-7,13-diene diterpene with an equatorial carboxylic acid at C-4 instead a methyl group. It is the main component (50 per cent) of the gum rosin (colophonium) obtained from sap of pine trees and frequently used in adhesives and glues (Bugnet *et al.*, 2008).

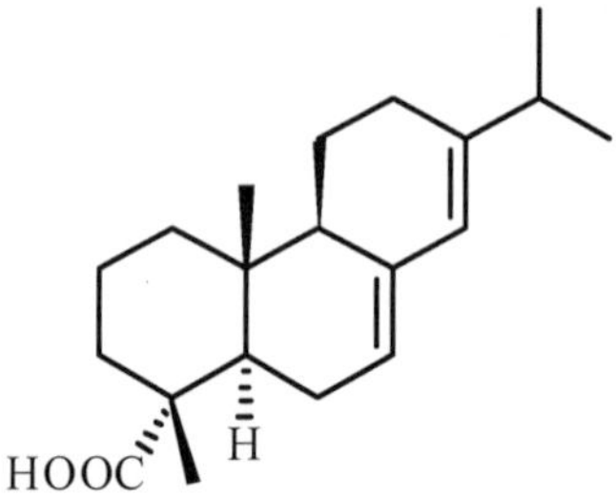

Figure 15.10: Abietic Acid Structure.

Abietic acid exhibit lower antistaphylococcal activity (MIC 64 μg/mL) against the MDR, possessing the TetK, MsrA and *NorA* efflux pumps, EMRSA-15 (resistant to erythromycin) and EMRSA-16 strains (resistant to erythromycin and norfloxacin) than totarol or ferruginol (Smith *et al.*, 2005). However, its activity against the most the strains tested is much higher than the reference antibiotic erythromycin (Smith *et al.*, 2005). Abietic acid was also assayed in combination with the antibiotics tetracycline, norfloxacin and erythromycin to test its modulatory activity, but no reduction in MIC activity was observed (Smith *et al.*, 2005).

The abietic acid and some derivatives did not show antimycotic activity against *Candida parapsilosis*, *C. krusei*, *C. tropicalis*, *C. albicans*, *Aspergillus fumigatus*, *A. flavus*, *A. niger*, and *A. terreus*. The only positive result was obtained when the carboxylic group was substituted by a formyl group, compound known as abietinal, and only against *A. fumigatus* (MIC 50 μg/mL) (González *et al.*, 2009). The same can be said about the antiviral activity of abietic acid and some derivatives (González *et al.*, 2009 and Agudelo-Gómez *et al.*, 2012).

The abietic acid belongs to a big family of natural TNF-α inhibitors (Iqbal *et al.*, 2013), and its anti-inflammatory effect is due to suppressive activity of TNF-α and COX-2 induction at the protein level in LPS stimulated macrophages and its action as activator of PPARγ in RAW264.7 macrophages (Takahashi *et al.*, 2003).

An *in vivo* study on experimental inflammation induced by flogogens of protein and non-protein nature, the moderated anti-inflammatory properties of abietic acid were confirmed being the best result obtained at a dose of 50 mg/kg. At this dose, its activity was about 1.4 times greater than the diclofenac activity at the recommended dose of 8 mg/kg, in the non-protein formalin-induced inflammation model (Kazakova *et al.*, 2013). However, and in opposition to diclofenac, abietic acid did not cause the development of erosive and ulcerative changes in the gastrointestinal tract that is an important advantage. Furthermore, the acute toxicity in mice showed that abietic acid is a low-toxic substance with a LD_{50} of 15200 mg/kg (Kazakova *et al.*, 2013). Studies with tetrahydroabietic acid proved that it also inhibit the production of NO, PGE2 and cytokines (IL-1β, IL-6, TNF-α) in LPS-activated in RAW264.7 macrophages through the same mechanism (Kim *et al.*, 2010).

The abietic acid showed cytotoxicity against HeLa cell lines (IC_{50} 14.9 μg/mL) and a selectivity index of 3.5. The substitution of the C-18 carboxylic group by a formyl or hydroxyl groups originates more active derivatives with identical selectivity index (González *et al.*, 2009). However, when the carboxylic group was methylated, the cytotoxicity and the selectivity increased significantly (IC_{50} 3.6 µg/mL, SI 13.7), but not enough to achieve the values of the reference compound vincristine (IC_{50} 0.05 µg/mL, SI 22) (González *et al.*, 2009).

Anticonvulsant agents are essentials to the treatment of epilepsy, a human brain disorder. Abietic acid, in a *in silico* study (Linear Discriminant Analysis based on 2D descriptors) was identified as a potential new anticonvulsant agent and its activity, by oral and intraperitoneal administration, was confirmed by a Maximal Electroshock Test (active at 30 and 100 mg/kg). These results indicate that it can be a good candidate for structural optimization and development of new anticonvulsant compounds (Talevi *et al.*, 2007).

Abietic acid, when pure is considered as a non-contact allergen while colophonium, the mixture containing abietic acid derivatives, is referred as causing contact dermatitis (Nilsson *et al.*, 2008; Bugnet *et al.*, 2008; Vandebuerie *et al.*, 2014). In fact abietic acid is oxidised to the allergen compound 15-hydroperoxyabietic acid when exposed to air (Karlberg *et al.*, 2007).

Abietic acid exhibit a strong *in vivo* antiulcer effect at a dose of 10 mg/kg in the indomethacin-induced ulceration model with an effect about 1.8 times greater than the effect of carbenoxolone at a dose of 50 mg/kg (Kazakova *et al.*, 2013). In the same test, the synthetic abietic acid derivative (7*R*,8*S*)-epoxy-(13*R*,17*R*)-trioxolane abietic acid (**4**) (Figure 15.19) showed an even higher activity at 10 mg/kg (Kazakova *et al.*, 2013). In the aspirin-induced ulceration the abietic acid causes an effect comparable with that of carbenoxolone at a dose of, respectively, 10 and 50 mg/kg (Kazakova *et al.*, 2013).

Abietic acid show similarity with thiazolidinedione, a drug involved in regulation of lipid metabolism, that causes suppression of TNF-α through PPARγ activation and up regulates the expression of adipocyte fatty acid-binding protein and lipoprotein lipase in 3T3-L1 adipocytes. This effect suggests that abietic acid can be used in control functions of adipocytes and as anti-atherogenic agent (Takahashi *et al.*, 2003).

An *in vivo* study proved that abietic acid has also an anti-obesity effect by the adipogenesis regulation (Hwang *et al.*, 2011). It was shown that the oral administration of abietic acid (40 mg/kg/day) decreased significantly the serum triglyceride, insulin and leptin concentrations, and also the body and adipose tissue weights.

Abietic acid exhibits inhibitory activity against testosterone 5α-redutase (IC_{50} 56±22 µM). A critical analysis of this result indicated that the error associated to the IC_{50} value is unacceptable and that the inhibitory activity of abietic acid is much lower than that of the clinically used drug, finasteride (IC_{50} 0.06 µM) (Roh *et al.*, 2010). These aspects should be considered by the authors especially when they chose the paper title.

4-*epi*-Abietinol

4-*epi*-Abietinol, also known as 4-*epi*-abietol, is a 19-hydroxyl derivative of the abieta-7,13-diene. This compound is a minor constituent of *Juniperus* species but the axial hydroxymethylene group seems to be of great significance in some biological activities.

The levels of SGPT, ALP and bilirubin in rats were significantly reduced upon administration of 4-*epi*-abietinol (62, 46, 63 per cent respectively), being the results comparable to those obtained with silymarin. Therefore the reduction of 32 per cent in SGOT level was weaker than the reduction produced by silymarin (52 per cent) (Alqasoumi and Abdel-Kader, 2012). Thus it seems that 4-*epi*-abietinol can be an effective agent in the liver protection, being its hepatoprotective activity higher than that of sugiol, although its exact mechanism of action is not known.

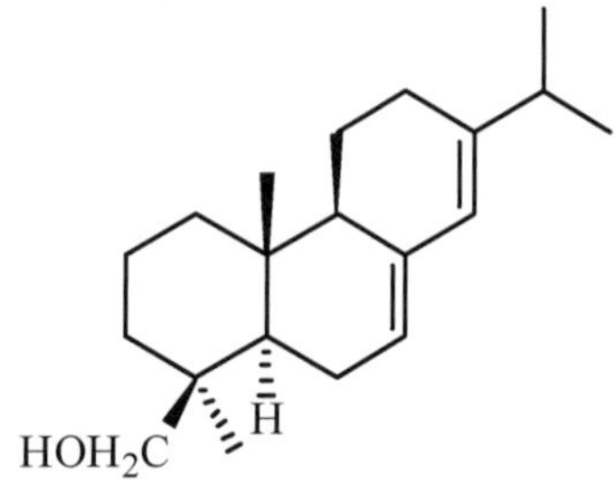

Figure 15.11: 4-*epi*-Abietinol Structure.

Communic Acid

Communic acid is a bicycle diterpene with a labdane skeleton containing an axial carboxyl group at C-4 and three double bonds: $\Delta^{8(17)}$ an exocyclic double bond, Δ^{12} a double bond that can has a *Z* (*cis*-communic acid) or a *E* (*trans*-communic acid) configuration; and a Δ^{14} double bond. It is found in many plants from Cupressaceae family, predominating in the genus *Juniperus* (Barrero *et al.*, 2012), and *trans*-communic acid is the most isomer abundant in nature.

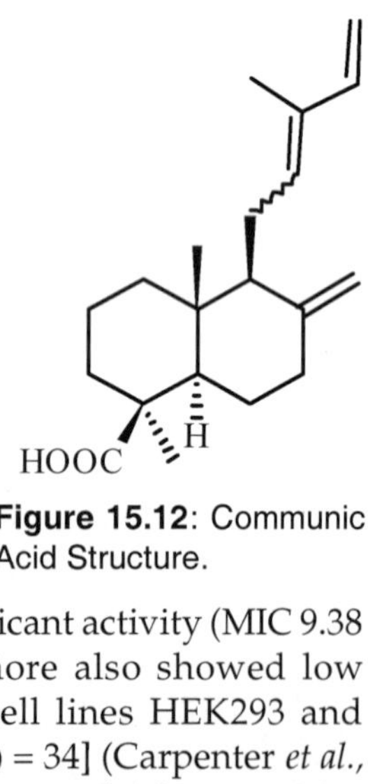

Figure 15.12: Communic Acid Structure.

The *trans*-communic acid was considered inactive (MIC > 100 μg/mL) against virulent type strain *Mycobacterium tuberculosis* H37Rv (Gordien *et al.*, 2009), while an isomeric mixture [*cis*- and *trans*-communic acids (3:2)] showed significant activity (MIC 9.38 μg/mL) against the attenuated strain H37Ra, furthermore also showed low cytotoxicity (IC_{50} 152.6 μg/mL) against noncancerous cell lines HEK293 and favourable therapeutic indexes [IC_{50}(HEK293)/IC_{50}(H37Ra) = 34] (Carpenter *et al.*, 2012). Misfortune is the fact that the authors did not present results for a positive control and consequently conclusions are impossible.

The conjunction of some low selectivity indexes with unfavourable miLog *P* displayed by communic acids as well as other diterpenes, such as totarol and ferruginol (miLog P> 5), do not contribute to their use in antimycobacterial therapeutics. However they may disclose novel modes of action that can be exploited in the development of new antituberculosis drugs. Also they are useful as chirons (contraction of "chiral synthon") for the synthesis of quassinoids, abietane antioxidants, ambrox and other perfume fixatives.

(*Z*)-8α-Hydroxylabda-13(16),14-dien-19-yl coumarate

(Z)-8α-Hydroxylabda-13(16),14-dien-19-yl coumarate, like communic acid (Figure 15.12), presents a bicyclic diterpene structure. However, there are significant differences: the axial C-4 hydroxymethylene group esterified with a *cis*-*p*-coumarate moiety instead of a carboxylic group; the α-hydroxyl group at C-8 instead of an exocyclic double bond; the unsaturated systems at $\Delta^{13(16)}$ and Δ^{14}.

The (Z)-8α-hydroxylabda-13(16),14-dien-19-yl coumarate when applied in log phase, exhibits a significant cytotoxic activity against HeLa tumor cell line (IC_{50} 15.3 μM) with higher selectivity index (IC_{50} > 176 μM against non-tumor Vero cells). Its cytotoxicity decreases significantly, in intensity and selectivity, when applied in lag phase (Moujir *et al.*, 2008).

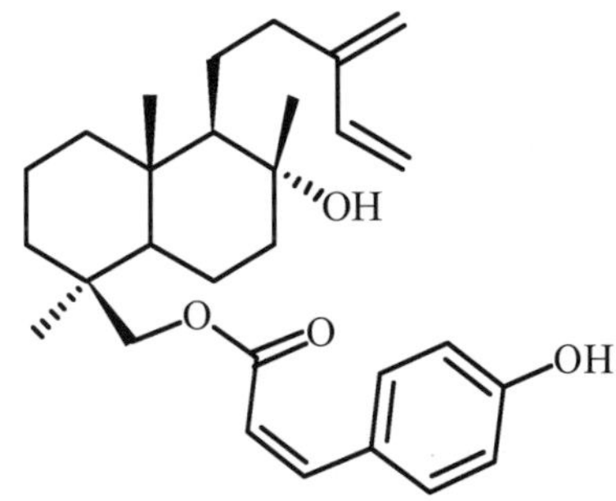

Figure 15.13: (*Z*)-8α-Hydroxylabda-13(16),14-dien-19-yl Coumarate Structure.

Shikimic Acid

Shikimic acid is a six membered highly functionalized carbocyclic ring with three asymmetric centres (3,4,5-trihydroxy-1-cyclohexene-1-carboxylic acid). It is known for its intervention in the biosynthesis of the aromatic amino acids (the shikimic acid pathway) and is particularly abundant in *Illicium anisatum* species (Ghosh *et al.*, 2012). Shikimic acid is a high valued enantiomerically pure building block for the synthesis of biologically important compounds, *e.g.* GS4104 (Tamiflu®) a neuramidase inhibitor used to treat antiviral infections.

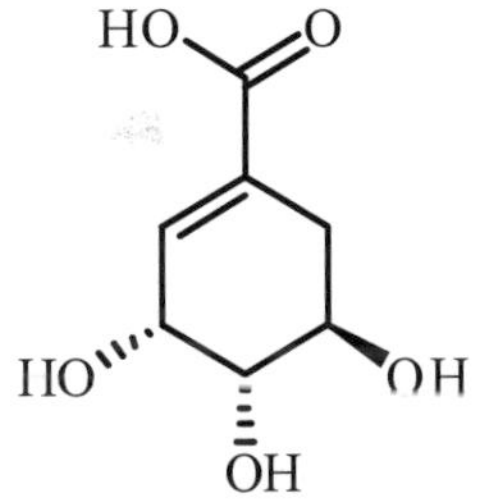

Figure 15.14: Shikimic Acid Structure.

The administration of shikimic acid to diabetic rats, during 8 days, showed that the blood glucose levels (24 per cent), malondialdehyde levels in kidney tissues (63–64 per cent) and liver enzymes (AST, ALT, ALP) were decreased (Orhan *et al.*, 2012a). This is the most recent study showing that shikimic acid might be beneficial for diabetes and its complications.

Umbelliferone

Umbelliferone is the common name of the lactone 7-hydroxycoumarin (also known as 7-hydroxychromen-2-one, hydrangine and skimmetine). Umbelliferone is present in many species of the Apiaceae (Umbelliferae) family and was isolated from the genus *Juniperus* for the first time from *J. communis* in 1980 (Seca and Silva, 2006).

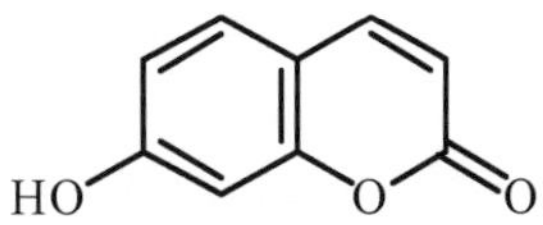

Figure 15.15: Umbelliferone Structure.

Escherichia coli O157 cause a large number of foodborne outbreaks worldwide and for which no effective therapy has been devised because antibiotics and anti-inflammatory drugs increase the risk of developing haemolytic uremic syndrome (Pennington, 2010). On the other hand, *E. coli* is able to form biofilms which are difficult to eradicate because of their inherent tolerance to physical and chemical antimicrobial treatments. In this context, the antibiofilm ability of umbelliferone and other coumarin derivatives against *E. coli* O157:H7 strain were measured and the results showed that the umbelliferone at concentrations up to 50 μg/mL exhibit high antibiofilm activity without inhibiting planktonic cell growth (Lee *et al.*, 2014). The hydroxylation pattern of the coumarin nucleus significantly affects the antibiofilm activity, being umbelliferone the most active (Lee *et al.*, 2014), thus this coumarin has potential to be used in antivirulence strategies against *E. coli* O157:H7 infections.

It seems that coumarin nucleus is important in anti-inflammatory drugs (Bansal *et al.*, 2013). Naturally, umbelliferone and some their synthetic derivatives (Figure 15.19) were subjected to anti-inflammatory evaluations. Umbelliferone showed ability to selectively inhibit COX-2 activity (IC_{50} < 1 μM) (Kaur *et al.*, 2012). Compounds **5** to **7** (Figure 15.19) inhibit considerably the growth of inflamed mouse macrophage RAW 264.7 cells (IC_{50} 50-78 μM); their interaction with human serum albumin were also evaluated (Yeggoni *et al.*, 2014). The results indicated that umbelliferone is a good synthon to develop coumarin-inspired drugs.

Asthma is a chronic inflammatory disorder based on an aberrant immune response to non-pathogenic that causes contraction in the smooth muscle of the airway and blocking of airflow (Gillissen and Paparoupa, 2014). Several umbelliferone derivatives were obtained, by semi-synthesis, and evaluated on the contraction induced by carbachol in the trachea rat rings. The results showed that umbelliferone is the less active (EC_{50} 449 μM) but the activity increases when the 7-hydroxyl group is substituted by an alkoxyl group, such as in 7-propoxyl-derivative (**8**) (Figure 15.19) (EC_{50} 133 μM), with a similar activity level to the positive control used theophylline (Sánchez-Recillas *et al.*, 2014). The authors evaluated other derivatives from which 6,7-diethoxycoumarin (**9**) (EC_{50} 42 μM) and 7-ethoxy-4-methylumbelliferone (**10**) (EC_{50} 80 μM) were the most active ones. Actually, compound (**9**) was 4-times more active than theophylline (Sánchez-Recillas *et al.*, 2014).

In a carrageenan-induced paw oedema *in vivo* assay, umbelliferone showed marked attenuation of induced oedema right from the 1st h of drug administration (10 mg/kg i.p. administration) and remained significant up to 5 h, with a maximum effect of 66.13 per cent (Rauf *et al.*, 2014).

Since 2004 that the umbelliferone cytotoxic activity is well known and its *in vitro* ability to inhibit the proliferation of a number of human malignant cell lines was demonstrated (Madari and Jacobs, 2004).

Kaur *et al.* (2012) showed that umbelliferone (at 20-600 μM) protect DNA against damage induced by H_2O_2 and 4NQO. The authors suggest that its antigenotoxic activity may be due to its radical scavenging activity, although the umbelliferone DPPH scavenging activity is moderate. Rezaee *et al.* (2014) also demonstrated that umbelliferone did not show any genotoxicity against DNA.

The antihyperglycemic effect of umbelliferone was also evaluated in normal and streptozotocin (STZ)-diabetic rats. The Ramesh research group (Ramesh and Pugalendi, 2006a) observed that the administration of umbelliferone at 30 mg/kg dose for 45 days, significantly decrease the blood glucose and glycosylated hemoglobin levels, while increase plasma insulin and liver glycogen levels, an effect that is comparable with reference drug glibenclamide at 0.6 mg/kg. Given that treatment with antioxidant reduces diabetic complications the same research group evaluated the antioxidant power of umbelliferone in STZ-diabetic rats and concluded that its antioxidant activity is similar to glibenclamide (Ramesh and Pugalendi, 2006b). Umbelliferone also minimize the risk of diabetic complications bringing to near normalcy the membrane fatty acid composition and fluidity of liver and kidney cells of the STZ-diabetic rats (Ramesh *et al.*, 2007).

During chronic hyperglycemia, the non-enzymatic glycation process between a reducing sugar and a free amino group of proteins, also known as a Maillard reaction, leads to the formation of AGE. AGE formation and increased protein glycation are strongly implicated in diabetic complications and age-related diseases. More recently, it was demonstrated that umbelliferone exhibit strong inhibitory activity of AGE (IC_{50} 2.95 µM) compared to the reference drug value (IC_{50} 932.66 µM of amino-guanidine) (Jung *et al.*, 2012).

The α-glucosidase and protein tyrosine phosphatase 1B are therapeutic targets for the treatment of diabetes (Fan *et al.*, 2013). Although umbelliferone appears to be an excellent anti-diabetic drug, it does not inhibit α-glucosidase (IC_{50} 633.94 µM; IC_{50} 130.52 µM of acarbose, the positive control used) neither protein tyrosine phosphatase 1B (IC_{50} 274.86 µM; IC_{50} 4.06 µM of ursolic acid, the positive control used) (Islam *et al.*, 2013).

Deoxypodophyllotoxin

Deoxypodophyllotoxin is an aryltetralin cyclolignan being the main lignan constituent of *Anthriscus sylvestris* (L.) Hoffm. and the most potent cytotoxic compound isolated from *Juniperus* species. It was isolated for the first time in 1880 from the North American plant *Podophyllum peltatum* L. (American podophyllum) (Khaled *et al.*, 2013) and is structurally closely related to podophyllotoxin (**11**) (Figure 15.19), the precursor of etoposide (**12**) (Figure 15.19), the most widely prescribed anticancer drug in the world due to its ability to inhibit the enzyme DNA topoisomerase II (Ketron and Osheroff, 2014). In spite of the impressive clinical efficacy of the deoxypodophyllotoxin and podophyllotoxin derivatives, their therapeutic use is often hindered by poor water solubility, acquired drug resistance and metabolic inactivation, but deoxypodophyllotoxin can be a leader for cytotoxic drug synthesis and development (Khaled *et al.*, 2013).

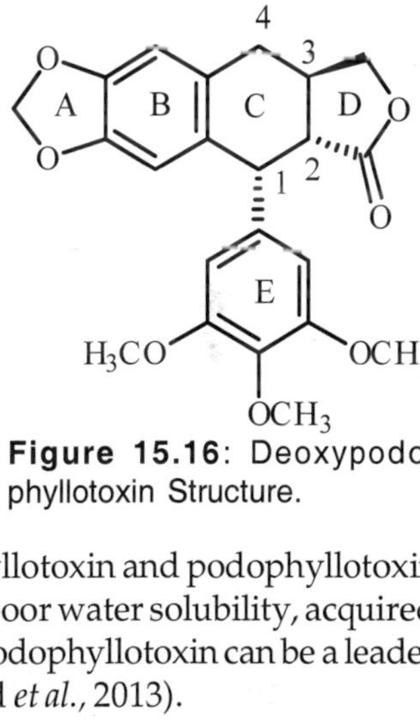

Figure 15.16: Deoxypodophyllotoxin Structure.

Deoxypodophyllotoxin exhibited remarkably potent cytotoxicity toward HL-60 cells by inducing apoptosis even at low concentration (2 ng/mL) (Muto *et al.*, 2008). Wu *et al.* (2013) showed that deoxypodophyllotoxin significantly inhibits the proliferation of H460 cells *in vitro* and the growth of H460 xenografts *in vivo* as well as the drug-resistant cell line H460/Bcl-xL providing a new potential choice for clinical cancer therapy. Jiang *et al.* (2013) demonstrate that deoxypodophyllotoxin, in addition to its potent antimitotic activity, also exerts potent anti-angiogenic and vascular disrupting effects *in vitro, ex vivo* and/or *in vivo*, while Yang *et al.* (2014) showed its potent activity against the ependymoma cell line EphB2-EPD (IC_{50} 1.93 nM). Deoxypodophyllotoxin is not readily available for commercial purposes because it is scarce in nature and requires cumbersome extraction procedures. Thus, several new deoxypodophyllotoxin derivatives were synthetized to found potent antitumor agents as well as compounds with fewer side effects. Huang *et al.* (2012) found that from the several synthetic derivatives tested 4′-*O*-(5-FU-acetic)-L-phenylalanine-4-deoxyl-4′-*O*-demethylpodophyllic ester (**13**) (Figure 15.19) is the most active against HL-60, A549, HeLa and SiHa cell lines with IC_{50} value of 0.023, 0.56, 0.83 and 0.76 μM respectively. These values are lower than the ones obtained for deoxypodophyllotoxin, etoposide and 5-fluorouracil (5-FU).

In 2013 several deoxypodophyllotoxin derivatives were synthetized and proved to be good candidates for cancer therapeutic drugs. 4β-(Benzoylthioureido)-4-deoxypodophyllotoxin (**14**) (Figure 15.19) inhibited the catalytic activity of topoisomerase II at 100 μM, much lower concentration than that required by etoposide (500 μM) (Zhao *et al.*, 2013). It was also cytotoxic against HCT116, A549, KB, and HepG2 cell lines with IC_{50} values from 0.1 to 0.3 μM (ten folder less than etoposide) (Zhao *et al.*, 2013). 4β-[*N*-(4‴-Acetyloxyphenyl-1‴-carbonyl)-4″-aminoanilino]-42-*O*-demethyl-4-desoxypodophyllotoxin (**15**) (Figure 15.19), displayed a wide range of cytotoxicity against human tumor cell lines (SGC-7901, KB, PC-3, A2780, A549, HCT116 and HepG2) with IC_{50} values ranging from 0.82 to 4.88 μM, much less than the IC_{50} values of etoposide (4.18–39.43 μM) (Yang *et al.*, 2013). Finally, 4β-*N*-(4-nitrophenylpiperazinyl)-4′-*O*-demethyl-4-deoxypodophyllotoxin (**16**) (Figure 15.19) was found to be more active than etoposide against HepG2 and HCT-8 cell lines, being particularly active against HeLa and A549 (IC_{50} value of 0.07 and 0.16 μM respectively, 67 and 93 fold lower than the etoposide IC_{50}) (Liu *et al.*, 2013). Unfortunately none of the derivatives mentioned was tested against non-tumor cell lines consequently their selectivity was not evaluated.

Whilst the anticancer and antiviral properties of the deoxypodophyllotoxin are well known, it exhibit lower antimycobacterial activity and presenting lower therapeutic index against the H37Ra strain of *Mycobacterium tuberculosis* than for example communic acid (Carpenter *et al.*, 2012). Although this activity level has lower clinical interest, this is the first report of antimycobacterial activity for deoxypodophyllotoxin.

Amentoflavone

Amentoflavone is a flavonoid dimer composed by two apigenin units linked by a C-C bond at 8 and 3' positions, belongs to the biflavonoid family of compounds which are mainly distributed in the Gymnosperms and Angiosperms and that have shown a variety of biological properties, including anticancer, antimicrobial activities.

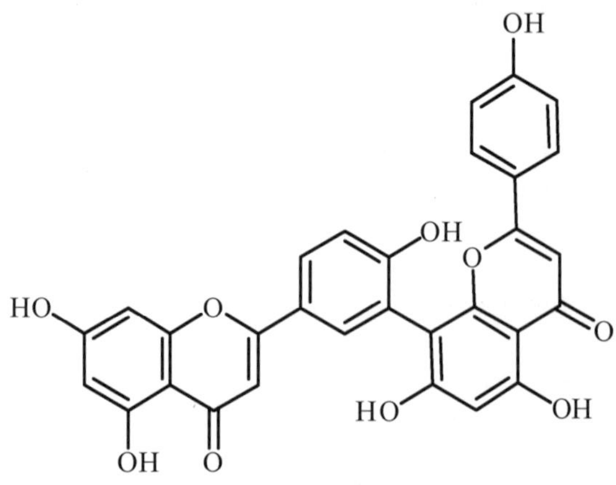

Figure 15.17: Amentoflavone Structure.

Amentoflavone showed potent antifungal activity (MIC 5 µg/mL), against *Saccharomyces cerevisiae* and *Candida albicans* which was near to the level of the reference amphotericin B (MIC 2.5 µg/mL) (Jung *et al.*, 2006). Later the same research group showed that the entry of amentoflavone into the *Candida albicans* cells is not mediated by cellular function, which requires cellular energy consumption such as ATP-dependent transporter, thus its mode of action is energy-independent (Jung *et al.*, 2007). More recently, it was demonstrated that amentoflavone causes apoptotic morphological changes in *Candida albicans* cells and the apoptotic death is associated with the mitochondrial dysfunction (Hwang *et al.*, 2012).

Amentoflavone showed to be more active than ferruginol (Figure 15.4) towards the inhibition of SARS-CoV 3CLpro (IC_{50} 8.3 µM) with a non-competitive inhibition type (K_i 13.8 µM). It is also more effective than the corresponding monomer flavone apigenin (IC_{50} 280.8 µM) (Ryu *et al.*, 2010), although less active than the peptide-derived 3CLpro inhibitors, one of the more effective 3CLpro inhibitors classes of the compounds (Thanigaimalai *et al.*, 2013). Amentoflavone also showed ability to inhibit the virus Coxsackievirus B3 (CVB3), a human pathogen that causes acute and chronic infections like myocarditis, dilated cardiomyopathy, aseptic meningitis and pancreatitis (Wilsky *et al.*, 2012).

The development of rat paw oedema carrageenan-induced can controlled through a pre-treatment with amentoflavone, being its inhibitory effect identical to that of nimesulide, although amentoflavone peak inhibitory effect was achieved with 100 mg/kg while for nimesulide was 50 mg/kg. Amentoflavone, at the concentration used in peak inhibitory effect, showed strong inhibition of TNF-α and also inhibits both COX and 5-LOX pathways of the arachidonate metabolism (Ishola *et al.*, 2013). In the same year, Oh *et al.* (2013), showed that amentoflavone, at 200 µg/mL, in LPS-induced RAW264.7 cell, clearly suppresses the production of NO and PGE2 and in particular strongly inhibited nuclear translocation of c-Fos through the inhibition of its upstream signalling enzyme ERK, a modulator of various inflammatory diseases. Another evidence of the amentoflavone inhibition of the inflammatory mediators iNOS and COX-2 production of the pro-inflammatory cytokines, such as TNF-α, IL-1β and IL-6, and of the NF-κB signal transduction pathway is the result of Sakthivel and Guruvayoorappan (2013) study. These authors showed that a pre-treatment with amentoflavone (10 mg/kg b.wt) exhibits protective effect, in *in vivo*, against acetic acid induced ulcerative colitis (inflammatory disorder affecting the colon and rectum). Furthermore the results are not significantly different from those obtained with sulfasalazine at 100 mg/kg.

From some natural bioflavonoids, amentoflavone showed to be the best cytotoxic compound against A549, HL-60 and CNE2 (IC_{50} 32-86 µM), being more active against K562 and PC-9 with IC_{50} value of 5.25 and 6.41 µg/mL respectively (9.7 and 11.9 µM) (Li *et al.*, 2014). The authors referred that the chemotherapeutic anti-cancer drug adriamycin hydrochloride (the trade name of doxorubicin) was used as the positive control, however its IC_{50} value is not displayed, so it is not possible to make a proper assessment of the cytotoxicity amentoflavone impact. It is interesting to verify that amentoflavone, in the antiproliferative assay against a large number of cancer cell lines (HL-60, U937, THP-1, Jurkat, KATO III, HCT-15 and HepG2) and also against human normal skin fibroblast cell lines, seems to be much less active once it exhibits a $IC_{50} > 50$ µM for all (Tung *et al.*, 2013). Several inhibitors of FAS have been used to study the loss of FAS function in tumor cells, especially in breast cancer. Among them, amentoflavone showed to be a potent inhibitor of FAS, 54.4 per cent of inhibition at 50 µM in FAS-overexpressed SK-BR-3 breast cancer cells, while, at same dose, cerulenin decreased FAS activity by 57.0 per cent (Lee *et al.*, 2009). Amentoflavone is able to activate apoptosis in FAS-expressed SK-BR-3 cells by stimulation of caspase-3 and is able to inhibit the SK-BR-3 and LNCaP cancer cells proliferation (at 75 µM the cell viability was 33 per cent) without affect the cell proliferation in FAS-non-expressed NIH-3T3 normal cells (90 per cent of cell viability at 75 µM) (Lee *et al.*, 2009). Later the same research group demonstrated that amentoflavone can suppress FAS expression at the protein and mRNA levels. It can also suppress HER2 activation and modulate Akt, mTOR, and JNK phosphorylation in SKBR3 cells (Lee *et al.*, 2013).

Amentoflavone gave positive results on the *in vitro* Ames test, but showed no mutagenicity in the *in vivo* test (mouse micronucleus test) (Cardoso *et al.*, 2006). These apparently contradictory results could be explained by the *in vivo* amentoflavone metabolism, generating metabolites that are no longer reactive with DNA. Thus, mutagenicity data obtained *in vitro* and *in vivo* in animal studies do not necessarily prove mutagenic risks to humans.

Amentoflavone produce, *in vivo* and at 50 mg/kg, significant mild central and peripheral analgesic effect and this effect could be the result of its ability to interfere with the synthesis or release of the endogenous substances or desensitization of the nerve fibres involved in the pain transmission pathway (Ishola *et al.*, 2013). Although this amentoflavone effect is lower than the effect of morphine at lower concentration (10 mg/kg), the addictive effects of morphine have to be taken into consideration.

The radical scavenging capacity of amentoflavone was assayed using DPPH (IC_{50} 0.92 µM) and ABTS (IC_{50} 30.8 µM) assays and its scavenging capacity is similar to the α-tocopherol capacity (IC_{50} 0.3 and 32.1 µM respectively) (Qiao *et al.*, 2014). This DPPH assay result is not in agreement with previously published results (Silva *et al.*, 2008) that described amentoflavone as a poor radical scavenger ($IC_{50} > 75$ µM; IC_{50} 20.8 µM to trolox). Unfortunately these contradictory results are not as rare as we would like and could be eliminated if more than one positive reference compound was used by the authors in these biological studies.

The ferrous metal ion chelating activity of amentoflavone (IC_{50} 20.1 µM) is much lower than α-tocopherol (IC_{50} 2.4 µM) (Qiao *et al.*, 2014). On the other hand, amentoflavone exhibited significant cardioprotective effect at 15 µM by inhibiting the H_2O_2-induced intracellular level of ROS in H9c2 cell (Qiao *et al.*, 2014).

The reduced contents of GSH induced by glutamate were recovered, the activities of antioxidant enzymes (SOD, GR) in response to high concentration of glutamate were preserved, the increased production of ROS was clearly attenuated and the phosphorylation of ERK1/2 induced by glutamate insult was clearly prevented by pre-treatment with amentoflavone at 50 µM. Thus amentoflavone scavenges ROS and exerts protective effect against oxidative damage induced by glutamate via maintaining the activities of antioxidant enzymes and/or inhibiting ERK1/2 activation (Jeong *et al.*, 2014).

Hinokiflavone

Hinokiflavone is also a biflavonoid like amentoflavone but the two apigenin units are coupled with a 6-*O*-3' bond. It is less abundant in the genus *Juniperus* but also exhibit interesting biological activities.

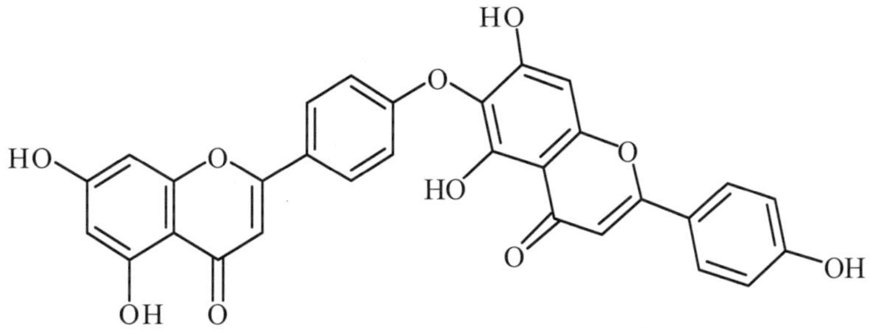

Figure 15.18: Hinokiflavone Structure.

The ADAMTS-5 inhibitors can stop the expression of ADAMTS-5, an important aggrecanase that cleaves the proteoglycan aggrecan in cartilage thereby acting as potential therapeutic drugs for inflammatory arthritis. An *in silico* study (ligand based pharmacophore model, dynamic simulations, 3D-QSAR, docking analysis, virtual screening with natural compounds) showed that the hinokiflavone is an excellent potential ADAMTS-5 inhibitor, with a glide score of -8.47 kcal/mol (Suganya *et al.*, 2011). Naturally, *in vitro* and *in vivo* studies are essential to prove its potential as an osteoarthritis drug.

An attractive target anticancer therapy is MMP-9 due to its vital role in the metastatic process. From a very recent *in silico* study (Kalva *et al.*, 2014), the hinokiflavone showed to have a good glidescore, binding free energy of –26.54 kJ/mol and with a stable interaction with S1 loop of MMP-9 compared with the known inhibitors of MMP-9. *In vitro* assay showed that the concentration value to inhibit the MMP-9 activity in 50 per cent was 43.08 μM, while its cytotoxic effect on the proliferation of MCF-7 cell lines was IC_{50} 1.857 mM (Kalva *et al.*, 2014). Thus hinokiflavone is able to inhibit MMP-9 *in vitro*, suggesting that it might possess antimetastatic potential.

Hinokiflavone treatment (started 5 days prior to CCl_4 administration and continued till the end of the experiment) showed a hepatoprotective effect, reducing elevated levels of SGOT, SGPT, ALP and bilirubin, closely comparable to silymarin, a reference drug, at the same dose (20.7 mmol/kg). Histopathological appearance of liver cells of rats treated with CCl_4 and hinokiflavone showed good recovery with absence of necrosis and fatty depositions (Alqasoumi *et al.*, 2013).

Conclusion

This short review present the most recent biological activities reported for the most abundant secondary metabolites of the genus *Juniperus*, mainly the abietatriene derivatives (totarol, ferruginol, and sugiol) but also of some minor metabolites that are reported in the literature as having high pharmacological potential (amentoflavone

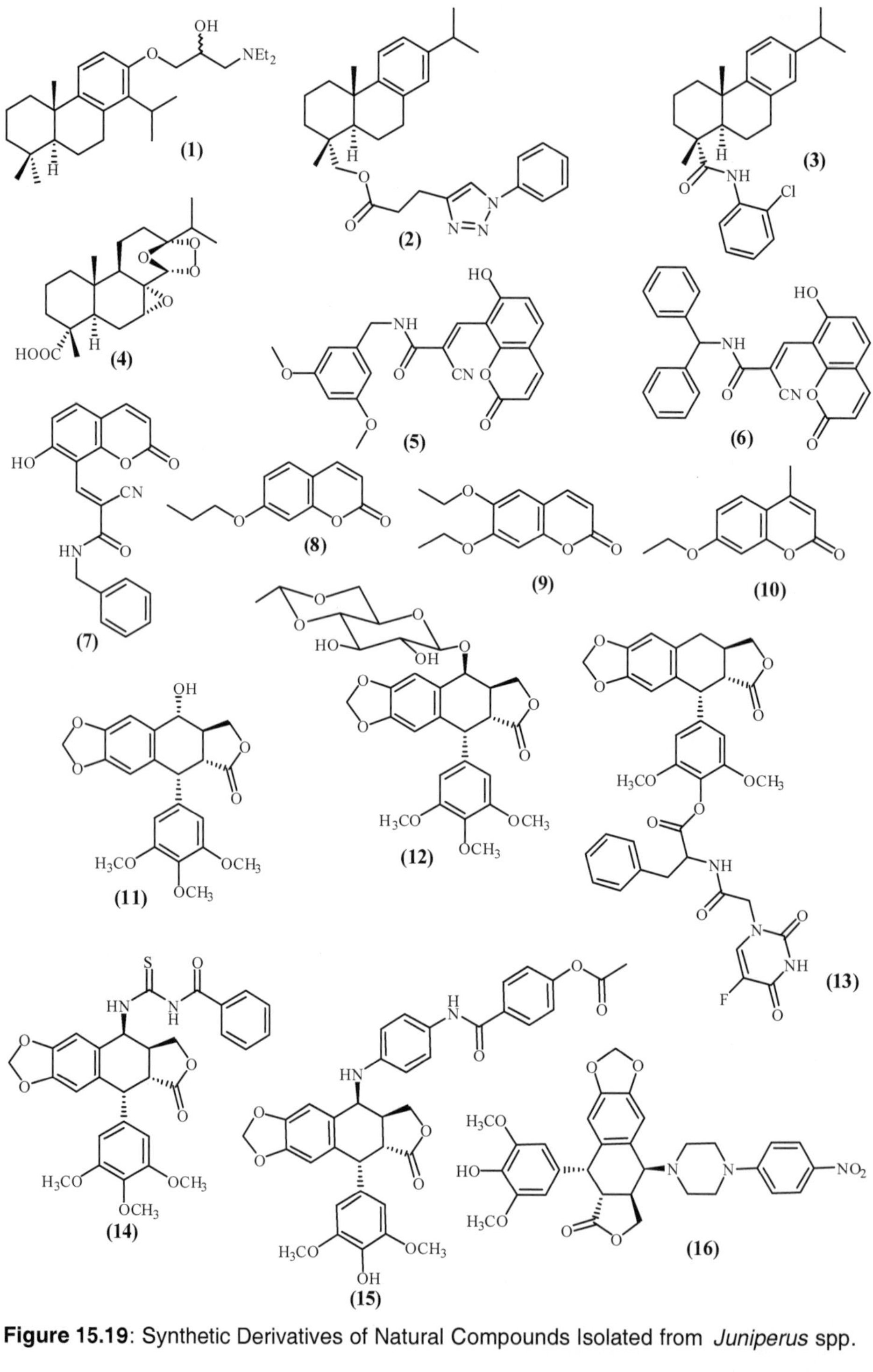

Figure 15.19: Synthetic Derivatives of Natural Compounds Isolated from *Juniperus* spp.

and deoxypodophyllotoxin). It is important to highlight that not always the most abundant metabolite is the most active compound or the responsible for the medicinal potential of the plant. This inference can be taken analysing the cases of sugiol and deoxypodophyllotoxin.

We tried to describe the most promising and/or valuable results but it is clearly that several data published are not undoubted. There is an urgent call for the scientific community, headlines common in newspapers or magazines are not suitable for scientific papers. For instance results where a positive control was not used cannot be considered valid, as well as cytotoxic results without selectivity evaluations. This review evidently shows that more studies on the bioactivities of the secondary metabolites from the genus *Juniperus* are needed.

Abbreviations

A2780: Human ovarian cancer cells
A549: Human non-small-cell lung tumor
ABTS: 2,2′-Azinobis(3-ethylbenzothiazoline-6-sulfonic acid)
ADAMTS-5: A disintegrin and metalloproteinase with thrombospondin motifs
AGE: Advanced glycation end products
AGS: Human gastric carcinoma cell line
Akt: Protein kinase B
ALP: Alkaline phosphatase
ALT: Alanine transaminase
ATCC: American Type Culture Collection
ATP: Adenosine triphosphate
AST: Aspartate aminotransferase
BHT: Butylated hydroxytoluene
b.wt: Body weight
c-Fos: Proto-oncogene
CHO: Chinese hamster ovary cell line
CNE2: Human nasopharyngeal carcinoma line
COX: Cicloxigenase
CVB3: Coxsackievirus B3
3D-QSAR: Quantitative structure–activity relationship 3D
DPPH: 1,1-Diphenyl-2-picrylhydrazyl radical
DNA: Deoxyribonucleic acid
EMRSA-15: Epidemic methicillin-resistant *Staphylococcus aureus* strain
EMRSA-16: Epidemic methicillin-resistant *Staphylococcus aureus* strain
EphB2-EPD: Ependymoma cell line
EPI: Efflux pump inhibitor

ERK: Extracellular signal-regulated kinase
ERK1/2: Extracellular signal-regulated kinase 1 and 2
EtBr: Ethidium bromide
FAS: Fatty acid synthase
5-FU: 5-Fluorouracil
GR: Glutathione reductase
GSH: Reduced state of glutathione
H37Ra: Avirulent *Mycobacterium tuberculosis* strain
H9c2: Rat heart-derived embryonic myocytes cell line
H460: Human non-small cell lung carcinoma
H460/Bcl-xL: Human non-small cell lung carcinoma drug-resistant
HCT116: Colon carcinoma cell line
HCT-15: Human colon adenocarcinoma colorectal
HeLa: Human cervix cancer cell line
HIV: Human immunodeficiency virus infection
HCV: Hepatitis C virus
HEK293: Noncancerous human embryonic kidney cell line
HepG2: Human hepatocellular carcinoma
HER2: Human epidermal growth factor receptor 2
5-HETE: 5-Hydroxyeicosatetraenoic acid
HL-60: Human acute promyelocytic leukaemia cell line
HHV-1: Herpes simplex virus type 1
HHV-2: Herpes simplex virus type 2
IC_{50}: The concentration causing 50 per cent inhibition of cell viability of the control culture
IL-1β: Interleukin-1β also known as catabolin
IL-6: Interleukin-6
INH: Isoniazid
iNOS: Inducible nitric oxide synthase
J82: Malignant human urothelial cell line
JNK: c-Jun N-terminal Kinases
Jurkat: Acute T cell leukemia
K562: Human erythroleukemia cell line
KATO III: Stomach cancer cell line
KB: Oral squamous carcinoma cells
LD_{50}: Amount of the substance required to kill 50 per cent of the test population
LNCaP: Androgen-sensitive human prostate adenocarcinoma cell line

5-LOX: 5-Lipoxygenase
LPS: Lipopolysaccharide
LTB4: Leukotriene B4
MCF-7: Breast cancer cell line
MIC: Minimum inhibitory concentration
MMP-9: Matrix metalloproteinase-9
MRC-5: Human fetal lung fibroblast cells
mRNA: Messenger RNA
mTOR: Mammalian target of rapamycin
NF-κB: Nuclear factor κB
PANC-1: Human pancreatic carcinoma, epithelial-like cell line
PC-3: Human prostate cancer cells
PC-9: Human lung-cancer cell line resistant to gefitinib.
PGE2: Prostaglandin E2
PPARγ: Peroxisome proliferator-activated receptor-γ
RAW264.7: Murine monocyte/macrophage line derived from ascitic tumor induced with Abelson leukaemia virus
RNS: Reactive nitrogen species
ROS: Reactive oxygen species
SAR: Structure-activity relationship
SARS-CoV: Human coronavirus that causes SARS (severe acute respiratory syndrome)
SiHA: Human cervix uteri cancer cell line
SGC-7901: Human gastric carcinoma
SGPT: Serum glutamic pyruvic transaminase
SGOT: Serum glutamic oxaloacetic transaminase
SKBR3: Human breast adenocarcinoma cell line
SK-MES-1: Human Caucasian lung squamous carcinoma
SOD: Super oxide dismutase
3T3-L1: Mouse 3T3 preadipocytes cells not contact inhibited
THP-1: Promyelocytic leukemia cell line
TNF-α: Tumor necrosis factor-α
U937: Promonocytic leukemia
VZV: Varicella zoster virus

Acknowledgements

We would like to thank Fundação para a Ciência e a Tecnologia (FCT, Portugal), the European Union, QREN, FEDER, COMPETE, for funding the Organic Chemistry

Research Unit (QOPNA) (project PEst-C/QUI/UI0062/2013; FCOMP-01-0124-FEDER-037296) and University of Aveiro and University of Azores.

References

Aboul-Ela, M., El-Shaer, N., and El-Azim, T.A. (2005). Chemical constituents and hepatotoxic effect of the berries of *Juniperus phoenicea*, Part II. *Natural Product Sciences*, **11**: 240-247.

Achour, S., Abourazzak, S., Mokhtari, A., Soulaymani, A., Soulaymani, R., and Hida, M. (2011). Juniper tar (cade oil) poisoning in new born after a cutaneous application. *BMJ Case Reports*, doi: 10.1136/bcr.07.2011.4427

Adams, R.P. (2014). Junipers of the World: the genus *Juniperus*. 4th Edition, Trafford Publishing, USA.

Adams, R.P., Hsieh, C.-F., Murata, J., and Pandey, R.N. (2002). Systematics of *Juniperus* from eastern Asia based on random amplified polymorphic DNAs (RAPDs). *Biochemical Systematics and Ecology*, **30**: 231-241.

Aggarwal, S., Verma, A., Shukla, R., Batra, S., Bhardwaj, T.R., and Kumar, M. (2014). An overview of phytotherapeutic approaches for the treatment of benign prostatic hyperplasia. *Mini-Review in Medicinal Chemistry*, **14**: 257-270.

Agudelo-Gómez, L.S., Betancur-Galvis, L.A., and González, M.A. (2012). Anti HHV-1 and HHV-2 activity *in vitro* of abietic and dehydroabietic acid derivatives. *Pharmacologyonline*, **1**: 36-42.

Ali, S.A., Rizk, M.Z., Ibrahim, N.A., Abdallah, M.S., Sharara, H.M., and Moustafa, M.M. (2010). Protective role of *Juniperus phoenicea* and *Cupressus sempervirens* against CCl_4. *World Journal of Gastrointestinal Pharmacology and Therapeutics*, **1**: 123-131.

Alqasoumi, S.I., and Abdel-Kader, M.S. (2012). Terpenoids from *Juniperus procera* with hepatoprotective activity. *Pakistan Journal of Pharmaceutical Sciences*, **25**: 315-322.

Alqasoumi, S.I., Farraj, A.I., Abdel-Kader, M.S. (2013). Study of the hepatoprotective effect of *Juniperus phoenicea* constituents. *Pakistan Journal of Pharmaceutical Sciences*, **26**: 999-1008.

Anjos, O., Nunes, D., and Caldeira, I. (2013). First evaluation of a traditional Portuguese alcoholic beverage, prepared with maceration of juniper berries. *Ciência e Técnica Vitivinícola*, **28**: 59-69.

Atkins, B.L., and Gottlieb, T. (2014). Skin and soft tissue infections caused by nontuberculous mycobacteria. *Current Opinion in Infectious Diseases*, **27**: 137-145.

Awale, S., Lu, J., Kalauni, S.K., Kurashima, Y., Tezuka, Y., Kadota, S., and Esumi, H. (2006). Identification of arctigenin as an antitumor agent having the ability to eliminate the tolerance of cancer cells to nutrient starvation. *Cancer Research*, **66**: 1751-1757.

Bailly, C. (2014). Cell-targeted cytotoxics: A new generation of cytotoxic agents for cancer treatment. *Phytochemistry Reviews*, **13**: 171-181.

Bajpai, V.K., Sharma, A., Kang, S.C., and Baek, K.-H. (2014). Antioxidant, lipid peroxidation inhibition and free radical scavenging efficacy of a diterpenoid compound sugiol isolated from *Metasequoia glyptostroboides*. *Asian Pacific Journal of Tropical Medicine*, **7**: 9-15

Bansal, Y., Sethi, P., and Bansal, G. (2013). Coumarin: a potential nucleus for anti-inflammatory molecules. *Medicinal Chemistry Research*, **22**: 3049-3060.

Barrero, A.F., Quílez Del Moral, J.F., Herrador, M.M., Akssira, M., Bennamara, A., Akkad, S., and Aitigri, M. (2004). Oxygenated diterpenes and other constituents from Moroccan *Juniperus phoenicea* and *Juniperus thurifera* var. *africana*. *Phytochemistry*, **65**: 2507-2515.

Barrero, A.F., Herrador, M.M., Arteaga, P., Arteaga, J.F., and Arteaga, A.F. (2012). Communic acids: Occurrence, properties and use as chirons for the synthesis of bioactive compounds. *Molecules*, **17**: 1448-1467.

Benzina, S., Harquail, J., Jean, S., Beauregard, A.P., Colquhoun, C.D., Carroll, M., Bos, A., Gray, C.A., Robichaud, G.A. (2014). Deoxypodophyllotoxin isolated from *Juniperus communis* induces apoptosis in breast cancer cells. *Anti-Cancer Agents in Medicinal Chemistry*, in press DOI: 10.2174/1871520614666140608150448

Brieger, K., Schiavone, S., Miller Jr., F.J., and Krause, K.-H. (2012). Reactive oxygen species: From health to disease. *Swiss Medical Weekly*, doi: 10.4414/smw.2012.13659.

Buglass, A.J., McKay, M., and Lee, C.G. (2010). Distilled spirits. In: Handbook of Alcoholic Beverages: Technical, Analytical and Nutritional Aspects. Buglass, A.J. (Ed.), Vol. 1. John and Wiley, Pg. 535.

Bugnet, L.D., Sanchez-Politta, S., Sorg, O., and Piletta, P. (2008). Allergic contact dermatitis to colophonium contaminated socks. *Contact Dermatitis*, **59**: 127-128.

Cardoso, C.R.P., Cólus, I.M.D.S., Bernardi, C.C., Sannomiya, M., Vilegas, W., and Varanda, E.A. (2006). Mutagenic activity promoted by amentoflavone and methanolic extract of *Byrsonima crassa* Niedenzu. *Toxicology*, **225**: 55-63.

Carpenter, C.D., O'Neill, T., Picot, N., Johnson, J.A., Robichaud, G.A., Webster, D., and Gray, C.A. (2012). Anti-mycobacterial natural products from the Canadian medicinal plant *Juniperus communis*. *Journal of Ethnopharmacology*, **143**: 695-700.

Chang, C.-I., Chen, W.-C., Shao, Y.-Y., Yeh, G.-R., Yang, N.-S., Chiang, W., and Kuo, Y.-H. (2008). A new labdane-type diterpene from the bark of *Juniperus chinensis* Linn. *Natural Product Research*, **22**: 1158-1162.

Chen, Y.-C., Li, Y.-C., You, B.-J., Chang, W.-T., Chao, L.K., Lo, L.-C., Wang, S.-Y., Huang, G.-J., and Kuo, Y.-H. (2013). Diterpenoids with anti-inflammatory activity from the wood of *Cunninghamia konishii*. *Molecules*, **18**: 682-689.

Chow, Y.-L., and Erdtman, H. (1962). The chemistry of the natural order Cupressales. 43. The structure and configuration of hinokiol and hinokione. *Acta Chemica Scandinavica*, **16**: 1296-1300.

Ciesla, W.M. (1998). Non-wood forest products from conifers. Food and Agriculture Organization of the United Nations. Rome, ISBN 92-5-104212-8. pp. 13.

Clarkson, C., Musonda, C.C., Chibale, K., Campbell, W.E., and Smith, P. (2003). Synthesis of totarol amino alcohol derivatives and their antiplasmodial activity and cytotoxicity. *Bioorganic and Medicinal Chemistry*, **11**: 4417-4422.

Cragg, G.M., and Newman, D.J. (2013). Natural products: A continuing source of novel drug leads. *Biochimica et Biophysica Acta -General Subjects*, **1830**: 3670-3695.

Elias, R.B., and Dias, E. (2009). Gap dynamics and regeneration strategies in *Juniperus-Laurus* forests of the Azores Islands. *Plant Ecology*, **200**: 179-189.

Enomoto, H., Yoshikuni, Y., Yasutomi, Y., Ohata, K., and Sempuku, K. (1977). Hypocholesterolemic action of tricyclic diterpenoids in rats. *Chemical and Pharmaceutical Bulletin*, **25**: 507-510

European Pharmacopoeia. (2008). European directorate for the quality of medicines and health care (6th ed., Vol. 3, p. 2206). Strasburg: Council of Europe.

Falasca, A., Melck, D., Paris, D., Saviano, G., Motta, A., and Iorizzi, M. (2014). Seasonal changes in the metabolic fingerprint of *Juniperus communis* L. berry extracts by ^{1}H NMR-based metabolomics. *Metabolomics*, **10**: 165-174.

Fan, S.-Y., Zeng, H.-W., Pei, Y.-H., Li, L., Ye, J., Pan, Y.-X., Zhang, J.-G., Yuan, X., and Zhang, W.-D. (2012). The anti-inflammatory activities of an extract and compounds isolated from *Platycladus orientalis* (Linnaeus) Franco *in vitro* and *ex vivo*. *Journal of Ethnopharmacology*, **141**: 647-652.

Fan, W., Liu, Q., and Tian, H.-Q. (2013). New progress in the research and development of anti-diabetic drugs. *Chinese Journal of New Drugs*, **22**: 2503-2509.

Fedeli, U., Avossa, F., Guzzinati, S., Bovo, E., and Saugo, M. (2014). Trends in mortality from chronic liver disease. *Annals of Epidemiology*, http: //dx.doi.org/10.1016/ j.annepidem.2014.05.004

Foss, M.H., Eun, Y.-J., Grove, C.I. Pauw, D.A., Sorto, N.A., Rensvold, J.W., Pagliarini, D.J., Shaw, J.T., and Weibel, D.B. (2013). Inhibitors of bacterial tubulin target bacterial membranes *in vivo*. *Medicinal Chemistry Communications*, **4**: 112-119.

Gaspar-Marques, C. Simões, M.F., Valdeira, M.L., and Rodríguez, B. (2008). Terpenoids and phenolics from *Plectranthus strigosus*. *Natural Product Research*, **22**: 167-177.

Ghosh, S., Chisti, Y., and Banerjee, U.C. (2012). Production of shikimic acid. *Biotechnology Advances*, **30**: 1425-1431.

Gillissen, A., and Paparoupa, M. (2014). Inflammation and infections in asthma. *Clinical Respiratory Journal*. in press DOI: 10.1111/crj.12135.

González, M.A., Correa-Royero, J., Agudelo, L., Mesa, A., and Betancur-Galvis, L. (2009). Synthesis and biological evaluation of abietic acid derivatives. *European Journal of Medicinal Chemistry*, **44**: 2468-2472.

Gordien, A.Y., Gray, A.I., Franzblau, S.G., and Seidel, V. (2009). Antimycobacterial terpenoids from *Juniperus communis* L. (Cuppressaceae) *Journal of*

Ethnopharmacology, **126**: 500–505

Guerrero, E., Abad, A., Montenegro, G., Del Olmo, E., López-Pérez, J.L., and San Feliciano, A. (2013). Analgesic and anti-inflammatory activity of podophyllotoxin derivatives. *Pharmaceutical Biology*, **51**: 566-572.

Huang, W.-T., Liu, J., Liu, J.-F., Hui, L., Ding, Y.-L., and Chen, S.-W. (2012). Synthesis and biological evaluation of conjugates of deoxypodophyllotoxin and 5-FU as inducer of caspase-3 and -7. *European Journal of Medicinal Chemistry*, **49**: 48-54

Hwang, K.-H., Ahn, J.-Y., Kim, S., Park, J.-H., and Ha, T.-Y. (2011). Abietic acid has an anti-obesity effect in mice fed a high-fat diet. *Journal of Medicinal Food*, **14**: 1052-1056.

Hwang, I., Lee, J., Jin, H.-G., Woo, E.-R., and Lee, D.G. (2012). Amentoflavone stimulates mitochondrial dysfunction and induces apoptotic cell death in *Candida albicans*. *Mycopathologia*, **173**: 207-218.

Innocenti, M., Michelozzi, M., Giaccherini, C., Ieri, F., Vincieri, F.F., and Mulinacci, N. (2007). Flavonoids and biflavonoids in Tuscan berries of *Juniperus communis* L.: Detection and quantitation by HPLC/DAD/ESI/MS. *Journal of Agricultural and Food Chemistry*, **55**: 6596-6602.

Iqbal, M., Verpoorte, R., Korthout, H.A.A.J., and Mustafa, N.R. (2013). Phytochemicals as a potential source for TNF-α inhibitors. *Phytochemistry Review*, **12**: 65-93.

Ishola, I.O., Chaturvedi, J.P., Rai, S., Rajasekar, N., Adeyemi, O.O., Shukla, R., and Narender, T. (2013). Evaluation of amentoflavone isolated from *Cnestis ferruginea* Vahl ex DC (Connaraceae) on production of inflammatory mediators in LPS stimulated rat astrocytoma cell line (C6) and THP-1 cells. *Journal of Ethnopharmacology*,**146**: 440-448.

Islam, M.N., Jung, H.A., Sohn, H.S., Kim, H.M., and Choi, J.S. (2013). Potent α-glucosidase and protein tyrosine phosphatase 1B inhibitors from *Artemisia capillaris*. *Archives of Pharmacal Research*, **36**: 542-552.

Jaiswal, R., Beuria, T.K., Mohan, R., Mahajan, S.K., and Panda, D. (2007). Totarol inhibits bacterial cytokinesis by perturbing the assembly dynamics of FtsZ. *Biochemistry*, **46**: 4211-4220.

Jazayeri S.B., Amanlou A., Ghanadian N., Pasalar P., and Amanlou M. (2014). A preliminary investigation of anticholinesterase activity of some Iranian medicinal plants commonly used in traditional medicine. *Journal of Pharmaceutical Sciences*, **22**: e17.

Jeong, E.J., Seo, H., Yang, H., Kim, J., Sung, S.H., and Kim, Y.C. (2012). Anti-inflammatory phenolics isolated from *Juniperus rigida* leaves and twigs in lipopolysaccharide-stimulated RAW264.7 macrophage cells. *Journal of Enzyme Inhibition and Medicinal Chemistry*, **27**: 875-879.

Jeong, E.J., Hwang, L., Lee, M., Lee, K.Y., Ahn, M.-J., and Sung, S.H. (2014). Neuroprotective biflavonoids of *Chamaecyparis obtusa* leaves against glutamate-induced oxidative stress in HT22 hippocampal cells. *Food and Chemical Toxicology*, **64**: 397-402.

Jiang, Z., Wu, M., Miao, J., Duan, H., Zhang, S., Chen, M., Sun, L., Wang, Y., Zhang, X., Zhu, X., and Zhang, L. (2013). Deoxypodophyllotoxin exerts both anti-angiogenic and vascular disrupting effects. *The International Journal of Biochemistry and Cell Biology*, **45**: 1710-1719.

Jung, H.J., Sung, Y.S., Yeo, S.-H., Kim, H.S., Lee, I.-S., Woo, E.-R., and Lee, D.G. (2006). Antifungal effect of amentoflavone derived from *Selaginella tamariscina*. *Archives of Pharmacal Research*, **29**: 746-751.

Jung, H.J., Park, K., Lee, I.-S., Kim, H.S., Yeo, S.-H., Woo, E.-R., and Lee, D.G. (2007). S-Phase accumulation of *Candida albicans* by anticandidal effect of amentoflavone isolated from *Selaginella tamariscina*. *Biological and Pharmaceutical Bulletin*, **30**: 1969-1971.

Jung, H.A., Park, J.J., Islam, M.N., Jin, S.E., Min, B.-S., Lee, J.-H., Sohn, H.S., and Choi, J.S. (2012). Inhibitory activity of coumarins from *Artemisia capillaris* against advanced glycation endproduct formation. *Archives of Pharmacal Research*, **35**: 1021-1035.

Kalva, S., Azhagiya Singam, E.R., Rajapandian, V., Saleena, L.M., and Subramanian, V. (2014). Discovery of potent inhibitor for matrix metalloproteinase-9 by pharmacophore based modeling and dynamics simulation studies. *Journal of Molecular Graphics and Modelling*, **49**: 25-37.

Kaneko, N., Hasegawa, S., and Hirose, Y. (1985). Terpenoids from seeds of *Abies firma*. *Phytochemistry*, **24**: 185-186.

Karlberg, A.-T., Bråred-Christensson, J., Börje, A., Harambasic, E., and Matura, M. (2007). Methyl esterification of 15-hydroperoxyabietic acid does not affect the patch-test result in colophonium allergic patients. *Contact Dermatitis*, **56**: 355-356.

Kaur, P., Kumar, M., Singh, B., Kumar, S., and Kaur, S. (2012). Amelioration of oxidative stress induced by oxidative mutagens and COX-2 inhibitory activity of umbelliferone isolated from *Glycyrrhiza glabra* L. *Asian Pacific Journal of Tropical Biomedicine*, S120-S126.

Kazakova, O.B., Smirnova, *I.E.*, Tkhu, H.D.T., Nguen, T.T., Apryshko, G.N., Zhukova, O.S., Medvedeva, N.I., Nazyrov, T.I., Tret'yakova, E.V., Chudov, I.V., Ismagilov, A.F., Suponitsky, K.Yu., Kazakov, D.V., Safarov, F.E., and Tolstikov, G.A. (2013). Synthesis, structure, and pharmacological activity of (7*R*,8*S*)-epoxy-(13*R*,17*R*)-trioxolane abietic acid. *Russian Journal of Bioorganic Chemistry*, **39**: 202-210.

Ketron, A.C., and Osheroff, N. (2014). Pytochemicals as anticancer and chemopreventive topoisomerase II poisons. *Phytochemistry Reviews*, **13**: 19-35.

Khaled, M., Jiang, Z.-Z., and Zhang, L.-Y. (2013). Deoxypodophyllotoxin: A promising therapeutic agent from herbal medicine. *Journal of Ethnopharmacology*, **149**: 24-34.

Khan, M., Khan, A., Rehman, N., and Gilani, A.H. (2012). Pharmacological explanation for the medicinal use of *Juniperus excelsa* in hyperactive gastrointestinal and respiratory disorders. *Journal of Natural Medicines*, **66**: 292-301.

Khare, C.P. (2007). Indian medicinal plants: An illustrated dictionary, Spinger-Verlag Berlin/Heidelberg.

Kim, N.-H., Son, Y., Jeong, S.-O., Hur, J.M., Bang, H.S., Lee, K.-N., Kim, E.-C., Chung, H.-T., and Pae, H.-O. (2010). Tetrahydroabietic acid, a reduced abietic acid, inhibits the production of inflammatory mediators in RAW264.7 macrophages activated with lipopolysaccharide. *Journal of Clinical Biochemistry and Nutrition*, **46**: 119-125.

Kim, M.B., O'Brien, T.E., Moore, J.T., Anderson, D.E., Foss, M.H., Weibel, D.B., Ames, J.B., and Shaw, J.T. (2012). The synthesis and antimicrobial activity of heterocyclic derivatives of totarol. *ACS Medicinal Chemistry Letters*, **3**: 818-822.

Koruk, S.T., Ozyilkan, E., Kaya, P., Colak, D., Donderici, O., and Cesaretli, Y. (2005). Juniper tar poisoning. *Clinical Toxicology*, **1**: 47-49.

Kunwar, R.M., Nepal, B.K., Kshhetri, H.B., Rai, S.K., and Bussmann, R.W. (2006). Ethnomedicine in Himalaya: a case study from Dolpa, Humla, Jumla and Mustang districts of Nepal. *Journal of Ethnobiology and Ethnomedicine*, **2**: e27.

Kusari, S., Lamshöft, M., and Spiteller, M. (2009). *Aspergillus fumigatus* Fresenius, an endophytic fungus from *Juniperus communis* L. Horstmann as a novel source of the anticancer pro-drug deoxypodophyllotoxin. *Journal of Applied Microbiology*, **107**: 1019-1030.

Kusari, S., Zühlke, S., and Spiteller, M. (2011). Chemometric evaluation of the anti-cancer pro-drug podophyllotoxin and potential therapeutic analogues in *Juniperus* and *Podophyllum* species. *Phytochemical Analysis*, **22**: 128-143.

Lee, J.S., Lee, M.S., Oh, W.K., and Sul, J.Y. (2009). Fatty acid synthase inhibition by amentoflavone induces apoptosis and antiproliferation in human breast cancer cells. *Biological and Pharmaceutical Bulletin*, **32**: 1427-1432.

Lee, J.S., Sul, J.Y., Park, J.B., Lee, M.S., Cha, E.Y., Song, I.S., Kim, J.R., and Chang, E.S. (2013). Fatty acid synthase inhibition by amentoflavone suppresses HER2/neu (erbB2) oncogene in SKBR3 human breast cancer cells. *Phytotherapy Research*, **27**: 713-720.

Lee, J.-H., Kim, Y.-G., Cho, H.S., Ryu, S.Y., Cho, M.H., and Lee, J. (2014). Coumarins reduce biofilm formation and the virulence of *Escherichia coli* O157: H7. *Phytomedicine*. http: //dx.doi.org/10.1016/j.phymed.2014.04.008

Lesjak, M.M., Beara, I.N., Orèiæ, D.Z., Ristiæ, J.D., Anaèkov, G.T., Božin, B.N., and Mimica-Dukiæ, N.M. (2013). Chemical characterisation and biological effects of *Juniperus foetidissima* Willd. 1806 *LWT - Food Science and Technology*, **53**: 530-539.

Lesjak, M.M., Beara, I.N., Orèiæ, D.Z., Petar, K.N., Simin, N.D., Emilija, S.D., and Mimica-Dukiæ, N.M. (2014). Phytochemical composition and antioxidant, anti-inflammatory and antimicrobial activities of *Juniperus macrocarpa* Sibth. et Sm. *Journal of Functional Foods*, **7**: 257-268.

Li, S., Zhao, M., Li, Y., Sui, Y., Yao, H., Huang, L., and Lin, X. (2014). Preparative isolation of six anti-tumor biflavonoids from *Selaginella Doederleinii* Hieron by high-speed counter-current chromatography. *Phytochemical Analysis*, **25**: 127-133.

Liu, J.-F., Sang, C.-Y., Qin, W.-W., Zhao, J., Hui, L., Ding, Y.-L., and Chen, S.-W. (2013). Synthesis and evaluation of the cell cycle arrest and CT DNA interaction properties of 4β-amino-4′-O-demethyl-4-deoxypodophyllotoxins. *Bioorganic and Medicinal Chemistry*, **21**: 6948-6955.

Loizzo, M.R., Tundis, R., Conforti, F., Saab, A.M., Statti, G.A., and Menichini, F. (2007). Comparative chemical composition, antioxidant and hypoglycaemic activities of *Juniperus oxycedrus* ssp. *oxycedrus* L. berry and wood oils from Lebanon. *Food Chemistry*, **105**: 572-578.

Lourenço, A.M., Ferreira, L.M., and Branco, P.S. (2012). Molecules of natural origin, semi-synthesis and synthesis with anti-inflammatory and anticancer utilities. *Current Pharmaceutical Design*, **18**: 3979-4046.

Luetkemeyer, A.F., Havlir, D.V., Currier, J.S. (2013). CROI 2013: Complications of HIV disease, viral hepatitis, and antiretroviral therapy. *Topics in Antiviral Medicine*, **21**: 62-74.

Madari, H., and Jacobs, R.S. (2004). An analysis of cytotoxic botanical formulations used in the traditional medicine of ancient Persia as abortifacients. *Journal of Natural Products*, **67**: 1204-1210.

Mao, K., Hao, G., Liu, J., Adams, R.P., and Milne, R.I. (2010). Diversification and biogeography of *Juniperus* (Cupressaceae): variable diversification rates and multiple intercontinental dispersals. *New Phytologist*, **188**: 254-272.

Miceli, N., Trovato, A., Marino, A., Bellinghieri, V., Melchini, A., Dugo, P., Cacciola, F., Donato, P., Mondello, L., Güvenç, A., De Pasquale, R., and Taviano, M.F. (2011). Phenolic composition and biological activities of *Juniperus drupacea* Labill. berries from Turkey. *Food and Chemical Toxicology*, **49**: 2600-2608.

Moerman, D.E. 2009. Native American medicinal plants: an ethnobotanical dictionary. Timber Press, Portland.

Mossa, J.S., El-Feraly, F.S., and Muhammad, I. (2004). Antimycobacterial constituents from *Juniperus procera*, *Ferula communis* and *Plumbago zeylanica* and their *in vitro* synergistic activity with isonicotinic acid hydrazide, *Phytotherapy Research*, **18**: 934-937.

Moujir, L.M., Seca, A.M.L., Silva, A.M.S., and Barreto, M.C. (2008). Cytotoxic activity of diterpenes and extracts of *Juniperus brevifolia*. *Planta Medica*, **74**: 751-753.

Moujir, L.M., Seca, A.M.L., Araujo, L., Silva, A.M.S., and Barreto, M.C. (2011). A new natural spiro heterocyclic compound and the cytotoxic activity of the secondary metabolites from *Juniperus brevifolia* leaves. *Fitoterapia*, **82**: 225-229.

Muto, N., Tomokuni, T., Haramoto, M., Tatemoto, H., Nakanishi, T., Inatomi, Y., Murata, H., and Inada, A. (2008). Isolation of apoptosis and differentiation-inducing substances toward human promyelocytic leukemia HL-60 cells from leaves of *Juniperus taxifolia*. *Bioscience, Biotechnology and Biochemistry*, **72**: 477-484.

Nilsson, U., Berglund, N., Lindahl, F., Axelsson, S., Redeby, T., Lassen, P., and Karlberg,

A.-T. (2008). SPE and HPLC/UV of resin acids in colophonium containing products. *Journal of Separation Science*, **31**: 2784-2790.

Oh, J., Rho, H.S., Yang, Y., Yoon, J.Y., Lee, J., Hong, Y.D., Kim, H.C., Choi, S.S., Kim, T.W., Shin, S.S., and Cho, J.Y. (2013). Extracellular signal-regulated kinase is a direct target of the anti-inflammatory compound amentoflavone derived from *Torreya nucifera*. *Mediators of Inflammation*, DOI: 10.1155/2013/761506.

Okasaka, M., Takaishi, Y., Kashiwada, Y., Kodzhimatov, O.K., Ashurmetov, O., Lin, A.J., Consentino, L.M., and Lee, K.-H. (2006). Terpenoids from *Juniperus polycarpus* var. *seravschanica*. *Phytochemistry*, **67**: 2635-2640.

Orhan, N., Orhan, *I.E.*, and Ergun, F. (2011a). Insights into cholinesterase inhibitory and antioxidant activities of five *Juniperus* species. *Food and Chemical Toxicology*, **49**: 2305-2312.

Orhan, N., Berkkan, A, Orhan, D.D., Aslan, M., and Ergun, F. (2011b). Effects of *Juniperus oxycedrus* ssp. *oxycedrus* on tissue lipid peroxidation, trace elements (Cu, Zn, Fe) and blood glucose levels in experimental diabetes. *Journal of Ethnopharmacology*, **133**: 759-764.

Orhan, N., Aslan, M., Pekcan, M., Orhan, D.D., Bedir, E., and Ergun, F. (2012a). Identification of hypoglycaemic compounds from berries of *Juniperus oxycedrus* subsp. *oxycedrus* through bioactivity guided isolation technique. *Journal of Ethnopharmacology*, **139**: 110-118.

Orhan, N., Akkol, E., and Ergun, F. (2012b). Evaluation of anti-inflammatory and antinocieptive effects of some *Juniperus* species growing in Turkey. *Turkish Journal of Biology*, **36**: 1203-1232.

Oztürk, M., Tümen, I., Uốur, A., Aydoốmuþ-ztürk, F., and Topçu, G. (2011). Evaluation of fruit extracts of six Turkish *Juniperus* species for their antioxidant, anticholinesterase and antimicrobial activities. *Journal of the Science of Food and Agriculture*, **91**: 867-876.

Pennington, H. (2010). *Escherichia coli* O157. *Lancet*, **376**: 1428-1435.

Pertino, M.W., Verdugo, V., Theoduloz, C., and Schmeda-Hirschmann, G. (2014). Synthesis and antiproliferative activity of some novel triazole derivatives from dehydroabietic acid. *Molecules*, **19**: 2523-2535.

Qiao, Y., Sun, W.-W., Wang, J.-F., and Zhang, J.-D. (2014). Flavonoids from *Podocarpus macrophyllus* and their cardioprotective activities. *Journal of Asian Natural Products Research*, **16**: 222-229.

Ramesh, B., and Pugalendi, K.V. (2006a). Antihyperglycemic effect of umbelliferone in streptozotocin-diabetic rats. *Journal of Medicinal Food*, **9**: 562-566.

Ramesh, B., and Pugalendi, K.V. (2006b). Antioxidant role of Umbelliferone in STZ-diabetic rats. *Life Sciences*, **79**: 306-310.

Ramesh, B., Viswanathan, P., and Pugalendi, K.V (2007). Protective effect of umbelliferone on membranous fatty acid composition in streptozotocin-induced diabetic rats. *European Journal of Pharmacology*, **566**: 231-239.

Rauf, A., Khan, R., Khan, H., Pervez, S., and Pirzada, A.S. (2014): *In vivo* antinociceptive and anti-inflammatory activities of umbelliferone isolated from *Potentilla evestita*. *Natural Product Research*, DOI: 10.1080/14786419.2014.901317

Renouard, S., Lopez, T., Hendrawati, O., Dupre, P., Doussot, J., Falguieres, A., Ferroud, C., Hagege, D., Lamblin, F., Laine, E., and Hano, C. (2011). Podophyllotoxin and deoxypodophyllotoxin in *Juniperus bermudiana* and 12 other *Juniperus* species: Optimization of extraction, method validation, and quantification. *Journal of Agricultural and Food Chemistry*, **59**: 8101-8107.

Rezaee, R., Behravan, E., Behravan, J., Soltani, F., Naderi, Y., Emami, B., and Iranshahi, M. (2014). Antigenotoxic activities of the natural dietary coumarins umbelliferone, herniarin and 7-isopentenyloxy coumarin on human lymphocytes exposed to oxidative stress. *Drug and Chemical Toxicology*, **37**: 144-148.

Roh, S.-S., Park, M.-K., and Kim, Y.U. (2010) Abietic acid from resina pini of *Pinus* species as a testosterone 5α-reductase inhibitor. *Journal of Health Science*, **56**: 451-455.

Ryu, Y.B., Jeong, H.J., Kim, J.H., Kim, Y.M., Park, J.-Y., Kim, D., Naguyen, T.T.H., Park, S.-J., Chang, J.S., Park, K.H., Rho, M.-C., and Lee, W.S. (2010). Biflavonoids from *Torreya nucifera* displaying SARS-CoV 3CLpro inhibition. *Bioorganic and Medicinal Chemistry*, **18**: 7940-7947.

Sakthivel, K.M., and Guruvayoorappan, C. (2013). Amentoflavone inhibits iNOS, COX-2 expression and modulates cytokine profile, NF-κB signal transduction pathways in rats with ulcerative colitis. *International Immunopharmacology*, **17**: 907-916.

Samoylenko, V., Dunbar, D.C., Gafur, Md.A., Khan, S.I., Ross, S.A., Mossa, J.S., El-Feraly, F.S., Tekwani, B.L., Bosselaers, J., and Muhammad, I. (2008). Antiparasitic, nematicidal and antifouling constituents from *Juniperus* berries. *Phytotherapy Research*, **22**: 1570-1576.

Sánchez-Recillas, A., Navarrete-Vázquez, G., Hidalgo-Figueroa, S., Rios, M.Y., Ibarra-Barajas, M., and Estrada-Soto, S. (2014). Semisynthesis, *ex vivo* evaluation, and SAR studies of coumarin derivatives as potential antiasthmatic drugs. *European Journal of Medicinal Chemistry*, **77**: 400-408.

Sassi, A.B., Harzallah-Skhiri, F., Bourgougnon, N., and Aouni, M. (2008). Antiviral activity of some Tunisian medicinal plants against *Herpes simplex* virus type 1. *Natural Product Research*, **22**: 53-65.

Seca, A.M.L., and Silva, A.M.S. (2006). The chemical composition of the *Juniperus* genus (1970-2004). *In*: Recent Progress in Medicinal Plants, Vol. 16, Phytomedicines, Ed. By Govil, J.N. and Singh, V.K., Studium Press LLC, Houston, USA, pp.401-522.

Seca, A.M.L., and Silva, A.M.S (2008). The chemical composition of hexane extract from bark of *Juniperus brevifolia*. *Natural Product Research*, **22**: 975-983.

Seca, A.M.L., Silva, A.M.S., Bazzocchi, I.L., and Jimenez, I.A. (2008). Diterpene constituents of leaves from *Juniperus brevifolia*. *Phytochemistry*, **69**: 498-505.

Seca, A.M.L., and Silva, A.M.S (2010). A new 42,7-epoxy-8,32-oxyneolignan from the acetone extract of *Juniperus brevifolia* leaves. *Phytochemistry Letters*, **3**: 126-128.

Semiz, G., Isik, K., and Unal, O. (2007). Enek Pekmez production from *Juniper* "fruits" by native people on the Taurus Mountains in southern Turkey. *Economic Botany*, **61**: 299-301.

Sepúlveda, B., Astudillo, L., Rodríguez, J.A., Yáñez, T., Theoduloz, C., and Schmeda-Hirschmann, G. (2005). Gastroprotective and cytotoxic effect of dehydroabietic acid derivatives. *Pharmacological Research*, **52**: 429-437.

Sharanappa, R., and Vidyasagar, G.M. (2013). Anti-*Candida* activity of medicinal plants. A review. *International Journal of Pharmacy and Pharmaceutical Sciences*, **5**: 9-16.

Silva, B.A., Malva, J.O., and Dias, A.C.P. (2008). St. John's Wort (*Hypericum perforatum*) extracts and isolated phenolic compounds are effective antioxidants in several *in vitro* models of oxidative stress. *Food Chemistry*, **110**: 611-619.

Skalli, S., Chebat, A., Badrane, N., and Bencheikh, R.S. (2014). Side effects of cade oil in Morocco: An analysis of reports in the Moroccan herbal products database from 2004 to 2012. *Food and Chemical Toxicology*, **64**: 81-85.

Smith, E., Williamson, E., Zloh, M., and Gibbons, S. (2005). Isopimaric acid from *Pinus nigra* shows activity against multidrug-resistant and EMRSA strains of *Staphylococcus aureus*. *Phytotherapy Research*, **19**: 538-542.

Smith, E.C.J., Kaatz, G.W., Seo, S.M., Wareham, N., Williamson, E.M., and Gibbons, S. (2007a). The phenolic diterpene totarol inhibits multidrug efflux pump activity in *Staphylococcus aureus*. *Antimicrobial Agents and Chemotherapy*, **51**: 4480-4483.

Smith, E.C.J., Williamson, E.M., Wareham, N., Kaatz, G.W., and Gibbons, S. (2007b). Antibacterials and modulators of bacterial resistance from the immature cones of *Chamaecyparis lawsoniana*. *Phytochemistry*, **68**: 210-217.

Smith, E.C.J., Wareham, N., Zloh, M., and Gibbons, S. (2008). 2 β-Acetoxyferruginol- A new antibacterial abietane diterpene from the bark of *Prumnopitys andina*. *Phytochemistry Letters*, **1**: 49-53.

Suganya, R.P., Kalva, S., and Saleena, L.M. (2011). Hinokiflavone from *Juniperus* as therapeutic lead against osteoarthritis by inhibiting ADAMTS-5. *International Journal of Bioscience, Biochemistry and Bioinformatics*, **1**: 16-20.

Tacon, C., Guantai, E.M., Smith, P.J., and Chibale, K. (2012). Synthesis, biological evaluation and mechanistic studies of totarol amino alcohol derivatives as potential antimalarial agents *Bioorganic and Medicinal Chemistry*, **20**: 893-902.

Takahashi, N., Kawada, T., Goto, T., Kim, C.-S., Taimatsua, A., Egawa, K., Yamamoto, T., Jisaka, M., Nishimura, K., Yokota, K., Yu, R., and Fushikia, T. (2003). Abietic acid activates peroxisome proliferator-activated receptor-γ (PPARγ) in RAW264.7 macrophages and 3T3-L1 adipocytes to regulate gene expression involved in inflammation and lipid metabolism. *Federation of European Biochemical Societies Letters*, **550**: 190-194.

Talevi, A., Cravero, M.S., Castro, E.A., and Bruno-Blanch, L.E. (2007). Discovery of anticonvulsant activity of abietic acid through application of linear discriminant analysis. *Bioorganic and Medicinal Chemistry Letters*, **17**: 1684-1690.

Thanigaimalai, P., Konno, S., Yamamoto, T., Koiwai, Y., Taguchi, A., Takayama, K., Yakushiji, F., Akaji, K., Chen, S.-E., Naser-Tavakolian, A., Schön, A., Freire, E., and Hayashi, Y. (2013). Development of potent dipeptide-type SARS-CoV 3CL protease inhibitors with novel P3 scaffolds: Design, synthesis, biological evaluation, and docking studies. *European Journal of Medicinal Chemistry*, **68**: 372-384.

The Plant List database, http: //www.theplantlist.org/tpl1.1/search?q=Juniperus. Accessed 7-07-2014.

Tung, N.H., Uto, T., Sakamoto, A., Hayashida, Y., Hidaka, Y., Morinaga, O., Lhieochaiphant, S., and Shoyama, Y. (2013). Antiproliferative and apoptotic effects of compounds from the flower of *Mammea siamensis* (Miq.) T. Anders. on human cancer cell lines. *Bioorganic and Medicinal Chemistry Letters*, **23**: 158-162.

Ulubelen, A., and Topcu, G. (1992). Abietane diterpenoids from *Salvia pomifera*. *Phytochemistry*, **31**: 3949-3951.

Uprety, Y., Asselin, H., Boon, E.K., Yadav, S., and Shrestha K.K. (2010). Indigenous use and bioefficacy of medicinal plants in the Rasuwa District, Central Nepal. *Journal of Ethnobiology and Ethnomedicine*, **6**: e3.

Van Auken, O.W. and Smeins, F. (2008) Western North American *Juniperus* communities: Patterns and causes of distribution and abundance. In: Western North American *Juniperus* communities. A dynamic vegetation type. Ed. Van Auken, O.W. Ecological Studies Vol. 196, pp 3-18.

Vandebuerie, L., Aerts, C., and Goossens, A. (2014). Allergic contact dermatitis resulting from multiple colophonium-related allergen sources. *Contact Dermatitis*, **70**: 117-127.

WHO (2013). Global tuberculosis report 2013. World Health Organization, Geneva, Switzerland. ISBN 978 92 4 156465 6

WHO (2014). Web page http: //www.who.int/mediacentre/factsheets/fs312/en/ (accessed May 2014).

Wilsky, S., Sobotta, K., Wiesener, N., Pilas, J., Althof, N., Munder, T., Wutzler, P., and Henke, A. (2012). Inhibition of fatty acid synthase by amentoflavone reduces coxsackievirus B3 replication. *Archives of Virology*, **157**: 259-269.

Woo, K.W., Choi, S.U., Park, J.C., and Lee, K.R. (2011). A new lignan glycoside from *Juniperus rigida*. *Archives of Pharmacal Research*. **34**: 2043-2049.

Wu, M., Jiang, Z., Duan, H., Sun, L., Zhang, S., Chen, M., Wang, Y., Gao, Q., Song, Y., Zhu, X., and Zhang, L. (2013). Deoxypodophyllotoxin triggers necroptosis in human non-small cell lung cancer NCI-H460 cells. *Biomedicine and Pharmacotherapy*, **67**: 701-706.

Yang, X.-C., Qian, S.-J., Wang, L., Liao, S.-D., Cao, J., Hu, Y.-Z., He, Q.-J., Zhu, H., and Yang, B. (2013). GL3, a novel 4β-anilino-42-*O*-demethyl-4-

desoxypodophyllotoxin analog, traps topoisomerase II cleavage complexes and exerts anticancer activities. *Translational Oncology*, **6**: 75-82.

Yang, J., Liang, Q., Wang, M., Jeffries, C., Smithson, D., Tu, Y., Boulos, N., Jacob, M.R., Shelat, A.A., Wu, Y., Ravu, R.R., Gilbertson, R., Avery, M.A., Khan, I.A., Walker, L.A., Guy, R.K., and Li, X.-C. (2014). UPLC-MS-ELSD-PDA as a powerful dereplication tool to facilitate compound identification from small-molecule natural product libraries. *Journal of Natural Products*, **77**: 902-909.

Yeggoni, D.P., Gokara, M., Mark Manidhar, D., Rachamallu, A., Nakka, S., Reddy, C.S., and Subramanyam, R. (2014). Binding and molecular dynamics studies of 7hydroxycoumarin derivatives with human serum albumin and its pharmacological importance. *Molecular Pharmaceutics*, **11**: 1117-1131.

Zaidi, S.F.H., Awale, S., Kalauni, S.K., Tezuka, Y., Esumi, H., and Kadota, S. (2006). Diterpenes from "Pini Resina" and their preferential cytotoxic activity under nutrient-deprived condition. *Planta Medica*, **72**: 1231-1234.

Zhao, W., Pu, J.-X., Du, X., Su, J., Li, X.-N., Yang, J.-H., Xue, Y.-B., Li, Y., and Sun, H.-D. (2011). Cytotoxic diterpenoids from *Isodon adenolomus*. *Chinese Journal of Natural Medicines*, **9**: 253-258.

Zhao, Y., Wu, Z., Zhang, Y., and Zhu, L. (2013). HY-1 induces G2/M cell cycle arrest in human colon cancer cells through the ATR-Chk1-Cdc25C and Weel pathways. *Cancer Science*, **104**: 1062-1066.

Zheng, C., and Fanta, C.H. (2013). Non-tuberculous mycobacterial pulmonary infection in the immunocompetent host. *Monthly Journal of the Association of Physicians*, **106**: 307-315.

Bioactive Phytochemicals: Perspectives for Modern Medicine Vol. 3 (2015) *Pages* **411–435**
Editor: **V.K. Gupta**
Published by: **DAYA PUBLISHING HOUSE, NEW DELHI**

16

Bioactive Phytochemicals: An Overview

Sumangala K Bhat[1*] and Vivek Kempraj[2]

ABSTRACT

Phytochemicals have been recognized as highly resourceful natural products throughout the world and employed for diverse applications with more focus on their therapeutic effects. Phytochemicals comprise heterogeneous chemical entities and capable of exerting modulatory effect on living organisms through wide ranging mechanisms and broad spectrum of effects. Analysis of the types of phytochemicals, strategies for discovery of bioactive compounds, their bioactivity and applications has been attempted in the first part of this article. Phytochemistry research, product development and current status of practical utility of research outcomes in the field of therapeutics against microbial diseases and cancer as well as biopesticides have been assessed. Lacunae in phytochemical research have been identified and recommendations for orientation of research focus towards practical application is suggested.

Keywords: Phytochemicals, Bioactivity, Antibiotics, Chemotherapeutics, Biopesticides.

Introduction

Phytochemicals comprise highly diverse group of compounds produced by plants through their metabolic activity. Plant defense against pathogens, parasites and pests often trigger production of these compounds involved in plant protection. The defense molecules belong to a broad category of functional compounds and capable of exerting modulatory influence on animals at cellular and organism levels. More than 10000 bioactive phytochemicals have been reported, of which the flavonoids predominate

1 Acharya Institute of Technology, Department of Biotechnology, Dr Sarvepalli Radha Krishna Road, Soldevanahalli, Bangalore – 560 107, Karnataka, India

2 Biowave Resources, #643, 6th Block, SMV Layout, Bangalore – 560 056, Karnataka, India

* *Corresponding author*: E-mail: bhat.sumangala@gmail.com

the list (Hairborne, 1993). Owing to their multiple activities and applications on various fields, secondary metabolites of plants, fungi, algae and animals (Bidlack, 2000) have elicited interest among traditional healers, scientists, agriculturists and of late, the modern medical practitioners. Accordingly, phytochemicals have found their applications in various domains of human interest. This has made this group of compounds an inseparable part of human civilizations world over. Every geographical region has its own ethnic knowledge and specific uses of plant resources of the area as source of phytochemicals, particularly in traditional healing practices. Parallel to the evolution of modern equipments and techniques for the analysis and identification of phytochemicals, there is resurgence of research interest on these compounds from the scientific community during recent years (Uma Shankar *et al.*, 2008). This has paved the way for the discovery of immense number of phytochemicals and their multitudes of applications in domains other than direct drugs such as drug precursors or reference molecules for derivation of synthetic drugs, and as pharmacological probes (Salim *et al.*, 2008).

Most of the phytochemicals are concerned with regulation of enzymes involved in cell metabolism and mechanisms of defense against physicochemical factors and plant pathogens. They are capable of exerting pleiotropic effects on animal cells (Russo *et al.*, 2010a). Some of the popular natural products of plant origin used as drugs comprise compounds like cocaine, quinine, curare, digitalis (Balandrin and Klocke, 1988). Status of plant derived compounds in modern medicine has been analyzed in several reviews during recent times (Fowler, 2006; Gurib-Fakin, 2006; Jones *et al.*, 2006). This review attempts to analyze various dimensions of the bioactivity of phytochemicals and their applications with focus on therapeutics for microbial diseases and cancer as well as their status as biopesticides.

Phytochemicals

Types of Phytochemicals

Types of phytochemicals identified from plants have been classified into different chemical groups based on their molecular structure and functional attributes. Table 16.1 illustrates the major phytochemicals and their bioactivities. Different approaches have been evolved for the discovery of bioactive phytochemicals over the years. Ethnobotonical, chemical ecology and anatomical approaches are some of the important strategies employed for the purpose (Duke *et al.*, 2000). Of these, chemical ecology and anatomical approaches contribute greatly towards understanding the distribution of bioactive compounds across the plant kingdom and their interactions. Isolation and identification of bioactive phytochemicals involve integration of bioassays, analytical processes and bio and chemoinformatics. The recently evolved strategy, Quantitative Structure-Activity Relationship (QSAR) has enhanced the output of phytochemical research through the rapid optimization of their activity on focused areas.

Many plants have evolved specialized structural and functional attributes for segregation, sequestering or secretion of bioactive components such as glandular trichomes, laticifers, idioblasts, resin canals, nectarines and epidermal secretary cells (Duke *et al.*, 2000). Hydrocarbons, aromatics and alkaloids represent the major broad

Table 16.1: Major Phytochemicals and their Bioactive Properties

Phytochemicals	*Examples*	*Bioactivities*	*Reference*
		Hydrocarbons	
Saturated Hydrocarbons	α-Pentene	Antimicrobial, Insecticidal, Anti-inflammatory	Cseke *et al.*, 2006
	β-Pinene	Antimicrobial, Insecticidal, Anti-inflammatory	Cseke *et al.*, 2006
	n-Heptane	Repellent, Prevents infection, Antiviral	Cseke *et al.*, 2006
Unsaturated Hydrocarbons	Falcarinol	Neurotoxin, Anticancer, Antimicrobial	Lund and White, 1990
	Wyerone acid	Antimicrobial	Nawar and Kuti, 2003
	Safynol	Antimicrobial	Redl *et al.*, 1994
		Functionalized Hydrocarbons	
Halogenated Hydrocarbons	Laurencin	Antitumor, Antimicrobial	Irie *et al.*, 1965
	Rogioloxepane A	Antitumor	Guella *et al.*, 1992
	Laurallene	Antitumor	Fukuzawa and Kurosawa, 1979
	Prepinnaterpene	Antitumor	Fukuzawa *et al.*, 1985
	Laurencial	Antitumor	Miyashita *et al.*, 1998
	Kumausallene	Antibacterial, Antitumor	Suzuki *et al.*, 1983
Alcohols	Ceryl alcohol	Antimicrobial	Cseke *et al.*, 2006
	1-Hexenol	Kairomones	Clark, 1990
	Cis-3-Hexen-1-ol	Kairomones, Attractants	Clark, 1990
Sulfides and Glucosinolates	Allyl iso-thioglucosinolate	Anticancer, Antitumor	Johnson, 2003
Aldehydes and Ketones	Nootkatone	Aroma compounds, Antimicrobial	Moshonas, 1971
	Citral	Aroma compounds, Antimicrobial	Moshonas, 1971
	Octanal	Aroma compounds, Antimicrobial	Moshonas, 1971
	Sinensal	Antimicrobial	Moshonas, 1971

Contd...

Table 16.1–*Contd...*

Phytochemicals	*Examples*	*Bioactivities*	*Reference*
Esters	Ethyl butyrate	Flavour compounds	Cseke *et al.*, 2006
	Ethyl acetate	Flavour compounds, Antimicrobial	Cseke *et al.*, 2006
	Ethyl valerate	Flavour compounds	Cseke *et al.*, 2006
	Propyl butyrate	Flavour compounds	Cseke *et al.*, 2006
Fatty Acids	Linolenic acid	Cardioprotectant	De Lorgeril and Salen, 2004
	α-Linolenic acid	Cardioprotectant, Neuroprotectant	Youdim *et al.*, 2000
	Arachidonic acid	Health of cells and nerves	Cseke *et al.*, 2006
		Terpenes	
Hemiterpenes	Tiglic acid	Antiparasitic, Antimicrobial	Holopainen, 2004
	Angelic acid	Insect repellent	Holopainen, 2004
	Furoic acid	Insect repellent	Holopainen, 2004
Monoterpenes	Thujone	Blocks GABA gated chloride channels	Sirisoma *et al.*, 2001
	Carvone	Antifungal	McGeady *et al.*, 2002
	3-Carene	Anesthetic	Librowski *et al.*, 2004
	Eucalyptol	Anti-inflammatory, Anesthetic, Anticancer	Moteki *et al.*, 2002
Sesquiterpenes	Farnesol	Cancer chemopreventive activity	Crowell and Gould, 2004
	Artemisinin	Antimalarial	Haynes and Vonwiller, 1994
	Santonin	Antihelminthic	Ceske *et al.*, 2006
	Helenalin	Antitrypanosomic	Hoet *et al.*, 2004
Diterpenes	Zoapatanol	Abortifacient	Dong *et al.*, 1989
	Clerodanes	Antifeedant	Krishna Kumari *et al.*, 2003
	Podolactones	Antileukemic	Barrero *et al.*, 2003
	Nigilactones	Antileukemic	Shrestha *et al.*, 2001
	Marrubiin	Vasorelaxant	El Bardai *et al.*, 2003

Contd...

Table 16.1–*Contd...*

Phytochemicals	*Examples*	*Bioactivities*	*Reference*
Triterpenes	Phytosterols	Cardioprotectant	Kris-Etherton *et al.*, 2002
	Glycyrrhizins	Artifical sweetener, Expectorant, Bactriostatic, Antiviral	Fenwick *et al.*, 1990; Bo *et al.*, 2002; Utsunomya *et al.*, 1997
	Ginsenoside	Immunostimulant, Antinociceptive	Naj *et al.*, 2000
Tetraterpenes	Lycopene	Anticancer	Cseke *et al.*, 2006
	β-carotene	Anticancer, Antibacterial, Eye protectant	Cseke *et al.*, 2006
		Aromatics	
Tetraoyrroles	Phytochromes	Colouring agents	Jacobi *et al.*, 2000; Warren, 2004
		Phenols	
Phenylpropanoids	Eugenol	Analgesic, Insecticidal	Samuelsson, 2001
	Galangin	Antibacterial	Cushine *et al.*, 2003
	Rotenone	Estrogenic, Insecticidal, Antifungal, Piscicidal	Geissman and Crout, 1969; Budavari, 2001
	Genistein	Estrogenic, Antifungal, Anticancer	Cornwell *et al.*, 2004; Rivera-Vargas *et al.*, 1993, Kaufman *et al.*, 1997
	Quercetin	Antioxidant	Graefe *et al.*, 1999
	Silybin	Antihepatotoxic	Sridar *et al.*, 2004
	Silymarin	Antihepatotoxic, Anticancer, Anti-inflammatory	Katiyar, 2005
Tannins	Corilagin	Anti-HIV	Notka *et al.*, 2004
	Gerilagin	Anti-HIV	Notka *et al.*, 2004
Quinones	1,4-Benzenediol	Antibacterial, Insecticidal	Cseke *et al.*, 2006
		Alkaloids	
	Reserpine	Antihypertensive	Cordell, 1981
	Vinblastine	Antitumor	Cordell, 1981
	Atropine	Muscle relaxant	Cordell, 1981

Contd...

Table 16.1–*Contd...*

Phytochemicals	*Examples*	*Bioactivities*	*Reference*
	Cocaine	CNS	Cordell, 1981; Flynn, 1991
	Strychnine	Nerve stimulant	Cordell, 1981
	Quinune	Antimalarial	Honigsbaum, 2002
	Morphine	Analgesic	Bercovitch *et al.*, 1999
	Colchicine	Anti-inflammatory, Anticancer	Jordan, 2002; Nakagawa-Goto *et al.*, 2005
	Protopine	Spasmolytic, Anticholinergic, Antiarrythmic	Ustunes *et al.*, 1988; Paul *et al.*, 2003
	Berberine	Antibacterial	Birdsall and Kelly, 1997; Taylor and Greenough, 1989
	Paclitaxel	Anticancer	Cseke *et al.*, 2006
	Codeine	Analgesic, Antitussive	Balandrin and Klocke,1988

categories of phytochemicals exhibiting influence on biochemical pathways at cellular level and modulating the physiological functions of living organisms. Current article attempts to analyze bioactivity based applications of phytochemicals in general with focus on their potential as antibiotics, anticancer drugs and as agents for plant protection.

What is Bioactivity?

Bioactivity refers to the modulatory influence of the material on biological activities of living organism at cellular, tissue or organism level. Most of the phytochemicals are known to exhibit bioactive properties on wide range of organism including man. The modulatory effect of bioactive phytochemicals includes both positive and negative aspects and hence can be exploited in a favourable manner depending on the context of desired outcomes. Types as well as mechanism of bioactivities of phytochemicals are diverse.

Types and Applications of Bioactivity

Bioactivities exhibited by plants are highly diverse with reference to mechanism of action, intensity and effects on organisms concerned. Bioactive phytochemicals have been extensively employed in pharmaceuticals and pest management products (Duke *et al.*, 2000). Pharmaceuticals like salicylic acid and morphine and pesticides such as azadirachtin, pytrethroids and rotenone are pioneers in the list of phytochemicals in practical use (Butterworth and Morgan, 1968; Lydon and Duke, 1989; Duke, 1991; Robbers *et al.*, 1996; Pachlatko, 1998). Other range of activities includes neuroprotectant, cardioprotectant, growth stimulant, cellular communication and so on (Table 16.1). Apart from these, they have also been used as colouring agents, flavouring agents and cosmetics. Therefore, phytochemicals represent a versatile group of highly resourceful compounds and much more work needs to be done for understanding unknown activities of these compounds.

Contribution of Phytochemicals to Antibiotic Therapeutics

Pathogens and parasites constitute a major cause of illness among man, animals and plants. Microorganisms comprising viruses, bacteria and fungi represent predominant groups of pathogens challenging human health. Intricate association between microbial pathogens and human hosts often lead to chronic infections. This has warranted focused attempt towards discovery and development of antibiotic drugs. High levels of research and development attempts have resulted in the discovery and evolution of multiple generations of antibiotic drugs over the last six decades. Most of the antibiotic drugs are of synthetic origin and often comprise single active ingredient. This factor has favored the tendency of developing resistance to the drugs by many of the pathogens. Therefore, effective life span of the antibiotic drugs remains to be short (Cowan, 1999). Multi drug resistant (MDR) pathogens pose real challenge in clinical world during recent years (Reddy *et al.*, 2009).

Phytochemicals have been explicitly explored for their antimicrobial potential by large number of investigators (Cowan, 1999; Duke, 1985; Thomson, 1978) and an extensive list of plants have been categorized as having antimicrobial potential. Most of the studies comprise reports of antimicrobial activity of crude extracts, latex or groups of secondary metabolites. Major groups of secondary metabolites with proved antimicrobial activity include phenolics and polyphenols, quinones, flavones and flavonoids, tanins, coumarins, terpenoids, alkaloids, and sugars (Cowan, 1999). Some of the available literatures on bioactive antimicrobials from plants report definite identity of single active compounds of plant origin (Table 16.2). While considering the extent of success achieved in developing phytochemicals derived antibiotic drugs, the resource appears to be under underexplored at advanced levels of research beyond *in vitro* trials on pathogenic organisms. From among the hundreds of antimicrobial plants reported (Schultes, 1978), only less than 50 active compounds have been identified. The compounds which have reached the level of drugs in clinical use are even less (Table 16.2). Therefore there is an urgent requirement towards focused research on development of known compounds of antimicrobial potentials from plants to formulations for clinical trials. However, many of the active fractions of plants are in practical application for the treatment of diseases caused by pathogenic microorganisms in alternative medicines like ayurveda (Bharadwaj *et al.*, 2005; Biradar *et al.*, 2008).

Contribution of Phytochemicals to Cancer Chemotherapeutics

Cancer is one of the major diseases causing morbidity and death among human beings world over. Accordingly, prevention and treatment of cancer has been in the frontiers of medical research, leading to wide range of approaches on this domain. Chemotherapy is an important basic approach adopted in cancer treatment. Large number of chemotherapeutic agents of heterogeneous origin are in current use for the treatment of cancer (Adjei, 1999; Chabner and Roberts, 2005; Newman *et al.*, 2008; DeVita Jr. and Chu, 2014). Plants have been extensively explored for their prospective use as source for anticancer components during the last few decades (Aggarwal *et al.*, 2008). Natural compounds are considered as a promising category of anticancer agents due to their multiple targets on cancer cells accompanied by limited toxic effect on healthy cells (Russo *et al.*, 2010a). Phytochemicals have been reported to exert multiple effects on cancer cells to prevent or inhibit various phases of carcinogenesis. Phytochemicals function through wide spectrum of mechanisms yielding preventive as well as curative effect on cancer. Induction of apoptosis, antiproliferative activity, antiangiogenic activity and modulation of the expression of oncogenes are some of the key mechanisms to name (Liu, 2004). Most of the phytochemicals have been known to elicit multiple influences on cancer synergistically and lead to preventive/inhibitory effect on different phases of tumerogenesis (Liu, 2004; Seeram *et al.*, 2005; Neto, 2007; Russo *et al.*, 2010b; Ugbogu *et al.*, 2013). Table 16.3 illustrates anticancer phytochemical lead compounds identified and their status of application in cancer treatment. Unlike the antibiotic therapeutics from phytochemicals, a major portion of the identified anticancer compounds have been put into practical use as chemotherapeutic drugs. But still, need for identification of new active compounds and developmental research for evolving the identified compounds to clinical formulations deserves directed focus.

Table 16.2: Major Phytochemical Antibiotics Leads and Status of their Current Applications

Compound	*Natural source*	*Activity*	*Status*	*Reference*
Eugenol	*Pimenta dioica*	Bacteria	C, T	Martinez *et al.*, 1996
Phloretin	*Phloretin*	Bacteria	R	Hunter and Hull, 1993
Withafarin A	*Withania somniferum*	Bacteria, fungi, protozoa	T, R	Hunter and Hull, 1993
Berberine	*Berberis vulgaris*	Bacteria, protozoa	T, R	McDevitt *et al.*, 1996; Omulokoli *et al.*, 1997
Catechols	*Piper betel*	Bacteria, fungi, protozoa	T, R	Ghoshal *et al.*, 1996
Piperine	*Piper nigrum*	Bacteria, fungi, protozoa	T, R	Ghoshal *et al.*, 1996
Fructose	*Vaccinium* spp.	*E. coli*	–	Ofek *et al.*, 1996
Terebinthone	*Schinus terebinthifolius*	Bacteria, fungi, protozoa	R	Ofek *et al.*, 1996
Protoanemonin	*Ranunculus bulbosus*	Bacteria, fungi, protozoa	R	Ofek *et al.*, 1996
Salicylic acid	*Anacardium pulsatilla*	*P. acnes*	C, T, R	Himejima and Kubo, 1991
Anthemic acid	*Matricaria chamomilla*	Bacteria, helminthes	R	Bose, 1958; Hamburger and Hostettmann, 1991; Scheel, 1972
Capsaicin	*Capsicum annuum*	Bacteria	R	Cichewicz and Thorpe, 1996; Jones and Luchsinger 1986
Fabatin	*Vicia faba*	Bacteria	R	Navarro *et al.*, 1996
Allicin	*Allium sativum*	Bacteria, fungi, protozoa	R	Naganawa *et al.*, 1996; San-Blas *et al.*, 1993; San-Blas *et al.*, 1989; Yoshida *et al.*, 1987
Colchicine	*Gloriosa superba*	Bacteria, fungi, protozoa	C, R	Naganawa *et al.*, 1996; San-Blas *et al.*, 1993; San-Blas *et al.*, 1989; Yoshida *et al.*, 1987
Hydrastine	*Hydrastis canadensis*	Bacteria, Protozoa	R	Freiburghaus *et al.*, 1996; Stange *et al.*, 1993
Asiatocoside	*Centella asiatica*	*M. leprae*	R	Vijaya *et al.*, 1995
Catechin	*Camellia sinensis*	Bacteria	T, R	Kadota *et al.*, 1997

Contd...

Table 16.2–*Contd...*

Compound	*Natural source*	*Activity*	*Status*	*Reference*
b-Resercyclic acid	*Cannabis sativa*	Bacteria and viruses	T, R	Suresh *et al.*, 1997
Trichorabdal A	*Rabdosia trichocarpa*	*Helicobacter pylori*	R	Suresh *et al.*, 1997
Lawsone	*Lawsonia*	*M. tuberculosis*	R	Perrett *et al.*, 1995
Alpinumisoflavone	*Millettia thonningii*	Schistosoma	R	Keating and O'Kennedy, 1997
Glabrol	*Glycyrrhiza glabra*	Bacteria	R	Hufford *et al.*, 1993
Helanins	*Arnica montana*	Bacteria	R	Hufford *et al.*, 1993
Quercetin	*Quercus rubra*	Bacteria	R	Hufford *et al.*, 1993
Petalostemumol	*Petalostemum*	Bacteria, fungi	R	Ali-Shtayeh *et al.*, 1997
Carvacrol	*Satureja montana*	Bacteria, fungi, Protozoa	R	Kubo *et al.*, 1994
Totarol	*Podocarpus nagi*	Bacteria	R	Kubo *et al.*, 1992
Nagilactone	*Podocarpus nagi*	Fungi	R	Kubo *et al.*, 1992, Kubo *et al.*, 1993
Curcumin	*Curcuma longa*	Bacteria, protozoa	C, T, R	Apisariyakul *et al.*, 1995
Ajoene	*Allium sativum*	Bacteria, fungi	R	San-Blas *et al.*, 1993; San-Blas *et al.*, 1989; Yoshida *et al.*, 1987
Camphor	*Cinnamomum camphora*		Fungi	R *unpublished

C: Commercially available; T: Traditionally used; R: Still under research and development.

Table 16.3: Major Phytochemical Anticancer Leads and Status of their Current Application

Sl.No.	*Compound*	*Natural Source*	*Status*	*Reference*
1.	Genistein	*Pueraria montana*	R	Kaufman *et al.*, 1997
2.	Daidzein	*Glycine max*	R	Kaufman *et al.*, 1997
3.	Paclitaxel	*Taxus brevifolia*	C, R	Walker and Croteau, 2001
4.	β-carotene	*Daucus carota*	R, S	
5.	Lycopene	*Solanum lycopersicum*	C, R, S	Suth, 2003
6.	Hypericin	*Hypercin perforatum*	R	Cellarova *et al.*, 1995
7.	Pseudohypericin	*Hypercin perforatum*	R	Cellarova *et al.*, 1995
8.	Hyperforin	*Hypercin perforatum*	R	Cellarova *et al.*, 1995
9.	Camptothecin	*Camptotheca accuminata*	C, R, T	Liu and Adams, 1996
10.	Etoposide	*Linum* spp.	R	Petersen and Alfermann, 2001
11.	Docetaxel	*Taxus brevifolia*	C, R	Pazdur *et al.*, 1993
12.	Homoharringtonine	*Cephalotaxus harringtonia*	R	Ohnuma and Holland, 1985
13.	Anthraquinone	*Hemerocallis fulva*	R	Cichewicz *et al.*, 2004
14.	Resveratrol	*Vitis vinifera*	C, R, S	Jang *et al.*, 1997
15.	Lapachol	*Tabebuia* spp.	R	Cassady and Douros, 1980
16.	Podophyllotoxin	*Podophyllum peltatum*	R	Cassady and Douros 1980
17.	Vinca alkaloids	*Catharanthus roseus*	C, R, T	Cassady and Douros, 1980
18.	Clerodane	*Croton oblongifolius*	R	Roengsumran *et al.*, 2002
19.	Colchicine	*Autumn crocus*	C, R	Stimanek *et al.*, 1990
20.	Falcarinol	*Panax ginseng*	C, R, S	Dembitsky, 2006

R: Research and development; C: Commercially available; T: Traditionally used; S: Nutritional supplement

Contribution of Phytochemicals to Biopesticides

Plant protection is a key element for the success of agriculture and hence has its origin parallel with agriculture. Pest management strategies have a long history and reached a crucial turning point during last decade. Eco friendly solution for plant care is in high demand as the environmental risks associated with the chemical pesticides were deciphered from time to time (Seiber, 1991; Fishel, 2005; Koushik *et al.*, 2010; Kesavachandran and Mudiam, 2010). Several alternative strategies and products have been evolved for plant care and the domain of this research gained momentum during the recent past. Among these, phytochemicals derived compounds represent novel tools and deserve focused attention.

Botanical pesticides have their origin during 1940s and later got sidelined due to the spectacular brands of synthetic chemicals, which ruled the plant protection portfolio for more than three decades. However, alarming revelations came to the fore on the hazardous environmental risks associated with these pesticides during later years. It has been reported that the environmental problems caused by the highly xenobiotic pesticides like organochlorines lace the food with residues (Gonzalez *et al.*, 1977; Parmar and Devkumar 1993). Some other studies have concluded that hardly 0.1 per cent of the agrochemicals used in crop protection reach the target pest leaving the remaining 99.9 per cent to enter the environment to cause hazards to non-target organisms including humans (Pimentel and Levitan, 1986). These facts have acted as the driving force for evolving alternate means for pest management. Accordingly, a wide range of strategies has entered into plant protection scenario of which biopesticides represent one of the promising options. The term "bio-pesticide" refers to any pesticide of biological origin, *i.e.* viruses, bacteria, pheromones, other compounds of plant or animal origin (Sinha and Biswas, 2008).

Table 16.4 illustrates the major compounds proved to have potential use in pest management applications. The compounds reported in this category belong to a wide range of distinct chemical entities. Apart from the profound chemical diversity, phytochemicals exhibit diversity with reference to their mechanism of action on target pests. Individual phytochemical components or their combinations interfere with normal feeding, reproduction, development and behavior of the pests in general. Owing to the diversity and heterogeneous composition of phytochemical fractions, development of resistance by the pests gets hampered unlike in the case of synthetic pesticides (Ntalli Menkissoglu-Spiroudi, 2011). In addition to this, difference in mechanisms of action of phytochemicals (Table 16.4) enables them to be effective on pests/their life stages, less affected by other pesticides. Diverse nature of phytochemicals will further add ample scope for development of novel formulations and modes of application of pest management products derived from them.

Phytochemicals and Bioactivities Identified from some Plants and Fungi

This section deals with the phytochemials identified from different plants and mushrooms by the authors and their colleagues during the last 6 years and the status of research and developmental work attained so far. Various streams of investigation have confirmed the role of active compounds from *Annona squamosa, Cyperus rotundus, Coriandrum sativum* and *Syzygium aromaticum* in pest management (Table 16.5). Some of the identified compounds have been developed into commercial formulations as well. Antibacterial and antifungal activities of active compound from *Piper betle, Agaricus bisporus*, and *Pleurotus ostreatus* have been confirmed on pathogenic bacteria and fungi affecting plants, animals and human beings (Ramya *et al.*, 2013; Bhat *et al.*, Unpublished) (Table 16.5). Active compounds isolated from *Calotropis procera* and *C.gigantea* have exhibited antimitotic and anticancer activities under *in vitro* conditions (Table 16.5). These outcomes depict the commendable impact of the phytochemical research on diversified domains of applications.

Discussion and Conclusion

The status of phytochemicals as source for antibiotics and anticancer drugs as well as biopesticides has been reviewed in the current article. Antibiotics are one of the important groups among the drugs in clinical practice and health care. As of now, the contribution of phytochemicals to this portfolio appears to be meager despite immense number of reports of antimicrobial activities of crude/partially purified

Table 16.4: Major Phytochemical Biopesticides and Status of their Use

Sl.No.	*Compound*	*Natural Source*	*Mechanism of Activity*	*Status of Use*	*Reference*
1.	Azadirachtin	Neem	Ecdysteroid and JH receptor inhibition	Extensively used as biopesticide	Mordue *et al.*, 2000
2.	Pyrethrins	Chrysanthemum	Neurotoxin	Not used extensively recently	Narahashi, 1971
3.	Rotenone	*Pachyrhizuserosus* and other Fabaceae members	Inhibits transfer of electron from complex to ubiquinone in ETC	Banned its usage commercially	Hayes, 1991
4.	Camphene	*Eucalyptus globulus*	Neurotoxin, Reproductive toxicity	Chlorinated Camphene compounds are banned	PAN Pesticide database
5.	Nicotine	Nightshade family plants	acetylcholine receptor agonist	Banned its usage commercially	Narahashi *et al.*, 2000
6.	Anabasine	*Nicotiana glauca*	Neurotoxin	Banned it usage commercially	Mann and Kaufman, 2012
7.	Ryanodine	*Ryania speciosa*	Calcium channel inhibitor	Usage banned commercially	Wikipedia.org
8.	Physostigmine	*Physostigmav enenosum*	Acetyl cholinesterase inhibitor	Usage Banned	Katzung *et al.*, 2009
9.	Skimmianine	Rutaceae family plants	Acetyl cholinesterase inhibitor	Usage banned as insecticide	Yang *et al.*, 2011

Table 16.5: Phytochemicals and Bioactivities Identified from some Plants and Fungi

Sl.No.	*Natural source*	*Compounds Identified*	*Reported Bioactivity*	*Status of Use*	*Reference*
1.	*Annona squamosa*	Ethyl oleate, Iso-octyl phthalate	Pest management	R, C	Kempraj and Bhat, 2011
2.	*Cyperus rotundus*	Cyprene, Cyerotundon	Pest management	R	Kempraj and Bhat, 2008
3.	*Coriandrum sativum* (Coriander)	Linalool	Pest management	R	Bhat and Kempraj, 2008
4.	*Syzygium aromaticum* (Clove)	EugenolIso-Eugenol	Pest management	R, C	Bhat and Kempraj, 2009
5.	*Calotropis* spp.(Milk weed)	Calactin, Calotropin, Cymarin, Asceplin	Anti-cancer, Anti-mitotic	R	Bhat and Sharma, 2013; Bhat *et al.*, 2013
6.	*Piper betle* (Betel vine)	Safrole, Eugenol, Benzoic acid	Antifungal	R	Unpublished
7.	*Agaricus bisporus* (Button mushroom)	Camphor	Antibacterial; antifungal*	R	Ramya *et al.*, 2013;* Unpublished
8.	*Pleurotus ostreatus* (Oyster mushroom)	Camphor	Antibacterial; antifungal*	R	Ramya *et al.*, 2013; *Unpublished

R: Research and development; C: Commercially available; T: Traditionally used; S: Nutritional supplement botanical extracts. The advantage of phytochemicals over synthetic counterparts as candidates for dug development on various grounds such as their heterogeneity, complex interactions and non toxicity collectively contribute towards extra edge of these compounds as pre drug molecules. Considering these facts, emphasis needs to be provided to advanced aspects of drug development research on identified pre drug phytochemicals, preferably in combination of two or more compounds synergistically for development of novel antibiotic therapeutics.

Phytochemicals have established a firm identity among the spectrum of chemotherapeutic agents in current use for cancer therapy. Further, several reports have confirmed multiple mechanisms of action involved in the process of prevention or inhibition of cancer by phytochemicals (Jang *et al.*, 1997; Petersen and Alferman, 2001; Cichewicz *et al.*, 2004). In addition, many reports have suggested the synergistic and complementary roles of the consortia of antioxidant phytochemicals in fruits and vegetables in prevention of carcinogenesis (Liu, 2004; Neto, 2007; Aggarwal *et al.*, 2008). These facts indicate the promising future for phytochemicals in anticancer drug discovery research at basic, advanced and practical levels at an aggressive rate.

Use of phytochemicals as crude extract or purified fraction(s) for pest management has long history across the world. Reasonably good number of compounds of plant origin have established as successful biopesticides. Azhadirachtin is the pioneer molecule in the range and still being used extensively against wide spectrum of pests (Mordue *et al.*, 2000). Pyrethrin represents another successful compound among biopesticides (Narahashi, 1971). Rotenone and few other compounds though formulated for practical use, later got withdrawn due to certain environmental issues (Narahashi *et al.*, 2000; Mann and Kaufman, 2012; Katzung *et al.*, 2009; Yang *et al.*, 2011). A new range of compounds non-toxic to higher animals comprising higher fatty acids, acetogenins, etc. have been identified during recent years for their prospective use in pest management programs (Bhat and Kempraj, 2008; Kempraj and Bhat, 2008; Bhat and Kempraj, 2009). However, details on their long term success and about commercial and environmental aspects are yet to be envisaged. The ongoing discussion on applications of phytochemicals on various fields has emphasized the need for focused research leading to real time utility of the outcomes. As the distribution of useful phytochemicals across plant kingdom is uneven and standardization of extraction methods for high purity and high yield demand long time and extensive resources, low cost alternative source for plentiful supply of the compounds need to be invented for attaining real success of this strategy.

References

Adjei, A. A. (1999). A review of the pharmacology and clinical activity of new chemotherapy agents for the treatment of colorectal cancer. *Br. J Clin. Pharmacol.*, **48**: 265–277.

Aggarwal, B. B., Kunnumakkara, A.B., Harikumar, K. B., Tharakan, S.T., Sung, B., and Anand P. (2008). Potential of spice-derived phytochemicals for cancer prevention. *Planta Med.*, 1560-1569.

Ali-Shtayeh, M.S., Al-Nuri, M.A., Yaghmour, R.M.R., and Faidi, Y.R. (1997). Antimicrobial activity of *Micromeria nervosa* from the Palestinian (area. *J. Ethnopharmacol.*, **58**: 143–147.

Apisariyakul, A., Vanittanakom, N., and Buddhasukh D. (1995). Antifungal activity of turmeric oil extracted from *Curcuma longa* (Zingiberaceae). *J. Ethnopharmacol.*, **49**: 163–169.

Balandrin, M.F., and Klocke, J. A. (1988). Medicinal and aromatic plants I. In: Biotechnology in agriculture and forestry Vol 4. (Ed. Y. P. S. Bjaj), Springer-Verlag, Berlin, Heidelberg, pp 1-4.

Barrero, A.F., Quilez, J.F., and Herrador, M. (2003). Podolactones: a group of biologically active norditerpe- noids. *Stud Nat Prod Chem.*, **28**: 453–516.

Bercovitch, M., Waller, A., and Adunsky, A. (1999). High dose morphine use in the hospice setting. A database survey of patient characteristics and effect on life expectancy. *Cancer*, **86**: 871–877.

Bharadwaj, S., Achliya, G. S., Meghre, V. S., Wadodkar, S.G., and Dorle, A.K. (2005). *In vitro* antibacterial activity of Takrarishta – an ayurvedic formulation. *Indian J. Traditional Knowledge*, **4(3)**: 325-328.

Bhat, S. K., and Kempraj, V. (2008). Evaluation of acaricidal potential of essential oils of plants against coconut mite. *Indian coconut J.*, **LI (1)**: 5-8.

Bhat, S. K., and Kempraj, V. (2009). Biocidal potential of clove oils against *Aedes albopictus* – A comparative study. *Afr. J. Biotechnol.*, **8(24)**: 6933-6937.

Bhat, S. K., and Sharma, A. (2013). Therapeutic potential of cardiac glycosides of *Calotropis gigantea* for breast cancer. *Int. Res. J. Pharmacy*, **4(6)**: 164 – 167.

Bhat, S.K., Singhal, K., Shruti Priya and Pal, S. (2013). Evaluation of antimitotic effect of *calotropis procera* l on *Allium cepa* L. *Int. J. Pharmacy*, **3(2)**: 356-359.

Bidlack, W. R. (2000). Preface. In: Bidlack, W. R., Omage S. T., Meskin, M. S., and Topham D.K. W.(Eds.), Phytochemicals as bioactive agents. CRC Press LLC, Florida, USA.

Biradar, Y. S., Jagatap, S., Khandelwal, K.R., and Singhania, S. S. (2008). Exploring of antimicrobial activity of Triphala *Mashi* – an ayurvedic formulation. *Evid. Based Complement. Alternat. Med.*, **5(1)**: 107- 113.

Birdsall, T., and Kelly, G. (1997). Berberine: therapeutic potential of an alkaloid in several medicinal plants. *Altern Med Rev.*, **2**: 94–103.

Bo, T., Li, K.A., and Liu, H. (2002). Fast determination of flavonoids in *Glycyrrhiza radix* by capillary zone electrophoresis. *Anal Chim Acta.*, **458**: 345–354.

Bose, P. K. (1958). On some biochemical properties of natural coumarins. *J. Indian Chem. Soc.*, **58**: 367–375.

Buckingham, J. (2005). *Dictionary of Natural Products* on CD-ROM, v. 13: 1. Chapman and Hall/CRC Press, Boca Raton, Florida.

Budavari, S. (Ed.). (2001). *The Merck Index*. 13th ed. Merck and Co, Whitehouse Station, New Jersey.

Butterworth J., and Morgan E. (1968). Isolation of a substance that suppresses feeding in locusts. *Chemical communications* (London), 1: 23. doi: 1039/c19680000023.

Cassady, J.M., and Douros, J.D. (1980). Anticancer Agents Based on Natural Product Models, Academic Press, New York, 1980.

Cellárová, E., Kimakova, K., Daxnerova, Z., and Martonfi, P. (1995). *Hypericum perforatum* (St. John's wort): *in vitro* culture and production of hypericin and other secondary metabolites. In *Biotechnology in Agriculture and Forestry*, Vol. 33, *Medicinal and Aromatic Plants VIII*, Y.P. Bajaj (Ed.). Springer-Verlag, Heidelberg, pp. 261–275.

Ceske Leland J., Ara Kirakosyan, Peter B Kaufman, Sara L Warber, James A Duke, and Harry L Brielmann. (2006). *Natural product from plants*, ISBN 0-8490-2976-0.

Chabner, B. A., and Roberts, T. G. (2005). Chemotherapy and the war on cancer. *Nature Rev. Cancer*, **5**: 65-72.

Cichewicz, R. H., and Thorpe, P. (1996). The antimicrobial properties of chile peppers (*Capsicum* species) and their uses in Mayan medicine. *J. Ethnopharmacol.*, **52**: 61–70.

Cichewicz, R.H., Zhang, Y., Seeram, N.P., and Nair, M.G. (2004). Inhibition of human tumor cell proliferation by novel anthraquinones from daylilies. *Life Sci.*,**74**: 1791–1799.

Clark, G.S. (1990). Leaf alcohol. *Perfumer and Flavorist*, **15**: 47–52.

Cordell, G. (1981). *Introduction to Alkaloids: A Biogenetic Approach*. Wiley and Sons, New York.

Cornwell, T., Cohick, W., and Raskin, I. (2004). Dietary phytoestrogens and health. *Phytochemistry*, **65**: 995–1016.

Cowan, M.M. (1999). Plant products as antimicrobial agents. *Clin. Microbiol. Rev.*, **12(4)**: 564–582.

Crowell, P.L., and Gould, M.N. (2004). Cancer chemopreventive activity of monoterpenes and other isoprenoids. *Cancer Chemoprevention*, **1**: 371–378.

Cushnie, T.P., Hamilton, V.E., and Lamb, A.J. (2003). Assessment of the antibacterial activity of selected flavonoids and consideration of discrepancies between previous reports. *Microbiol Res.*, **158**: 281–289.

De Lorgeril, M., and Salen, P. (2004). A-linolenic acid and coronary heart disease. *Nutr Metab Cardiovasc Dis.*, **14**: 162–169.

Dembitsky, V.M. (2006). Anticancer activity of natural and synthetic acetylenic lipids. *Lipids*, **41**: 883.

DeVita, Jr. V. T., and Chu, E. (2014). A history of cancer chemotherapy. *Caner Res.*, **68(21)**: 8642 – 8653.

Dong, X., Hamburger, M.O., Cordell, G.A., and Fong, H.H.S. (1989). Studies on zoapatle. IX. HPLC analysis of *Montanoa* species for pharmacologically active constituents. *Planta Medica,* **55**: 185–187.

Duke, J. A. (1985). Handbook of medicinal herbs. CRC Press, Inc., Boca Raton, Fla.

Duke, S.O. (1991). Plant Terpenoids as Pesticides. In *Toxicology of Plant and Fungal Compounds. Handbook of Natural Toxins, Vol. 6.,* R.F. Keeler and A.T. Tu, Eds., Marcel Dekker, New York, pp. 269-296.

Duke, S.O., Rimando A.M., Dayan F. E., Canel C., Wedge D.E., Tellez M. R. Schrader, K.K., Weston L.A., Smillie T. J., Paul R. N., and Duke M. V. (2000). Strategies for the discovery of bioactive Phytochemicals. In: Phytochemicals as bioactive agents, Eds: Bidlack, W. R., Omaye, S. T., Meskin, M. S., Topham D. K. W. CRC Press, Florida, USA, pp. 1-20.

El Bardai, S., N. Morel, M. Wibo, N. Fabre, G. Llabres, B. Lyoussi, and J. Quetin-Leclercq. (2003). The vasorelaxant activity of marrubenol and marrubiin from *Marrubium vulgare. Planta Medica,* **69**: 75–77.

Fenwick, G.R., J. Lutomski, and C. Nieman. (1990). Liquorice, *Glycyrrhiza glabra* L.– Composition, uses and analysis. *Food Chem.,* **38**: 119–143.

Fishel, F. M. (2005) (revised 2011). Pesticide effects on non target organisms. University of Florida IFAS Extension document PI - 85[http: / /edis.ifas.ufl.edu. accessed on 30/5/11].

Flynn, J. (1991). *Cocaine: An In-depth Look at the Facts, Science, History, and Future of the World's Most Addictive Drug*. Birch Lane, New York.

Fowler, M.W. (2006). Plants, medicines and man. *J Sci Food Agric.,* **86**: 1797- 1804.

Freiburghaus, F., Kaminsky, R., Nkunya, M. H. H., and Brun, R. (1996). Evaluation of African medicinal plants for their *in vitro* trypanocidal activity. *J. Ethnopharmacol.,* **55**: 1–11.

Fukuzawa, A., and E. Kurosawa. (1979). Constituents of marine plants. Part XXXVI. Laurallene, a new bromoallene from the marine red alga *Laurencia nipponica* Yamada. *Tet Lett.,* **30**: 2797–2800.

Fukuzawa, A. *et al.* (1985). Structure of a new bromoditerpene, prepinnaterpene, from the red alga *Laurencia pinnata* Yamada. *Chem Lett.,* **8**: 1263.

Geissman, T.A., and Crout, D.H.G. (1969). *Organic Chemistry of Secondary Plant Metabolism*. Freeman Cooper, San Francisco, California.

Ghoshal, S., Krishna Prasad, B. N., and Lakshmi, V. (1996). Antiamoebic (activity of *Piper longum* fruits against *Entamoeba histolytica in vitro* and *in vivo. J. Ethnopharmacol.,* **50**: 167–170.

Gonzalez, R. H., Buyckx, E. J., and Brader, L. (1970). In *Natural Products and the Protection of Plants* (ed. Marini-Bettolo, G. B.), Elsevier Scientific and Publishing Company, New York, 1977, pp. 687–707.

Graefe, E.U., Derendorf, H., and Veit, M. (1999). Pharmacokinetics and bioavailability of the flavonol quercetin in humans. *Int J Clin Pharmacol Ther.*, **37**: 219–233.

Guella, G., Mancini, I. Chiasera, G., and Pietra, F. (1992). On the unusual propensity by the red seaweed *Laurencia microcladia* of Il Rogiolo to form C15 oxepanes: isolation of rogioloxepane A, B, and C, and their likely biogenetic acyclic precursor, prerogioloxepane. *Helv Chim Acta.*, **75**: 310–322.

Gurib-Fakin, A. (2006). Medicinal plants: Tradition of yesterday and drugs of tomorrow. *Mol Aspects Med.*, **27**: 1- 93.

Hairborne, J.B. (1993). *The Flavonoids Advances in Research since 1986*; Chapman and Hall: London, UK, 1993; pp. 1–676.

Hamburger, H., and Hostettmann, K. (1991). The link between phytochemistry and medicine. *Phytochemistry*, **30**: 3864–3874.

Hayes, W.J. (1991). *Handbook on Pesticides, Volume 1*. Academic Press. ISBN 0123341612.

Haynes, R.K., and Vonwiller, S.C. (1994). Extraction of artemisinin and artemisinic acid: preparation of artemether and new analogues. *Transactions of the Royal Society of Tropical Medicine and Hygiene*, **88 (Suppl. 1)**: 23–26.

Himejima, M., and Kubo, I. (1991). Antibacterial agents from the cashew *Anacardium occidentale. J. Agric. Food Chem.*, **39**: 418–421.

Hoet, S., Opperdoes, F., Brun, R., and Quetin-Leclercq, J. (2004). Natural products active against African trypanosomes: a step towards new drugs. *Nat Prod Rep.*, **21**: 353–364.

Holopainen, J.K. (2004). Multiple functions of inducible plant volatiles. *Trends in Plant Sci.*, **9**: 529–533. http: //www.uku.fi/~holopain/Holopainen-Trends-2004-revised.pdf.

Honigsbaum, M. (2002). *The Fever Trail: In Search of the Cure for Malaria*. Farrar, Straus, and Giroux, New York.

Hufford, C. D., Jia, Y., Croom, E. M. Jr., Muhammed, I., Okunade, A. L., Clark, A. M., and Rogers, R. D. (1993). Antimicrobial compounds from *Petalostemum purpureum. J. Nat. Prod.*, **56**: 1878–1889.

Hunter, M. D., and Hull, L. A. (1993). Variation in concentrations of phloridzin and phloretin in apple foliage. *Phytochemistry*, **34**: 1251–1254.

Irie, T., Susuki, M., and Masamune, T. (1965). Constituents from marine plants. II. Laurencin, a constituent from *Laurencia* species. *Tet Lett.*, 1**6**: 1091–1092.

Jacobi, P.A., DeSimone, R.W., Ghosh, I., Guo, J., Leung, S.H.m and Pippin, D. (2000). New syntheses of the C,D-rings of pyrromethenones of phytochrome and phycocyanin. *J Org Chem.*, **65**: 8478–8489.

Jang, M., Cai, L., Udeani, G.O., Slowing, K.V., Thomas, C.F., Beecher, C.W., Fong, H.H., Farnsworth, N.R., Kinghorn, A.D., Mehta, R.G., Moon, R.C., and Pezzuto, J.M. (1997). Cancer chemopreventive activity of resveratrol, a natural product derived from grapes. *Science*, **275**: 218–220.

Johnson, I.T. (2003). Glusosinolates in the human diet. Bioavailability and implications for health. *Phytochem Rev.*, **1**: 183–188.

Jones, W.P., Chin, Y.W., and Kinghorn, A.D. (2006). The role of pharmacognosy in modern medicine and pharmacy. *Curr Drug Targets,* **7**: 247 – 264.

Jones, S. B., Jr., and Luchsinger, A. E. (1986). Plant systematics. McGraw- Hill Book Co., New York, N.Y.

Jordan, M.A. (2002). Mechanism of action of antitumor drugs that interact with microtubules and tubulin. *Curr Med Chem Anti-Canc Agents,* **2**: 1–17.

Kadota, S., Basnet, P., Ishii, E. Tamura, T., and Namba, T. (1997). Antibacterial activity of trichorabdal from *Rabdosia trichocarpa* against *Helicobacter pylori. Zentbl. Bakteriol.,* **286**: 63–67.

Katiyar, S. (2005). Silymarin and skin cancer prevention: anti-inflammatory, antioxidant and immunomodulatory effects (Review). *Int J Oncol.,* **26**: 169–176.

Katzung, B. G., Masters, S., and Trever, A. (2009). *Basic and Clinical Pharmacology*. McGraw Hill. p. 110. ISBN 978-0-07-160405-5.

Kaufman, P.B., Duke, J.A., Brielmann, H., Boik, J., and Hoyt, J.E. (1997). A comparative survey of leguminous plants as sources of the isoflavones, genistein and daidzein: implications for human nutrition and health. *J Altern Complement Med.,* **3**: 7–12.

Kempraj, V., and Bhat, S. K. (2008). Ovicidal and larvicidal activities of *Cyperus giganteus* Vahland *Cyperus rotundus* Linn. essential oils against *Aedes albopictus* (Skuse). *Nat. Product Rad.,* **7 (5)**: 420-425.

Keating, G. J., and O'Kennedy, R. 1997. The chemistry and occurrence of coumarins, p. 348. *In* R. O'Kennedy and R. D. Thornes (ed.), Coumarins: biology, applications and mode of action. John Wiley and Sons, Inc., New York, N.Y.

Kempraj, V., and Bhat, S. K. (2008). Ovicidal and larvicidal activities of *Cyperus giganteus* Vahl and *Cyperus rotundus* Linn.essential oils against *Aedes albopictus* (Skuse). *Nat. Product Rad.,* **7 (5)**: 420-425.

Kempraj, V., and Bhat, S.K. (2011). Acute and reproductive toxicity of *Annona squamosa* to *Aedes albopictus*. *Pesticide Biochem. Physiol.,* **100**: 82-86.

Kesavachandran, C., and Mudiam, (2010). Adverse sub-clinical health effects in pesticide-exposed population: challenges and need for developing non-invasive clinical biomarkers. *Curr. Sci.,* **99(12)**: 1643.

Koushik, A., Sharma, H. R., Jain, S., Dawra, J., and Koushik, C. P. (2010). Pesticide pollution of River Ghaggar in Haryana, India. *Environ. Monit. Assess.,* **169**: 61-69.

Kris-Etherton, P.M., Hecker, K.D. Bonanome, A. Coval, S.M., Binkoski, A.E., Hilpert, K.F. Griel, A.E., and Etherton, T.D. (2002). Bioactive compounds in foods: their role in the prevention of cardiovascular disease and cancer. *Am J Med.,* **113 (Suppl 9B)**: 71–88.

Krishna Kumari, G.N., S. Aravind, J. Balachandran, M.R. Ganesh, S. Soundarya Devi, S.S. Rajan, R. Malathi, and K. Ravikumar. (2003). Antifeedant neo-clerodanes from *Teucrium tomentosum* Heyne (Labiatae). *Phytochemistry,* **64**: 1119–1123.

Kubo, I., Muroi, H., and Kubo, A. (1994). Naturally occurring anti-acne agents. *J. Nat. Prod.,* **57**: 9–17.

Kubo, I., Muroi, H., and Himejima, M. (1992). Antibacterial activity of totarol and its potentiation. *J. Nat. Prod.,* **55**: 1436–1440.

Kubo, I., Muroi, H., and Himejima, M. (1993). Combination effects of antifungal nagilactones against *Candida albicans* and two other fungi with phenylpropanoids. *J. Nat. Prod.,* **56**: 220–226.

Librowski, T., Vetulani, J., and Nalepa, I. (2004). Carane derivative stereoisomers of different local anaesthetic and antiplatelet activity similarly potentiate forskolin-stimulated cyclic AMP response and bind to β-adrenoceptors in the rat brain cortex. *J Pharm Pharmacol.,* **56**: 1429–1434.

Liu, R H. (2004). Potential synergy of phytochemicals in cancer prevention: Mechanism of action. *J Nutrition,* 3479S- 3485S.

Liu, Z., and J. Adams. (1996). Camptothecin yield and distribution within *Camptotheca accuminata* trees cultivated in Louisiana. *Can J Bot.,* **74**: 360–365.

Lydon, J., and Duke, S.O. (1989). The Potential of Pesticides from Plants. In *Herbs, Spices, and Medicinal Plants: Recent Advances in Botany, Horticulture, und Pharmacology, Vol. 4,* L.E.Craker and J.E. Simon, Eds., Oryx Press, Phoenix, AZ, pp. 1-41.

Lydon, J., and Duke, S.O. (1989). The Potential of Pesticides from Plants. In *Herbs, Spices, and Medicinal Plants: Recent Advances in Botany, Horticulture, und Pharmacology, Vol. 4,* L.E.Craker and J.E. Simon, Eds., Oryx Press, Phoenix, AZ, pp. 1-41.

Mann, R.S., and Kaufman, P.E. (2012). Natural product pesticides: Their development, delivery and use against insect vectors. *Mini-Reviews in Organic Chemistry,* **9**: 185-202.

Martinez, M. J., Betancourt, J., Alonso-Gonzalez, N., and Jauregui, A. (1996). Screening of some Cuban medicinal plants for antimicrobial activity. *J. Ethnopharmacol.,* **52**: 171–174.

McDevitt, J. T., Schneider, D. M., Katiyar, S. K., and Edlind, T. D. (1996). Berberine: a candidate for the treatment of diarrhea in AIDS patients, abstr. 175. *In* Program and Abstracts of the 36th Interscience Conference on Antimicrobial Agents and Chemotherapy. American Society for Microbiology, Washington, D.C.

McGeady, P., Wansley, D.L., and Logan, D.A. (2002). Carvone and perillaldehyde interfere with the serum- induced formation of filamentous structures in *Candida albicans* at substantially lower concentrations than those causing significant inhibition of growth. *J Nat Prod.,* **65**: 953–955.

Miyashita, K., A. Tanaka, H. Shintaku, and Iwata, C. (1998). Regiospecific bromination-cyclization of spirocyclic cyclohexanones and its application to the synthesis of (+-)-laurencial. *Tetrahedron*, **54**: 1395–1406.

Mordue (Luntz), A., Jennifer, and Nisbet, Alasdair J. (2000). Azadirachtin from the neem tree *Azadirachta indica*: its action against insects. *Anais da SociedadeEntomológica do Brasil*, **29(4)**: 615-632.

Moshonas, M.G. (1971). Analysis of carbonyl flavor constituents from grapefruit oil. *J Agric Food Chem.*, 19: 769–770.

Moteki, H., Hibasami, H., Yamada, Y., Katsuzaki, H., Imai, K., and Komiya, T. (2002). Specific induction of apoptosis by 1,8-cineole in two human leukemia cell lines, but not in a human stomach cancer cell line. *Oncol. Rep.*, **9**: 757–760.

Naganawa, R., Iwata, N., Ishikawa, K., Fukuda, H., Fujino, T., and Suzuki, A. (1996). Inhibition of microbial growth by ajoene, a sulfur-containing compound derived from garlic. *Appl. Environ. Microbiol.*, **62**: 4238–4242.

Naj, J.J., Hahn, J.H., Chung, S., Kim, Y.I., and Nah, S.Y. (2000). Effects of ginsenosides, active components of ginseng, on capsaicin-induced pain-related behavior. *Neuropharmacology,* **39**: 2180–2184.

Nakagawa-Goto, K., Chen, C.X., Hamel, E., Wu, C.C., Bastow, K.F., Brossi, A., and Lee, K.H. (2005). Antitumor agents. Part 236: synthesis of water-soluble colchicine derivatives. *Bioorg Med Chem Lett.*, 15: 235–238.

Narahashi, T. (1971). Mode of action of pyrethroids. *Bull. Wld. Hlth. Org.*, **44**: 337-345.

Narahashi, T.1., Fenster, C. P., Quick, M. W., Lester, R. A. J., Marszalec, W., Aistrup, G. L., Sattelle, D. B., Martin, B. R., and Levin, E. D. (2000). Symposium overview: Mechanism of action of nicotine on neuronal acetylcholine receptors, from molecule to behavior. *Toxicol. Sci.*, **57 (2)**: 193-202. doi: 10.1093/toxsci/57.2.193.

Navarro, V., Villarreal, M. L., Rojas, G., and Lozoya, X. (1996). Antimicrobial evaluation of some plants used in Mexican traditional medicine for the treatment of infectious diseases. *J. Ethnopharmacol.*, **53**: 143–147.

Nawar, H. F., and Kuti, J.O. (2003). Wyerone acid phytoalexin synthesis and peroxidase activity as markers for resistance of broad beans to chocolate spot disease. *J Phytopathol.*, **151**: 564–570.

Neto, C. C. (2007). Cranberry and its phytochemicals: A review of *in vitro* anticancer studies. *J Nutrition*, 186S- 193S.

Newman, R. A., Yang, P., Pawlus, A. D., and Block, K. I. (2008). Cardiac glycosides as novel cancer therapeutic agents. *Mol. Intervent.*, **8(1)**: 36-49.

Notka, F., Meier, G., and Wagner, R. (2004). Concerted inhibitory activities of *Phyllanthus amarus* on HIV replication *in vitro* and *ex vivo*. *Antiviral Res.*, **64**: 93–102.

Ntalli, N.G., and Menkissoglu-Spiroudi (2011). Pesticides of Botanical Origin: A Promising Tool in Plant Protection. In: Pesticides - Formulations, Effects, Fate, (Ed. Stoytcheva, M.), InTech, [Open Access Publisher, ISBN 978-953-307-532-7] January 2011.

Ofek, I., Goldhar, J., and Sharon, N. (1996). Anti-*Escherichia coli* adhesin activity of cranberry and blueberry juices. *Adv. Exp. Med. Biol.*, **408**: 179–183.

Ohnuma, T., and J.F. Holland. (1985). Homoharringtonine as a new antileukemic agent. *J Clin Oncol.*, **73**: 604–606.

Omulokoli, E., Khan, B., and Chhabra, S. C. (1997). Antiplasmodial activity of four Kenyan medicinal plants. *J. Ethnopharmacol.*, **56**: 133–137.

Pachlatko, J.P. (1998). Natural products in crop production. *Chimia*, **52**: 29-47.

PAN Pesticide database, http: //www.pesticideinfo.org/ Detail_Chemical.jsp?Rec_Id=PC36180

Parmar, B. S., and Devkumar, C. (1993). in *Botanical and Biopesticides*, West Vill Publishing House, New Delhi, 1993, pp. 197–199.

Paul, L.D., Springer, D., Staack, R.F., Kraemer, T., and Maurer, H.H. (2003). Cytochrome P450 isoenzymes involved in rat liver microsomal metabolism of californine and protopine. *Eur J Pharmacol.*, **485**: 69–79.

Pazdur, R. *et al.* (1993). The taxoids: paclitaxel (Taxol®) and docetaxel (Taxotere®). *Canc Treat Rev.*, **19**: 351–386.

Perrett, S., Whitfield, P. J., Sanderson, L., and Bartlett, A. (1995). The plant molluscicide *Millettia thonningii* (Leguminosae) as a topical antischistosomal agent. *J. Ethnopharmacol.*, **47**: 49–54.

Petersen, M., and A.W. Alfermann. (2001). The production of cytotoxic lignans by plant cell cultures. *Appl Microbiol Biotechnol.*, **55**: 135–142.

Pimentel, D., and Levitan, L. (1986). Pesticides: amounts applied and amounts reaching pests. *Biosciences*, **36**: 86-91

Ramya, R., Satish, K., Shubhashree Rao, Manasa, D.A., Gaganashilpa, Sandhya, S., and Bhat, S.K. (2013). Comparative evaluation of antimicrobial activity of fresh and dried samples of mushrooms. *Int. J. Recent Scientific Res.*, **4(12)**: 1946-1948.

Reddy, P., Chadaga, S., and Noskin, G.A. (2009). Antibiotic considerations in the treatment of multidrug-resistant (MDR) pathogens: a case-based review. *J Hosp Med.*, **4(6)**: E8-15.

Robbers, J.E., Speedie, M.K., and Tyler, V.E. (1996). *Pharmacognosy and Pharmacobiotechnology.* Williams and Wilkins, Baltimore, 337 pp.

Roengsumran, S. *et al.* (2002). Croblongifolin, a new anticancer clerodane from *Croton oblongifolius, Planta Med.*, **68**: 274–277.

Russo, M., Spagnuolo,C., Tedesco, I., and Russo, G.L. (2010). Potential synergy of phytochemicals in cancer prevention: Mechanism of action. *Toxins*, **2**: 517-551.

Russo, M., Spagnuolo, C., Tedesco, I., and Russo, G. L. (2010). Phytochemicals in cancer prevention and therapy: Truth or dare? *Toxins*, **2**: 517-551.

Redl, K., Breu, W., and Davis, B. (1994). Anti-inflammatory active polyacetylenes from *Bidens campylotheca*. *Planta Medica*, **60**: 58–62.

Rivera-Vargas, L.I., Schmitthenner, A.F., and Graham, T.L. (1993). Soybean flavonoid effects on and metabolism by *Phytophthora sojae*. *Phytochemistry,* **32**: 851–857.

Salim, A.A., Chin, Y.-W., and Kinghorn, A.D. (2008). Drug discovery from plants. In: Biactive molecules and medicinal plants. Rmawat K.G. and Merillon, J. M. (Eds), Springer, pp 1 - 18.

Schultes, R. E. (1978). The kingdom of plants, p. 208. *In* W. A. R. Thomson (ed.), Medicines from the Earth. McGraw-Hill Book Co., New York, N.Y.

Seeram, N. P., Adams, L. S., Henning, S. M., Niu, Y., Zhang, Y., Nair, M.G., and Heber, D. (2005). *In vitro* antiproliferative, apoptotic and antioxidant activities of punicalagin, ellagic acid and a total pomegranate tannin extract are enhanced in combination with other polyphenols as found in pomegranate juice. *The J Nutr. Biochem.,* **16(6)**: 360-367.

Seiber, J. (1991). Paper-Overview of the Problem of Pesticides in Ground Water: Factors which Influence Fate Processes, California EPA.

Sinha, B., and Biswas, I. (2008). Potential of biopesticide in Indian agriculture vis-à-vis rural development. In: India, Science and Technology, 2008. NISTADS, CSIR, 2008 pp. 340 -343. [http: / /www.nistads.res.in/indiasnt2008/accessed on 6/ 1/2011].

Stimanek, V. *et al.* (1990). Phytochemical studies of Turkish Colchicum and Merendera species. *Herb. Hung.,* **29**: 64.

Samuelsson, G. (2001). *Drugs of Natural Origin: A Textbook of Pharmacognosy*. 4th ed., Swedish Pharmaceutical Press, Stockholm, Sweden, p. 149.

San-Blas, G., San-Blas, F.F,. Gil Marino, L., and Apitz-Castro, R. (1989). Inhibition of growth of the dimorphic fungus *Paracoccidioides brasiliensis* by ajoene. *Antimicrob. Agents Chemother.,* **33**: 1641–1644.

San-Blas, G., L. Marino, F. San-Blas, and R. Apitz-Castro. 1993. Effect of ajoene on dimorphism of *Paracoccidioides brasiliensis. J. Med. Vet. Mycol.,* **31**: 133–141.

Scheel, L. D. (1972). The biological action of the coumarins. *Microbiol. Toxins,* **8**: 47–66.

Shrestha, K., Banskota, A.H., Kodata, S., Shrivastava, S.P., Strobel, G., and Gewali, M.B. (2001). An antiproliferative norditerpene dilactone, Nagilactone C, from *Podocarpus neriifolius. Phytomedicine,* **8**: 489–491.

Sirisoma, N.S., Hold, K.M., and Casida J.E. (2001). ?- and ?-thujones (herbal medicines and food additives): synthesis and analysis of hydroxyl and dehydro metabolites. *J Agric Food Chem.,* **49**: 1915–1921.

Sridar, C., Goosen, T.C., Kent, U.M., Williams, J.A., and Hollenberg, P.F. (2004). Silybin inactivates cytochromes P450 3A4 and 2C9 and inhibits major hepatic glucuronosyltransferases. *Drug Metab Dispos.,* **32**: 587–594.

Stange, R. R., Jr., Midland, S. L., Eckert, J. W., and Sims, J. J. (1993). An antifungal compound produced by grapefruit and Valencia orange after wounding of the peel. *J. Nat. Prod.,* **56**: 1627–1629.

Suresh, B., Sriram, S., Dhanaraj, S. A., Elango, K., and Chinnaswamy, K. (1997). Anticandidal activity of *Santolina chamaecyparissus* volatile oil. *J. Ethnopharmacol.*, **55**: 151–159.

Suth, Y. J. (2003). Cancer chemoprevention with dietary phytochemicals. *Nat. Rev. Cancer*, **3(10)**: 768-780.

Suzuki, T., Koizumi, K., Suzuki, M., and Kurosawa, E. (1983). Constituents of marine plants. 56. Kumausallene, a new bromoallene from the marine red alga *Laurencia nipponica* Yamada. *Chem Lett.*, **10**: 1639–1641.

Taylor, C.E., and Greenough, W.B. (1989). Control of diarrheal diseases. *Annu Rev Public Health,* **10**: 221–244.

Thomson, W. A. R. (ed.). (1978). Medicines from the Earth. McGraw-Hill Book Co., Maidenhead, United Kingdom.

Ugbogu, A. E., Akubugwo, E. I., Iweala, E.J. J., Uhegbu, F. O., Chinyere, G. C., and Obasi, N. A. (2013). Role of phytochemicals in chemoprevention of cancer: A review. *Int J Pharmaceutical and Chemical Sci.*, **2(2)**: 566-575.

Uma Shaanker, R., Ramesha, B.T., Ravikanth, G., Gunaga, R.P., Vasudev, R., and Ganeshaiah, K.N. (2008). Chemical profiling of *Nothapodytes nimmoniana* for camptothecin, an important anticancer alkaloid: towards the development of a sustainable production system. In: Biactive molecules and medicinal plants. Rmawat K.G. and Merillon, J. M. (Eds), Springer, pp 198-210.

Ustunes, L., Laekeman, G.M., Gozler, B., Vlietinck, A. J., Ozer, A., and Herman, A.G. (1988). *In vitro* study of the anticholinergic and antihistaminic activities of protopine and some derivatives. *J Nat Prod.*, **51**: 1021–1022.

Utsunomiya, T., Kobayashi, M. Pollard, R.B., and Suzuki. (1997). Glycyrrhizin, an active component of licorice roots, reduces morbidity and mortality of mice infected with lethal doses of influenza virus. *Antimicrob Agents Chemother.*, **41**: 551–556.

Vijaya, K., Ananthan, S., and Nalini, R. (1995). Antibacterial effect of the aflavin, polyphenon 60 (*Camellia sinensis*) and *Euphorbia hirta* on *Shigella* spp.–a cell culture study. *J. Ethnopharmacol.*, **49**: 115–118.

Walker, K., and R. Croteau. (2001). Taxol biosynthetic genes. *Phytochemistry,* **58**: 1–7.

Warren, M. (2004). *Tetrapyrroles,* Landes Bioscience, Georgetown, Texas.

Wikipedia, en.wikipedia.org/wiki/Ryanodine

Yang, Zhong-duo., Zhang, Dong-bo., Ren, Jin., Yang, Ming-jun (2011). Skimmianine, a furoquinoline alkaloid from Zanthoxylumnitidum as a potential acetylcholinesterase inhibitor. *Medicinal Chemistry Research,* **21** (6): 722.

Yoshida, S., Kasuga, S., Hayashi, N., Ushiroguchi, T., Matsuura, and Nakagawa, S. (1987). Antifungal activity of ajoene derived from garlic. *Appl. Environ.Microbiol.*, **53**: 615–617.

Youdim, K.A., Martin, A., and Joseph, J.A. (2000). Essential fatty acids and the brain: possible health implications. *Int J Dev Neurosci.*, **18**: 383–399.

Bioactive Phytochemicals: Perspectives for Modern Medicine Vol. 3 (2015) *Pages* **437–447**
Editor: **V.K. Gupta**
Published by: **DAYA PUBLISHING HOUSE, NEW DELHI**

17

New Phyto-Enzymes of Therapeutic and Industrial Values

Subhabrata Sengupta[1*], Abhishek Mukherjee[1] and Subhasree Sengupta[1]

ABSTRACT

Plant enzymes have a little share in global enzyme market except for a few obtained from edible fruits or cereals (papain, bromelian, ficin, malt extract etc). Food industries have obligation to use enzymes from edible sources although plant enzymes are costly than microbial enzymes. Research on plant enzymes remained confined within those on germinating cereals as a source of amylase for brewing process. Sengupta et al. (2002) first reported profuse production of extracellular saccharifying amylase by the plant Tinospora cordifolia Miers. Before this invention, presence of huge extracellular amylase by any plant biomass was not known. T. cordifolia is a succulent climbing shrub, grows wild throughout the year producing huge biomass. The medicinal plant grows in different parts of India and is used for the treatment of various diseases including diabetes. The fresh plant stem (100 g) contains 30,000-50,000 units of extractable amylase. The amylase purified, was a 40k Da thiol protein. The plant amylase was superior to fungal amylase in terms of digestion of cereals, stability in stomach pH ranges set during digestion, excellent acid pH stability and wide substrate specificities. Further study by the same group reported presence of a number of disaccharidases in the same plant, useful for the treatment of disaccharidase deficiency diseases including lactose intolerance. The fresh plant stem (100 g) contains acid maltase, iso-maltase, sucrase, acid lactase (ß-galactosidase), cellobiase, trehalase at average amounts of 400,130, 370, 3500, 35 and 40 U respectively. The enzyme composition is similar to that reported to be present per gram of human intestinal mucosa. Lactase present was an acid lactase (optimum at pH 4.0), similar to the type linked with human lactose intolerance. A multi-substrate specific sucrase-

1 Department of Biotechnology, Heritage Institute of Technology, Anandapur, P.O. East Kolkata Township, Chowbaga Road, Kolkata – 700 107, India

* *Corresponding author*: E-mail: s.sengupta@heritageit.edu; profs_sengupta@yahoo.com

maltase has been purified from the crude enzyme. Disaccharidases enzyme mixture may be useful for enzyme therapy in disaccharidase deficiency disease. The crude enzyme is practically non toxic to mice up to oral dose of 1.5 g/Kg body. The study suggests that plant biomass should be explored more intensely to find useful enzymes which would be more acceptable than microbial enzyme in terms of safety and as a product of low cost Green technology suitable for our country with wide plant biodiversity.

Keywords: *Tinospora cordifolia*, Thiol amylase, Plant amylase, Plant disaccharidase, Disaccharide intolerance, Sucrase-maltase, Plant acid lactase.

Introduction

Plant enzymes have a little share in global enzyme market in spite of having more acceptability than microbial enzyme in food and pharmaceutical industries for various reasons (Jach *et al.*, 2010). Plant proteases (bromelain, papain, ficin etc.) are commercially used in brewing and food processing (De Roos *et al.*, 2007; Ross and Kang, 2008). Germinated cereals as a source of amylase have a commercial market and are used mainly for brewing processes. Use of amylase in industries is next to that of highest selling alkaline protease (Negi and Banerjee, 2006) and commercial amylases are mostly obtained from microbial sources like *Bacillus* and *Aspergillus* species (Sivaramakrishnan *et al.*, 2006). Amylases have been detected in many plants and are classified as family I (extra cellular), family II (cytosolic) and family III (plastidal) (Stanley *et al.*, 2005). But these enzymes are present in low amounts, unsuitable for commercial production. Actually, production of substantial amount of any useful enzyme by plant biomass was not widely known. We first reported the presence of huge amount of extra-cellular saccharifying amylase in *Tinospora cordifolia* Miers stem, a non-cereal non-leguminous plant of Meninspermaceae family (Sengupta *et al.*, 2002). The plant is a succulent climbing shrub, indigenous to and found widely distributed in India. It grows wild on unconditioned soil throughout the year and produces huge biomass in a short period. The plant is extensively used in folk and traditional medicine. Indian Ayurvedic system of medical treatment prescribes aqueous extract of the plant for the treatment of various diseases like diabetes, debility, hepatitis, dyspepsia, jaundice etc.

Tinospora cordifolia Amylase

Tinospora cordifolia amylase is present extra-cellularly in the gummy plant matter distributed between the bark and stick. Crude aqueous extract of *T. cordifolia* stem contained 450 ± 50 U of amylase/g of fresh tissue which is about 50 per cent of the amount reported for malted barley (Douglas *et al.*, 1983). Amyalse is best extracted with buffer [pH 5- 6] at 50°C. Presence of a reducing agent (10 mM cysteine), $CaCl_2$ (10mM) and EDTA (10mM) are required to be present in the buffer for the safe storage of enzyme. Gum is removed from the plant extract by ethanol precipitation at 15 per cent (v/v) concentration. Crude amylase is more than 90 per cent recovered from the concentrated extract by ethanol precipitation (4 volumes). The lyophilized stable enzyme preparation contained about 90,000 - 1,10,000 U/g of solid (Mukherjee *et al.*, 2012).

Properties of Crude Amylase

T.cordifolia amylase, showed optimum activity at a pH range close to that of fungal enzyme but exhibited catalytic activity over a wide pH range (4- 7.5), compared to those of fungal and pancreatic enzymes used in various pharmaceutical preparations. The pH and thermo stability of crude amylase were similar or even better than commercial amylases of fungal origin *T.cordifolia* crude amylase showed optimal activity on starch in the range of 60° – 65°C and $t_{1/2}$ at 62 °C was 30 min. These values for extracellular *A. oryzae* amylase were 50 °C and $t_{1/2}$ at 55 °C was 30 min.

The stability of amylase in acid pH is highly beneficial for its use as digestive enzyme. An ideal digestive amylase requires being stable and active over a wide pH range that occurs in normal human digestion. *A. oryzae* amylase, commonly used in pharmaceutical preparation showed poor acid stability and low activity at pH 3.0 and 7.0 while *T. cordifolia* amylase had 30 per cent and 70 per cent activity at pH 3.0 and 7.0 respectively. The inactivation kinetics at pH 3, determined for various amylases showed that *T. cordifolia* amylase retained more than 50 per cent activity over a period of 4 hours compared to loss of full activity of other amylases in 30 min (Mukherjee *et al.*, 2012; Mukherjee *et al.*, 2010).

Purification and Physico-chemical Properties of the Unique Thiol Amylase

T. cordifoia amylase was reported in a patent by Sengupta *et al.* (2002). Affinity purification recovered optimum amount of enzyme from the plant extract. Amylase was precipitated out using 2 per cent (w/v) glycogen. The amylase-glycogen complex was subjected to ammonium sulfate precipitation and the enzyme was purified through gel filtration (Bio-Gel P-60) column. The glycogen precipitated method recovered about 58 per cent of enzyme activity and final 5.84 fold purification recovered about 33-35 per cent of enzyme activity with a specific activity of 546.20 U/mg of protein (Mukherjee *et al.*, 2010). The molecular weight of *T.cordifolia* amylase was found to be 43KDa on both SDS PAGE and HPGPLC (Mukherjee *et al.*, 2010), the molecular weight was similar to that of several other amylases purified from different source except 28 KDa protein purified from *B. licheniformis* (Krishnan and Chandra, 1983). Purified amylase from *T. cordifolia* is active in the pH range of 4 –7, with optimal activity at 6.0 and is stable in pH range of 4-7. It is optimally active between 55-65° C and activity lowers sharply beyond 65°C (Mukherjee *et al.*, 2010).

Amylases are generally metallo-enzyme that requires the presence of a metal cation co-factor for expression of their full activity. It was apprehended that the enzyme could tightly bind Ca^{2+} sufficiently for its optimal activity similar to that of pancreatic amylase (Levitzki and Steer, 1974). 5mM $CaCl_2$ could not improve the enzyme as such but when the enzyme was subjected to dialysis for 48 hours against 1mM EDTA, Ca^{2+} improved both the activity and thermostability of the enzyme (Mukherjee *et al.*, 2010). Activity of purified *T.cordifolia* α-amylase was inhibited by heavy metal ions like Hg^{2+}, Ag^{+} and Cd^{2+} similar to that of tulip amylase (Ranwala and Miller, 2000). But metal ions like Fe^{3+}, Zn^{2+}, Mg^{2+} and Mn^{2+} did not have much effect on the activity of the enzyme. The enzyme was highly sensitive to Hg^{2+} ion and 0.2mM Hg^{2+} completely inhibited the enzyme activity (Mukherjee *et al.*, 2010).

Purified amylase from *T. cordifolia* was strongly inhibited by SH reacting reagents (DTNB > PCMB > N-ethylmalemide > iodoacetic acid > iodoacetamide) (Mukherjee *et al.*, 2010), unlike cereal α-amylases which are usually insensitive to SH reacting reagents (Zeigler, 1988). However, loss of about 90 per cent of activity after 10 min of incubation of the enzyme with 5 mM DTNB was regained within 20 min by the addition of 5 mM cysteine. SH group present in enzyme protein (43 KDa) was estimated (by Ellman's reagent) to be 3 groups/mole (Mukherjee *et al.*, 2010). *T. cordifolia* amylase was suggested to be a thiol enzyme whose thiol groups are possibly involved in the exhibition of catalytic activity. Tulip α-amylase was also reported to be inhibited by DTNB and N-ethylmalemide (Ranwala and Miller, 2000). It has been reported that α-amylase from poplar leaves was reversibly inactivated by oxidation in absence of reducing agents (Witt and Sauter, 1996). Although it is known that cereal amylases are usually unaffected by SH reagents, however, α-amylase purified from germinated common millet (*Panicum milaceu*) seeds was inhibited by iodoacetic acid and PCMB.

Purified α amylase from *T.cordifolia* was completely inactivated at 0.4 per cent (w/v) of SDS while it remained about 30 per cent active at a concentration of 8M urea and 4M guanidine–HCL (Mukherjee *et al.*, 2010). Activity of *Tinospora cordifolia* amylase was not affected by proteolytic digestion of the native protein by trypsin, chymotrypsin, pepsin and proteinase K (Mukherjee *et al.*, 2010), similar to that for *B. subtilis*, and *A.oryzae* amylases. Human salivary amylase however was relatively less stable and activity was lost by proteolytic digestion (Stein and Fischer, 1958). The purified *T.cordifolia* amylase displayed a Km and V_{max} of 4.1 mg/mL and 0.13 µmole of maltose equivalent/min respectively for soluble starch (Mukherjee *et al.*, 2010). Km values (mg/mL) obtained were: 4.5, 4.7, 7.5 and 2.7 for gelatinized corn flour, wheat flour, rice flour and gram flour respectively. The purified enzyme showed a Km value (mg/mL) of 4.3 and 10.0 for amylopectin and glycogen respectively (Mukherjee *et al.*, 2010). The V_{max} value [µ mole of maltose equivalent/min] obtained for various substrates were as follows: 0.130 (gelatinized corn flour), 0.200 (gelatinized rice flour), 0.118 (gelatinized wheat flour), 0.108 (gelatinized gram flour), 0.137 (amylopectin) and 0.25 (glycogen) (Mukherjee *et al.*, 2010).

The Novel Thiol Enzyme from the Plant

Unlike other α-amylases from cereals, fungi and bacteria, *T.cordifolia* amylase hydrolyzed soluble starch and amylopectin equally and partially hydrolyzed dextran and glycogen. The hydrolysis rate for glycogen was half than that obtained for soluble starch (Sengupta *et al.*, 2008; Sengupta *et al.*, 2013). The enzyme was inactive upon pullulan and had no isoamylase activity. The purified enzyme hydrolyzed soluble starch completely into maltose as major product with some maltodextrins and little amount of glucose. It must be mentioned here that barley amylase hydrolyzes amylopectin at half the rate than that for soluble starch and is practically inactive on glycogen (Schwimmer and Balls, 1949). *T. cordifolia* amylase is capable of endo-hydrolyzing dextran, amylopectin and glycogen (as mentioned earlier) as evident by gel-filtration chromatography analysis and TLC of the enzyme-digested sample. The stem-bark contains (U/100 g of fresh tissue) 10000 ± 1000, 40000 ± 2000, and 22000

± 2000 of dextran hydrolyzing, amylopectin hydrolyzing and glycogen hydrolyzing activities respectively. The purified enzyme is also capable of degrading sephadex G50, sepahdex G75, sephadex G100 and gum arabic (Sengupta *et al.*, 2013). Dextran hydrolyzing activity can effectively be used as food enzyme for use in food processing, particularly in sugar mill for the improvement of yield and quality of cane sugar.

Comparative study of various cereal meal hydrolysis using *T.cordifolia* and *A.oryzae* amylase was undertaken in the investigation which showed that the plant amylase hydrolyzed the gelatinized cereal flours more efficiently than fungal enzyme. The DE (Dextrose Equivalent) obtained for different cereal meals using *T.cordifolia* amylase was almost twice than that obtained by using fungal enzyme.

The ability of some plant amylase to hydrolyze both soluble starch and amylopectin was reported for amylases from pea leaves and potato tuber (Zeigler, 1988; Witt and Sauter, 1996). However, these enzymes are present in very low amount, completely unsuitable for commercial exploitation.

Use of amylase for starch saccharification has the ultimate objective of producing either maltose or glucose preferably from both amylose and amylopectin fractions of cereal starches. The goal is not always achieved by the use of a single enzyme – Amylase, which produces maltose as a main end product but with reasonable amount of undigested limit dextrin. The yield of maltose or glucose is enhanced by the use of maltase, isomaltase, pullulanse or isoamylase from other sources. It was very rarely observed that those enzymes are co-produced with amylase from the same source.

We observed that crude preparation of *T.cordifolia* could hydrolyze soluble starch and amylopectin liberating about 65 per cent glucose (about 75 per cent of total reducing sugar). The enzyme preparation also excellently hydrolyzed various cereal meals into glucose as major end product. The DE obtained for hydrolysis of corn, gram and wheat flour by the crude enzyme preparation were about 81-85, while the purified amylase could reach to a DE of about 42-44, indicating maltose as main end product (Mukherjee *et al.*, 2012).

While studying the physicochemical properties of crude maltase present in the extract, it was observed that hydrolysis of maltose entered a static phase at a product (glucose) concentration of about 12-13 mg/mL, suggesting the possibility of an end product inhibition. While studying the kinetics of starch hydrolysis using higher substrate concentration it was found that though amount of reducing sugar was high, yet the yield of glucose decreased with the increase in substrate concentration (20 per cent w/v corn starch). Possibly this may have occurred because of end product inhibition of the disacchridases. Complete hydrolysis of starch into glucose in a single step using a single enzyme package has much biotechnological significance for operational simplicity.

In brewing technology where barley malt amylase plays a significant role, a term 'Diastatic power' (DP) is used. It is the measure of the level of activity of starch-hydrolyzing enzymes and is a term that refers to the combined activity levels of β-amylase, α-amylase, limit dextrinase, and α-glucosidase. The result of the action of these enzymes during brewing is to break down starch into component sugars that are readily fermented into alcohol by yeast. This variation in α-amylase and limit dextrinase combined with that of β-amylase provides an opportunity for barley breeders to produce divergent malting varieties that better fulfill brewers' ferment ability requirements (Evans *et al.*, 2003).

Tinospora cordifolia Disaccharidases

Tinospora cordifolia extract hydrolyses various disaccharides like maltose, sucrose, isomaltose and a trisaccharide, raffinose. The respective activities in the crude extract as amylase : maltase : isomaltase : sucrase were 450±50: 3.0±0.5: 1.5±0.5: 25±5 U/g of fresh stem (Sengupta *et al.*, 2013). However, these disaccharidases were recovered to the extent of about 50 per cent by ethanol precipitation (while recovering 90 per cent amylase activity). The presence of disaccharidases along with amylase in the plant extract is very useful for complete hydrolysis of starch into glucose by amyalse. The simultaneous production of maltase, isomaltase and α-amylase are highly beneficial for production of glucose directly from starch. (Matsushimo, 1960) purified taka maltase from taka amylase of *Aspergillus oryzae* and studied its physico-chemical properties. Maltase and other glucosidases were also reported from several amylase-producing bacteria like *Bacillus amyloliquefacians* and *B. licheniformes* (Fogarty *et al.*, 1985; Moore and Priest, 1987). Cereals like rice and corn, which have considerable amylase activities, are also known to contain α-glucosidase activities (Nakai *et al.*, 2007; Matsui *et al.*, 1981).

Enzymes Mimicking Human Carbohydrate Digestive Enzymes

It is very interesting to note that mammalian digestive system contains sucrase-isomaltase and maltase-glucoamylase complex in the small intestine brush-border membrane (Nichols *et al.*, 2003; Naim *et al.*, 1988). These enzyme complexes ensure the complete breakdown of dietary starch into glucose, which can then be absorbed into the blood stream. Since absorption cannot take place until monosaccharides are produced, sucrase-isomaltase deficiency leads to increased luminal disaccharides and consequent osmotic diarrhea (Belmont *et al.*, 2002). Isomaltase accounts for approximately half the digestion of maltotriose and maltose. Sucrase accounts for the 100 per cent breakdown of sucrose (Johnson and Byrne, 2003). Generally, sucrase from *Saccharomyces cerevisiae* (commercially known as Sacrosidase) is given orally to treat the subjects suffering from sucrose-isomaltse deficiency (Treem *et al.*, 1993). It appears that *T.cordifolia* mimics the mammalian digestive system and thus the traditional use of the plant extract to treat indigestion (as mentioned in Ayurveda) has a strong scientific background.

Enzymatic Production of Glucose from Starch

In commercial process of starch hydrolysis various enzymes, like pullulanase, isoamylase and isomaltase are used along with α-amylase. As already mentioned saccharifying α-amylases, used as the major enzyme, cannot hydrolyse α-1, 6 glucosidic branch points of amylopectin and hydrolysis of α-1,4 branch of amylopectin also varies with different enzymes. Hydrolysis of both α-1,4 and 1,6 glucosidic linkages of starch by amyloglucosidase is not much encouraged as the reaction rate lowers with the shortening of oligosaccharide chain length and accumulation of iso-oligosaccharides by reverse reaction.

Useful Enzymes for Human Disaccharidase Deficiency Therapy

In human, disaccharidase deficiency is a genetic disorder occurring in a reasonable percentage throughout the global populations. Disaccharidases are enzymes of the small intestine, which are essential for normal carbohydrate digestion. Whole human small intestine was reported to contain amylase : maltase : isomaltase : lactase : cellobiase : dextranase: trehalase as 2288 : 1240 : 341: 415 : 79 : 41: 48 Units respectively/g of fresh mucosa (Sengupta *et al.*, 2013). The "disaccharide intolerance," results when there is a deficiency of the disaccharidases in the small intestine. Disaccharide intolerance seems to be relatively common and sometimes presents a serious clinical picture, especially in infants. Therefore, it is important that the clinician be able to recognize this syndrome. There are phenomena in disaccharide intolerances such as hereditary multiple enzyme defects and acquired deficiency of single enzyme activity. Enzyme therapy by oral supplementation of disaccharidase enzymes to control deficiency syndromes was not attempted because of unavailability of disaccharidase enzymes (in a commercial amount). Unfortunately microorganisms are poor producers of disaccharidases.

Most commercial saccharifying enzymes were found to less effective because of poor disaccharidase content. *Tinospora cordifolia* has been found to produce huge extracellular amylase. Extensive study has already been carried out by this laboratory on this amylase and it was strongly suggested that the amylase was a better digestive enzyme than the fungal enzyme (*A.niger*) - globally used in all digestive pharmaceutical preparations (Mukherjee *et al.*, 2012).

Commercial Enzyme Preparation

The aqueous extract obtained by blending of plant stem hydrolyzed many disaccharides namely sucrose, maltose, isomaltose, lactose, raffinose, melezitose, trehalose and cellobiose other than starch. Enzyme activity varied from 11 per cent to 0.8 per cent of that of starch hydrolyzing activity (100 per cent). All the enzymes were present in the space between the bark and core stick of the stem and activities could leach out from stem slices but best recovered by the blending of stem at 40 °C in acetate buffer pH 5.0. Stable commercial preparations of disaccharidases were obtained by lyophilization of aqueous extract, ethanol precipitation or lyophilization of the whole stem. Ethanol precipitation did not affect amylase activity but caused more than 50 per cent loss of disaccharidase activities. Enzyme stabilizing chemicals like glycerol, mannitol, sorbitol, NaCl did not improve stability of concentrated enzyme solution kept at 40 °C. $CaCl_2$, cysteine and EDTA improve the storage stability appreciably. Storage stability of the raw material was not satisfactory and needed processing within short time. But fresh stem cut into small pieces and lyophilized retained more or less same activity over a period of 18 months studied.

Properties of Crude Disaccharidases

Sucrase, maltase and isomaltase present in the crude enzyme were all active in the acid pH range 2–6, optimum being pH 4-5. Disaccharidases were optimally active at 50 °C. Lactase which had some β–galactosidase activity had optimum activity in the pH range of 2–4. All disaccharidases were excellently stable in acid pH 2–6 but not 100 per cent thermostable beyond 40 °C (Sengupta *et al.*, 2013).

Purification of Disaccharidases

Major disaccharidases (maltase and sucrase) were purified by the steps involving DEAE – sephadex ion exchange chromatography, gel filtration on Biogel P-100 column and HPGPLC on Biosuite 125 column. Specific activities of maltase and sucrase were 30.7 and 310 U/mg protein respectively obtained by 22.6 and 17.2 folds purifications. Amylase and lactase present in the crude enzyme as well as small amount of sucrase were always remained bound to DEAE – sephadex column. Maltase and rest of sucrase washed out of the column were always co-eluted during Biogel–P100 and HPGPLC during subsequent purification. The purified protein was suggested to be homodimeric multi substrate specific sucrase – maltase having 23 per cent homology to human α-glucosidase in N terminal sequence. The similarity varied from 9–18 per cent with those of multi substrate specific α-glucosidase of plant and micro organisms. Sucrase and maltase activity of the purified protein showed identical activity – pH activity – temperature profiles. Both had optimum activities at pH 4.0 – 5.0 and temperature 50 °C. The enzyme had low activity beyond pH 7.0. Both activities were stable throughout pH 2–7. Maltase – sucrase activities were similarly sensitive to SDS, urea and guanidine – HCl. Activities were reduced to 10 per cent in presence of 0.1 per cent SDS. Urea and guanidine – HCl slowly lowered the enzyme activities till 8M and 4M concentrations respectively. Activities were insensitive to the presence of Zn^{2+}, Ca^{2+}, Mn^{2+}, Mg^{2+} while Ni^{2+}. Hg^{2+}, Pb^{2+}, Ag^{+} and Cu^{2+} inhibited enzyme activities in decreasing order. 5 mM DTNB, 50 mM iodoacetic acid, 50 mM iodoacetamide and 10 mM H_2O_2 did not inhibit the enzyme activities. PCMB (1mM) inhibited 90 per cent of enzyme activity, while 50 mM EDAC inhibited 85 per cent of enzyme activity and 10 mM NBS inhibited 75 per cent of enzyme activities during 50 min of incubation. Involvement of tryptophan and –COOH group in active site formation were indicated. Since the enzyme activities were not inhibited by Ellman's reagent (DTNB), the protein was excluded to be a thiol enzyme. The effects of Hg^{2+} ion and PCMB (both known to be thiol inhibitor) on enzyme activity were reinvestigated. The kinetics of inhibition by both followed a competitive fashion of inhibition. It was concluded that the enzyme was a non thiol protein but contained an active site susceptible to interact with mercury compound as reported earlier for other non thiol protein. The purified enzyme was free from amylase, inulinase, dextranase, glycogenase, dextrinase and lactase activities present in crude extract. The enzyme hydrolyzed sucrose, maltose, melezitose, isomaltose, 1-O-methyl–α-D–glucoside, maltotriose, p-nitrophenyl-α-D-glucoside, maltotetraose and trehalose with specific activities as 310, 30.7, 22.5, 15, 12, 10, 10, 8 and 4 units per mg protein respectively. Enzyme activities were not destroyed by pepsin, trypsin and chymotrypsin.

In the toxicity evaluation *T.cordifolia* protein, the highest oral dose of 200 mg/kg body weight did not show any mortality and did not alter basic blood pictures of experimental rats under acute and sub-acute toxicity tests.

Conclusion

The studies carried by the laboratory strongly suggest that the renewable biomass (of *Tinospora cordifolia*) might be a useful source of many enzymes of pharmaceutical and commercial interests. Intensive research is desired to be carried out to find new non toxic plant sources, not only as an alternative source of the conventional microbial enzymes but also for novel type enzymes not produced by microorganisms. Plant enzyme production has no upstream processing cost and the technology used is an environmental friendly green technology.

References

Belmont, J.W., Reid, B., Taylor, W., Baker, S.S., Moore, W.H., Morriss, M.C., Podrebarac, S.M., Glass, N., and Schwartz, I.D. (2002). Congenital sucrase-isomaltase deficiency presenting with failure to thrive, hypercalcemia, and nephrocalcinosis. *BMC Pediatrics,* **2**: 4.

De Roos, A., Grassin, C., Herweijer, M., Kragh, K.M., Poulsen, C.H., Soe, J.B., Sorensen J.F., and Wilms J. (2007). Industrial enzymes: Enzymes in food applications. *In*: Enzymes in Industry: Production and Applications, Ed. By Aehle, W, Wiley-VCH, Weinheim, Germany, pp. 123-131.

Douglas, C., Doehlert, and Duke, S.H. (1983). Specific determination of α-amylase activity in crude plant extracts containing β amylase. *Plant Phsiol.,* **71**: 229-234.

Evans, D.E., Van Wegen, B., Ma, Y.F., and Eglinton, J. (2003). The impact of the thermostability of á-amylase, B-amylase and limit dextrinase on potential wort fermentability. *J. Am. Soc. Brew.Chem.,* **61**: 210-218.

Fogarty, W.M., Kelly, C.T., Kadam, S.K. (1985).Separation and characterization of an Ü glucosidase and maltase from *Bacillus amyloliquificiens. Can.J of Microbiol.,* **31**: 670 -674.

Jach, G., Soezer, N., Schullehner, K., Lalla, B., Welters, P., and Mueller A. (2010). Phytomining of plant enzymes for biotechnological use of fats and oils. *Eur. J. Lipid. Sci. Tech.,* 1**12**: 75–86.

Johnson, L. R., and Byrne, J.H. (2003). Essential Medical Physiology, 3rd ed., Elsevier Academic Press, London. 534 pp.

Krishnan, T., and Chandra, A.K.(1983). Purification and characterization of α-amylase from *Bacillus licheniformis* CUMC305. *Appl Environ Microbiol.,* **46**: 430–437.

Levitzki, A., and Steer, M. L. (1974). The allosteric activation of mammalian α-amylase by chloride. *Eur. J. Biochem.,* **41**: 171-180.

Matshushima, T. (1960). Studies on taka maltase I. Purification and properties of taka – maltase from taka diastase. *J Biochem,* **46**: 830–836.

Matsui, H., Yazawa, I., and Chiba, S. (1981).Purification and substrate specificity of sweet corn α-glucosidase. *Agric.Bio. chem.,* **45**: 887-894.

Moore, J., and Priest, F.G. (1987). Synthesis of two distinct Ü glucosidase activities in *Bacillus licheniformis. Letter in Appl.Microbio.,* **4**: 1-3.

Mukherjee, A., Ghosh, A.K., and Sengupta, S. (2010). Purification and characterization of a thiol amylase over produced by a non-cereal non-leguminous plant, *Tinospora cordifolia. Car. Res.,* **345**: 2731–2735.

Mukherjee, A., Sengupta, S., and Sengupta, S. (2012). Evaluation of *Tinospora Cordifolia* amylase as a commercial digestive enzyme of plant origin. *J Herbs Spices Med. Plants*, **18**: 56-76.

Naim, H.Y., Sterchi, E.E., Lentze, M.J. (1988). Structure, biosynthesis, and glycosylation of human small intestinal maltase-glucoamylase. *J Biol Chem.*, **263**: 19709-19717.

Nakai, H., Ito, T., Hayashi, M., Kamiya, K., Yamamoto, T., Matsubara, K., Kim, Y.M., *et al.* (2007). Multiple forms of α-glucosidase in rice seeds (*Oryza sativa* L., var.Nipponbare). *Biochimie*, **89**: 49–62.

Negi, S., and Banerjee, R. (2006) Amylase and protease production from A. awamori. *Food Technol. Biotechnol.*, **44**: 257–261.

Nichols, B.L., Avery, S., Sen, P., Swallow, D.M., Hahns, D., and Sterchis, E. (2003). The maltase-glucoamylase gene: Common ancestry to sucrase-isomaltase with complementary starch digestion activities. *PNAS*, **100**: 1432 – 1437.

Ranwala, A.P., and Miller, W.B. (2000). Purification and characterization of an endoamylase from tulip (*Tulipa gesneriana*) bulbs. *Physiologia Plantarum*, **109**: 388-395.

Ross, M. R., and. Kang, Y.M. (2008). Enzyme composition for improving food digestion. U.S. Patent. 20080199448.

Schwimmer, S., and Balls, A.K. (1949). Isolation and properties of crystalline α- amylase from germinated barley. *J. Biol. Chem.*, **179**: 1063-1074.

Sengupta, S., Mukherjee, A., and Sengupta, S. (2008). A process for the preparation of a complete enzyme composition from the plant *Tinospora cordifolia* useful for hydrolysis of starch into glucose as the major end product. Indian Patent Application No.1989/Kol/2008; Publication date: 29.04.2011.

Sengupta, S., Mukherjee, A., and Sengupta, S. (2013). A process for the production of dextran, amylopectin and glycogen endo-hyrolase enzyme composition from the plant, *Tinospora cordifolia.* Indian Patent Application No.895/Kol/2013

Sengupta, S., Mukherjee, A., Ray, L., and Sengupta, S. (2013). *Tinospora cordifolia,* a novel source of extracellular disaccharidases, useful for human disaccharidase deficiency therapy. *Phytother Res.*, **27**: 725-730.

Sengupta, S., Naskar, A.K., Jana, M.L., and Naskar, P. (2002). Process for the preparation of α-amylase from *Tinospora cordifolia* Miers, useful for starch saccharification. US Patent 6379721.

Sivaramakrishnan, S., Gangadharan, D., Nampoothiri, K. M., Soccol, C.R., and Pandey, a.(2006). α-amylases from microbial sources- an overview on recent developments. *Food Technol. Biotechnol.*, **44**, 173–184.

Stanley, D., Farnden, K.J.F., and MacRae, E.A. (2005). Plant α-amylases: functions and roles in carbohydrate metabolism: Review. *Biol. Bratislava*, **60**: 65-71.

Stein, E.A., and Fischer, E.H.(1958). The resistance of α-amylases towards proteolytic attack. *J. Biol. Chem.*, **232**: 867-879.

Treem, W.R., Ahsan, N., Sullivan, B., Rossi, T., Holmes, R., Fitzgerald, J., Roy, P., Hyams, J. (1993). Evaluation of liquid yeast derived sucrase enzyme replacement in patient with sucrase isomaltase deficiency.*Gastroenetorology*, **105**: 1061-1068.

Witt, W., and Sauter, J.J. (1996). Purification and chratcerization of α-amylase from poplar leaves. *Plant Physiol.*, **41**: 365 –372.

Witt, W., and Sauter, J.J. (1996). Purification and properties of a starch granule-degrading α-amylase from potato tubers. *J.Exp. Bot.*, **47**: 1789-1795.

Zeigler, P. (1988). Partial purification and characterization of the major endoamylase of mature pea leaves. *Plant. Physiol.*, **86**: 659-666.

Bioactive Phytochemicals: Perspectives for Modern Medicine Vol. 3 (2015) *Pages* **449–464**
Editor: **V.K. Gupta**
Published by: **DAYA PUBLISHING HOUSE, NEW DELHI**

18

Efficiency of Garlic Derived Phytochemicals against Advanced Metabolic Disorders: New Directions

Mohd. Mazid[1*]

ABSTRACT

Currently natural products are attaining more popularity to combat various physiological threats including oxidative stress, cardiovascular complexities, cancer insurgence and immune dysfunction. The use of traditional remedies may encounter more frequently due to a broad myriad of scientific evidence in their remedic favour. Spices are a dried seed, fruit, roots, bark or vegetable substance. Spices possess a variety of phytochemicals that gaining wide attention for their well-recognized potential health benefits against advanced physiological threats in present scenarios. Among the spices, garlic (Allium sativum L.) holds a unique position for its recognized therapeutic potential. The potent remedic role of garlic recognized particularly with respect to aged-garlic extract (AGE) has been the subjects of much research interest as well as emergent focus for a large number of reviews. This review investigates the cardiovascular related health potential of garlic, examining the role of their bioactive chemicals like thiosulfinate organosulphur volatiles, vinyldithiins, ajoenes, and water soluble organosulphur compounds. In this review, much emphasis given to evidences for health benefits is based on potentialities of bioactive constituents to ameliorate oxidative stress, active participation in cardiovascular cure and their prospective as immune boosters.

***Keywords*:** Garlic, Organosulphur, Oxidative stress, Physiological threats, Phytochemicals, Spice.

1 Plant Physiology Section, Department of Botany, Faculty of Life Sciences, Aligarh Muslim University, Aligarh – 202002, U.P., India

* *Corresponding author*: E-mail: mazidmohd@gmail.com

Introduction

Globally, unhealthy diets and physical inactivity are two of the most leading causes of major chronic diseases. According to the WHO, non-communicable chronic disorders, such as heart diseases, stroke, cancer, chronic respiratory diseases, diabetes, are by far the principle leading cause of mortality in the world reporting 60 per cent of all death (Wei *et al.*, 1998). In 2004, the 192 member states of the WHO endorsed the global strategy on diet, physical activity and health addressing two main risk factors. Diet is a central pivotal link with human health and food rich in phytochemicals often associated with proper functionality of immune system. Food levels are widely used to convey the health benefits of conventional foods or a component of food to the consumer. The increasing amount of health information available regarding the health benefits of food has resulted in consumer interest in the health issues and has become a leading factor in purchasing decisions. Many consumers try to eat healthier foods, use natural medicines, and make life style changes in the quest to feel good, maintain body weight, reduce the risk of chronic disease, and live healthier longer lives. Thus, it is now widely accepted that the ageing and age related disease are in part caused by free radical reactions or free radical induced reactions. The arrest of ageing and stimulation of rejuvenation of the human body is also being sought.

Moreover, countries around the world are monitoring the prevalence of chronic "life style" disorders and also, developing strategies to treat, prevent and minimize the incidence of disease in future times. Health professionals are promoting dietary changes; including the increased consumption of plant food materials to compact nutritional deficiencies is chronic disease risk. Over the last 30 years the uses of herbs and natural products has gained more popularity and these are being consumed backed by epidemiological evidence. Similarly trends have been observed and the growth rate of therapeutics in Europe has been repeated to be greater than those pharmaceuticals (Chang *et al.*, 2008). Therefore, medicinal herbs have been used in primary health care over many countries before the advent of modern medicine. Over the last 20 years, there has been an international resurgence of medicinal herbs in all cultures of world, especially in the Asia which has an enhanced interest in natural system of cure and the questioning of an over-dependence on synthetic drugs to maintain health. Moreover, today, there has been an impressive gain in individual life expectancy with parallel increase in age-related chronic diseases of the cardiovascular, brain and immune systems. These can cause loss of autonomy, dependence and high social cost for individual and society. Several epidemiological studies have thrown that a diet rich in plant food may reduce the development of certain chronic diseases such as cardiovascular related diabetes, atherosclerosis, cancer, arthritis, rejuvenation of stain and disease associated with cerebral aging (Kandil *et al.*, 1988; Rahman, 2000), one such spice (food) is garlic.

Garlic (*Allium sativum* L.)

Garlic is one of the most ancient medicinal plants and believed to have originated free central Asia 6000 years ago. Garlic based remedies were functioning in India some 6000 years ago and its inclusion in Chinese has started 2000 years ago. As early as 1550 B.C. Egyptians feed garlic to pyramids construction crews to give them extra vigor (Rivlin, 2001). It acquired a reputation in the folk fore of many cultures over the centuries as a formidable prophylactic and therapeutic medicinal agent. Garlic belongs to the family Liliaceae (Alliance) and is cultivated worldwide for the flashy segments (cloves) of its bulbs. It is believed to have originated in central Asia and to date the genus Allium comprises over 600 known species, which include *Allium cepa* (onion), *Allium porrum* (leek) and *Allium oprasum* (chives). Garlic even form aoristic times, has been used in all parts of the world not only as a spice or a food, but also for treatment of many diseases. Its uses have been inscribed on the walls of ancient Egyptian places of workshop and pyramids. Its importance has often been highlighted in the spirituals (Napoli *et al.*, 2000).

The famous herbal doctors Hippocrates, Paracelsus and Lonicerus recognized garlic as a diuretic, an emmen gouge, and used it for the treatment for stomach chills, flatulence, colic etc (Stoll and See back, 1948). Garlic has been investigated extensively for health benefits, resulting in more than1000 publications over the last decades alone, and it is considered one of the best preventive towards, based on its potent and varied effects. During the last two decade more scientific research and clinical trials to determine the effect of garlic consumption were widely studied and now the medicinal use of garlic is common. Healthful properties of garlic are common. Healthful properties of garlic are legion and over a thousand scientific reports enumerated its functional activities which include free radical scavenging activities, immune stimulation, curing cardiovascular diseases, anticancer and anti-infectious properties (Borek, 2005).

Chemical Composition

Garlic has been used historically for medicinal purposes, particularly for treatment of diseases associated with ageing (Rahman, 2006). AGE contains potent antioxidant activity and is prepared from natural garlic that is aged for 20 months reduced its harsh irritating taste and odour. However, this AGE has a greater concentration of organosulphur compounds such as SAC which is potent antioxidant and free radicals scavenger (Imai *et al.*, 1994). In spite of tuts, some non-S-Leping compounds of AGE like allixin also play a therapeutic role in metabolism and diabetes treatment. Although numerous studies have demonstrated the antioxidant properties of AGE, its ability to inhibit formation of advanced glycation end (AGE) products and CML (carboxyl-methyl–lysine, a non-cross linked AGE products derived from oxidation process) *in vitro*. SAC has Amadori activity and inhibited formation of cross linked AGE products but was not as effective as pyridoxamine at higher concentration adopted.

Result of Ahmed *et al.* (2005) demonstrates that AGE protected against glycation -induced protein fragmentation probably because of its ability to chelate transition metal therefore preventing anti-oxidative glycation and glycol-oxidation reaction. AGE may also inhibit AGE products because of its antioxidant properties as has been reported for green tea (Robertson *et al.*, 2002) also, AGE inhibited formation of methyl-glyoxal derived AGE products and may also act by blocking conversion of dicarbonyl intermediates to AGE. Results of Ahmad *et al.* (2005) also, show that AGE posses Amadorin activity. AGE has more potent antioxidant capacity compared to other garlic preparations because of high concentration of SAC but S-allyl mercaptocystein, selenium and allexin, all of which are stable, bioavailable antioxidant (Imai *et al.*, 1994; Borek., 2001). Potential health benefits of garlic, has its origin in antiquity, but still there is a need to unveil the details of these benefits (King *et al.*, 1988).

Moreover, epidemiological, clinical, and preclinical studies have shown the close relation between dietary habits of garlic appear to be true today and its use as a dietary supplement is recommended in many centuries (Naaz *et al.*, 2003; Kodera *et al.*, 2002). However, garlic has been a subject of considerable interest as a medicine worldwide since ancient times. Several lines of evidence through both *in vitro* and *in vivo* studies have revealed pharmacological potential of garlic. *In vitro* studies demonstrated its antimicrobial (Abdullah *et al.*, 1989), antithrombotic, anticancer, anti-platelets aggregation and antioxidant activities (Carson, 1987). *In vivo* studies, both in animal model and human clinical traits, have demonstrated its beneficial effects in a number of pathological conditions also, including hyperlipidermia, cardiovascular disorder and arteriosclerosis etc.

Chemistry of Garlic

Garlic is a vegetable of the Allium genus and is characterized by a high content organosulphur compounds and flavonoids. Variation in processing yields quiet different preparation because of the complex chemistry of garlic. The chemistry of the Allium species has been dominated by many sulphur containing compounds that give them a characteristic flavour or odour. However, a variety of components, including non-sulphur compounds, work synergistically to provide various health benefits. The garlic bulb contains approximately 65 per cent water, 28 per cent carbohydrates, 2.3 per cent organo-sulphur compounds, 2 per cent protein, 1.2 per cent free amino acids (arginine mainly), and 1.5 fibre. Therapeutic properties of garlic often attributed to allicin and its derivatives (Mader, 1990; Milner, 2001). Compounds of garlic work synergistically to produce various effects, but, because of garlic chemical complexity, processing methods yield preparations with differing efficacy and safety.

Sulphur-based Compounds

Garlic is rich in such kinds of compounds, which contribute to its characteristic flavour and taste and even to its beneficial effects. The major S-containing compounds in inactive garlic are glutamyl-S-allyl-L-cysteine, S-allyl-L-cystiene and S-allyl-L-cystiene sulphoxides (allin). The compounds act as precursors of several compounds. It was first scientifically demonstrated 170 years ago by the Wertheim (1844-45), who also determined that these compounds have the bane formula of C H and S. It took almost 50 years before Semmler (1892), fractionally distilled this type of oil and identified specific compounds. He found also that oil contains 60 per cent diallyl disulphide, 20 per cent di-allyltrisulphide, 10 per cent diallyltetrasulphide and 6 per cent allyl propyl disulfide tetra-sulfide and6 per cent allyl propyl disulfide. Stern *et al.* (2002) results were surprisingly similar to what is found today except that the allyl propyldisulfide content was later not produced by garlic (Stener and Lin, 1994). These diallyl sulfides are not actually found in whole or crushed garlic cloves but are produced during steam distillation and during the storage of crushed garlic.

Organosulphur Volatiles

Produced garlic containing a wider variety of organosulphur volatiles than the intact garlic cloves. The main volatiles that have been identified in distributed garlic and garlic essential oil including (diallyl sulphides) diallyl trisulphide methylallyl disulphide, methyl trisulphide, methyl allyl trisulphide, vinyl dithins, and ajoenes. All the volatiles usually formed constituents of steam distilled garlic oil soluble extracts of garlic but with varied composition.

The main sulphides in garlic oil are DAS (57 per cent), allyl methyl.

Garlic: (*Allium sativum* L.)

Kingdom - Plantae

Subkingdom - Tracheobionta- Vascular plants

Superdivision - Spermatophyta - Seed plant

Division - Magnoliophyta-flowering plant

Class - Liliopsida-Monocotyledons

Subclass - Liliideae

Order - Lilales

Family - Liliaceae (Alliaceae - lily family)

Genus-*Allium* L. (Onion)

Species-*Allium sativum* L.-Cultivated garlic

Reactive Oxygen Species, Oxidative Stress-aged Garlic Extract

Reactive oxygen species (ROS) and oxidative stress are implicated in CVD, cancer and various other forms of dementia including Alzheimer's disease (AD) (Borek, 2004). Oxidative damage to DNA, proteins, lipids and other molecules rank high as a major cause in the onset and development of these diseases. ROS including free radicals ($OH^{\bullet -}$, H_2O_2 and $O_2^{\bullet -}$), are by-products of normal metabolism and increase during infection and inflammation, hyperhomocysteinemia and exposure to exogenous sources, including nitrogenous oxide metabolite pollutants, smoking certain drugs (*e.g.*, acetaminophene and radiation). Garlic ranks highly among foods that help prevent disease, largely due to its high content of organosulphur compounds and antioxidant activity. Fresh garlic, however, may cause indigestion, and its pungent odour that lingers on the breath and skin can be a social deterrent. The majority of the diseases associated with old age are initiated by free radicals. Since, garlic has strong antioxidant properties and epidemiological studies support the fact that diets rich in antioxidants may prevent some of the above mentioned chronic diseases.

Thus, garlic is reported to decrease serum cholesterol and triglycerides levels inhibit platelet aggregation and increase blood circulation. Studies of Steiner *et al.* (1996) found that allixin (a constituent of AGE), a phytoalexin of garlic is a good candidate for the developments of synthetic metal complexes with anti-diabetic effects (Kodera *et al.*, 2002). Allixin (3-hydroxy-5-methoxy-6-methyl-2-pentyl-4H-pyran-4-one), a non-sulphur compound with a γ-pyrone structure, was the first compound isolated from garlic as a phytoalexin, a product induced in plants by continuous stress. Among several induction methods, Kodera *et al.* (2002) have found that allexin crystals can be induced at an extremely high concentration (1400 ng mg-1wet garlic weight) on the surface of garlic after approximately two years of storage at room temperature in a dark room. These disagreeable effects of fresh garlic are due to allicin, an oxidant reduced upon cutting or chewing the clove. The arrest of ageing and stimulation of rejuvenation of the human body is being investigated intensively and garlic has also been investigated for this purpose. Garlic consumption may be beneficial by the elderly as it has strong antioxidant properties since, it is known that antioxidant can modulate the immune system (Fukushima *et al.*, 2000). Therefore, additional research is needed to further investigations of anti-oxidative properties of garlic and other potential role in human health and disease.

Role of Age in Ageing

Ageing is a progressive decline in the efficiency of biochemical and physiological processes after the reproduction phase of life. Free radical theory of ageing postulates that ageing is caused by free radical reactions which may be involved in production of the ageing changes associated with the environment, disease and intrinsic factors of ageing process. Since, it is well accepted that oxidative free radical stress is an important contributor to the ageing process and too many age-related diseases, the focus must be on reducing oxidative stress *in vivo*. This is important because oxidative damage apparently increases with age and thus may overwhelm the natural repair systems in the olderly (Elliott and McGrath, 1994). One best way to neutralize free radical mediated oxidative stress in the elderly is to ingest diet rich in phytochemicals with antioxidant properties. These are widely present in plants products. Such two naturally occurring plants are soy and garlic and their potential in prevention of diseases associated with ageing is reviewed here.

Age in Cardiovascular Diseases

Coronary heart diseases (CHD) are the leading cause of death in North America and in most Western countries (Duraisamy *et al.*, 2003). Epidemiological studies have identified number of risk factors for the development of CHD which include elevated serum lipids increased plasma fibrinogen and coagulation factors, increased platelet activation, alternations in glucose metabolism (Durant *et al.*, 1995). There is strong epidemiological evidence that atherosclerosis-related conditions (Coronary artery disease, Ischemic stroke and peripheral artery disease) all increase with age (Fleischauer and Arab, 2001) and its effects are mainly evident in the muscular arteries. Ageing causes the changes in the structure and function of the vessels that leads to an increase in the incidence of certain CHD causing enhancement of both morbidity and mortality. Enhanced oxidative stress with ageing may also play an important role in the increased prevalence of atherosclerosis in older individuals. Evidence from both *in vitro* and *in vivo* studies suggests that oxidation of LDL may contribute to early atherosclerotic lesion formation (Horie *et al.*, 1989) and there is also a continuous increase in LDL hydroxyl fatty acids content with age in healthy, olderlys individuals (Masamoto, 2002). Oxidised LDL elicits pro-atherogenic properties like increased smooth muscles proliferation (Koba *et al.*, 1999), cytotoxicity to vascular endothelial cells, smooth muscles cells and fibroblasts (Lau *et al.*, 1987) together with the induction of apoptotic cell death in vascular endothelial cells (Napoli *et al.*, 2000).

There are a strong evidence that nutritional factors contribute to the etiology of the condition and that dietary modifications, together with life-style modification are important in the treatment of patients (Lawson, 1996). Populations with diets rich in carbohydrates tend to have reduced risk for CHD. It appears that intact fruits, vegetables, spices and whole grains are the best sources of carbohydrate, most recommended in diets to reduce the risk of CHD (Liu and Yeh, 2002). A positive correlation has been established between CHD death rate and plasma cholesterol level, and among other things, the latter is due to too high a consumption of saturated fat. Above these foods have been shown to decrease serum LDL-cholesterol and triglycerides (Major factor for CHD) and affect other risk factors.

Moreover, garlic has been used to treat a variety of CHD over the years. Various garlic preparations (extract) have been shown to reduce diet-induced hypercholesteromia in rats and rabbits (Liu and Yeh, 2001). Among the various extracts, Aged-garlic extract (AGE/GEX) supplementation has been shown to be effective in lowering plasma cholesterol and triglycerides and LDL-cholesterol in hyperlipidermia subjects (Steiner *et al.*, 1996), whilst it had no effect in nor-lipidemic subjects (Rahman and Billinton, 2000). In addition, it also demonstrates a wide variety of biological activities like hepatoprotective, neuroprotective and antioxidative activities (Imai *et al.*, 1994). These additional biological effects may be due to conversion compounds that are formed during AGEs long term extraction process, called the ageing processes. According to many studies of AGE, garlic extraction results in greater and more resistant efficiency and safety compared with raw garlic, dehydrated garlic powder, or other preparations with in a dosage range of 1-7.2 g/d, AGE has been shown to lower plasma cholesterol in humans (Milner, 2001). Moreover, studies show that as little as 1.8 g to as much as 10g/d of AGE is effective in enhancing human immune responses (Abdullah *et al.*, 1989). Age has been treated in several clinical traits and show no certain dictions with several medications, including warfarin (Milner, 2006), aspirin and statins (Budoff *et al.*, 2004) adriamycin/doxysorubicin (Nagae *et al.*, 1994). Among the various garlic preparations, AGE has been proves to be safe in toxification studies such as acute and chronic toxicity tests (Amagase *et al.*, 2001). However, the above meta-analysis excluded the results of several clinical studies of the effects of AGE on cholesterol. AGE has consistent effects on risk factors for CHD, including cholesterol and others (Ruddok *et al.*, 2005; Rahman *et al.*, 2000).

In addition, SAC is another characteristic compound present in AGE and provide protection against oxidation, free radicals and CHD. The pharmacokinetics of SAC is well-established *in vivo* (Nagae *et al.*, 1994). SAC is detected in the blood, and its blood concentration and other pharmacokinetic parameters are well-associated with doses of orally administered SAC in animal studies. Because SAC is present in garlic preparations and has many biological effects in addition to its bioavailability, it must be one of the active substances in garlic preparations and account for at least a portion of garlic in biological activities. Thus, the standardization of garlic preparations using SAC as a biological marker is scientifically reasonable and well justified. In various studies, blood SC level was measured in the subjects as a compliance marker. The blood SAC level in the group taking supplements was significantly higher than that of the placebo group (Budoff *et al.*, 2004). It is clear that SAC is bio available because it was absorbed into the blood and is therefore active in the human body.

Age as Antioxidant

ROS or free radicals have been implicated in mediating various pathological processes such as cancer, ischemia, inflammatory disease, diabetes, and atherosclerosis. Garlic has been reported to be effective against diseases of which ROS are anti-oxidative efficacy of various garlic preparations differs according to variations in chemical structures and standardization. ROS are involved in signal transduction pathways leading to nuclear factor κB (NF-κB) activation that has been implicated in the regulation of gene transcription. Studies suggest that garlic may work by reducing ROS or interacting with them to minimize the negative impact on the body. LDL oxidation has been recognized as playing an important role in initiation and progression of atherosclerosis. Allicin, free AGE and its constituent SAC have a similar preventive effect against Cu^{+2}-initiated oxidation of LDL taken from the human subjects who consume AGE. Ruddok *et al.* (2005) investigated and found clear supportive data that AGE and SAC significantly present membrane damage, loss of cell viability and lipid per oxidation in bovine pulmonary artery endothelial cells (PAECs) exposed to oxidized LDL. AGE and SAC inhibited both lactate-dehydrogenase release and lipid per oxidation induced by H2O2. These data indicate that the anti-oxidative capabilities of AGE and SAC may be useful in preventing of atherosclerosis.

Furthermore, Budoff *et al.* (2004) showed that AGE increases intracellular glutathione levels, glutathione disulphide reductase, and SOD activity in PAECs, whereas the level of glutathione disulphide decreased. These results suggest that the anti-oxidative effect of AGE may be due to its modulation of the glutathione redox cycle and SOD activity in vascular endothelial cells. Budoff *et al.* (1996) also examined effects of AGE and its thioallyl components on rat brain ischemia using a middle cerebral artery occlusion model and a transient global ischemia model. Also, Horie *et al.* (1989) demonstrated that AGE prevents the formation of thiobarbituric acid-reactive substances and fluorescent substances during lipid per oxidation of rat liver microsomes. AGE inhibited the emission of liver-level chemiluminescence and the early formation of thiobarbituric acid-reactive substances in a liver microsomal fraction inhibited by t-butyl hydro peroxide. Wei and Lau (1998) and Yamaguchi *et al.*, 2000) observed that AGE suppression of H_2O_2 and $O_2^{\bullet-}$ generation and also enhances cellular antioxidant enzymes thus protecting vascular endothelial cells from oxidative injury. Weiss *et al.* (2006) provided evidence that oxidative stress that includes AGE (1ml/kg) restored the reduced GSH levels, decreased free radicals and MDA, as well as myeloperoxidase activity, AGE scavenges oxidants, enhances enzymes activity and GSH levels, and inhibits lipid peroxidation and production of inflammatory prostaglandins (Borek, 2004). In conclusion, AGE are effective tool in amelioration of oxidative stress and related discrepancies but care should be taken not to use it in excess quantities and opinions and consulting a physician should be taken in account before its use.

Moreover, AGE and its main constituents have been reported to scavenge the t-butyl-hydro-peroxide radical and hence prevent lipid peroxidation of liver microsomes (Imai *et al.*, 1994). It has also been shown to modulate the production and function of both endothelial derived relaxing factor (NO) and constricting factors (endothelial-1) in rat isolated pulmonary arteries and reduce blood pressure in hypercholesteromic subjects (Steiner *et al.*, 1996). AGE may at least partly prevent a decrease in NO production. AGE may at least partly present a decrease in bio available NO and endothelium-derived hyper-polarizing factor during acute hyper-homo-cysteinemia (Weiss *et al.*, 2006). Homocysteine in plasma exists in two forms (1) Free homocysteine and (2) Protein bound and amount of total homocysteine is considered as a marker of atherosclerosis. AGE can decrease plasma total homocysteine concentration by 30 per cent without changing the protein-bound/free homocysteine ratio. AGE efficiency in reducing cholesterol synthesis is additive with statins, which inhibit 3-hydroxy-3-methylglutaryl-CoA reductase at a transcriptional level. AGE can also temporarily increase by 30-40 per cent (Ankari and Mirelman, 1999), the synthesis of constitutive NO, a protective factor against myocardial ischemic reperfusion injury, risk factor in CHD and dementia following stroke. Age has been found to inhibit the progression of coronary-artery calcification (Budoff *et al.*, 2004; Augusti, 1996), thus reducing the risk of a myocardial infarct.

The garlic extract might enhance glucose utilization because it significantly decreased the blood glucose level in glucose-loaded rates. It may be due to restoration of delayed insulin response or due to inhibition of intestinal absorption of glucose. This coiled be due to potentiating of the insulin effect of plasma by increasing the pancreatic secretion of insulin from existing β-cells or its release from bound insulin. Hypoglycaemia effects of garlic, attributed mainly to allicin-type compounds (Amagase *et al.*, 2006). The hypoglycaemic potency of garlic has been attributed to the sulphur compounds [di (2-propenyl) disulphide and 2-propenyl propyl disulphide, respectively].The mechanism of hypoglycaemic action probably involves direct to indirect stimulation of insulin secretion (Carson, 1987). Further, it is also suggested that these disulphide compounds have the effect of sparing insulin from-SH inactivation by reacting with endogenous thiol containing molecule such as cysteine, glutathione, and serum albumins (Augusti, 1996).

Age in Diabetes

Diabetes is a condition where there is too much sugar (glucose) in the blood. It results when people either don't produce enough insulin or have high levels of insulin in their blood, which is not working properly. It is of two types. Type 1 diabetes is most common in children and young adults but it can occur at any age. It occurs when the pancreas no longer produces insulin and treatment involves lifelong insulin injections. Type 2 diabetes is the most common form, affecting both adults and, an increasing number of children and young people, particularly in populations which are sedentary and overweight. In this case, the pancreas does not produce enough insulin. The prevalence of type 2 diabetes mellitus (type 2 DM) has been increasing rapidly worldwide (Weiss *et al.*, 2006); thus, knowledge of risk factors and protective factors associated with type 2 DM is essential for the development of prevention strategies. Yet, a healthy life style can totally prevent or dramatically reduce the risk of type-2 diabetes (Weber *et al.*, 2001). Diabetes mellitus is a common endocrine disorder characterized by hyperglycemias and long-term complications affecting the eyes, nerves, blood vessels, skin and kidneys. Increased glycation of proteins and accumulation of advanced glycation products (AGEPs) have been implicated in the pathogenesis of diabetic complications. Glycation and AGEP formation are also accompanied by formation of free radicals via auto-oxidation of glucose and glycated proteins. Compounds with combined antiglycation and antioxidant properties may offer therapeutic potential.

Present number of diabetic worldwide is 150 million and this and this is likely to increase to 300 million or more by the year 2025 (Uesugi *et al.*, 2001). Many herbal medicines have been recommended for the treatment of diabetes (Stener and Lin, 1994). Frequently, plant drugs are considered to be less toxic and more free from side effects than synthetic ones. Of which DM (is a metabolic disorder characterized by chronic hyperglycemia and hyperlipidermia that predisposes affected individuals to long term micro and macrovascular complications. Hyper-glycemia causes increased protein glycation and the formation of advanced glycation end products which underlie the complications of diabetes and ageing. Glycation is accompanied by metal-catalysed oxidation of glucose and Amadori products to form free radicals capable of proteins fragmentation. Glycation products involving dicarbonyl intermediates such as 3-deoxyglycosome and methyl glyoxal to for caplumes, heterogeneous, florescent and cross linked structures. Accumulation of glycation products in body tissue are believed to be responsible for the long term complications of diabetes and ageing (Ahmad, 2005). Indeed, diabetes mellitus and ageing are associated with a build-up of tissue advanced glycation food products, increased oxidative stress and decline in antioxidant status (Amagase, 2006). The involvement of advanced glycation end products in diabetes complications and ageing has promoted a search for compounds capable of inhibiting their formation. Recent studies suggest that compounds with combined antiglycation and antioxidant properties after maximum protection against glucose -induced cellular damage (Duraisamy *et al.*, 2003).

Recent studies suggest that AGE inhibits formation of AGEPs *in vitro* and formation of glycation derived free radicals. SAC, a key component of AGE, is a potent oxidant and can inhibit AGEP formation as well (Ahmad *et al.*, 2006). Glucose and Amadori products can undergo auto-oxidation in the presence of transition metals to generate free radicals. Auto oxidation of glucose (auto-oxidative glycation) generates a ketoimine capable of reacting with proteins to form AGEPs and also generates free radicals such as $O_2^{\bullet-}$ radicals in the process. Similarly, Amadori products undergo metal-catalysed oxidation (glucose oxidation), generating reactive dicarbonyl compounds capable of forming AGEPs and free radicals (Hunt *et al.*,

1993). Free radicals can damage proteins, lipids and nucleic acid and might contribute towards tissue damage in diabetes (Bonnefunt-Rousselot, 2002). Adiponectin is a protein hormone produced and secreted exclusively by adipocytes that regulates the metabolism of lipids and glucose (Amagase *et al.*, 2001). The hormone is known to influence the body's response to insulin and its levels are generally reduced under type 2 DM. The monitoring of adipo-nectin is thus essential for evaluating compounds with anti-metabolic syndrome effects. Adiponectin is an adipocytokine, which is synthesized and released by adipocytes, abundantly present in plasma and leads to enhanced insulin action, indicating that this adipocytikine maintain sensitivity and glucose homeostasis. However, adiponectin levels are reduced in patients with increased insulin resistance due to conditions such as obesity, type 2DM and hypertension. Thus, adipocytokine is considered as a good biomarker to assess efficiency for developing therapeutics for type 2DM (Amagase *et al.*, 2001). It is already known that thiazolidinedione derivatives (TDZs) increase the adiponectin level as potential insulin-sensitizing therapeutics (Bathena *et al.*, 2002). However, TDZs are associated with edema, body weight gain, longestive heart failure, osteoporosis and liver dis-function in type 2DM patients (Bathena *et al.*, 2002).

Furthermore, garlic is a gift from nature and has been used globally for thousands of years for culinary and medicinal purposes in most of races. The garlic bulk is the most commonly used part of this plant, where plenty of the low molecular weight D-containing compounds as allicin, dialkylsulphides, dithiis, allin and S-alkylcysteine have been found for many years. Allixin, an unusual non-sulphur compound was found from the bulb with unique biological properties. Allixin, with a hudroxy-γ-pyrone structure, is also a good ligand for several metal ions. Allixin is an interesting compound with several unique biological properties such as antidiabetic, inhibition of alfatoxinB1DNA binding activity, neurotropic activity, and inhibition activity for the growth of Helicobacter pylori (Kodera *et al.*, 2002). By using this unique allixin, the physico-chemical and biological studies on metallo-allixinate complexes have been performed with the great help of Kodrea and the Wakunaga Pharmaceuticals Co. Ltd. Allixin is a natural pyrone derivative and its vanadyl and zinc complexes were found to be very efficient in lowering high blood glucose levels in animals models in both type-1 and type -2 diabetes (Stener and Lin, 1994; Kodera *et al.*, 2002; Lawson, 1996).

Moreover, pyrone derivatives form O, O-coordinated complexes with metal ions. Recently, it was also found that the zinc complexes of the S, O analogues to pyrone derivatives (such as thioxomaltol or 1, 2-dimethyl-3-hydroxypyrimidine-4-thione can be considered as more efficient potential drug candidates for the treatment of diabetes. The characteristic metal complexes with these compounds, helpful in treatment of diabetes and metabolic syndrome in experimental animals. Studies of Milner, (2006) found that both vanadyl-and zinc-allixin complexes ameliorates diabetes and metabolic syndrome and finally opened a new research field for role of metal therapeutics and a suitable drug designs of allixins, enhanced the biological and pharmaceutical activities of the original vanadyl and zinc complexes. Metallo-allixinate complexes are now evolving in a new metallomics world, and the fruitful outcome may offer a novel medicine with high quality of antidiabetic and anti-metabolic syndrome activity for humans in the near future.

Conclusion

Nature sometimes gives us valuable crops containing compounds with significant pharmaceuticals values. Among the group of crops, spices have a significant place in terms of medicinal values. Garlic respectively belongs to spice group of plants. Garlic is the generous gifts from nature to us and have been used globally for thousands of years for culinary and medicinal purposes in most races. The overall benefits of spices have historically been associated with their macronutrient composition, such as protein and carbohydrate (starch), although there are now sufficient evidence to suggest that non-nutritional bioactive compounds play a significant role. Despite a large volume of literature, there are still the need for additional work around the substantiation of the health benefits of different metabolites and the potential synergistic effects between the different classes of bioactive. There are good evidence that levels of these bioactive in the plant are the subject to manipulation. There appears to be significant natural variation both between and within the different species of the spices and the opportunity to enhance the concentrations through plant breeding or the application of agronomic practices. Garlic has been widely studied for its chemical structure, evaluated in several clinical trials for its beneficial effects in particular, its hypocholestermic, and antiatherosclerosis, antibiotic and anticancer properties. In case of garlic, garlic bulk is the most commonly used part of the plant, where plenty of low molecular weights-containing compounds as allicin, dialkylsulfides, dithiis, alliin and S-alkylcysteine have been found for many years. Of which, allixin, an unusual non-sulphur hydroxyl-γ-pyrone structure, also a good ligand for several metal ions. Recently, allixin based metal complexes (*e.g.*, vanadyl-and zinc-allixin complexes) are now used in treatment of diabetes and various other metabolic disorders. Today, the detailed biological and pharmaceutical properties of the complexes need further research before aiming in clinical use in diabetes, CVD and cancers treatment and open a new metallomic world for treatment of such disorders in human in near future. In this way, garlic is seen as the staple food because of their nutritious nature and provides most of the ingredients that help to improve health. All of this could encourage more consumers who are concerned about their health against chronic disorders to consider eating more garlic in diet.

References

Abdullah, T. H., Kirkpatrick, D. V., and Carter, J. (1989). Enhancement of natural killer cell activity in AIDS with garlic. *Journal of Oncology*, **21**: 52-3.

Ahmed, N. (2005). Advanced glycation endproducts - role in pathology of diabetic complications. *Diabetes Research Clinical Practical*, **67**: 3-21.

Amagase, H. (2006). Clarifying the real bioactive constituents of garlic. *Journal of Nutrition*, **136 (3)**: 716-725.

Amagase, H., Petesch B.L., Matsuura, H., Kasuga, S., and Itakura, Y. (2001). Intake of garlic and its bioactive components. *Journal of Nutrition*, **131 (3)**: 955-962.

Ankari, S., and Mirelman, D. (1999). Antimicrobial properties of allicin from garlic. *Microbes and Infection*, **2**: 125-129.

Augusti, K. T. (1996). Therapeutic values of onion (*Allium cepa*) and garlic (*Allium sativum*). *Indian Journal of Experimental Biology*, **34**: 634-640.

Bhathena, S. J., Ali, A. A., and Mohammed, A. (2002). Differential effects of dietary flaxseed protein and soy protein in triglyceride and uric acid levels in animal models. *Journal of Nutritional Biochemistry*, **13**: 684-9.

Block, E. (1992). The organosulphur chemistry of the genus Allium-implications for the organic chemistry of sulphur. *Angew Chem Int Ed Engl*, **31**: 1135-78.

Bonnefont-Rousselot, D. (2002). Glucose and reative oxygen species. *Current Opinion in Clinical Nutrition and Metabolic Care*, **5**: 561-8.

Borek, C. (2004). Antioxidants and radiation therapy. *Journal of Nutrition*, **134**: 3207S-9S.

Borek, C. (2004). Dietary antioxidants and human cancer. *Integrated Cancer Therapy*, **3**: 333-341.

Budoff, M.J., Takasu, J., Flores, F.R., Niihara, Y., Lu, B., Lau. B.H., Rosen, R.T., and Amaagse, H. (2004). Inhibiting progression of coronary circulation using aged garlic extract in patients receiving statin therapy: a preliminary study. *Preverse Medicos*, **39**: 985-991.

Carson, J. F. (1987). Chemistry and biological properties of onion and garlic. *Food Review International*, **3**: 71-103.

Chang, J.S., Wendt, T., Qu W., Kong, L., Zou, Y. S., Schmidt, A. M., and Yan, S. F. (2008). Oxygen deprivation triggers up-regulation of early growth response-1 by the receptor for advanced glycation end products. *Circular Research*, **102**: 905-913.

Dorant, E., Van den Brandt, P.A., and Goldbohm, R. A. (1995). Allium vegetables consumption, garlic supplement intake and female breast carcinoma incidence. *Breast Cancer Research Treatment*, **33**: 163-170.

Duraisamy, Y., Gaffney, J., Slevin, M., Smith, C.A., Williamson, K., and Ahmed N. (2003). Amino-salicylic acid reduces the anti-proliferative effect of hyper-glycemia, advanced glycation end-products and glycated basic fibroblast with factor in cultured bovine aortic endothelial cells: comparison with aminoguanidine. *Molecular Cell Biochemistry*, **246**: 143-153.

Elliott, R.J., and McGrath, L.T. (1994). Calcification of the human thoracic aorta during aging. *Calicif Tissue International*, **54**: 268-273.

Fleischauer, A.T., and Arab, L. (2001). Garlic and cancer: A critical review of the epidemiologic literature. *Journal of Nutrition*, **131**: 1032S-1040S.

Fukushima, S., Araki, T., and Tohno, Y. (2005). Optical measurement of age-related calcification in human blood vessels. *Journal of Physiology Anthropological Application and Human Science*, **24**: 493-496.

Horie, T., Murayama, T., Mishima, T., Itoh, F., Minamide, Y., Fuwa, T., and Awazu S. (1989). Protection of liver microsomal membranes from lipid peroxidation by garlic extract. *Planta Medico*, **55**: 506-8.

Imai, J., Ide, N., Nagae, S., Moriguchi, T., Matsura, and H., Itakura, Y. (1994). Antioxidant and radical scavenging effects of aged garlic extract and its constituents. *Planta Medicos*, **60**: 417-420.

Kandil, O. M., Abdullah, T.H., Tabuni, A.M., and Elkadi, A. (1988). Potential role of *Allium sativum* in natural cytotoxicity. *Arch AIDS Research*, **1**: 230-1.

King, H., Aubert, R. E., and Herman, W. H. (1998). Global burden of diabetes, 1995-2025: Prevalence, numerical estimates, and projections. *Diabetes Care*, **21**: 1414-1431.

Kodera, Y., Suzuki, A., Imada, I., Kasuga, S., Sumioka, I., Kanezawa, A., Fujikawa, M., Nagae, S., and Masamoto, K. (2002). Physical, chemical, and biological properties of S-allylcysteine, an amino acid derived from garlic. *Journal of Agricultural and Food Chemistry*, **50**: 622-32.

Lau, B. H. S., Lam, F., and Wang-Cheng, R. (1987). Effect of odour modify garlic preparation on blood lipids. *Nutritional Research*, **7**: 139-149.

Lawson, L. D. (1996). The composition and chemistry of garlic cloves and processed garlic (2 ed.). In H. P. Koch and L. D. Lawson (Eds.). Garlic: The science and therapeutic application of Allium sativum L. and related species (pp. 37-39). Baltimore: Williams and Wilkins.

In: Koch, H. P., Lawson, L. D. (Eds.). Garlic The Science and Therapeutic Application of *Allium sativum* L. and related species. Williams and Willkins Press, USA. pp. 37-107.

Liu, L., and Yeh, Y. Y. (2002). S-alkyl cysteines of garlic inhibit cholesterol synthesis by deactivating HMG-CoA reductase in cultured rat hepatocytes. *Journal of Nutrition*, **132**: 1129-34.

Liu, L., and Yeh, Y.Y. (2001). Water-soluble organosulphur compounds of garlic inhibit fatty acids and triglycerides synthesis in cultured rat hepatocytes. *Lipids*, **36**: 395-400.

Mader, F. H. (1990). Treatment of hyperlipidermia with garlic-powder tablets. *Arzneim-Forsch*, **10**: 3-8.

Milner, J. A. (2001). Mechanism by which garlic and allyl sulphur compounds suppress carcinogen bioactivation. Garlic and carcinogenesis. *Advances in Experimental Medicine and Biology*, **492**: 69-81.

Milner, J. A. (2006). Preclinal the real bioactive constituents of garlic. *Journal of Nutrition*, **136**: 716S-25S.

Naaz, A., Yellayi, S., and Zakroczymski, M. A. (2003). The soy isoflavones genistein decreases adipose deposition in mice. *Endocrinology*, **144**: 3315-20.

Nagae, S., Ushijima, M., Hatono, S., Imai, J., Kasuga, S., Matsurra, H., Itakura, Y., and Higashi, Y. (1994). Pharmacokinetics of the garlic compound S-allyl cysteine. *Planta Medicos*, **60**: 214-217.

Napoli, C., Quehenberger, O., De Nigris, F., Abete, P., Glass, C.K., and Palisinki, W. (2000). Mildly oxidixed low density lipoprotein activates multiple apoptotic signalling pathways in human coronary cells. *FASEB Journal,* **14**: 1996-2007.

Rahman, K., and Lowe, G. M. (2006). Garlic and cardiovascular diseases. *A critical review. Journal of Nutrition,* **13**: 736-740.

Rahman, K., and Billington, D. (2000). Dietary supplementation with aged garlic extract inhibits-ADP-induced platelet aggregation in human. *Journal of Nutrition,* **130**: 2666-5.

Rivlin, R. (2001). Historical perspective on the use of garlic. *Journal of Nutrition,* **131**: 951S-954S.

Robertson, K. M., O'Donnell, L., Simpson, E. R., and Jones, M. E. (2002). The phenotype of the aromatase knockout mouse reveals dietary phyto-estrogens impact significantly on tests function. *Endrochrinology,* **43**: 2913-21.

Ruddok, P. S., Liao, M., and Foster, B.C. (2005). Garlic natural health products exhibit variable constituents levels and antimicrobial activity against *Neisseria gonorrhoeae, Staphylococcus aureus* and *Enterococcus faecalis. Pyhtotherapy Research,* **19 (4)**: 327-334.

Steiner, M., Kham, A.H., Holbert, D., and Lin, R.I.S. (1996). A double-blind crossover study in moderately hyper-cholestermic men that compared the effect of aged garlic extract and placebo administration on blood lipids. *American Journal of Clinical Nutrition,* **64**: 866-870.

Stener, M., and Lin, R. (1994). Cardiovascular and lipid changes in response to aged garlic extract ingestion. *Journal of American College of Nutrition,* **13**: 524.

Stern, D.M., Yan, S.D., Yan, S.F., and Schmidt, A. M. (2002). Receptor for advanced glycation endproducts (RAGE) and the complications of diabetes. *Ageing Research Review,* **1**: 1-15.

Stoll, A., and Seebeck, E. (1948). Allium compounds.1.Allin the true mother compound of garlic oil. *Helv Chim Acta,* **31**: 189-210.

Uesugi, T., Toda, T., Tsuji, K., and Ishida, H. (2001). Comparative study on reduction of bone loss and lipid metabolism abnormality in overiectomized rats by soy isoflavones, daidzin, genistin and glycitin. *Biology Pharma Bulletin,* **24**: 368-72.

Weber, K.S., Setchell, K. D., Stocco, D.M., and Lephart, E.D. (2001). Dietary soy-phytoestrogens decrease testosterone levels and prostate weight with altering LH, prostate 5 α-reductase or testicular steroidogenic acute regulatory peptide levels in adult male Sprague-Dawley rats. *Journal of Endocrinology,* **170**: 591-9.

Wei, Z., and Lau, B.H.S. (1998). Garlic inhibits free radical generation and augments antioxidant enzyme activity in vascular endothelial cells. *Nutritional Research,* **18**: 61-70.

Wei, Z., and Lau, B. H. S. (1998). Garlic inhibits free radical generation and augments antioxidant enzymes activity in vascular endothelial cells. *Nutritional Research*, **18**: 61-70.

Weiss, N., Ide, N. Abahji, T., Nill, L., Keller, C., and Hoffmann, U. (2006). Aged garlic extract improves homocysteine-induced endothelial dysfunction in macro- and microcirculation. *Journal of Nutrition*, **136**: 750S-754S.

Yamaguchi, F., Ariga, T., Yoshimura, Y., and Nakazawa H. (2000). Antioxidative and anti-glycation activity of garcinol from *Garcinia indica* fruit rind. *Journal of Agriculture and Food Chemistry*, **48**: 180-5.

Bioactive Phytochemicals: Perspectives for Modern Medicine Vol. 3 (2015) *Pages* **465–485**
Editor: **V.K. Gupta**
Published by: **DAYA PUBLISHING HOUSE, NEW DELHI**

19

Potential of Pulse Derived Phytochemicals against Advanced Physiological Disorders: A Critical Review

Mohd. Mazid[1*]

ABSTRACT

Soyabean is an annual plant widely cultivated for both medicinal and culinary uses. The seeds of this herb have been known through the ages for their medicinal value. Presently natural herbal products are attracting attention against a number of metabolic and physiological complexities including cardiovascular disorders, cancer and immunity based dysfunctions as a herbal healer. The use of pulse derived phytomedicine may encounter rapidly due to a broad spectrum of scientific proofs in their remedic behaviour. Pulses are the seeds of legumes. Pulses possess a variety of phytochemicals that gaining wide attention for their well-recognized potential health benefits against advanced physiological threats in present scenarios. Among pulses, the most studied pulse is soybean (Glycine max L.), traditionally recognized as an herbal medicinally used pulse rather than as an oil seed or an ordinary crop. The plant of soyabean is quite nutritious, being high in proteins, ascorbic acid, niacin, and potassium. Also, Soyabean is very rich in some amino acids, as its content of lysine and isoleucine is lower than fenugreek. It holds a unique and peculiar status for its recognized therapeutic capacity. The potent remedic roles recognized especially with respect to isoflavones amount and quality have been the subjects of more research value as well as emergent target for a number of research papers and review articles. Present article investigates the cardiovascular associated health potential of soy, observing the role of their bioactive products like isoflavones, phytosterols, resistant starch, carbohydrate, alkaloids, and saponins. Here,

---

1 Plant Physiology Section, Department of Botany, Faculty of Life Sciences, Aligarh Muslim University, Aligarh – 202002, U.P., India

* *Corresponding author*: E-mail: mazidmohd@gmail.com

much emphasis given to evidences for health benefits is based on strong activities of bioactive constituents to combat oxidative stress, active participation in cardiovascular cure and their prospective as immune stimulators. These preliminary studies not only suggest alternative and cheaper remedies for the pharmaceutical industries also.

Keywords: Isoflavones, Oxidative stress, Physiological disorders, Soybean, Phytochemicals, Diabetes.

Introduction

The World Health Organization (WHO) has estimated that up to 80 per cent of all diseases and sickness in the world is caused by inadequate sanitation, polluted water or unavailability of water. About 1.8 million people are forced to use contaminated water (Cheesbrough,1984), which are polluted with either industrial waste like pharmaceutical wastes or domestic waste. Diet is a pivotal link with human health and food rich in phytochemicals often associated with proper functionality of immune system. Food levels are widely used to convey the health benefits of conventional foods or a component of food to the consumer. The increasing amount of health information available regarding the health benefits of food has resulted in consumer interest in the health issues and has become a leading factor in purchasing decisions. Many consumers try to eat healthier foods, use natural medicines, and make life style changes in the quest to feel good, maintain body weight, reduce the risk of chronic disease, and live healthier longer lives. Globally, unhealthy diets and physical inactivity are two of the leading causes of major chronic diseases. According to the WHO, non-communicable chronic diseases, such as heart diseases, stroke, cancer, chronic respiratory diseases, diabetes, are by far the leading cause of mortality in the world reporting 60 per cent of all death (Alfred *et al.*, 2001). In 2004, the 192 member states of the WHO endorsed the global strategy on diet, physical activity and health (Alfred *et al.*, 2001), addressing two main risk factors. Countries around the world are monitoring the prevalence of chronic "life style" diseases and developing strategies to treat, prevent and reduce the incidence of disease in future years. Health professionals are promoting dietary changes; including the increased consumption of plant food to compact nutritional deficiencies is chronic disease risk.

Medicinal herbs have been used in primary health care over many countries before the advent of modern medicine. Over the last 20 years, there has been an international resurgence of medicinal herbs in all cultures of world, especially in the Asia which has an enhanced interest in natural system of cure and the questioning of an over-dependence on synthetic drugs to maintain health. Moreover, today, there has been an impressive gain in individual life expectancy with parallel increase in age-related chronic diseases of the cardiovascular, brain and immune systems. These can cause loss of autonomy, dependence and high social cost for individual and society. It is now accepted that the ageing and age related disease are in part caused by free radical reactions. The arrest of ageing and stimulation of rejuvenation of the human body is also being sought. Over the last 20 years the uses of herbs and natural products has gained popularity and these are being consumed backed by epidemiological evidence. Similarly trends have been observed and the growth rate of therapeutics in Europe has been repeated to be greater than those pharmaceuticals (Alhasan *et al.*, 2000). Several epidemiological studies have thrown that a diet rich in plant food may reduce the development of certain chronic diseases such as cardiovascular related diabetes, atherosclerosis, cancer, arthritis, rejuvenation of stain and disease associated with cerebral aging (Allred *et al.*, 2006; Boydak *et al.*, 2002), one such food is soybean.

Pulses

The world food supplies are usually debated in terms of cereals being the dominant commodities, but there exists a second group of crops, the pulses (legume grains).The pulses by virtue of having almost twice the amount of protein in comparison with cereals, make a major contribution to human diet in developing countries of tropical and sub-tropical areas where their nutritional contribution is of paramount importance as a large segment of the population in these areas has limited access to food of animal origin. Eleven primary pulses have been recognized by the Food and Agriculture Organization (FAO) of the United Nations at global level. These pulses include dry beans (common bean, *Phaseolus vulgaris* L.; lima bean, *Phaseolus lunatus* L.; tepary bean, *Phaseolus acutifolius* A. Gray; scarlet runner bean, *Phaseolus coccineus* L.; black gram, *Vigna mungo* L. Hepper; green gram, *Vigna radiata* L. Wilczek; moth bean, *Vigna aconitifolia* Jacq Marechal; rice bean, *Vigna umbellata* Thumb Ohwi and Ohashi and adzuki bean, *Vigna angularis* Willd Ohwi and Ohashi), dry broad bean (*Vicia faba* L.), dry peas (*Pisum* spp.) dry cowpea (*Vigna unguiculata* L. Walp), pigeon pea (*Cajanus cajan* L. Millspaugh), chickpea (*Cicer arietinum* L.), lentil (*Lens culinaris* Medik or *Lens esculenta* Moench), bambara groundnut (*Vigna subterranean* L. Verdc.), lupines (*Lupinus* spp.), common vetch (*Vicia sativa* L.) and minor pulses (lablab, *Lablab purpureus* L. Sweet; jack beans, *Canavalia ensiformis* L.DC.; sword bean, *Canavalia gladiate* Jacq. DC.; winged bean, *Psophocarpus teragonolobus* L.DC.; velvet bean, *Mucuna pruriens* L. DC. and yam bean, *Pachyrhizus erosus* L. Urb.). As far as our country is concerned, 12 different pulse crops, namely chickpea, pigeon pea, lentil, black gram, green gram, lablab, moth bean, horse gram (*Dolichos uniflorus* Lam.), pea (*Pisum sativum* L.), grass pea, (*Lathyrus sativus* L.), cowpea (*Vigna unguiculata* L. Walp.) and faba bean (*Vicia faba* L.), are cultivated (Nene, 2006).

Background and Taxonomic History

Soybean (*Glycine max* L.)

Soybean originated in China over 13,000 years ago where they were considered one of the most important crops in the area and also evident from Chinese writings dating back to 2800 B.C., in which it is mentioned as one of the five principal and sacred crops. But the good news about soy's culinary versatility and exceptional health benefits is a relatively recent phenomenon in the west. It made first appearance in the US in the 18th century, planted by an American who brought then back from China. American farmers began planting soybeans in the 19th century. Interest in the nutritional benefits of soybeans has steadily increased since then, in the past few years, a true groundswell of interest has occurred. This has come about in response to the scientific research that is supporting the numerous ways that soy can promote health. It is very nutritive and used as a protein adjunct to starchy diets. It is given as preventive diet to antherosclerosis patients because of its rich phosphorus (P) content. Whole germinated seeds are used as a prophylactic against deficiency diseases, scurvy in particular in famine affected areas.

It was introduced to India in about 1880 and is now being cultivated in Madhya Pradesh (3600, 00 t), Maharashtra (67000 t), Rajasthan (370,000 t) and to some extent in Uttar Pradesh, Karnataka, Himachal Pradesh, Assam and Manipur. *Glycine max* L. is essentially a sub-tropical plant but its cultivation extends to tropical and temperate regions up to latitude 52 C. It will successes on nearly all types of soil, but grows best on deep fertile soils with high calcium content. It is essentially a short-day- plant. It is the most widely grown and utilized legume in the world and one of the most well researched, health promoting food available today. Like other beans, it grows in pods, featuring edible seeds. It provides each of the nutrients which are good, very good or excellent sources according to our Food Rating System (FRS). There are several factors for its low productivity of chickpea in our. A few of these are described here (i) more than 75 per cent of Indian farmers own small or marginal holdings of less than two hectares, (ii)severe drought results in sudden decline in chickpea area and ultimately productivity, (iii) even, otherwise, the farmer does not give the same weightage to pulses(including chickpea) as to cereals, (iv) excessive cold conditions adversely affect productivity, (v) most of the area under chickpea is rain-fed, (vi) use of poor quality seed diminishes productivity further, (vii) low or no use of fertilizers due to scarcity of funds, (viii) generally, farmers are ignorant of precise doses of fertilizers recommended by the Agriculture Department for a particular cultivar and region, the techniques of cultivation of high yielding varieties, post-harvest technology and poor processing and storage facilities, (ix) about one third of flowers produced do not develop into fruits, (x) pest and diseases cause considerable losses, (xi) sudden excessive rain soon after sowing or at flowering does great harm, (xii) an early hot summer shortens the growing period, hastens maturity and ultimately reduces yield and (xiii) hailstorms at ripening causes much damage.

Composition of Soybean

Pulses have traditionally played a major role in providing food nutrition particularly in the Indian sub-continent and other developing countries. Traditionally, pulses were consumed with minimal processing, and consumers were interested primarily with size shape and colour characteristics. As the countries of the Indian subcontinent developed, a greater emphasis was placed on processing characteristics, which included hydration and cooking times as well as dehulling and splitting efficiency. This pulse represents the current status for the majority of markets that consume pulse grains as a staple diet. Market traits represent basic quality characteristics, the underlying chemical characteristics are based on protein and starch composition and phenolic compounds that affect the taste and colour of the seed coat and cotyledons. The nutritional properties of pulse have been investigated extensively and have been reported to impart physiologically beneficial effects in humans. Pulse grains are high in protein, carbohydrates, and dietary fibre and are a rich source of other nutritional components (Collerchio *et al.*, 2006). Pulse grains contain a large number of bioactive compounds which have a metabolic benefit when consumed on a regular basis (Guillon *et al.*, 2002). Demand has increased regarding the use of pulses for human consumption either to extract a functional compound to incorporate this in to cereal-based products or to extract phytocompounds which are bioactive and can be used as nutraceutical products. Considerable genetic variation has been reported in the chemicals composition of the pulses both between and within species. In addition, chemical composition is modified by environmental factors during plant development, and many of the phytochemicals are secondary metabolites produced during the seed development and seed maturation. Soybean is an excellent source of molybdenum. They are also a very good source of protein and manganese. In addition, soybean is a good source of iron, phosphorus, dietary fibre, omega-3 fatty acids, magnesium, cupper, vitamins B_2, and potassium. In addition to the full array of nutrients, soybean also posses carbohydrates, sugar, soluble and insoluble fibre, sodium, vitamins minerals, fatty acids, amino acids, oxalate and more.

Furthermore, soybean is regarded as equal in protein quality to animal foods. Just one cup of soybean provides 57.2 per cent of the Daily Value (DV) for protein for less than 300 calories and only 2.2 grams of saturated fat. Soy protein tends to lower cholesterol levels, while consuming protein from animals sources tends to raise them, since they also include saturated fat and cholesterol. In addition to healthy protein, some of soybeans nutritional high points include a good deal of well-absorbed iron; 49.1 per cent of the DV for iron in that same cup of soybean; pulse 37 per cent of the DV for natures relaxant, magnesium; and 41.2 per cent of the DV for essential omega-3 fatty acids. Soybean attain a good position among other pulse crops due to naturally occurring plant products (isoflavones) posses various potent biological activities in human health. In fact, most of investigations on soybean's active principles have focused on the isoflavones, in which two most important are genitein and daidzen; Genistein has been consistently linked to lower incidence of prostate cancer. This not only induced chemicals that block cell cycling, thus preventing the proliferation of cancerous cells in the prostrate, but at self-destruct sequence the body uses to eliminate worn-out or abnormal cells. Other one is, daidzen has also demonstrated protective action against prostate cancer.

Because of the intense interest in soybean, commercial soy preparations have over the years become available. Soy foods contain complex mixtures of bioactive compounds that interest with one another to promote health, while the partially purified isoflavones-containing products consumed in the U.S, may have lost many of the biologically active components in whole soy foods. These partially purified isoflavones-containing products may not have the same health benefits as whole soy foods. Soy foods may offer special benefits for the heart and bones of premenopausal women's; several studies indicate a beneficial synergy between isoflavones, the weakly estrogenic compounds in soy, and the body's own estrogens in decreasing cholesterol and increasing bone mass. In addition, the texture of soy is so adoptable that they can be processed in a host of different ways making it easy for you to enjoy them in your daily diet. There are fresh soy (edamame) dried soy seeds, soy milk, soynuts, tofu, tempeh soy flour, natto, miso.... the list goes on and on. A variety of soy commercially eaten in the Asian diet contains isoflavones including tofu, miso, soymilk, soybeans sprout and a fermented soy food called natto. Almost 75 per cent of the women's reported eating miso soup daily and of these 34 per cent are three or more cups of misso soup per day. More than 45 per cent reported eaten soy foods other than miso daily.

Chemistry of Soybean

The nutritional importance of soybean are numerous, it can be a valuable source of energy. The energy content of soybean has been found to be between 403Kcal/100 gm. The energy of pulses came from the nutrient supply of protein, fat and carbohydrate. Soy contains a large number of bioactive compounds which have a metabolic benefit when consumed on a regular basis (Guillon *et al.*, 2002). Most pulse species contain about 1 per cent fat, while soybean has very high fat content about, 30 per cent (Davis *et al.*, 1968). Soy also contains linolenic acid, which is an omega-3-fatty acid. This fatty acid is currently being studied for its ability to reduce the risk of heart disease and cancer. Potential of certain classes of soybean phytochemicals, including starch, phytosterols, isoflavones, saponins, alkaloids, and bioactive carbohydrates, is discussed below in reference to their influence on human health.

Phytosterols

They are structural components of the plant-cell membranes. In soybean, they are present in small quantities, and the most common are β-sitosterol (Tharanathan and Mahadevamma, 2003) compersterol (Peterson *et al.*, 1997), and stigmas-sterol (Guillon and Champ, 2002). These compounds are also abundant as sterol glycosides and esterify sterol glycosides. Epidemiological data indicates that the consumption of soy grains lowers the mortality rate from CVD (Kushi *et al.*, 1999). Elevated levels of serum low-density lipoprotein (LDL) cholesterol is a major cause of CVD and studies have shown that every reduction in cardiovascular mortality (Shepherd *et al.*, 1995). The consumption of soy has been reported to lower serum cholesterol and increase the saturation level of LDL cholesterol by partially interrupting the entrohepatic circulation of the bile acids and increasing the cholesterol saturation by increasing the hepatic secretion of cholesterol.

Resistant Starch (RS)

Soy is high in RS and retains their functionality even after cooking. There are a strong inverse relation between the intake of starch and the risk of colorectal cancer (Cassidy *et al.*, 1994). RS is the proportion of starch that is not hydrolyzed as it passes through the gastro-intentional tract (Englyst *et al.*, 1992). It can be considered a probiotic and acts as a substrate for microbiological fermentation, producing short-chain fatty acids, methane and carbon dioxide, conferring benefits to human colonic health and to a lesser extent can impact lipid and glucose metabolism. The production of these fermentation products from the consumption of RS is less than that from the consumption of non-oligosaccharides (Christl *et al.*, 1992). As a food ingredient, RS has a lower calorific (8 KJ/g); however, it can be incorporated in to a wide range of mainstream food products such as backed products without affecting processing properties/the overall disappearance and taste of the products (Douglas *et al.*, 2006).

Saponins

They consist of a triterpene/steroid nucleus with mono-or oligosaccharides attached to this core. They have great structural diversity and have long been considered undesirable due to toxicity and their haemolytic activity. The most common in soy is soy saponins, classified in to group AB and E saponins on the basis of the chemical structure of the steroid nucleus. Soya saponins have reported for their better taste (Shi *et al.*, 2004). The literature suggests that soysaponins may possess anticancer activity (Zhu *et al.*, 2006 and Fung *et al.*, 2001), and be beneficial for hyperlipidermia (Shi *et al.*, 2004 and Alzorriz *et al.*, 1999). The adjuvant properties of certain saponins have been utilized in vaccines for many years (Rajput *et al.*, 2007). Additional mechanistic studies indicates that there is evidence for saponins regulation of the apoptosis pathway enzymes (AKT, Bcl and ERK1/2) leading to PCD of cancer cells (Ellington *et al.*, 2006; Xiao *et al.*, 2007). Research on colon cancer cells suggests that it is the lipophilic saponins cores that may be responsible for the biological activity. The *in vitro* fermentations carried out by these authors also suggest that colonic micro flora hydrolyze soysaponins to the aglycones, potentially enhancing the activity of the soysaponins (Gurfinkel and Rao, 2003).

Isoflavones

Isoflavones are secondary vegetable substances which can act as estrogens in the body and have protective functions. The estrogens effects of isoflavones are much less powerful than the estrogens hormones. They also have been isolated from a wide variety of soybean or other leguminous plants. There has been enormous interest in their biological activity. Chemically, they are based on phenylchromen. They are transferred by bacteria in the intestinal flora during digestion. In order to obtain a regular absorption of isoflavones, the intake of isoflavones rich food or isoflavones supplements must be spread during the day. The best way to consume isoflavones is in the form of soy or soy foods, so you can benefit from other healthy components of soy. Soy contains many types of isoflavones, but the most beneficial are genitein and daidzen. Isoflavones are fairly stable. Under normal cooking conditions, isoflavones are not destroyed. The chemical structure of isoflavones is very similar to that of our own estrogens. Because of this similarity in structure of isoflavones can interfere with the action of our own estrogens. Sometimes, isoflavones will reduce the effects of estrogens because they complete with the same receptor sites on our cells. Some of the risk of excess estrogens can be lowered in this way. They can also increase the estrogens activity.

Recently, there has been attention focused on a different class of isoflavones, the glyceollins, which have been reported from soy. These are biosynthetically related to pterocarpan and probably derive from the condensation of pterocarpan and a C-5-terpene. Five of the most reported isoflavones are Genistein (Panozzo and Materne, 2007), daidzen (Cassidy *et al.*, 1994), coumestrol (Englyst *et al.*, 1992), for monoetin (Christl *et al.*, 1992) and biochanin A (Topping *et al.*, 2003). There are many biological activities associated with the isoflavones, including a reduction in osteoporosis and the prevention of cancer and CVD, and they can be used for the treatment of symptoms of menopause. The potential health benefits of isoflavones for humans have been the subjects of several reviews that have analysed clinical, animal, and *in vitro* evidence for biological activity (Trock *et al.*, 2006; Kostelac *et al.*, 2003). Trock *et al.* (2006) conclude that there are a small inverse correlation between soy intake and breast cancer but note that data limitations cannot rule out the possibility that this result is an artefact of the analysis. One of the recommendations of the conference was to encourage future studies to reduce the heterogeneity of soy exposure data on the literature and provide more detail regarding not only total soy food but also nutrient content, such as the level of isoflavones (Martinez *et al.*, 2006).

Research in several areas of healthcare has shown that consumption of isoflavones may play a role in lowering risk for disease. They can fight against diseases on several fronts. The following potential health benefits are attributed to isoflavones: (1) CHD (2) Cancer (3) Diabetes. Bhathena *et al.* (2004) observed significant effect of isoflavones on body weight in obese rats. However, there was no effect food intake. In genetically obese mice and in aromatise knock out (ER-deficient) mice, isoflavones have been reported to reduce body weight (Robertson *et al.*, 2002; Aoyama *et al.*, 2000). In ovariectomized mice the isoflavones, genitein had no significant effect on body weight/food intake (Leterme *et al.*, 2002). A decrease in body weight was observed only with high intake of genitein (Leterme *et al.*, 2002). Leterme *et al.* (2002) did not observe any decrease in muscle weight in mice fed genitein (Leterme *et al.*, 2002). Thus, the effect of isoflavones appears to be tissue specific and may also depends on species and gender. Previous studies of Leterme *et al.* (2002) have shown no significant difference in body weight or tissue weight between rats fed casein or soy protein concentrate (Bhathena *et al.*, 2002; Bhathena *et al.*, 2003). Thus, it appears that isoflavones but not the type of protein affects the body weight or the tissue weights. The striking findings of Bhathena *et al.* (2004) are the significant reduction in all fat depots by isoflavones. Adipose tissue metabolism is under the control of estrogens and the studies of Bhathena *et al.* (2004) show that soy isoflavones have several effects even though phytoestrogens have several fold less estrogenic and anti-estrogenic effect than the endogenous estrogen estradiol. In addition, genistein has been shown to decrease lipoprotein lipase mRNA in parametrical fat pads indicating anti linolenic effect. Other isoflavones, daidzen and glycetin also affect adipose tissue weight (Messina *et al.*, 2002). Several previous studies in human and animals have suggested that isoflavones affect the endocrine system or circulating hormones that may affect obesity or lipid metabolism. For example, Moon *et al.* (2006) have repeated that phytoestrogens from soy decreased plasma testosterone and androstenedione in rats. A 3-years breeding study demonstrated that levels of isoflavones are related to both environmental and genetic elements that would be susceptible to selection (Mebrahtu *et al.*, 2004), and these genomic regions have been identified (Kassem *et al.*, 2004). This is an active area of research; for example, U.S. Agriculture research service has initiated research project working to isoflavones to enhance content in plants (Ofuya and Akhidue, 2005).

Uses

The cultivation has several benefits for the farming community and land and society. These include, among others, (i) reduction of fertilizer costs as farmers do not need to supply N, (ii) natural rejuvenation of the soil as the crop fixes N, (iii) lower water usage as the crop does not require extensive irrigation, (iv) reduction in carbon dioxide (CO_2) emission as these is a reduced need for fertilizers and subsequently fossil fuels that are used to manufacture fertilizers, and (v) reduction in greenhouse gases as the crop absorbs CO_2 for photosynthesis and lowers nitrous oxide level in the atmosphere by their ability to fix N. It is an important pulse crop. It is used in various ways. The important uses are given below.

Immature green pods and young tender leaves are cooked and eaten as vegetables especially in India and Nepal. The leaves are used in salads and sauces. Chickpea seeds are eaten fresh as green vegetables, parched, fried, roasted and boiled and as snack food, sweet and condiments. The floor obtained after grinding the seeds, can be used as soup, dal and to make bread. The seeds (boiled or germinated) after preparing with pepper, salt and lemon can be used as a side dish. A small portion of canned chickpea is also used to produce fermented food. It is a good source of minerals and vitamins. Soyabean husks, green or dried stems and leaves and even seed are used for stock feed.

Seeds have 61 per cent carbohydrates that breakdown more slowly during digestion and thus the seeds have a glycaemic index of less than half that of wheat and whole (canned) white bread. Seeds contain 2-3 times more protein than cereal grains, and thus can specifically be used to treat protein mal-nutrition and Kwashiorkor disease in children. Moreover, the protein contains balanced amino acids, *i.e.* S amino acids are limited and lysine content is high. Soyabean is, therefore, an ideal companion to cereals which are known to be higher in S-amino acids but limited in lysine. Soyabean contains higher lipid content than other pulses. The lipid content comprises 59-60 per cent poly-unsaturated, 14-20 per cent mono-unsaturated and 18-24 per cent saturated fatty acids. Soyabean, therefore, contains mostly of the beneficial kind (mono-unsaturated and poly-unsaturated) of fat rather than saturated fats that have been linked to heart and circulatory diseases.

The green preparations are rich in several vitamins, including folate, vitamins A, C, K and β-carotene, and other various health-beneficial Phytochemicals such as carotenoids. By virtue of containing 0.02 to 6.00 mg/g phenolics, the seed proved as a potent agent for the treatment and prevention of cancer, cardiovascular disease, hypertension, hypercholesterolemia, atherosclerosis, bacterial and viral infection, diarrhoea, ulcers, inflammation and allergies.

Soybean: Scientific Classification

Kingdom-Plantae

Sub-kingdom-Tracheobionta

Super-division-Spermatophyta

Division-Magnoliophyta-Angiosperms

Order-Fabales

Family-Fabaceae

Sub-family- Fabiodeae

Genus-*Glycine*

Species-*Glycine max* L. cultivated soybean

Reactive Oxygen Species (Oxidative Stress) and Soy (Isoflavones)

Reactive oxygen species and oxidative stress are implicated in CVD, cancer and various forms of dementia including Alzheimer's disease (AD) (Panozzo and Materna, 2007). Oxidative damage to DNA, proteins, lipids and other molecules rank high as a major cause in the onset and development of these diseases. ROS including free radicals ($OH^{\bullet-}$, H_2O_2 and $O_2^{\bullet-}$), are by-products of normal metabolism and increase during infection and inflammation, hyperhomocysteinemia and exposure to exogenous sources, including nitrogenous oxide metabolite pollutants, smoking certain drugs (*e.g.*, acetaminophene and radiation). The majority of the diseases associated with old age are initiated by free radicals. Genistein and daidzen are the important components of soy seeds like other phytoestrogens, which have been demonstrated to have strong antioxidative properties. The soy yogurt enriched with blue berries inhibited the activity of various enzymes such as angiotensin-1 converting enzyme (ACE-1), which plays a role in the construction of blood vessels and is a target of blood pressure-lowering medications (ACE-inhibitors). Plain soy yogurt had higher phenols content (phenols are potent anti-oxidants to and are sometimes even more potent than vitamins antioxidants) and high levels of antioxidant activity. However, some of the anti-oxidative effects *in vivo* may be predominantly the results of other phenolic components and not ACE inhibitors (Mitchell, 2001). Although a small number of studies have identified certain ACE inhibitors containing drugs as having antioxidative properties, further research is needed to characterize ACE inhibitors isolated from pulse seeds. Moreover, most of the antioxidative studies described above have been performed *in vitro*. Further research should be undertaken to examine antioxidative potentialities *in vivo,* with and without encapsulation. Therefore, additional research is needed to further investigations of antioxidative properties of garlic and soy and other potential role in human health and disease.

Biochemistry of Ageing: Role of Isoflavones

Ageing is a progressive decline in the efficiency of biochemical and physiological processes after the reproduction phase of life. Free radical theory of ageing postulates that ageing is caused by free radical reactions which may be involved in production of the ageing changes associated with the environment, disease and intrinsic factors of ageing process. Since, it is well accepted that oxidative free radical stress is an important contributor to the ageing process and too many age-related diseases, the focus must be on reducing oxidative stress *in vivo*. This is important because oxidative damage apparently increases with age and thus may overwhelm the natural repair systems in the elderly (Peterson *et al.*, 2000). One best way to neutralize free radical mediated oxidative stress in the elderly is to ingest diet rich in phytochemicals with antioxidant properties. These are widely present in plants products. Such two naturally occurring plants are soy and garlic and their potential in prevention of diseases associated with ageing is reviewed here.

Role of Isoflavones in Cardiovascular Diseases (CVD)

Coronary heart diseases (CHD) are the leading cause of death in North America and in most Western countries (Pisulewska and Pisulewska, 2000). Epidemiological studies have identified number of risk factors for the development of CHD which include elevated serum lipids increased plasma fibrinogen and coagulation factors, increased platelet activation, alternations in glucose metabolism (Wood, 2001). There are strong epidemiological evidence that atherosclerosis-related conditions (Coronary artery disease, Ischemic stroke and peripheral artery disease) all increase with age (Roy *et al.*, 2010) and its effects are mainly evident in the muscular arteries. Ageing causes the changes in the structure and function of the vessels that leads to an increase in the incidence of certain CHD causing enhancement of both morbidity and mortality. Enhanced oxidative stress with ageing may also play an important role in the increased prevalence of atherosclerosis in older individuals. Evidence from both *in vitro* and *in vivo* studies suggests that oxidation of LDL may contribute to early atherosclerotic lesion formation (Sakurai *et al.*, 1996) and there is also a continuous increase in LDL hydroxyl fatty acids content with age in healthy, olderly individuals (Salim-ur-Rehman *et al.*, 2007). Oxidised LDL elicits pro-atherogenic properties like increased smooth muscles proliferation (Sarkar *et al.*, 2006), cytotoxicity to vascular endothelial cells, smooth muscles cells and fibroblasts (Sing *et al.*, 2006) together with the induction of apoptotic cell death in vascular endothelial cells (Napoli *et al.*, 2000). There is strong evidence that nutritional factors contribute to the etiology of the condition and that dietary modifications, together with life-style modification are important in the treatment of patients (Tsukamoto *et al.*, 1995). Populations with diets rich in carbohydrates tend to have reduced risk for CHD. It appears that intact fruits, vegetables, pulses and whole grains are the best sources of carbohydrate, most recommended in diets to reduce the risk of CHD. A positive correlation has been established between CHD death rate and plasma cholesterol level, and among other things, the latter is due to too high a consumption of saturated fat. Above these foods have been shown to decrease serum LDL-cholesterol and triglycerides (Major factor for CHD) and affect other risk factors. Epidemiological data suggests that a regular intake of soy may contribute to lowering of the plasma cholesterol level. In numerous clinical trials, consumption of soy has shown to significantly reduce serum lipid levels. Total serum cholesterol was reduced by 7 per cent, LDL-cholesterol by 6 per cent and serum tri-acylglycerols by more than 17 per cent with no significant changes in HDL-cholesterol in a recent meta-analysis of 11 clinical trials investigating the effects of soy intake on serum lipids (Sarkar *et al.*, 2006).

Soy protein is rich in phytoestrogens, notably the isoflavones genistein and daidzen (Sarkar *et al.*, 2006). Phytoestrogens are naturally formed environmental oestrogens that are synthesized from phenyl propanoid and simple phenols and have a similar structure to oestradiol. Epidemiological evidence suggests that population that consume soy products as a dietary staple have a lower incidence of cardiovascular disease than those in which soy protein consumption is minimal, and this has led to the suggestion that isoflavones may be dependency between soy intake and risk of coronary heart diseases has been reported in 40 to 70-year old women's in China, although population based studies of this nature cannot prove causality and may be confounded by other dietary influences. Moreover, recent studies have suggested that soy protein *per se* rather than dietary isoflavones may have biological effects that could reduce cardiovascular risk (Sarkar *et al.*, 2006). Studies in experimental animals in which cardiovascular responses to genistein and daidzein have been assessed are broadly supportive of a protective role of isoflavones. Studies of Xavier *et al.* (2004) suggests that the isoflavones content of soy protein has no influence on blood pressure in healthy rates fed a diet based on soy protein but influences small artery function like increased sensitivity to acetylcholine. Daidzen has been shown to improve aortic function through enhancement of the NOS (nitric oxide synthase) pathway in male rats (Zhu *et al.*, 1999), and in female ovariectomized rats genitein leads to improved acetylcholine-mediated relaxation. However, a recent report suggested soy protein consumption throughout life substantially reduced B.P and improved endothelial function and antioxidant gene expression in 12-to 16 month-old male rats. Soy isoflavones also appear to reduce cardiovascular disease risk via several distinct mechanisms. They inhibit the growth of cells that form artery clogging plaque. These arteries usually form blood clots which can lead to a heart attack. Several studies on soy and heart disease concluded that soy is definitely effective for improving cholesterol profile. There is some evidence that they are the active ingredient of soy responsible for improving cholesterol profile.

Moreover, the meta-analysis of Zulet *et al.* (1999) concluded the effects of soy protein intake on serum lipids. This study also suggests that soy protein is correlated with significantly decreases in serum cholesterol, LDL (bad cholesterol) and triglycerides. However, HDL (good cholesterol) did not increase by a significant amount.Soy isoflavones (genistein and daidzein) absorbed on the soy protein were suggested as the agent reducing serum cholesterol levels. On the basis of this research Technologies International (PTI) filed a petition with FDA in 1998 for a health claim that soy protein may reduce cholesterol and the risk of heart disease. The FDA granted the following heath claim for soy: 25 grams of soy protein a day, as a part of a diet low in saturated fat and cholesterol, may reduce the risk of heart disease (Leterme *et al.*, 2008). Now, there is growing evidence that the isoflavones may have a role to play in the treatment of metabolic disorders. A meta-analysis of 38 different controlled clinical traits concluded that soy protein intake led to decreased serum concentrations of total cholesterol, LDL cholesterol, and triglycerides. Genistein, daidzein and biochanin-A have been reported as oestrogen-related receptors (ERRα, ERRβ and ERRγ) bind and regulate transcription by estrogens response elements but do not bind endogenous estrogens. ERRα is involved in energy homeostasis and so is a widely target for the treatment of metabolic disorders (Ariazi and Jordon, 2006). Moreover, studies of Moon *et al.* (2006) has shown first time that the isoflavones component of dietary soy protein (principally genistein, daidzein and its metabolic equol) induces modest functional changes in small arteries from rat fed a balanced diet containing soy protein from conception to 6-months of age and also demonstrated that dietary isoflavones influence the distensibility and endothelium-dependent dilatation of resistance arteries. These modest functional changes could be associated with reduction in cardiovascular risk as they occurred in the presence of plasma genistein concentrations comparable to those reported in Japanese men consuming as standard soy rich Japanese diet (Sarkar *et al.*, 2006). However, dietary soy isoflavones may afford cardio protection during the course of ageing and in vascular disease. Previous studies of Chinese women's (age-50) and Japanese men (age-50) have shown an inverse association between soy protein consumption and Singh *et al.* (2006) claimed that these associations may be unrelated to the isoflavones content of the soy diet and that soy protein itself may have some hypotensive benefit. Results of experimental studies of Roy *et al.* (2010) on rats suggests that cholesterol lowering effects of a soy protein isolate were found partly explicable on the basis of the protein component rather than isoflavones content.

Furthermore, isoflavones have been implicated in reducing the mean arterial pressure in adult ovariectomized spontaneously hypersensitive rats fed a soy based diet compared with a casein base diet for 8 weeks whereas no effect was seen in normotensive ovariectomized animals (Xavier *et al.*, 2004). There are a modest effect of isoflavones elution from the soy protein on endothelial function are assessed by acetylcholine-induced relaxation in the small mesenteric arteries. As no difference observed that in endothelium-independent relaxation, it is unlikely that this resulted from greater NO smooth muscle sensitivity, but more probably was associated with greater NO bio-availability. Increased NO synthesis has been implicated in rats treated subcutaneously with daidzen (Xavier *et al.*, 2004). Isoflavones may also increase NO bioavailability by enhancement of antioxidant capacity. However, endothelium-derived hyper-polarizing factor (EDHF) is also very likely to play a role, since in rats EDHF accounts for 60-70 per cent of acetylcholine mediated relaxation in small mesenteric arteries (Taylor *et al.*, 2004), whereas acetylcholine mediated relaxation in aorta is almost exclusively due to NO. The divergence from the other reports which have shown enhancement by isoflavones of aortic endothelial function could partially be explained by the dose of isoflavones used (Singh *et al.*, 2006).

Role of Isoflavones in Diabetes

Diabetes is a condition where there is too much sugar (glucose) in the blood. It results when people either don't produce enough insulin or have high levels of insulin in their blood, which is not working properly. It is of two types. Type 1 diabetes is most common in children and young adults but it can occur at any age. It occurs when the pancreas no longer produces insulin and treatment involves lifelong insulin injections. Type 2 diabetes is the most common form, affecting both adults and, an increasing number of children and young people, particularly in populations which are sedentary and overweight. In this case, the pancreas does not produce enough insulin. The prevalence of type 2 diabetes mellitus (type 2 DM) has been increasing rapidly worldwide (Zulet *et al.*, 1999); thus, knowledge of risk factors and protective factors associated with type 2 DM is essential for the development of prevention strategies. Yet, a healthy life style can totally prevent or dramatically reduce the risk of type-2 diabetes. Diabetes mellitus is a common endocrine disorder characterized by hyperglycemias and long-term complications affecting the eyes, nerves, blood vessels, skin and kidneys. Increased glycation of proteins and accumulation of advanced glycation products (AGEPs) have been implicated in the pathogenesis of diabetic complications. Glycation and AGEP formation are also accompanied by formation of free radicals via auto-oxidation of glucose and glycated proteins. Compounds with combined antiglycation and antioxidant properties may offer therapeutic potential.

Present number of diabetic worldwide is 150 million and this and this is likely to increase to 300 million or more by the year 2025. Many herbal medicines have been recommended for the treatment of diabetes. Frequently, plant drugs are considered to be less toxic and more free from side effects than synthetic ones. Of which DM is a metabolic disorder characterized by chronic hyperglycaemia and hyperlipidermia that predisposes affected individuals to long term micro and macro-vascular complications. Hyperglycaemia causes increased protein glycation and the formation of advanced glycation end products which underlie the complications of diabetes and ageing. Glycation is accompanied by metal-catalysed oxidation of glucose and Amadori products to form free radicals capable of proteins fragmentation. Glycation products involving dicarbonyl intermediates such as 3-deoxyglycosome and methyl glyoxal to for caplumes, heterogeneous, florescent and cross linked structures. Accumulation of glycation products in body tissue are believed to be responsible for the long term complications of diabetes and ageing (Tsukamoto *et al.,* 2005).

Indeed, diabetes mellitus and ageing are associated with a build-up of tissue advanced glycation food products, increased oxidative stress and decline in antioxidant status. The involvement of advanced glycation end products in diabetes complications and ageing has promoted a search for compounds capable of inhibiting their formation. Recent studies suggest that compounds with combined antiglycation and antioxidant properties after maximum protection against glucose-induced cellular damage (Sarkar *et al.,* 2006).

Legumes have been indirectly linked to a protective role in the development of type 2DM as component of a prudent diet (Hu *et al.,* 2000), which is associated with a lower risk of type 2DM. Conversely, in another study, high consumption of soy was linked to a dietary pattern associated with an increased risk of type 2DM. The protective effect of soy isofalvones intake on type 2DM involve multiple biological pathways, including increased fibre content in the diet (Hu *et al.,* 2000), a reduction in the glycemic index of mixed meals (Jenkins *et al.,* 1988), or both. In addition, soybean are good sources of fibres and are rich in isoflavones which act as antioxidant in the body as well as have a low glycemic index (GI), important in controlling blood sugar levels. Now, it has been postulated that a diet high in isoflavones has be beneficial for the prevention of type 2 DM. However, data linking type 2DM risk and soy are limited (Zhou *et al.,* 2005). Soy alone may be associated with a lower risk of type 2DM. In animal models of obesity and diabetes, isoflavones has been shown to reduce serum insulin and insulin resistance (Bhathena *et al.,* 2002). In studies of human subjects with and without type 2DM, isoflavones appears to moderate hypoglycemia, reduce body weight, and hyperinsulinemia (Bhathena *et al.,* 2002). Studies of Bathena *et al.* (2002) also suggests that isoflavones intake was inversely associated with the type 2DM. Increasing intake of isoflavones helps to regulate blood sugar levels and reduces your cholesterol. In addition, eating more of isoflavones rich food in their unrefined or whole grain form can assist with weight control and insulin resistance as these foods are more filling and generally cause a slower rise in your blood sugar levels. A large study of Chinese women from shanghai found that among post-menopausal women, a regular intake of tofu and other soy products was strongly protective against type 2 diabetes (Messina *et al.,* 2004). Women who consumed the most soy had about a 50 per cent lower risk of having sugar detected in their urine-a powerful predicator of diabetes. The finding that soy isoflavones may guard against type-2 diabetes is consistent with previous report from a 20 year follow-up survey of finish and Datch population in the seven countries study, which showed that a high intake of isoflavones protects against type 2 diabetes. In a study of healthy menopausal women from Taiwan researchers found that a supplement of soy isoflavones taken daily from six months was equally effective as estrogens replacement therapy in lowering fasting blood glucose and insulin levels (Singh *et al.*, 2006), meaning it improved glucose tolerance reducing the risk of diabetes in these women. Besides, in another study of post-menopausal women with type 2 diabetes (Sarkar *et al.*, 2006), including foods rich in soy protein containing isoflavones daily for 3 months was shown to reduce fasting insulin and improve insulin resistance. Also, the level of HbA1C (is a measure of the average blood sugar levels over time) was reduced in the blood, suggesting that diabetes control was better in these women while they were taking the soy isoflavones food. Moreover, another study of men with type-2 diabetes found that soy isoflavones added to the diet lower LDL cholesterol and triglycerides. In addition, studies of Sarkar *et al.* (2006) in rats suggest that soy isoflavones may increase the production of adiponectin from fat tissue as compared to animal protein. Adipoprotein is one of the important proteins. Since its low levels in the body have been linked with insulin resistance and diabetes. It has been suggested that soy isoflavones may be one way to increase adiponectin, which has anti- diabetic properties. Further research in still needed to determine the exact role of soy isoflavones in preventing diabetes and reducing complications in people with these conditions. More studies are needed to fully understand the effect of soy intake on the development of type 2 DM and the underlying biological mechanism.

Soy isoflavones may reduce adiposity by inhibiting insulin secretion from pancreatic β-cells or by inhibiting lipogenesis and enhancing lipolysis in the liver and adipocytes (Bhathena *et al.*, 2002). Results from animal studies suggest that soy isoflavones intake improve insulin sensitivity and recent data suggest that isoflavones may exert antidiabetic effects in rats through peroxisome proliferators-activated receptors. Among post-menopausal women, dietary isoflavones and isoflavone supplementation have been associated with improved insulin resistance. However, epidemiologic evidence directly linking isoflavones intake with diabetes is limited (Classidy *et al.*, 1994). Adiponectin is a protein hormone produced and secreted exclusively by adipocytes that regulates the metabolism of lipids and glucose. The hormone is known to influence the body's response to insulin and its levels are generally reduced under type 2 DM. The monitoring of adipo-nectin is thus essential for evaluating compounds with anti-metabolic syndrome effects. Adiponectin is an adipocytokine, which is synthesized and released by adipocytes, abundantly present in plasma and leads to enhanced insulin action, indicating that this adipocytikine maintain sensitivity and glucose homeostasis. However, adiponectin levels are reduced in patients with increased insulin resistance due to conditions such as obesity, type 2DM and hypertension. Thus, adipocytokine is considered as a good biomarker to assess efficiency for developing therapeutics for type 2DM. It is already known that thiazolidinedione derivatives (TDZs) increase the adiponectin level as potential insulin-sensitizing therapeutics (Moller, 2001). However, TDZs are associated with edema, body weight gain, longestive heart failure, osteoporosis and liver disfunction in type 2DM patients.

In recent years, the isoflavones found in the soybean meal portion have documented for benefits in diabetic patients. These one now being expected and marketed as neutra-ceuticals in functional foods. Chemical structures, taste characteristics and localization of isoflavones in seed have been well studied. Of the total seed isolavones, 80-90 per cent was located in cotyledons, with the remainder in the hypocotyls. The hypocotyls had higher concentrations of isoflavones on a weight basic compared with cotyledons. In addition to potential medicinal applications isoflavones are reported to perform a number of physiological functions involved in the growth and development of soybean. For example, soybean isoflavones induce nod genes in *Bradyrizobium joponicum*, and they are associated with the response of soybeans to infection by *Phytophthora megasperma*. Because of these physiological responses, it has been assumed that isoflavones content might be difficult to control by genetic means. However, certain soybean cultivars have recently been identified that have remarkably low isoflavone contents in seeds. The isoflavones from whole seeds were isolated and identified. Daidzin, genistin malonyldaidzin, and malonyl gentisin were routinely detected, but other isoflavones (Aglycons and Acetyl forms) were present only in trace amount. The importance of isoflavones is widely appreciated and is currently the subject of intense research and discussion. Isoflavones appear to protect against hormone-related disorders such as breast cancer and prostate cancer. Many recent papers recognize the potential benefits of isoflavones components for reducing the risk of various cancers and for related pharmaceuticals roles (Takano *et al.*, 1993).

Conclusion

Nature sometimes gives us valuable crops containing compounds with significant pharmaceuticals values. Among the group of crops, pulses have a significant place in terms of medicinal values. Soybean belongs to pulse group of plants. This is the generous gifts from nature to us and has been used globally for thousands of years for culinary and medicinal purposes in most races. The overall benefits of pulses have historically been associated with their macronutrient composition, such as protein and carbohydrate (starch), although there is now sufficient evidence to suggest that non-nutritional bioactive compounds play a significant role. Despite a large volume of literature, there are still the need for additional work around the substantiation of the health benefits of different pulse metabolites and the potential synergistic effects between the different classes of bioactive. There are good evidence that levels of these bioactive in the plant are the subject to manipulation. There appears to be significant natural variation both between and within the different species of the pulses and the opportunity to enhance the concentrations through plant breeding or the application of agronomic practices. Soy is a good taste, versatile, economical and have many associated health benefits like decreased risk of obesity (diabetes), heart disease and prostate, colon and breast cancer-diseases which affect almost a good percentage of individuals in any country of world. It is logical that we should join forces in promoting soy consumption across the world. The nutritional profile of soy reveals that they are beneficial for the whole family to enjoy. In this way, soy is seen as a staple food because they are nutritious and provide most of the ingredients that help to improve health. While further research is still needed to determine the exact role of soy protein in preventing diabetes, CVD and cancer and reducing complications in people with this conditions. Finally, although progress in understanding the effects of soy on chronic disease risk has been made, this is still a relatively new field. Human clinical trials and ongoing research are investigating and substantiating the role of soy and garlic in CVD, diabetes and cancer. In this way, soy is seen as the staple food because of their nutritious nature and provides most of the ingredients that help to improve health. All of this could encourage more consumers who are concerned about their health against chronic disorders to consider eating more soy in diet.

References

Adams, K.F., Lampe, P.D., Newton, K.M., Ylvisikar, J. T., Feld, A., Myerson, D., Emerson, S.S., White, E., and Potter, J.D. (2005). Soy protein containing isoflavones does not decrease colorectal epithelial cell proliferation in a randomized controlled trial. *American Journal of Nutrition*, **82**: 1308-1319.

Alfred, C. D., Allred, K. F., Ju, Y. H., Virant, S. M., and Helferich, W.G. (2001). Soy diets containing varying amounts of genistein stimulate growth of estrogen-dependent (MCF-7) tumors in a dose-dependent manner. *Cancer Research*, **66**: 1241-1249.

Alhasan, S. A., Aranha, O., Sarkar, F. H. (2001). Genistein elicits pleiotrophic molecular effects on head and neck cancer cells. *Clinical Cancer Research*, **23**: 4174-4181.

Allred, C. D., Allred, K. F., Ju, Y.H., Goeppinger, T.S., Boue, S.M., Burow, M.E., McCoy, T., and Cline, J.M. (2006). Effects of soyabean glyceolins and estradiol in postmenopausal female monkeys. *Nutrition of Cancer Patients*, **56**: 74-81.

Alzorriz, M. A. Z., and Hernandez, J.A.M.(1999).Possible beneficial role of dietary chickpea (Cicer arietinum L.) var. macrocarpum or pharmacological treatment with B 3-adrenogic agonist. *Anal. Real. Acad. Farm*, **65**: 327-349.

Ariazi, E. A., and Jordon, V.C. (2006). Estrogen-related receptors as emerging targets in cancer and metabolic disorders.*Curr.Top.Med.Chem.*, **6**: 203-215.

Bhathena, S.J., Ali, A.A., and Mohammed. A.l. (2002). Differential effects of dietary flaxseed protein and soy protein in triglyceride and uric acid levels in animal models. *Journal of Nutritional Biochemistry*, **13**: 684-9.

Boydak, E., Alpaslan, M., Hayta, M., Gercek, S., and Simsek, M. (2002). Seed composition of soyabeans grown in the Harran Region of Turkey as affected by row spacing and irrigation. *Journal of Nutrition*, **50**: 4718-4720.

Cassidy, A., Albertazzi, P., and Lise, N. (2006). Critical review of health effects of soyabean phyto-oestrogens in post-menupausal women. *Proc. Nutr Soc.*, **65 (1)**: 76-92.

Cassidy, A., Bingham, S.A., and Cummings, J.H. (1994). Starch Intake and colorectal cancer risk: an international comparison. *British Journal of Cancer*, **69**: 937-942.

Christl, S. U., Mursgatroyed, P. R., Gibson, G. R., and Cummings, J.H. (1992). Production, metabolism, and excretion of hydrogen in the large intestine. *Gastroentrology*, **102**: 1269-1277.

Cheesbrough, M. (1984). Medical laboratory Manual for Tropical Countries, Tropical Health Technology, Butterworth, pp. 1-15.

Cotterchio, M., Boucher, B.A., Manno, M., Gallinger, S., Okey, A., and Harper, P. (2006). Dietary phyto-estrogen intake is associated with reduced colorectal cancer risk. *Journal of Nutrition*, **136**: 3046-3053.

Davis, J.N., Kucuk, O., and Sarkar, F.H. (2001). Genistein elicits pleiotropic molecular effects on head and neck cancer cells. *Clinical Cancer Research*, **7**: 4174-4181.

Douglas, G., Armitage, J. A., Taylor, P. D., Lawson, J.R., Mann, G. E., and Poston, L. (2006). Cardiovascular consequences of life-long exposure to dietary isoflavones in the rat. *Journal of Physiology*, **24**: 477-487.

Ellington, A.A., Berhow, M.A., and Singletary, K.W. (2006). Inhibition of Akt signalling and enhanced ERK1/2 activity are involved in induction of macro-autophagy by triterpenoid B-group soyasaponins in coan cancer cells. *Carcinogenesis*, **27**: 298-306.

Englyst, H.N., Kingman, S.M., and Cummings, J.H. (1992). Classification and measurement of nutritionally important starch fractions. *Europian Journal of Clinical Nutrition*, **46 (2)**: S33-50.

Fung, T. T., Willett W.C., Stampfer, M.J., Manson, J. E., and Hu, F. B. (2001).Dietary patterns and the risk of coronary heart disease in women. *Arch Intern. Med.*, **161 (15)**: 1857-62.

Guillon, F., and Champ, M.M. (2002). Carbohydrate fractions of Legumes: uses in human nutrition and potential for health. *British Journal of Nutrition*, **88**: S293-306.

Gurfinkel, D.M., and Rao, A.V. (2003). Soysaponins: the relationship between chemical structure and colon anti-carcinogenic activity. *Nature of Cancer*, **47**: 24-33.

Hu, F.B., Rimm, F.B., Stampfer M. J., Ascherio, A., Spiegelonman, D., and Willett W. C. (2000). Prospective study of major dietary patterns and risk of coronary heart disease in men. *Am J. Clinical Nutrition*, **72 (4)**: 912-21.

Hu, F.B., van Dam R.M., and Liu, S. (2001). Diet and risk of type [22] diabetes: the role of types of fat and carbohydrate. *Diabetologia*, **44 (7)**: 805-17.

Jenkins, D. J., and. David, G. (1983). Low glycemic index starchy foods in the diabetic diet. *American Journal of Clinical Nutrition*, **48 (2)**: 248-54.

Kassem, M. A., Meksem, K., Iqbal, M.J., Njiti, V.N., Banz, W.J., Winters, T.A., Wood, A., and Lightfoot, D.A. (2004). Definition of soyabean Genome regions that control seed phytoestrogen amount. *Journal of Biomedical Biotechnology*, **24**: 52-60.

Kerley, M.S., and Allee, G.L. (2003). Modifications in soyabean seed composition to enhance animal feed use and value: Moving from a dietary ingredient to a functional dietary component. *Ag-Bio- Forum*, **6 (1 and 2)**: 14-17.

Kostelac, D., Rechkemmer, G., and Briviba, K. (2003). Phytoestrogens modulate binding response of estrogen receptors α and β to the estrogen response element. *Journal of Agriculture and Food Chemistry*, **51**: 7632-7635.

Kushi, L. H., Meyer, K. A., and Jacobs, D. R., Jr. (1999). Cereals, legumes, and chronic disease risk reduction: evidence from epidemiologic studies. *American Journal of Clinical Nutrition*, **70**: 451S-458S.

Leterme, P. (2002). Recommendation by health organizations for pulse consumption. *British Journal of Nutrition*. **88 (3)**: S239-S242.

Martinez, M. E., Thomson, C.A., and Smith-Warner, S.A. (2006).A soy and breast cancer: the controversy continues. *Journal of Nature Cancer Instruments*, **98**: 459-431.

Mehrathu, T., Mohamed, A., Wang, C.Y., and Andebrhan, T. (2004).Analysis of isoflavones contents in vegetable soybeans. *Plant Foods Human Nutrition*, **59**: 55-61.

Messina, M., Gardner, C., and Barnes, S. (2002). Gaining insight into the health effects of soy but a long way still to go: Commentary on the fourth International Symposium on the Role of soy in preventing and treating chronic disease. *Journal of Nutrition*, **12(3)**: 237-249.

Mezei, O., Banz, W.J., Steger, R.W., Peluso, M. R., Winters, T.A., and Shay, N. (2003). Soy isoflavones exert antidiabetic and hypolipidemic effects through the PPAR pathways in obese Zucker rats and murine RAW 264.7 cells. *Journal of Nutrition*,**133 (5)**: 1238-43.

Mitchell, J. H. (2001). Phytoestrogens: Involvement in breast and prostate cancer. In R. E. C. Wildman (Ed.), Handbook of neutra-ceuticals and functional foods (pp. 99-108). CRC Press.

Moon, Y. J., Wang, X., Morris, M. E. (2006). Dietary flavonoids: effects on xenobiotics and carcinogenic metabolism. *Taxicol.*, **20**: 187-210.

Nene, Y.L. (2006). Indian pulses through the millennia. *Asian Agricultural – History*, **10**: 179-202.

Ofuya, Z. M., and Akhidue, V. (2005). The role of pulses in Human Nutrition: A Review. *Journal of Applied Science and Environtal Management*, **9 (3)**: 99-104.

Panozzo, J., and Materne, M. (2007). Developing quality pulses for a Sustainable Environment, Population and Community. Personal Communication.

Peterson, D.S., Sipsa, S., and Mackintosh, J.B. (1997). The Chemical composition and Nutritive Value of Australian Pulses. Grain Research and Development Corporation, Kingston ACT, Australia.

Pisulewska, E., and Pisulewski, P.M. (2000). Trypsin inhibitor activity of legume seeds as affected by the technique of harvest. *Animal Feed Science and Technology,* **86**: 261-265.

Rajput, Z. I., Hu, S. H., Xiao, C. W., and Arijo, A.G. (2007). Adjuvant effects of saponins on animal immune responses. *J. Zhejiang Univ. Sci., B.* **8**: 153-161.

Ricketts, M. L., Moore, D.D., Banz, W.J., Mezei, O., and Shay, N.F. (2005).Molecular mechanisms of action of the soy isoflavones includes activation of promiscuous nuclear receptors. A Review. *Journal of Nutritional Biochemistry,* **16**: 321-330.

Rochfort, S., and Panozzo, J. (2007). Phytochemicals for health, the role of pulses. *Journal of Agricultue and Food Chemistry,* **3**: 7981-7994.

Roy, F., Boye, J. I., and Simpson, B. K. (2010). Bioactive proteins and peptides in pulse crops: Pea, chickpea and lentil. *Food Research International,* **43**: 432-442.

Sakurai, H., Katoh, A., Kiss, T., Jakusch, T., and Hattori, M. (2010). Metallo-allixinate complexes with anti-diabetic and anti-metabolic syndrome activities. *Metallomics,* **2**: 670-682.

Salim-ur-Rehman, Nawaz, H., Ahmad, M.M., Hussain,S., Murtaza, A., and Shahid, S. H. (2007). Physico-chemical and sensory evaluation of ready to drink soy-cow milk blend. *Pakistan Journal of Nutrition,* **6 (3)**: 283-285.

Sarkar, F. H., Adsule, S., Padhye, S., Kulkarni, S., and Li, Y. (2006). The role of genistein and synthetic derivatives of isoflavones in cancer prevention and therapy. *Mini Review Medicinal Chemistry,* **6**: 401-407.

Shephered, J., Codde, S. M., Ford, I., Isles, C.G., Lorimer, A. R., McFarlane, P. W., McKillop, J.H., and Packhard, C. J. (1995).Prevention of coronary heart disease with pravastatin in men with hypercholestermia. *North England Journal of Medical,* **333**: 1301-1307.

Shi,J., Arunasalam, K.,Yeung, D., Kakuda,Y., Mittal, G., and Jinag, Y. (2004). Saponins from edible legumes: chemistry, processessing, and health benefits. *Journal of Medicinal Food,* **7**: 67-78.

Singh, A.V., Franke, A.A., Blackburn, G.L., and Zhou, J.R. (2006). Soy Phytochemicals prevent orthotopic growth and metastasis of bladder cancer in mice by alterations of cancer cell proliferation and apoptosis and tumur angiogenesis. *Cancer Research,* **66**: 1851-1858.

Tharanathan, R.N., and Mahadevanmma, S. (2003). Grain Legumes-a boon to human nutrition. *Trends Foods Science and Technology,* **14**: 507-518.

Topping, D. L., Fukusima, M., and Bird, A.R. (2003). Resistant starch as a prebiotic and symbiotic: state of art. *Proceeding of Nutritional Society,* **62**: 171-176.

Trock, B. J. Hilakivi-Clarke, L., and Clarke, R. (2006). Meta-analysis of soy intake and breast cancer risk. *Journal of Natural of Cancer Institute,* **98**: 430-431.

Tsukamoto, C., Shinji, S., Igita, K., Kudou, S., Kokubum, M., Okubo, K., and Kitamura, K. (1995). Factors affecting isoflavones content in soyabean seeds: Changes in isoflavones, saponins, and composition of fatty acids at different temperatures during seed development. *Journal of Agriculture and Food Chemistry*, **43**: 1184-1192.

Van Dam, R.M. Rimm, E.B., Willett, W.C., Stampfer, M.J., and Hu, F.B. (2002). Dietary patterns and risk for type 2 diabetes mellitus in U.S. men. *Ann Intern Med.*, **136 (3)**: 201-9.

Verma, S.K., Jain, V., and Verma, D. (2008). Garlic-"The spice of Life" : Composition, Cooking Chemistry and Preparations. *Journal of Herbal Medicine and Toxicology*, **2(2)**: 21-28.

Villegas, R., Gao, Y., Yang, G., Li, H., Elasy, T.A., Zheng, W., and Shu, X. U. (2008). Legume and soy food intake and the incidence of type-2 diabetets in the Shanghai Women's Health study. *American Journal of Clinical Nutrition*, **87**: 162-167.

Wood, C. E., Register, T.C., Franke, A.A., Anthony, M. S., and Cline, J. M. (2006). Dietary soy isoflavones inhibit estrogen effects in the postmenopausal breast. *Cancer Research*, **66**: 1241-1249.

Xavier, R., Rekha, K., and Bairy, K. L. (2004). Health Perspective of Pesticide Exposure and Dietary Management. *Malasian Journal of Nutrition*, **10 (1)**: 39-51.

Xiao, J.X., Huang, G.Q., Zhu, C.P., Ren, D.D., and Zhang, S. H. (2007). Morphological study on apoptosis Hela cells induced by soyasaponins. *Taxicol.*,

Zhu, J., Xiong, L., Yu, B., and Wu, J. (2005). Apoptosis induced by a new member of saponin family is mediated through caspase-8-dependent cleavage of Bcl-2. *Molecular Pharmacology*, **68**: 1831-1838.

Zou, K., Zhao, Y.Y., and Zhang, R.Y.A. (2006). A cytotoxic saponin from *Albizia julibrissin. Chemical Pharmacology. Bull. (Tokyo)*, **54**: 1211-1212.

Zulet, M.A., Macarulla, M.T., Portillo, M.P., NoelSuberville, C., Higueret, P., and Martinez, J.A. (1999). Lipid and glucose utilization in hypercholerstermic rats fed a diet containing heated chickpea (*Cicer arietinum* L.): a potential functional food. *International Journal of Vitaminal Nutritional and Chemical Research*, **69**: 403-411.

Bioactive Phytochemicals: Perspectives for Modern Medicine Vol. 3 (2015)
Editor: **V.K. Gupta**
Published by: **DAYA PUBLISHING HOUSE, NEW DELHI**

Pages **487–515**

20

Potential Bioactive Phytoconstituents and Synthesis of Modern Antimalarials: Historical Perspectives

Kaliyaperumal Karunamoorthi[1*]

ABSTRACT

Malaria is closely related to human history and affects mankind for centuries. Symptoms of malaria were described in numerous ancient medical literatures and treatises worldwide. It can be fatal, if not promptly diagnosed and treated. In the past, we have eliminated and eradicated this scourge in several industrialized nations, particularly from much of Europe, North America, Australia and much of the Middle East by 1970 through vector control interventions, particularly intra-domiciliary spraying of dichloro-diphenyl-trichloroethane (DDT) with effective larviciding and public health campaigns. However, early diagnosis, and prompt and effective treatment with chloroquine have played the pivotal role in the malaria eradication programme. Recent scientific advancements, discovery of new concepts as well as bio-molecular tools have significantly enriched our knowledge and understanding about malarial parasites and mosquito vectors. It has paved the way to formulate several potent anti-malarials and a prophylactic vaccine. World's most clinically advanced malaria vaccine candidate (RTS, S) is now within reach as early as 2015. However, currently the widespread multi-drug resistant Plasmodium strains is a matter of important concern, as the parasites have exhibited varied resistance profiles against almost all existing first-line antimalarials globally. It calls for development of low-cost resistance-proof antimalarials with new modes of action. In these perspectives this chapter delineates the global burden of malaria in terms of negative socio-economic, public health and clinical impact, importance of vector control interventions, and the role of anti-malarials in reducing the global malaria

1 Tropical and Infectious Diseases Unit, Department of Environmental Health, Faculty of Public Health and Tropical Medicine, Jazan University, Kingdom of Saudi Arabia.

* *Corresponding author*: E-mail: karunamoorthi@gmail.com

burden. It also describes on the history of a few potent anti-malarials, existing anti-malarials and the significance of developing cost-effective new antimalarials to prevent and combat malaria effectively in the near future.

Keywords: Malaria, Anti-malarials, Chloroquine, ACT, Traditional anti-malarial plants.

Introduction

Arthropod-borne diseases remain as a major public health threat to the mankind, which are responsible for over a million death and considerable morbidity worldwide, particularly in the resource-poor settings (Karunamoorthi, 2012). Since, the pre historical era mosquitoes are closely associated with mankind and even today it has been considered as one of the ancient deadliest public health enemies. They serve as a vector for the transmission of many dreadful diseases like malaria, filariasis, Japanese encephalitis, dengue and yellow fever (Karunamoorthi and Sabesan, 2013) and resource-limited Third World countries are the major victims of several mosquito-borne diseases (Karunamoorthi and Sabesan, 2010), particularly malaria.

Throughout human history, malaria has been considered as a world's most serious public health issue and has ruled humankind for nearly 500,000 years (Karunamoorthi, 2014a). It is caused by *Plasmodium* parasites and the infected person often experience fever, chills, and flu-like illness. Though it is a preventable and curable illness, if left untreated, it may cause severe complications ultimately death. It remains as a global public health issue nearly in 104 countries across the globe. It has been estimated that nearly half of the world population (3.4 billion people) is at the risk of malaria (Karunamoorthi *et al.*, 2013; World Malaria Report, 2013). WHO estimates that there were about 219 million cases of malaria in 2012 (with an uncertainty range of 154 million to 289 million) with more than 627 000 deaths. Most children die before celebrating their fifth birth day in Africa, as a child dies from malaria for every single minute there (World Malaria Report, 2013).

Malaria-in-Pregnancy

Despite the availability of effective interventions, it remains as one of the most important causes of maternal and childhood morbidity and mortality in sub Saharan Africa. Malaria-in-pregnancy imposes a serious threat to the mother, fetus and neonate, as pregnancy reduces a woman's immunity, increasing the risk of malaria infection (Karunamoorthi *et al.*, 2010). It includes spontaneous abortion, preterm delivery, low birth weight, still-birth (Menendez, 1995; Onwujekwe *et al.*, 2012; Karunamoorthi, 2012a), congenital infection and maternal death (Ruth and Lagerberg, 2008). Risk of anaemia in both mother and baby is higher in first and second pregnancies than in the later pregnancies (WHO, 2004; Malaria Consortium, 2007). Tragically, in Africa nearly eighty-percent of cases are treated at home (World Malaria Report, 2013) without proper medical supervision.

Malaria and Socio-economic Development

Malaria seriously affects the health and wealth of nations and individuals and it is often considered as a disease of poverty and a cause of poverty (Karunamoorthi,

2012a). The social burden of malaria in fact remains elusive. It is not a universal entity that can be measured or quantified, however it can be understood and linked to the outcomes such as morbidity and mortality (Jones and Williams, 2004). Malaria causes repeated work absenteeism resulting in short and long term losses in productivity as the main transmission periods coincide with the peak agricultural and harvesting seasons (Karunamoorthi and Bekele, 2009).

The direct costs of malaria include a combination of personal and public expenditures on both prevention and treatment of the disease (van Ballegoyen, 2005). At the micro level the personal expenditures include individual or family spending on insecticide-treated nets (ITNs), doctors' fees, antimalarials, transport to nearest health facilities, and support for the patient and an accompanying family member during hospital visits and stays (RBM, 1998). At the macro level the economic burden of malaria is estimated at an average annual reduction in economic growth of 1.3 per cent for those African countries with the highest burden with an estimated 12 billion US$ loss to the African continent's Gross Domestic Product (GDP) annually (World Malaria Report, 2009).

Malaria Control Interventions

Though malaria vaccines hold future promise, vector control and chemotherapy remain as the primary weapons for reducing the burden of malaria in individuals and populations (Elfawal *et al.*, 2012). In the past decade, we have significantly minimized the global burden of malaria and ultimately the malaria map has shrunken now by implementing integrated malaria control like vector control, access to early diagnosis and prompt effective case-management according to the local context and need. Vector control remains as a cornerstone to combat malaria (Karunamoorthi, 2011), and it includes intra-domiciliary low volume residual insecticide spraying, enhancing the personal or household protection by free-distribution of long-lasting insecticide treated nets (*LLINs*), and killing immature (larval stage) larva by applying larvicidal agents in the selected potential mosquito breeding sites (Karunamoorthi and Yirgalem, 2013) in the resource-limited settings. In fact, vector control heavily relies upon synthetic insecticides as a mainstay. Nevertheless, the indiscriminate and haphazard usages of insecticides pose potential environmental and health hazard (Karunamoorthi, 2012b; Karunamoorthi *et al.*, 2012). Besides it has led to the emergence of resistance also, which often undermines the potentiality of vector control. It is a potential threat to the global public health too (Karunamoorthi and Sabesan, 2013).

Anti-malarials: A Great Savior

Drugs are well-known as 'Magic Bullets' because of their speedy curative and healing properties to alleviate various diseases. It is one of the generous donations or great boons of modern scientific technologies, tools and advanced computational techniques to build a disease-free healthier society. Indeed, potent antimalarial could cure the patient and subsequently it can minimize the malaria related illness and deaths considerably. However, in the past decades, the efficacy of the existing most affordable antimalarials has declined remarkably and unfortunately there is no new drug developed and available at at the final stage (Karunamoorthi *et al.*, 2013).

Accordingly, currently our primary goal is: (1) preserving and enhancing the efficacy of existing potent antimalarials by combination therapies and, (2) parallely formulating new antimalarials from the various potential anti-malarial candidate plants. In the history of malaria until today over a thousand plant species have been identified and reported to possess varied degrees of anti-malarial properties by various researchers across the globe (Karunamoorthi *et al.,* 2013). However, the history of chloroquine and artemisinin development and synthesis from Cinchona and *Artemisia annua* plants is world-renowned, respectively. In these perspectives, this chapter becomes more significant and pertinent.

History of Synthesis of Modern Antimalarials

It has been estimated that nearly between 30,000 and 75,000 of plants possess medicinal properties (Pamplona-Roger, 2001). In the human history, the traditional and folk herbal medicinal system has played a pivotal role in the fight against various illnesses and disorders, particularly malaria by saving millions of lives and curing billions of debilitating episodes of malaria (Karunamoorthi, 2014a). To date, there are about1, 277 plant species from 160 families, listed to treat malaria related illness or fever (Willcox and Bodeker, 2004a). Evidently the world's potent antimalarial chemotherapy both Quinine and Artemisinin have been isolated and identified from cinchona tree bark in 1820 and from the leaves of the Artemisia annua in 1972, respectively (Karunamoorthi, 2014a).

Emergence of the Peruvian bark (*Cinchona* sp.) and also the synthesis of the important bio-active substance, called quinine, is one of the most important sagas in the history of medicine and therapeutics. It has saved millions of lives every year and has served as a potent anti-malarial for over five decades to treat malaria related illness with permitable human side-effects. Infact it is a discovery involved exploration, exploitation and secrecy (Lee, 2002a). Due to the emergence of multi-drug resistance strains of malarial parasites in 1972, artemisinin compound was isolated from *Artemisia annua* and this plant species has had many traditional uses in China for several millennia (Wright, 2005a).

Cinchona: The Tree of Fever

Indeed, for centuries there was no specific reliable drug for the treatment of malaria until the seventeenth century. Spanish colonisers brought back from Peru the tree bark called *Cinchona* sp., from which quinine was later extracted. Subsequently, in the twentieth century, synthetic alternatives to quinine were developed (Butler *et al.,* 2010). Quinine was used as a template for the synthesis of another potent anti-malarial called chloroquine (CQ) in 1940.

In the West, cinchona has been well-known as an anti-malarial agent in the traditional system of medicine for almost four-hundred years (Lee, 2002a). The first widely used antimalarial drug was quinine, a natural product extracted from the bark of the tree called *Cinchona calisaya*. However, synthetic derivatives of quinine, such as the 8-aminoquinoline primaquine and the 4-aminoquinoline chloroquine, can be traced back to the pioneering work of Ehrlich on methylene blue in the late nineteenth century. These drugs cause parasite death by blocking the polymerization of the toxic byproduct of haemoglobin degradation, haem, into insoluble and non-toxic pigment granules, resulting in cell lysis and parasite cell autodigestion (Olliaro and Yuthavong, 1999).

History of Chloroquine: An Incredible Chapter in Infectious Diseases Control

Discovery of chloroquine and its subsequent worldwide usage against malaria in the twentieth century produced one of the greatest public health advances ever achieved by a drug against an infectious disease (Wellems, 2002). In 1820, quinine (Figure 20.1) was isolated by the French scientists Pelletier and Caventou from the bark of the *Cinchona* spp. (Oliveira *et al.*, 2009). Quinine has a molecular formula of $C_{20}H_{24}N_2O_2$. It is (R)-(6-methoxyquinolin-4-yl)((2S,4S,8R)- 8-vinylquinuclidin-2-yl)methanol. Many physicians are familiar with the story of the Countess of Chinchón, wife of the Viceroy of Peru; it was claimed by Bado that she was cured of a certain ague by Cinchona bark sometime in the late 1620s or early 1630s (Jaramillo-Arango 1949). The genus Cinchona is said to have been named after the Spanish Countess of Chinchón (Garnham, 1966).

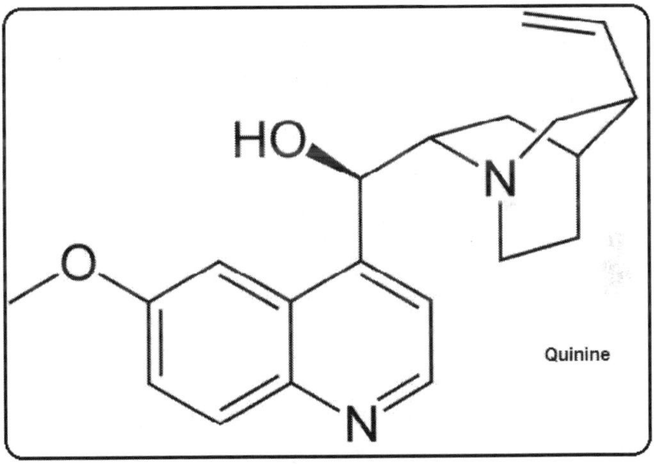

Figure 20.1: The Chemical Structure of Quinine.

The first definite written account of the medicinal properties of the bark appears to be that by Fray Antonio dela Calancha, an Augustinian missionary, in 1633, who wrote an account of 'the fever tree' which 'grows in Loja, Peru, the bark of which when made into a powder and given as a beverage, cured the tertian fevers'. He also described its widespread use in Lima, the capital of Peru (Paredes-Borja, 1946). In 1630, Juan Lopez, a missionary Jesuit, learned of the bark from Pedro Leiva, chieftain of the Malacatos tribe. He, and probably other Jesuits, took the knowledge of the bark and seeded back to their headquarters, St Paul's at Lima, then took it to Europe (Lee, 2002a), and used for centuries to treat human malaria with efficacy.

In the seventeenth-century, Rome had been one of the malarious zones where many cardinals died of the 'Malignant ague' (or malaria) while attending the papal congregations in the Eternal City. By the time of the Conclave of 1655, during which Alexander VII was elected as Pope, despite the availability of the Peruvian bark the 'Malignant ague' had not been recorded among the attendees and even Cardinal de Lugo died in 1660 due to the same malignant ague (malaria). Redi wrote some years later to the noted Jesuit Chircher that *'the whole World owes a debt of gratitude to those Fathers of your most venerable Order who were the very first, much to their glory, to bring the bark to Europe'*. We would now add 'and in particular to de Lugo and Puccerini' (Redi, 1966). Cinchona tree plantations were established an cultivated in Java and they were the main source of quinine supply until the Second World War (Krettli *et al.*, 2001).

In 1940, the world's most effective low-cost anti-malarial called chloroquine (Figure 20.2) was synthesized and administered to treat malaria related illness. The structure of quinine was established by Rabe in 1908, and its synthesis was accomplished in 1944 by Woodward and Doering (Oliveira *et al.*, 2009). However, its synthetic production is more complex as well as costlier, as it is obtained from the *Cinchona* spp., by extraction, although it grows wild in South America and cultivated in Java (Boulos *et al.*, 1997). Subsequently, chloroquine has became the chief alternative for quinine, during the Second World War and until recently, this was the only drug, used for the treatment of both complicated and uncomplicated malaria (Krettli *et al.*, 2001; Bharel *et al.*, 1996).

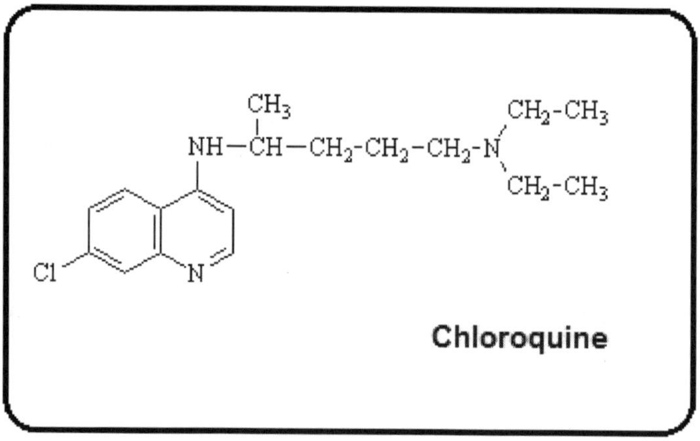

Figure 20.2: The Chemical Structure of Chloroquine.

Physical and Chemical Properties of Chloroquine

CQ Resistant: A Great Disaster in the War Against Malaria

Chloroquine was much closer to the ideal anti-malarial drugs and was administered to treat malaria for nearly five decades due to its high efficacy against all species of malaria parasites, and high tolerance (Krettli *et al.*, 2001). However,

P. falciparum, the most malignant of the four human malaria parasite species, showed foci of chloroquine resistance (CQR) in Southeast Asia and South America in the late 1950s, Papua New Guinea in the 1960s, and East Africa in the late1970s. The steady and unremitting spread of CQR from these foci could only be met by a few alternative drugs, all of which were more expensive encountering resistance problems of their own, or were less safe and more difficult to use than chloroquine itself (Wellems, 2002). Over the past three decades, the increasing prevalence of resistant strains of *P. falciparum* was the major factor responsible for the increase in mortality that occurred mainly in Africa (World Malaria Report, 2005).

Synthesis of other Potent Anti-malarials

Malaria has had an enormous impact on human history, not least in times of war. In the 1920s research workers in the Bayer laboratories of the IG Farbenindustrie consortium developed the 8-aminoquinoline plasmoquine (the forerunner of primaquine). They went on to develop the acridine dye, atebrin (mepacrine) and the 4-aminoquinolines, Resochin (developed at the end of the Second World War in America as chloroquine) and Sontochin. British attempts to match the advances achieved by the Germans were at first unproductive, partly because collaboration between academic and industrial organizations in the United Kingdom was beset by concerns over patent rights. However, with the outbreak of World War II, when supplies of antimalarials were scarce, ICI succeeded in the large-scale production of mepacrine (essential to prosecution of the war, particularly in the Far East) and also initiated a programme of collaborative research that eventually led to the discovery of proguanil (Paludrine) (Table 20.1); this, in its turn led to the diaminopyrimidine, pyrimethamine. A massive cooperative screening programme in the United States of America during World War II eventually bore fruit in the realization of the therapeutic potential of chloroquine, and in the later development of amodiaquine and primaquine (Table 20.1). Some of this work also influenced the subsequent discovery of mefloquine and halofantrine (Table 20.1) at the Walter Reed Army Institute of Research (Greenwood, 1995).

Artemisinin: A New Chapter in the Book of Malaria History

Artemisia (Qinghaosu): The Mysterious Chinese Aromatic Plant

Genus Artemisia is a member of Compositae (Astraceae) family, which comprises over three-hundred plant species. It is an annual, biennial and perennial herb (and shrubs) (Hyam and Pankhurst, 1995). *Artemisia annua* (sweet wormwood) was known to the Chinese herbal practitioners for at least more than thousand years ago but it was introduced into Western medicine only for the past forty years. A major difference between *Cinchona* and *Artemisia* plant species is that the active principle of the Artemisia called, artemisinin was rapidly isolated, synthesized and then modified to produce effective therapeutic entities than *Cinchona* plant species, and this is mainly due to the recent advancement of modern scientific techniques and efficiency of modern tools as well as computational pharmacological innovation (Lee, 2002b). In 1972, artemisinin-based compound was isolated from *A. annua*; this plant species has had many traditional uses in Chinese system of medicine for several millennia (Wright, 2005a).

Table 20.1: Review of Existing Principle Anti-malarials (Yarnell, 2014)

Drug	*Chemical Family*	*Malaria Life Cycle Targeted*	*Indications*	*Adverse Effects*
Quinine	Amino-alcohols	Fast-acting erythrocytic schizonticide	IV for cerebral malaria (or quinidine); childhood or pregnancy malaria unresponsive to other agents	Cinchonism, tachycardia, sinus arrhythmias, hypoglycemia
Chloroquine*	4-Aminoquinolines	Fast-acting erythrocytic schizontocide (mild gametocide)	Acute uncomplicated malaria; pregnancy and childhood malaria (note high resistance rates)	Pruritis, nausea, agitation (all uncommon)
Amodiaquine*	4-Aminoquinolines	Fast-acting erythrocytic schizontocide (mild gametocide)	Acute uncomplicated malaria; prevention in travelers	Nausea, pruritus, agranulocytosis and hepatotoxicity (long-term use)
Mefloquine	Amino-alcohols	Fast-acting erythrocytic schizontocide	Acute malaria; prevention in travelers	Sleep disturbance, nightmares, nausea, rash, myalgias, psychosis, arrhythmias, pneumonitis (rare)
Halofantrine	Amino-alcohols	Fast-acting erythrocytic schizontocide	Acute malaria not responding to other agents	Nausea, arrhythmias, elevated transaminases
Pyrimethamine	Diaminopyrimidine	Fast-acting erythrocytic schizonticide (mild tissue schizontocide)	Acute malaria; pregnancy malaria (usually with sulfadoxine)	Nausea, headache, mild anemia
Sulfadoxine	Sulfonamides and sulfones	Fast-acting erythrocytic schizontocide	Acute malaria; pregnancy malaria (usually with pyrimethamine)	Nausea, headache, mild anemia, hemolysis in G6PD deficiency, severe skin rashes (rare) – sulfa drug
Doxycycline	Antibiotics	Slow-acting erythrocytic schizontocide	Acute malaria (with fast-acting agents); prevention in travelers	Nausea, photosensitivity, esophagitis
Primaquine	8-Aminoquinoline	Tissue schizontocide; gametocidal	Infection with *P. vivax* or *P. ovale;* relapsing infection; low risk of reinfection; prevention in travelers to high *P. vivax* areas	Nausea, methemoglobinemia (self-limiting), hemolysis in G6PD deficiency
Artemisinins	Sesquiterpene lactones	Fast-acting erythrocytic schizontocide; gametocidal	General acute treatment; IV or rectal suppository for cerebral malaria	Minimal; transient mild nystagmus or ataxia (self limiting)

Contd...

Table 1.3–*Contd...*

Lumefantrine	Amino-alcohols	Long-acting erythrocytic schizontocide	Acute treatment (only combined with artemether) in Africa	Headache, dizziness, nausea
Dapsone	Sulfonamides and sulfones	Fast-acting erythrocytic schizontocide	Acute treatment not responding to other agents	Hemolytic anemia (especially in G6PD deficiency), methemoglobinemia, jaundice, nausea, headache, insomnia, psychosis, neuropathy (rare)
Atovaquone	Naphthoquinone	Fast-acting erythrocytic schizontocide	Acute uncomplicated malaria, always given in combination with proguanil	Nausea, mild elevated transaminases
Proguanil	Biguanides	Fast-acting erythrocytic schizonticide (mild tissue schizontocide)	Acute uncomplicated malaria, always given in combination with proguanil	Nausea, mild elevated transaminases

History of Artemisinin derivatives

In China, in the midst of antiquity around 2800 BC, Sheng Nung lived as an individual, who was known as the "Divine Ploughman" (Huang, 1998), and his works were later set down by an anonymous scribe in 101 BC. The demigod codified rules for the cultivation of crops such as rice and millet; and having tested many herbs himself, described those that were poisonous and those that might be useful in medicine. Amongst the herbs described by the Ploughman was Qinghaosu (Artemisia), an agent effective for the treatment of fever (Lee, 2002b).

In the 1960s China was fighting a war in the jungles of North Vietnam, a most malarious region, and the signs of chloroquine resistance were manifested. Consequently, in 1967 the Chinese government has established a large anti-malarial research programme in order to find an alternative for the replacement of ineffective chloroquine (Li, 2007) and this research initiative was unknown to the rest of the world. This research team consisted of more than five-hundred scientists from over sixty premier Chinese institutions, comprising of chemists, pharmacologists, medical entomologists and doctors. They were recruited by the Chinese government for the anti-malaria drug project, well-known as 'Project-523' (Butler *et al.*, 2010).

Mao Zedong, a great scholar had insisted that traditional Chinese medicine was a 'Great Treasure House', a phrase immortalized in the Little Red Book, and to be taken seriously (Taylor, 2005). The early studies in Qinghaosu established that the preparation was very active against malarial parsites and that the active herb in the preparation was almost certainly *A. annua* (Li *et al.*, 1982; Qinghaosu, 1979). Initial attempts to isolate the active principle or principles from the *A. annua* plant failed, but later in 1971, a great success was achieved by extracting with diethyl-ether at low temperature. The extract cured mice infected with *Plasmodium berghei* and, in 1972, further work culminated in the isolation of a crystalline compound called by the Chinese Qinghaosu (artemisinin) (Ying and Yu-Lin, 1998).

Artemisinin Chemical Structure

Chemical structure of the bio-active phyto-constituent called artemisinin was identified from the extract in the late 1970s and was found, totally unexpectedly, to be the sesquiterpene lactone peroxide. However, the pharmaceutical production of marketable anti-malarials began in 1986. Subsequently the World Health Organization (WHO) initiated to investigate artemisinin (Figure 20.3) and its derivatives in the early 1990s and has promoted them on a large-scale since 2004. Semi-synthetic derivatives, including arteether, artemether and sodium artesunate, are used increasingly more often (Wright, 2005b). Though they are effective against CQ-resistant *P. falciparum* as single therapeutic agents, a combination therapy with a second anti-malarials is recommended in order to minimize the risks of recrudescence as well as the development/emergence of resistant strains (World Malaria Report, 2005).

Isolation of artemisinine has inspired many research groups, since the early 80's, to look for new plant-based antimalarial drugs to potentially contain malaria (Krettli *et al.*, 2001). The first major hurdle in translating artemisinin into a global leader in malaria chemotherapy is its short half-life, which implies the need for

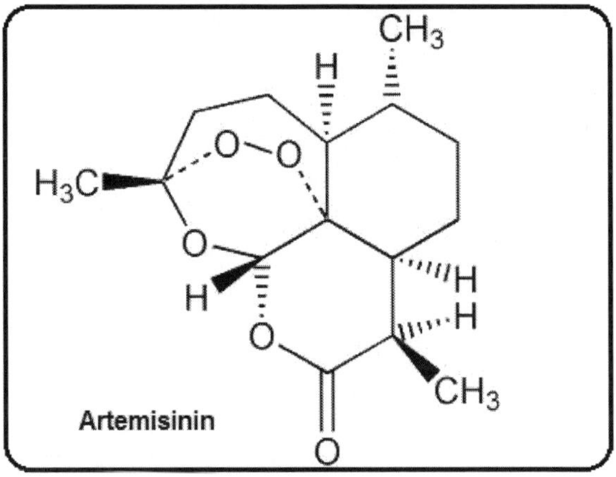

Figure 20.3: The Chemical Structure of Artemisinin.

repeated dosages, and potential problems with treatment adherence and subsequent drug resistance (Awofeso, 2011).

Chemical Constituents of *A. annua*

Artemisinin derivatives are sesquiterpenoides with an endoperoxide, which is the essential component of the anti-malarial property (White, 1999a). The chemical composition of *A. annua* consists of both the volatile and non-volatile phyto-constituents. The volatile components are mainly attributable to essential oils with the content of the latter being 0.2–0.25 per cent. The main compounds, which account for about seventy percent of the essential oils, appear to be camphene, β-camphene, isoartemisia ketone, 1-camphor, β-caryophyllene and β-pinene. In addition, other minor ingredients, such as artemisia ketone, 1,8-cineole, camphene hydrate, and cuminal are also found in the volatile parts of *A. annua*. The main non-volatile ingredients include sesquiterpenoids, flavonoids and coumarins, together with proteins (such as β-galactosidase, β-glucosidase) and steroids (*e.g.* β-sitosterol and stigmasterol) (Youyou *et al.*, 1981; Shilin *et al.*, 1989; Peigen, 2002).

The main chemical constituents of *A. annua* are sesquiterpenoids, including artemisinin, artemisinin I, artemisinin II, artemisinin III, artemisinin IV, artemisinin V, artemisic acid, artemisilactone, artemisinol and epoxyarteannuinic acid (Peigen, 2002; Qinghaosu, 1977; Ying *et al.*, 1982).

Physical and Chemical Properties of Artemisinin (International Pharmacopoeia, 2003)

Molecular formula:	$C_{15}H_{22}O_5$
Chemical name:	(3*R*,5α*S*,6*R*,8α*S*,9*R*,12*S*,12α*R*)-Octahydro-3,6,9-trimethyl-3,12- epoxy-12*H*-pyrano [4,3-*j*]-1,2-benzodioxepin-10(3*H*)-one
Relative molecular mass:	282.3
Description:	Colourless needles or a white, crystalline powder.

Solubility: Practically insoluble in water.

Storage: Artemisinin should be kept in a well-closed container, protected from light and stored in a cool place.

Melting range: 151-154°C

Artemisinin Derivatives

Artelinic acid, artemether, artemotil (arteether, β-arteether) artenimol (dihydroartemisinin, β-dihydroartemisinin) and artesunate, are considered to be about five times more potent than artemisinin (WHO, 2001a).

Artemisinin Compounds

Artemisinin compounds (collective term used for artemisinin and its derivatives) (WHO, 2001b) are effective against *P. falciparum* and *P. vivax,* including multidrug-resistant strains. Nevertheless, there is less information on the efficacy against the remaining other two human malaria parasites, namely *P. malariae* and *P. ovale,* but they are likely to be effective against these parasites too. Artemisinin compounds rapidly kill and clear the asexual blood stages of the parasites, which are responsible for the disease manifestations (blood schizonticidal activity); they have some adverse-effect on the gametocytes (the stage which is infective to mosquitoes ingesting a blood meal from an infected person), but have no effect has been observed on the hypnozoites, which lodge in the liver and can cause relapses in vivax and ovale malaria.

Toxicity Profile of Artemisinin

Artemisinin has no reported toxicity if taken in recommended doses for short periods in the treatment of malaria (Meshnick, 2002). The pollen is extremely allergenic and a cause of hay fever as its cousin ragweed (*Ambrosia artemisifolia*). In animal studies, artemisinin has been used in high oral doses in dogs and rabbits (Zhao and Song, 1990) and at 200-300 mg/kg BW in mice (Shuhua and Catto, 1989) without toxicity. In human beings, artemisinin has been effective against *Plasmodium* in doses of about 30 mg/kg BW, but it has a poor bio-availability and a short half-life of being quickly eliminated from the body (Titulaer *et al.*, 1990; Navaratman *et al.*, 1995). Artemisinin derivatives (dihydroartemisinin, artesunate, artemether, arteether) present better bioavailability and antimalarial activity than artemisinin, but have different safety margins than artemisinin. The bio-availability and half-lives also vary with the delivery system (intramuscular, intra-venous, intra-peritoneal, and oral).

Side-effects of Artemisinin

Artemisinin and its derivatives are generally reported as being safe and well tolerated, and the safety profile of ACTs may be largely determined by the partner drug (WHO, 2006a; Nosten and White, 2007). Studies of artemisinin derivatives in animals have reported significant neurotoxicity (brain damage), where as this is not observed in human studies (Price *et al.*, 1999). Animal studies have also shown adverse effects on the early development of the fetus, but the Artemisinin derivatives have not been fully evaluated during early pregnancy in human beings (Nosten and White, 2007). Other reported adverse events include gastrointestinal disturbance (stomach upset), dizziness, tinnitus (ringing in the ears), neutropenia (low levels of white blood cells), elevated liver enzymes (a marker for liver damage), and electrocardiographic (ECG) abnormalities (changes in cardiac conduction). Most studies however, have found no evidence of ECG changes, and only non-significant changes in liver enzymes (WHO, 2006a; Nosten and White, 2007). The incidence of type 1 hypersensitivity (allergic) reactions is reported to be approximately 1 in 3000 patients (Nosten and White, 2007).

Indeed the wide-spread *P. falciparum* multi-drug resistant strains have created severe set-back in the ongoing malaria control interventions. Accordingly, now artemisinin based combination therapy (ACT) is the drug of choice against both drug-resistant and cerebral malaria causing strains of *P. falciparum*. It has been estimated that roughly 500 million episodes of clinical malaria are there per year and the majority of which needs to be ideally treated with ACT (Karunamoorthi, 2014a). However, they are often inaccessible and unaffordable in the resource-limited settings. Besides, there are signs of resistance to artemisinin emerging in Thai-Cambodian border. Therefore, effective malaria control with existing anti-malarials is a matter of important concern and it calls for exploring for the low-cost and easily accessible plant-based potent anti-malarials from the traditional anti-malarial plants (Karunamoorthi and Tsehaye, 2012).

Other Existing Anti-malarials

The existing principle anti-malarials have been listed with their mode of actions and side-effects in the following table (Table 20.1). These drugs are mainly used both as chemo-prophylaxis and therapeutic agents in the form of monotherapy as well as combination therapies for the management of malaria related illness, and deaths worldwide.

Major Set-backs with Existing Anti-malarials

Anti-malarial Resistance

Drug resistance is a global public health challenge, affecting numerous diseases and no borders. Indeed, it is an evolutionary phenomenon resulting with several unavoidable consequences in terms of treating various life-style and life-saving related illnesses with existing potent therapeutic agents (Beith, 2008). In fact, anti-malarials play a crucial role in every phases of malaria elimination, including early control and subsequent stages of interruption of transmission and reinfection too. Currently, we have achieved meaningful malaria control and elimination than ever before by implementing the existing front-line interventions to reduce the malaria related illness ultimately death. Nevertheless, evolution and spread of multidrug-resistant strains of *P. falciparum* is a severe set-back to eliminate and eradicate malaria worldwide and to maintain and preserve what we have achieved currently (Karunamoorthi, 2011).

Definition of Anti-malarial Resistance

Antimalarial drug resistance has been defined as the "*ability of a parasite strain to survive and/or multiply despite the administration and absorption of a drug given in doses equal to or higher than those usually recommended but within tolerance of the subject"*. This definition was later modified to specify that the drug in question must *"gain access to the parasite or the infected red blood cell for the duration of the time necessary for its normal action"* (Bruce-Chwatt *et al.*, 1986).

Negative Impact of Resistance

Adequate and proper usage of anti-malarials is extremely important for reducing the high morbidity and mortality associated with malaria in non-immune migrants as well as travelers. It requires proper understanding on the epidemiology of drug resistance to design and implement effective national and international treatment policy. Anti-malarials are often administered in the form of chemotherapeutic, chemoprophylactic, and potent intermittent preventive agent. Nevertheless, widespread of multi-drug resistant strains has substantially limited treatment options. It is the greatest obstacle to control and eliminate/eradicate malaria worldwide (Wongsrichanalai *et al., 2002).*

Thai-Cambodian Border: An Epicenter of Anti-malarials Resistance

Thailand and its neighboring countries have been widely known as an epicenter of emergence of multi-drug resistant *Plasmodium* strains (World Health Organization, 2007). Interestingly, chloroquine resistance was first reported in this area in the 1970s, followed by resistance to other anti-malarials reported in the Thailand -Cambodian border area (World Health Organization, 2010). Resistance to chloroquine has spread rapidly through South America, Southeast Asia to East Africa and eventually to all endemic countries of the continent. A similar resistance process has happened to Sulfadoxine–Pyrimethamine (SP) exceptfor West-Africa where resistance to the drug in Africa is low, and is beginning to increase in East African countries where SP has replaced chloroquine as the first-line anti-malarial (FMoH-Nigeria, 2005).

Over past decade, as result of worldwide emergence and spread of muti-drug resistance strains of *P. falciparum,* artemisinin-based therapy (ACT) has became the first-line protocol for the management of *P. falciparum* infections worldwide (World Health Organization, 2010). Potency of ACT has been acknowledged worldwide, especially in areas where *P. falciparum* became highly resistant to other potent anti-malarials (Dondorp *et al.,* 2011). However, recently there has been an increasing public health concern regarding the emergence of *P. falciparum* resistance to artemisinins along the Thai-Cambodian border, as they possibly spread it to the rest of the world (Dondorp *et al.*, 2009). Several studies have also provided the evidence of resistant hotspots in some western provinces of Cambodia and certain eastern provinces of Thailand, and more recently there has been a serious suspicion of additional hotspots along the Thai-Myanmar border too (Vijaykadga *et al.*, 2006; Wongsrichanalai and Meshnick, 2008; Carrara *et al.*, 2009). The artemisinin-resistance situation remains critical in areas along the Thai-Cambodian border, where the incidence of falciparum infection is declining drastically (Dondorp *et al.*, 2009).

Consequences of anti-malarial resistance

- ☆ It increases morbidity and mortality, delays in initial therapeutic response and, increases the treatment-cost (FMoH-Nigeria, 2005).

- It may spread malaria to new areas and may cause re-emergence of malaria in areas where malaria had been previously eliminated/eradicated (Foster, 1991; Ridley, 1997).
- It may lead to the occurrence and severity of epidemics in some parts of the world. Population movement also introduces resistant parasites to areas previously free of drug resistance (Foster, 1991; Ridley, 1997).
- It increases the global cost of malaria control, including the cost of new anti-malarial development (Phillips and Phillips-Howard, 1996).
- Therapeutic failure requires consultation at a health facility for further diagnosis and treatment, resulting in loss of working days for adults, absence from school for children and increased cost to the health system (Talisuna *et al.*, 2004).

Therefore, there is an urgent need to preserve and prolong the efficacy of the existing antimalarials (FMoH-Nigeria, 2005). Combination therapy has been often advocated as the standard treatment to prevent as well as to delay the spread and development of resistance to antimalarial drugs (White *et al.*, 1999).

Counterfeit Anti-malarials

Besides drug resistance, the manufacturing, distribution and supply of fake antimalarials is a matter of important concern in the resource-limited malaria endemic settings. The counterfeiting of anti-malarials is one of the oldest professions and it represents a form of attack on global public health in which fake and substandard anti-malarials serve as *de facto* weapons of mass destruction, particularly in resource-poor settings, where malaria causes nearly 660,000 preventable deaths and threatens millions of lives annually. But then it has been estimated that fake anti-malarials itself contribute to nearly 450,000 preventable deaths every year. This crime against humanity is often underestimated or ignored (Karunamoorthi, 2014b).

This persistent threat has torn society by imposing severe menace in all spheres of clinical, socio-economic, and public health domains. The majority of victims often belong to the underprivileged sections of society. They primarily prefer self-medication from informal, private, pharmaceutical sectors owing to the inaccessibility and unaffordability of quality healthcare medicines. Fortunately, there is an unprecedented awareness among all stakeholders due to adverse repercussions of fake anti-malarials. An urgent and intensified effort is imperative in terms of multi-layered approaches and multi-disciplinary scientific research and policies to prevent a public health disaster (Karunamoorthi, 2014b).

In order to combat global counterfeiting, the following stringent measures to ensure the availability of lower-priced, genuine anti-malarials (Karunamoorthi, 2014b): (a) determining the actual extent of the problem; (b)community-based, anti-counterfeit campaigns; (c) strict law enforcement agencies against all perpetrators; (d) setting up quality drug surveillance systems; (e) developing affordable next generation anti-malarials; (f) removal of taxes and tariffs on anti-malarials and other commodities of malaria control; (g) sharing the knowledge and logistical information within and between the endemic countries; (h) launching and maintaining national and international databases; (i) establishing adequate analytical laboratories; (j) imposition of price controls; (k) post-market surveillance; (l) supply chain security for active pharmaceutical ingredients and medicinal products; and, (m) distribution of low-cost (ideally free) potent anti-malarial through health care facilities and community healthcare workers.

Importance of Novel Anti-malarials

Malaria case management encompasses prompt and effective treatment to minimize morbidity and mortality, reduce transmission and prevent the emergence and spread of antimalarial drug resistance (Upke *et al.,* 2013). Provision of early diagnosis and prompt treatment is extremely important for the management of both uncomplicated, and severe or complicated malaria and it is a vital component of programmatic strategies for malaria control and elimination. Though currently ACT is one of the most potent anti-malarial to combat malaria effectively, it often inaccessible and unaffordable in the resource-constrained settings. Besides, already a sign of resistance has been observed against artemisinin along the Thai-Combodian and Thai-Myanmar borders (Karunamoorthi and Tsehaye, 2012). It demands for exploring for the low-cost and easily accessible anti-malarials from various plant species as a potential source of antimalarials in the near future.

Lack of Accessibility to Potent Anti-malarials in the Rural Settings

Many malaria endemic countries have free ACT treatment policy; however, it is often not accessible to majority of the rural poor, particularly those living in the remote villages. An Ethiopian study indicated that over half of the Ethiopian population has to travel a minimum of ten kilometers to access the modern health care facilities (Bilal *et al.,* 2010). Unfortunately in malaria endemic countries many villages are not approachable by means of road and even if they travel, theyreach only a few health facilities supplies of ACT regularly (Karunamoorthi *et al.,* 2013a). In Ethiopia, the author has personally witnessed in many occasions the rural illiterate poor women to prepare plant-based anti-malarial quasi-drug mainly by using freely available traditional anti-malarial plants to treat fever, where the signs suggest as malaria. Irrespective of its anti-malarial properties, they are used to administer. It is purely because of the lack of accessibility and affordability of potent anti-malarial like ACT (Karunamoorthi *et al.,* 2013a). Therefore, the widespread scaling up of ACT with rapid diagnostic tests (RDTs) at the village level is extremely important to curtail malaria burden.

Free Supply of Potent Anti-malarials

A recent study estimated that one-third and nearly half of the anti-malarials are fake or substandard in the resource-constrained settings of sub-Saharan Africa and Southeast Asia, respectively (Karunamoorthi, 2014b). Since, malaria is a disease of poverty and a cause of poverty (Karunamoorthi, 2012a), majority of victims belong to low socio-economic status and are unable to access more expensive ACT. Consequently, they procure cheaper fake anti-malarials. An appropriate anti-malarial distribution policy, ideally low-priced or free genuine one (Ambroise-Thomas, 2012), would hamper the counterfeit industry. It is indeed a Herculean task, but this can be achieved with the pecuniary aid of international/national donors, malaria control partners, and non-governmental organizations (Karunamoorthi, 2014b).

In addition, though anti-malarials are produced at very low cost or donated for free, it can become expensive along the supply chain to the end user. Therefore, adequate measures must be identified and implemented to confront these barriers (Karunamoorthi, 2014b). Price must not be a barrier to save lives, particularly for malaria related illness which is preventable and curable too and the cost of anti-malarial must be as low as possible. Ideally, malaria treatment should be free in the public sector. If, for any reason, treatment cannot be free, then it should be subsidized to a level at which cost will not be a disincentive to the seeking of prompt and adequate treatment of malaria. At the national level, tariffs and taxes on locally manufactured and imported anti-malarials should either be waived altogether or reduced substantially. This will contribute to bringing down the treatment costs to affordable levels (FMoH-Nigeria, 2005).

Development of Affordable Novel Anti-malarials

Over centuries, more than a thousand plant species have been used as anti-malarial agents in the resource-poor settings. However, their clinical efficacy, quality, and safety are a matter of grave concern. Plant-derived compounds will still be an essential aspect of the therapeutic array of new anti-malarials (Karunamoorthi *et al.*, 2013). The cheaper anti-malarials can be formulated by forming a vibrant anti-malarial discovery pipeline by bringing all stakeholders, such as traditional healers, ethnobotanists, scientists, medical entomologists, pharmacists, universities, and research institutions to a common platform to isolate and identify lead compounds to develop the next generation of affordable anti-malarials to combat multidrug-resistant strains effectively (Karunamoorthi *et al.*, 2013a). As the world's potential anti-malarials, such as quinine and artemisinin, have been derived from the ancient herbal remedy for malaria, it has infact driven several researchers to develop and deploy an affordable anti-malarial to attack the various stages of malarial parasites (Karunamoorthi *et al.*, 2013a).

Traditional Anti-malarial Plants: A Repository of Modern Anti-malarials

Since malaria is a major public health issue in the resource-limited settings, where there is a fragile health care system, it quite often fails to meet the expectation of needy poor people. As a result, in order to address the antimalarial drug resistance catastrophe, a keen interest has been observed among the researches towards traditional system of medicine to explore with the possibilities of identifying the new affordable, accessible and potential anti-malarials from our age-old traditional system of medicine (Karunamoorthi *et al.*, 2014). There is a growing awareness/interest that herbs have a role to play in the global fight against malaria. As the traditional anti-malarial plants contain numerous bio-active molecules and secondary metabolites, these can optimally attack various stages of malaria parasites with multiple pathways, and thereby minimizing the already low (and purely theoretical) risk of resistance but also toxicity (by limiting the absolute dose of each herb necessary for efficacy) (Yarnell, 2014).

In the past two decades, a new class of anti-malarial agents is available. They are obtained from the sesquiterpene lactone artemisinin, which is found in the Chinese medicinal plant namely *A. annua*, and its principal metabolite dihydroartemisinin (Yarnell, 2014). Suggestions for sustainable combination therapy with *A. annua* using local herbal resources, or plants that are likely sustainable in many tropical climates, include *Cinchona* spp (Peruvian bark and the source of quinine and related antimalarial alkaloids), *Azadirachta indica* (neem) leaf or oil, *Vernonia amygdalina* (bitter leaf), *Argemone mexicana* (Mexican poppy), and *Curcuma longa* (turmeric). Other herbs proven effective in clinical trials may also be relevant in the specific geographic regions in which they grow (Yarnell, 2014).

Neem has not yet been shown to be effective for treating malaria patients in clinical trials. In animal trials, it is clearly shown antimalarial property, including killing gametocytes which would help to interrupt malaria transmission from infected people to new hosts (Udeinya *et al.*, 2006; Isah *et al.*, 2003). Empirically, an infusion of neem leaves has been effective at preventing and treating acute malaria, at least in some patients in Kenya. However, to authenticate it is efficacy further clinical trials are needed. Neem seed and leaf extracts are observed to be effective against malarial parasites (Khalid *et al.*, 1986, 1989). Components of the alcoholic extracts of leaves and seeds are effective against both chloroquine resistant and sensitive strains of malarial parasite (Badam *et al.*, 1987).

Neem seed extract and its purified fractions have been shown to inhibit growth and development of asexual and sexual stages of drug sensitive and resistant strains of the human malarial parasite *P. falciparum* (Dhar *et al.*, 1998). The gametocytocidal effect of neem fractions on gametocytes of *P. falciparum* is different from that of artemisinin, which affects preferentially young gametocytes only (Kumar and Zheng, 1990). Neem extracts have also exhibited significant level of antiretroviral properties (Udeinya *et al.*, 2004), and it has offered us an ideal opportunity to treat both human immunodeficiency virus (HIV) and malaria co-infection in many parts of the Third World countries (Yarnell, 2014), particularly in sub-Saharan Africa and South-East Asia, where HIV and malaria is one of the common phenomena.

Curcuminoids, a mixture of yellow, liphophilic molecules found in *Curcuma longa* (turmeric) often referred to as just curcumin, have shown synergist activity in enhancing the anti-malarial potency of artemisinins. In *P. berghei*-infected mice, a combination of 100 mg/kg of body weight of curcumin orally after a single intramuscular injection of arteether led to 100 per cent survival of the mice, compared with 100 per cent mortality with arteether injection alone after eleven to thirty-four days (Nandakumar *et al.*, 2006).

Mature leaves of *C. papaya* are widely used to treat malaria and splenomegaly while the fruit is often used against anaemia, which can also be caused by malaria (Adjanohoun, 1996). The petroleum ether extract of the seed rind of this species showed a considerable antimalarial activity, with an IC_{50} of 15.19 µg/ml (Bhat and Surolia, 2001). This clearly indicates that the papaya seeds contain the highly active antiplasmodial compounds. Moreover, Ngemenya *et al.* (2004) has also recorded the antiplasmodial activity of the leaves and seeds of *C. papaya* with IC_{50} of about 60 µg/

ml. In Ethiopia, it has been reported by Karunamoorthi and Tsehaye (2012) that the local residents are consuming the powder of the papaya seeds by mixing with honey orally as an antimalarial agent.

A study was carried out to evaluate the antimalarial activity of the methanolic seed extract of *C. papaya* on *Plasmodium berghei* infected mice. The seed extract of *C. papaya* showed a significant malaria parasitaemia suppressive activity. These activities are dose dependent and comparable to those of Chloroquine phosphate. The present finding justifies the inclusion of the seeds of *C. papaya* in the treatment of malaria by local herbalists. The seed extract therefore, if well purified and characterized, it may be used in treatment of very early plasmodiasis as well as a good prophylactic drug in human. This work is limited to animals, thus clinical trials in humans are recommended particularly, when *C. papaya* seeds are non-harmful/non toxic (Amazu *et al.*, 2009).

Recently, Melariri *et al.* (2011) demonstrated greater antiplasmodial activity of the crude ethyl acetate extract of *C. papaya* leaves with an IC_{50} of 2.96/0.14 μg/ml when compared to the activity of the fractions and isolated compounds. Yet the presence of alkaloids in the leaves of papaya could be the rationale why it is often being effectively administered as an anti-malarial agent (Ayoola and Adeyeye, 2010). However, so far there is no comprehensive report on the phyto-chemistry and mode of action of papaya with reference to its antiplasmodial activity. Therefore, further pharmacological and phytochemical investigations on papaya are required to be warranted to authenticate the claims or beliefs on the efficacy and safety concerns (Karunamoorthi and Tsehaye, 2012).

Essential oils of *Cymbopogon citratus* were found to produce 86.6 per cent suppression in growth of *P. berghei* while compared with chloroquine (Tchoumbougnang *et al.*, 2005). A study investigated the in vivo anti-plasmodial activity, when mice treated with a combination of *C. citratus* and *Vernonia amygdalina* extracts at a dose of 600 mg/kg each and this showed no parasitemia after treatment using the four-day suppressive test (Melariri *et al.*, 2011). The number of existing antimalarials is still inadequate especially in the face of parasite resistance. The results of these studies could help encourage more identification and validation of natural products which has shown antiparasitic properties thus facilitating the development of a new generation of antimalarials (Melariri *et al.*, 2011). Besides, there is an urgent need to determine whether combinations of these herbs with *A. annua* and other antimalarial herbs is effective acutely and at preventing recrudescence, as well as at preventing the spread of malaria (Yarnell, 2014).

Globally, over thousand plants have been used as potential antimalarials in the resource-poor settings due to fragile health-care systems and lack of accessibility and affordability of artemisinin-based combination therapies. Though many believe that the usages of medicinal plants are relatively safe, which have folklore reputations for antimalarial properties, many herbs may also be potentially toxic due to their intrinsic adverse side-effects. Therefore herbal-derived remedies need a powerful and deep assessment of their pharmacological qualities in order to establish their mode of action, safety, quality and efficacy (Karunamoorthi *et al.*, 2013a).

Current Development Efforts in Developing Plant-based New Antimalarials

In malaria endemic countries traditional medicinal plants are frequently used to treat malaria. The analysis of traditional medicines that are employed for treatment of malaria represents a potential for the discovery of lead molecules and hence for further development as potential antimalarial drugs ((Muthaura *et al.*, 2007). New drugs are required to combat the emergence of antimalarials resistance. The main goal of ethnopharmacology is to discover novel plant derived compounds, based on the indigenous use of medicinal plants, which can be developed into new pharmaceuticals. Historically, plants have proven to be a major source of drugs (Newman *et al.*, 2003), with two of the most widely used antimalarials originating from plants: the quinoline-based antimalarials are modeled on quinine, derived from the bark of the Peruvian *Cinchona* tree; and the endoperoxide-based antimalarials originated from artemisinin, rst isolated from the Chinese herbal medicine *A. annua* (Camacho *et al.*, 2000). In light of this historic success, there is every possibility that ethnopharmacological approaches could lead to new antimalarial agents (Phillipson and Wright, 1991).

ACTs have now been adopted globally as the first line of treatment. However, in the long term there will always be a need for new therapies no matter how carefully the current medicines are used, and then there is the constant threat of resistance (Wells, 2011). This is an early warning sign that new classes of anti-malarials are needed, and are an urgent priority. It takes at least ten years to move a molecule from late in the discovery phase to the completion of clinical trials. Herbal medicinal products carry one strategic advantage that in several cases we know that there is an activity in patients. Once the active ingredients are identified it is likely that medicinal chemistry will be needed to optimize it for clinical use (Wells, 2011).

Recommendations

It is mandatory that the new antimalarials meet the requirements of rapid efficacy, minimal toxicity and low cost (Karunamoorthi and Tsehaye, 2012). It can be achieved by the formulation of potent anti-malarials like choloroquine and artemeisinin from the traditional anti-malarial plants. It requires integrated and multivalent strategies like forming a vibrant anti-malarial discovery pipeline among all important stakeholders (Karunamoorthi *et al.*, 2013).

- ☆ Potent anti-malarials must be made affordable and available. To be affordable, they must cost 10 percents or less, in a day in both the public and private sectors, as chloroquine does (White, 2006).
- ☆ Anti-malarials must be highly effective, with acceptable adverse-effect profiles.
- ☆ Political willingness is another important issue for ensuring ready access to effective antimalarial drugs with affordable cost even to the remote area of the countries.
- ☆ An effective, reliable and affordable malaria vaccine shall be a breakthrough for the complete eradication of malaria; therefore, pursuing meaningful

active research could pave the way for the development of malaria vaccine (Karunamoorthi, 2014c).

- In Africa, where the mortality burden from malaria is the greatest, the majority of children die before they reach health facilities. Therefore, prompt access of ACTs means having treatment available as near to the home as possible so that it can be given within 48 hours of onset of symptoms.

Ideal Anti-malarial medicines of the Future

The ideal product profile of antimalarial medicines for large-scale deployment in malaria endemic countries includes the following properties:

- Must be highly effective in providing both clinical and parasitological cure.
- It should be very much safe, including in infancy and pregnancy.
- It must be resistance proof.
- Should have potent anti-gametocidal (transmission blocking) activity.
- Should be Effective against all malaria parasite species.
- Should be friendly to use as an intermittent preventive treatment agent.
- It has to be available in fixed-dose combinations.
- It should be of simple regimen (Ideally as single dose).
- It must have long shelf-life period (minimum of three-year).
- It has to be available in paediatric formulations and course-of-therapy packaging.

Conclusions

Malaria is one of the ancient diseases, which has killed millions of lives, even the death of Alexander the Great attributable to a relapse of the malaria or typhoid fever, which were rampant in ancient Babylon. Over centuries, mankind mainly depends on medicinal plants to alleviate various illnesses and has enhanced his immunity status by consuming various nutraceutical fruits. Therefore, the history of anti-malarial is as old as human history. Quinine remains as an important anti-malarial for almost 400 years after its effectiveness was first documented. Artemisinin derivatives are now considered as one of the ideal anti-malarials in terms of efficacy, safety, quality, and well-tolerability. Nevertheless, it is often inaccessible and unaffordable too. Besides, the issues like short-supply, emergence of resistance strains and fake anti-malarials are a matter of grave concern. In the light of the history of anti-malarials, the author believes that the low-cost, resistant proof potent anti-malarials can be quite obtainable from the natural warehouse of traditional anti-malarial plants in the future.

Acknowledgements

I sincerely would like to thank Mrs. L. Melita for her sincere assistance in editing this manuscript. I also would like to acknowledge my wife Mrs. K. Dhavamani and my kids Mr. Rohith and Ms. Mathivathani for their valuable support. Without their contribution, this study would have been impossible. My last but not least heartfelt thanks go to our colleagues from the School of Environmental Health Science, Faculty of Public Health, Jimma University, Jimma, Ethiopia, for their kind support and cooperation.

References

Adjanohoun, J.E., Aboubakar, N., Dramane, K., Ebot, M.E., Ekpere, J.A., Enoworock, E.G., Focho, D., Gbile, Z.O., Kamanyi, A., Kamsu, K. J., Keita, A., Mbenkum, T., *et al.* (1996). Organization of African Unity; Scientific, Technical and Research Commission, editor. Traditional Medicine and Pharmacopoeia: Contribution to ethno botanical and floristic studies in Cameroon.

Amazu, L.U., Ebong, O.O., Azikiwe, C.C.A., *et al.* (2009). Effects of the methanolic seeds extract of *Carica Papaya* on *plasmodium berghei* infected mice. *Asian Pacific Journal of Tropical Medicine*, **2(3)**: 1-6.

Ambroise-Thomas, P. (2012). The tragedy caused by fake antimalarial drugs. *Mediterranean Journal of Hematology and Infectious Diseases,* **4**: e2012027. DOI 10.4084/MJHID.2012.027.

Awofeso, N. (2011). Project 523: transformation of Artemisinin from traditional Chinese medicine to mainstream anti-malaria chemotherapy. *Spatula DD*, **1(2)**: 113-118

Ayoola, P.B., and Adeyeye, A. (2010). Evaluation of *Carica papaya* (Pawpaw) leaves. *International Journal of Research Review and Applied Sciences*, **5(3)**: 325-328.

Badam, L., Deolankar, R.P., Kulkarni, M.M., Nagsampgi, B.A., and Wagh, U.V. (1987). *In vitro* antimalarial activity of Neem (*Azadirachta indica* A. Juss) leaf and seed extract. *Indian Journal of Malariology,* **24**: 111-117.

Beith. A. (2008). Mapping Factors that Drive Drug Resistance (with a Focus on Resource-Limited Settings): A First Step towards Better Informed Policy. Drug Resistance Working Group Background Paper. Centre for Global Development. www.cgdev.org/drug_resistance. Accessed on 25th September 2013.

Bharel, S., Gulati, A., Abdin, M.Z., Srivastava, P.S., and Jain, S.K. (1996). Structure, biosynthesis and functions of artemisinin. *Fitoterapia,* 67: 387-399.

Bhat, P.G., and Surolia, N. (2001). *In vitro* antimalarial activity of extracts of three plants used in the traditional medicine of India. *American Journal of Tropical Medicine and Hygiene,* **65(4)**: 304-308.

Bilal, N.K., Herbst, C.H., Zhao, F., Soucat, A., and Lemiere, C. (2005). Health Extension Workers in Ethiopia: Improved Access and Coverage for the Rural Poor. Available at: http: //siteresources.worldbank.org/AFRICAEXT/Resources/258643-1271798012256/Health_Extension_Workers_Ethiopia.pdf (accessed on 29th May 2014).

Boulos, M., Dutra, A.P., Disanti, S.M., Shiroma, M., and Amato Neto, V. (1997). Avalia.o clínica do quinine para o tratamento da malária por *Plasmodium falciparum*. *Revista da Sociedade Brasileira de Medicina Tropical,* **30**: 211-213.

Bruce-Chwatt, L.J., Black, R.H., Creig, J.C., and Peters, W. (1986). Chemotherapy of malaria. World Health Organization, Geneva. Technical Reports Series No. 735.

Butler, A.R., Khan, S., and Ferguson, E. (2010). A brief history of malaria chemotherapy. *Journal of the Royal College of Physicians of Edinburgh,* **40**: 72-77.

Camacho, M.D.R., Croft, S.L., and Phillipson, J.D. (2000). Natural products as sources of antiprotozoal drugs. *Current Opinion in Investigational Drugs,* **2**: 47-62.

Carrara, V.I., Zwang, J., Ashley, E.A., Price, R.N., Stepniewska, K, *et al.* (2009). Changes in the treatment responses to artesunate-mefloquine on the northwestern border of Thailand during 13 years of continuous deployment. *PLoS One,* **4**: e4551.

Dhar, R., Zhang, K., Talwar, G. P., Garg, S., and Kumar, N. (1998). Inhibition of the growth and development of asexual and sexual stages of drug–sensitive and resistant strains of the human malaria parasite *Plasmodium falciparum* by Neem (*Azadirachta indica*) fractions. *Journal of Ethnopharmacology,* **61**: 31-39.

Dondorp, A.M., Fairhurst, R.M., Slutsker, L., Macarthur, J.R., Guerin, P.J., Wellems, T.E., Ringwald, P., Newman, R.D., and Plowe, C.V. (2011). The threat of artemisinin-resistant malaria. *New England Journal of Medicine,* **365**: 1073-1075.

Dondorp, A.M., Nosten, F., Yi, P., Das, D., Phyo, A.P., *et al.* (2009). Artemisinin resistance in *Plasmodium falciparum* malaria. *New England Journal of Medicine,* **361**: 455-467.

Elfawal, M.A., Towler, M.J., Reich, N.G., Golenbock, D., Weathers, P.J., *et al.* (2012). Dried whole plant *Artemisia annua* as an antimalarial therapy. *PLoS ONE,* **7(12)**: e52746. doi: 10.1371/journal.pone.0052746.

FMoH-Nigeria. (2005). National antimalarial treatment policy. Federal Ministry of Health, National Malaria and Vector Control Division, Abuja-Nigeria.

Foster, S.D. (1991). Pricing, distribution, and use of antimalarial drugs. *Bulletin of the World Health Organization,* **69**: 349-363.

Garnham, P.C.C. (1966). Malaria Parasites and Other Heamosporidia. Blackwell Scientific Publications, Oxford; pp1114.

Greenwood, D. (1995). Conflicts of interest: the genesis of synthetic antimalarial agents in peace and war. *Antimicrobial and Chemotherapy,* **36(5)**: 857-872. doi: 10.1093/jac/36.5.857.

Huang, K.C. (1998). The pharmacology of Chinese Herbs. 2nd edition Boca Raton,: CRC Press, 1-14.

Hyam, R., and Pankhurst, R. (1995). Plants and their Names: A Concise Dictionary. Oxford: Oxford University Press; pp40-41.

International Pharmacopoeia. (2003). 3rd edition. Volume 5. World Health Organization, Geneva, Switzerland.

Isah, A.B., Ibrahim, Y.K., and Iwalewa, E.O. (2003). Evaluation of the antimalarial properties and standardization of tablets of *Azadirachta indica* (Meliaceae) in mice. *Phytotherapy Research,* **17(7)**: 807-10.

Jaramillo-Arango, J. (1949). A critical review of the basic facts in the history of Cinchona. *Journal of Linnaean Society*, **53**: 1272-1309.

Jones, C.O.H., and Williams, H.A. (2004). The social burden of malaria: what are we measuring? *American Journal of Tropical Medicine and Hygiene,* **71(S2)**: 156-161

Karunamoorthi, K. (2011). Vector Control: A Cornerstone in the Malaria Elimination Campaign. *Clinical Microbiology and Infection*, **17(11)**: 1608-1616. DOI: 10.1111/j.1469-0691.2011.03664.x.

Karunamoorthi, K., and Bekele, M. (2009). Prevalence of malaria from peripheral blood smears examination: A 1-year retrospective study from the Serbo Health Center, Kersa Woreda, Ethiopia. *Journal of Infection and Public Health*, **2(4)**: 171-176.

Karunamoorthi, K., Deboch, B., and Tafere, Y. (2010). Knowledge and practice concerning malaria, insecticide-treated net (ITN) utilization and antimalarial treatment among pregnant women attending specialist antenatal clinics. *Journal of Public Health*, **18(6)**: 559-566.

Karunamoorthi, K., Kim, H., Jegajeevanram, K., Xavier, J., and Vijayalakshmi, J. (2014). Papaya: A gifted nutraceutical plant –a critical review of recent human health research. *International Journal of Genuine Traditional Medicine (TANG)* **4(1)**: e2: 1-17. DOI: http: / /dx.doi.org/10.5667/tang.2013.0028

Karunamoorthi, K., Mohammed, M., and Wassie, F. (2012). Knowledge and practices of farmers with reference to pesticide management: implications on human health. *Archives of Environmental and Occupational Health*, **67(2)**: 109-116.

Karunamoorthi, K., and Sabesan, S. (2010). Laboratory evaluation of Dimethyl phthalate treated wristbands against three predominant mosquito (Diptera: Culicidae) vectors of disease. *European Review of Medical and Pharmacological Science*, **14(5)**: 443-448.

Karunamoorthi, K., and Sabesan, S. (2013). Insecticide resistance in insect vectors of disease with special reference to mosquitoes: A potential threat to global public health. *Health Scope*, **2(1)**: 4-18. DOI: 10.5812/jhs.9840.

Karunamoorthi, K., and Tsehaye, E. (2012). Ethnomedicinal knowledge, belief and self-reported practice of local inhabitants on traditional antimalarial plants and phytotherapy. *Journal of Ethnopharmacology,* **141(1)**: 143-50. DOI: 10.1016/j.jep.2012.02.012.

Karunamoorthi, K.,Sabesan, S., Jegajeevanram, K., and Vijayalakshmi, J. (2013). The role of traditional anti-malarial plants in the battle against global malaria burden. *Vector Borne and Zoonotic Diseases,* **13**: 521-544. DOI: 10.1089/vbz.2011.0946.

Karunamoorthi, K. (2012). Yellow fever encephalitis: an emerging and resurging global public health threat in a changing environment: In Sergey Tkachev (Ed.) for the Encephalitis, InTech Publishers, Crotia. Available at: http: / / www.intechopen.com/books/encephalitis/yellow-fever-encephalitis-an-emerging-and-resurging-global-public-health-threat-in-a-changing-enviro.

Karunamoorthi, K. (2014b). The counterfeit anti-malarial is a crime against humanity: a systematic review of the scientific evidence. *Malaria Journal,* **13**: 209. doi: 10.1186/1475-2875-13-209.

Karunamoorthi, K. (2012a). Global Malaria Burden: Socialomics Implications. *Journal of Socialomics,* **1**: e108. DOI: 10.4172/jsc.1000e108.

Karunamoorthi, K. (2014a). *Cymbopogon citratus*: Phytotherapeutic Potentialities and their Efficacy in Traditional Systems of Medicine, In V. K. Gupta (Eds) for the special issue on Utilisation and Management of Medicinal Plants- Vol. 2. M/S Daya Publishing House, New Delhi, India. Available at: http: //astralint.com/indian-books/utilisation-and-management-of-medicinal-plants-vol-2/isbn-9788170358756.aspx

Karunamoorthi, K. (2014c). Malaria Vaccine: A Future Hope to Curtail the Global Malaria Burden. *International Journal of Preventive Medicine,* **5**: 529-538.

Karunamoorthi, K. (2012b). Medicinal and Aromatic Plants: A Major Source of Green Pesticides/Risk-reduced Pesticides. *Journal of Medicinal and Aromatic Plants,* **1**: *e137. doi: 10.4172/2167-0412.1000e137*

Khalid, S.A., Duddeck, H., and Gonzales–Sierra, M. (1989). Isolation and characterization of an antimalarial agent of the neem tree *Azadirachta indica. Journal of Natural Products,* **52**: 922–927.

Khalid, S.A., Farouk, A., Geary, T.G., and Jensen, J.B. (1986). Potential antimalarial candidates from African plant an *in vitro* approach using *Plasmodium falciparum. Journal of Ethnopharmacology,* **15**: 201–209.

Krettli, A.U., Andrade-Neto, V.F., Brandão, M.G.L., and Ferrari, W.M.S. (2001). The search for new antimalarial drugs from plants used to treat fever and malaria or plants ramdomly selected: a review. *Memórias do Instituto Oswaldo Cruz.,* **96(8)**: 1033-1042.

Kumar, N., and Zheng, H. (1990). Stage–specific gametocytocidal effect *in vitro* of the antimalaria drug qinghaosu on *Plasmodium falciparum. Parasitology Research,* **76**: 214-218.

Lee MR. (2002a). Plants against Malaria Part 1: Cinchona or The Peruvian bark. *Journal of the Royal College of Physicians of Edinburgh,* **32**: 189-196.

Lee MR. (2002b). Plants against malaria part 2: *Artemisia annua* (Qinghaosu or the sweet wormwood). The *Journal of the Royal College of Physicians of Edinburgh,* **32**: 300-305.

Li, G.Q., Guo, X.B., Jin, R, *et al.* (1982). Clinical studies on treatment of cerebral malaria with Qinghaosu and its derivatives. *Journal of Traditional Chinese Medicine,* **2**: 125-130. .

Li, Y. (2007). Editorial. Discovery and development of new antimalarial drug (artemisinin). Shanghai: Scientific and Technical Publishers.

Malaria Consortium (2007). *Malaria: A Handbook for Health Professionals.* Macmillian Publishers, London.

Melariri, P., Campbell, W., Etusim, P., and Smith, P. (2011). Antiplasmodial properties and bioassay-guided fractionation of ethyl acetate extracts from *Carica papaya* leaves. *Journal of Parasitology Research*, doi: 10.1155/2011/104954.

Menendez, C. (1995). Malaria during pregnancy: a priority area of malaria research and control. *Parasitology Today*, **11**: 178-183.

Meshnick, S.R. (2002). Artemisinin: mechanisms of action, resistance and toxicity. *International Journal for Parasitology*, **32**: 1655-1660.

Muthaura, C.N., Rukunga, G.M., Chhabra, S.C., Omar, S.A., *et al.* (2007). Antimalarial Activity of Some Plants Traditionally used in Meru district of Kenya. *Phytotheraphy Research*, **21**: 860-867.

Nandakumar, D.N., Nagaraj, V.A., Vathsala, P.G., *et al.* (2006). Curcumin-artemisinin combination therapy for malaria. *Antimicrobial Agents and Chemotherapy*, **50(5)**: 1859-1860.

Navaratman, V., Mansor, S.M., Chin, L.K., Mordi, M.N., Asokan, M., and Nair, N.K. (1995). Determination of artemether and dihydroartemisinin in blood plasma by high-performance liquid chromatography for application in clinical pharmacological studies. *Journal of Chromospheres*, **669**: 289-294.

Newman, D.J., Cragg, G.M., and Snader, K.M. (2003). Natural products as sources of new drugs over the period 1981-2002. *Journal of Natural Products*, **66**: 1022-1037.

Ngemenya, M.N., Tane, P., Berzins, K., and Titanji, V.P.K. (2004). Antiplasmodial Activity of some Medicinal Plants used in Cameroon: preliminary toxicity studies of highly active extracts; XIth Annual Conference of The Cameroon Bioscience Society; 16-18 December, 2004.

Nosten, F., and White, N.J. (2007). Artemisinin-based combination treatment of falciparum malaria. *American Journal of Tropical Medicine and Hygiene*, **77(6 S)**: 181-92.

Oliveira, A.B., Olabela, M.N., Braga, F.O.C., *et al.* (2009). Plant-derived antimalarial agents: new leads and efficient phytomedicines. Part I. Alkaloids. *Anais da Academia Brasileira de Ciências Academia Brasileira de Ciências*, **81(4)**: 715-740.

Olliaro, P.L., and Yuthavong, Y. (1999). An overview of chemotherapeutic targets for antimalarial drug discovery. *Pharmacological Theraphy*, **81**: 91-110.

Onwujekwe, *et al.* (2012). Patterns of case management and chemoprevention for malaria-in-pregnancy by public and private sector health providers in Enugu state, Nigeria. *BMC Research Notes*, **5**: 211.

Pamplona-Roger, M.D.G.D. (2001). Encyclopedia of Medicinal Plants. Education and Health library. Volume 1 and 2. ISBN 84-7208-157-5.

Paredes-Borja, V. (1946). Contribucion del Ecuador a la Materia Quimica: la Quina. Ecuador; (Three year II (January-December) pp. 217 et sequitur.).

Peigen, X. (2002). (ed.). [Modern Chinese Materia Medica], Vol. 3. Beijing, Chemical Industry Press.

Phillips, M., and Phillips-Howard, P.A. (1996). Economic implications of resistance to antimalarial drugs. *Pharmacoeconomics,* **10**: 225-238.

Phillipson, J.D., and Wright, C.W. (1991). Can ethnopharmacology contribute to the development of antimalarial agents? *Journal of Ethnopharmacology,* **32**: 155-165.

Price, R., van Vugt, M., Phaipun, L., Luxemburger, C., Simpson, J., McGready, R., *et al.* (1999). Adverse effects in patients with acute falciparum malaria treated with artemisinin derivatives. *American Journal of Tropical Medicine and Hygiene,* **60(4)**: 547-555.

Qinghaosu Antimalaria Coordinating Research Group. (1979). Antimalaria studies on Qinghaosu. *Chinese Medical Journal,* **12**: 811-816.

Qinghaosu. (1977). Qinghaosu anti-malarial coordinating research group. Ò»ÖÖÐÂÐÍµÄ±¶°ë ÝÆÄÚõ¥–ÇàÝïËØ[A new sesquterpenoid-artemisinin]. ¿ÆÑ§Í¨±¨ [Science Bulletin], **22**: 142.

Redi F. (1966). Opere de Francesco Redi. *Venice: Ertz,* 1712-1750.

Ridley, R.G. (2002). Medical need, scientific opportunity and the drive for antimalarial drugs. *Nature,* **415**: 686-693.

Roll Back Malaria (RBM). (1998). Economic costs of malaria. Available at: http: // www.rbm.who.int/cmc_upload/0/000/015/363/RBMInfosheet_10.htm (accessed on 15th February 2014).

Ruth, E., and Lagerberg, C.M.N. (2008). Malaria in Pregnancy, A literature Review. *Journal of Midwifery and Women Health,* **53**(3): 209-215.

Shilin, Y., Roberts, M.F., and Phillipson, D. (1989). Qinghaosu anti malarial coordinating research group. Methoxylated flavones and coumarins from *Artemisia annua. Phytochemistry,* **28**: 1509-1511.

Shuhua, X. and Catto, B.A. (1989). *In vitro* and *in vivo* studies of the effect of artemether on *Schistosoma mansoni. Antimicrobial Agents and Chemotherapy,* **33**: 1557-1562.

Talisuna, A.O., Bloland, P., and D'Alessandro, U. (2004). History, dynamics, and public health importance of malaria parasite resistance. *Clinical and Microbiology Reviews,* **17**: 235-254.

Taylor, K. (2005). Chinese medicine in early Communist China, 1945-63. London: Routledge Curzon.

Tchoumbougnang, F., Zollo, P.H.A., Dagne, E., and Mekonnen, Y. (2005). *In vivo* antimalarial activity of essential oils from *Cymbopogon citratus* and *Ocimum gratissimum* on mice infected with *Plasmodium berghei. Planta Medica,* **71**: 20-23.

Titulaer, H.A.C., Zuidema, J., Kager, P.A., *et al.* (1990). The pharmacokinetics of artemisinin after oral, intramuscular and rectal administration to volunteers. *Journal of Pharmacy and Pharmacology,* **42**: 810-813.

Udeinya, I.J., Brown, N., Shu, E.N., *et al.* (2006). Fractions of an antimalarial neem-leaf extract have activities superior to chloroquine, and are gametocytocidal. *Annals of Tropical Medicine and Parasitology,* **100(1)**: 17-22.

Upke, I.S., Moonasar, D., Raman, J., Barnes, K.I., Baker, L., and Blumberg, L. (2013). Case management of malaria: treatment and chemoprophylaxis. *South African Medical Journal,* **103(10)**: 793-798. doi: 10.7196/samj.7443.

van Ballegoyen, A.F. (2005). Roll back malaria: A WHO initiated network in the fight against malaria. Available at: http: //www.gppi.net/fileadmin/gppi/van_Ballegoyen_WHO_Malaria.pdf (accessed on 15th February 2014).

Vijaykadga, S., Rojanawatsirivej, C., Cholpol, S., Phoungmanee, D., Nakavej, A., and Wongsrichanalai, C. (2006). *In vivo* sensitivity monitoring of mefloquine monotherapy and artesunate-mefloquine combinations for the treatment of uncomplicated falciparum malaria in Thailand in 2003. *Tropical Medicine and International Health,* **11**: 211-219.

Wellems, T.E. (2002). Plasmodium chloroquine resistance and the search for a replacement antimalarial drug. *Science,* **298**: 124.

Wells, T.N.C. (2011). Natural products as starting points for future anti-malarial therapies: going back to our roots? *Malaria Journal,* **10(S1)**: S3.

White, N. (1999a) Antimalarial drug resistance and combination chemotherapy. *Philos Transaction of Royal Society of London Bulletin of Biological Science,* **354(1384)**: 739-749.

White, N.J., Nosten, F., Looareesuwan, S., *et al.* (1999). Averting a malaria disaster. *Lancet,* **353**: 1965-67.

White, N.J. (2006). Malaria - Time to Act. *New England Journal of Medicine,* **355(19)**: 1956-1957.

WHO. (2001a). The use of antimalarial drugs: Report of a WHO Informal Consultation 13-17 November 2000. Geneva, World Health Organization, 2001 (WHO/CDS/RBM/2001.33).

WHO. (2001b). Antimalarial Drug Combination Therapy. Report of a WHO Technical Consultation. Geneva: World Health Organization. WHO/CDS/RBM/2001.35.

WHO. (2006a). Guidelines for the treatment of malaria. WHO/HTM/MAL/2006.1108. Available at: http: //www.who.int/malaria/docs/TreatmentGuidelines 2006.pdf]. (accessed on 3rd January 2011).

World Malaria Report - 2009. World health Organization, Geneva, Switzerland.

World Malaria Report - 2013. The World Health Organization, Geneva, Switzerland.

Willcox, M., and Bodeker, G. (2004). Traditional herbal medicines for malaria. *British Medical Journal,* **329**: 1156-1159.

Wongsrichanalai, C., and Meshnick, S.R. (2008). Declining artesunate-mefloquine efficacy against falciparum malaria on the Cambodia-Thailand border. *Emerging Infectious Diseases,* **14**: 716-719.

Wongsrichanalai, C., Pickard, A.L., Wernsdorfer, W.H., and Meshnick, S.R. (2002). Epidemiology of drug-resistant malaria. *Lancet Infectious Diseases,* **2**: 209-218.

World Health Organisation. (2004). *A Strategic Framework for Malaria Prevention and Control During Pregnancy in the African Region. AFR/MAL/04/01*. WHO, Brazzaville.

World Health Organization. (2007). *Containment of malaria multi-drug resistance on the Cambodia-Thailand border. Report of an Informal Consultation*. WHO-Mekong Malaria Programme, Phnom Penh, Cambodia.

World Health Organization. (2010). *Guidelines for the treatment of malaria - 2nd edition*. World Health Organization, Geneva, Switzerland.

World Malaria Report - 2005. The World Health Organization, Geneva, Switzerland. 2005. Available at: http: / / rbm.who.int / wmr.2005 (Accessed on 31st December 2013).

Wright, C.W. (2005b). Plant derived antimalarial agents: New lead and challenges. *Phytochemistry Review*, **4**: 55-61.

Wright, C.W. (2005a). Traditional antimalarial and the development of novel antimalarial drugs. *Journal Ethnopharmacology*, **100**: 67-71.

Yarnell, E. (2014). *Artemisia annua* (Sweet Annie), Other *Artemisia* Species, Artemisinin, Artemisinin Derivatives, and Malaria. *Journal of Restorative Medicine*, **3**: 69-84.

Ying, L.I., and Yu-Lin, W.U. (1998). How Chinese scientists discovered Qinghaosu (Artemisinin) and developed its derivatives. What are the future perspectives? *Medecine Tropicale (Mars)*, **58(3S)**: 45-47.

Ying, T., Zhenxing, W., and Zhaohua W. (1982). [Study on chemical compositions of Herbal *Artemisia annua*]. [*Chinese traditional and Herbal Drugs*] **13**: 249-251.

Youyou, T. *et al.* (1981). [Studies on the constituents of *Artemisia annua* L.]. [*Acta Pharmaceutica Sinica*] **16**: 366-370.

Zhao, K. and Song, Z. (1990). The pharmacokinetics of dihydroqinghaosu given orally to rabits and dogs (chinese). *Acta Pharmaceutica Sinica*, **25**: 161-163.

Bioactive Phytochemicals: Perspectives for Modern Medicine Vol. 3 (2015)
Editor: **V.K. Gupta**
Published by: **DAYA PUBLISHING HOUSE, NEW DELHI**

21

Ethnopharmacological Review of Traditional Medicinal Plants for Anticancer Activity

Khyati Vadera[1], Darshana Patil[2] and Avinash Patil[1*]

ABSTRACT

Cancer is a major public health burden in both developed and developing countries. Cancer is a disease in which body cells become abnormal and divide without control. Cancer cells may invade nearby tissues and they may spread through the blood stream and lymphatic system to other parts of the body. Several synthetic agents are used to cure the disease but they have their toxicity and hence the research is going on to investigate the plant derived chemotherapeutic agents.

Anticancer activity is the effect of natural and synthetic or biological and chemical agents to reverse, suppress or prevent carcinogenic progression. Therefore an attempt is being made for evaluating anticancer properties of natural products from medicinal plants by using different in vitro and in vivo methods all over the world. Herbal medicines have a vital role in the prevention and treatment of cancer. With advanced knowledge of molecular science and refinement in isolation and structure elucidation techniques, various anticancer herbs has been identified, which execute therapeutic effect by inhibiting cancer- activating enzymes and hormones, stimulating DNA repair mechanism, promoting production of protective enzymes, inducing antioxidant action and enhancing immunity of the body. These herbs were found to posses anticancer, cytotoxic or antioxidant activity in various pre-clinical or clinical studies.

The search for anticancer agents from the plant sources such as Vincristine, Vinblastine and the isolation of cytotoxic Podophyllotoxins reduces white blood cell count causing bone

1 Birla College of Arts, Science and Commerce, Kalyan (W) – 421 304, M.S., India

2 Smt. C.H.M. College, Ulhasnagar, M.S., India

* *Corresponding author*: E-mail: dravinashpatil@rediffmail.com

marrow depression in rats. Roots, leaves, stem, root, bark and fruits of the plant herbs are used in the treatment of cancer. The dietary antioxidants having anti carcinogenic property are in demand. Identification and characterization of these anti-carcinogens in the diet can be used for reducing the risk of human cancer. Several anticancer agents including taxol, vinblastine, vincristine, the campothecin derivatives, Topotecan, etoposide and Irinotecan derived from epipodophyllotoxin are clinically used all over the world. Hence an attempt has been made to review the plants used previously and recently for treatment of cancer.

Keywords: Anticancer agents, Antioxidants, Cancer, Chemotherapeutic agents, Herbal medicines, *In vitro* methods, *In vivo* methods.

What is Cancer?

Cancer is a general term applied to series of malignant diseases that may affect different parts of body. These diseases are characterized by a rapid and uncontrolled formation of abnormal cells, which may mass together to form a growth of tumor, or proliferate through out the body, initiating abnormal growth at other sites. If the process is not arrested, it may progress until it causes the death of the organism (Tyler, 1994). Consequently cancer cells continue to divide even in situations in which normal cells will usually wait for a special chemical transduction signal. The tumor cells would ignore such stop signals that are sent out by adjacent tissues. A cancer cell also has the character of immortality even *in vitro*, whereas normal cells stop dividing after 50-70 generations and undergoes a programmed cell death (Apoptosis). Cancer cells continue to grow invading nearby tissues and metastasizing to distant parts of the body. Metastasis is the most lethal aspect of carcinogenesis (McNutt, 1995).

In the normal situations, the cells grow and divide as the body needs them. This process is disturbed when new cells form and old cells don't die when they should. These extra cell lumps together to form a growth or tumor. Broadly, two types of tumors exists *i.e.* benign and malignant. Benign tumors are not cancerous. They can usually be removed and generally don't grow back. Malignant tumors are cancerous in nature. The cells in malignant tumor are abnormal and divide randomly. The cells attack the tissue around them. The cells of malignant tumor can also enter the blood stream or lymphatic system to form new tumors. This type of spread is known as metastasis.

DNA is found in every cell in the body and regulates all of its activities. Cancer is caused by damage to DNA. The body is usually able to repair damaged DNA, but is unable to do so in cancer cells. Some people inherit damaged DNA, but in most cases DNA is damaged by their own lifestyle choices such as smoking, exposure to UV radiations or exposure to cancer causing substances (carcinogens) in the environment. While being infected with certain viruses, such as Human Papilloma Virus (HPV) and Human Immunodeficiency Virus (HIV), can increase the risk of cancer.

Cancer is classified into various stages on the basis of severity. There are multiple staging scales in use. Cancers are divided into five progressively more severe stages:

0, I, II, III and IV. Stage 0 cancer is cancer that is just beginning, involving just a few cells. Stages I, II, III and IV represent progressively more advanced cancers, characterized by large tumor sizes, more tumors, the aggressiveness with which the cancer grows and spreads, and the extent to which the cancer has spread to infect adjacent tissues and body organs (Kumar *et al.*, 2013).

Cancer in each person differs according to the person's exposure to pathogens and genetic constitutions which make each of them to react differently to the same diet (Bhishagratna, 1991). Ayurveda says that in cancer the aura is disturbed, allowing negative astral forces to enter in body. Cancer may be caused by environmental pollution, junk food, lethargy, lack of spiritual purpose, suppressed emotions and stagnation, past life karma also plays a role in disease. Cancer can also be caused by imbalance of the three doshas. Poor digestion allows for a build up of toxins in the body (Acharaya, 1979). Cancer originates due to a metabolic crisis, *i. e.* aggravation of vata forces, both interacting with one another resulting in proliferation (Badmaev and Majeed, 1995).

Causes of Cancer

Cancers may be caused in one of three ways, namely incorrect diet, genetic predisposition and via the environment. As many as 95 per cent of all cancers are caused by life style and may take as long as 20-30 years to develop (Kutluk and Kars, 1998). The major cause of cancer is smoking, dietary imbalances, hormones and chronic infections leading to chronic inflammation (Ames *et al.*, 1995). Modern medicine attributes most cases of cancer to changes in DNA that reduce or eliminate the normal controls over cellular growth, maturation and programmed cell death. These changes are more likely to occur in people with certain genetic backgrounds (as illustrated by the finding of genes associated with some cases of cancer and familial prevalence of certain cancers) and in persons infected by chronic viruses (*e.g.*, viral hepatitis may lead to liver cancer; propensity or viruses that may influence the risk of cancer, is often exposure to carcinogenic chemicals (including those found in nature) and/or to radiation (including natural cosmic and earthly radiation), coupled with a failure of the immune system to eliminate the cancer cells at an early stage in their multiplication. The immunological weakness might arise years after the exposure to chemicals or radiation. Other factors such as tobacco smoking, alcohol consumption, excess use of caffeine and other drugs, sunshine, infections from such oncogenic virus like cervical papillomaviruses, adenoviruses. Karposis sarcoma (HSV) or exposure to asbestos. These obviously are implicated as casual agents of mammalian cancers. However a large population of people is often exposed to these agents (McNutt, 1995).

Every type of cancer is different, and has a unique set of symptoms. Some of the types of cancers and symptoms associated with them are enlisted below: (Kumar *et al.*, 2013).

Cancer is one of the dreadful diseases of 20th century and moving vastly towards 21st century (Reddy *et al.*, 2003). It is a major public health problem in both developed and developing countries. (Parkin *et al.*, 2005; Shoeb, 2006). It has become one of the most devastating diseases, pose significant social and economic impacts on the health

Table 21.1: Different Types of Cancers and their Symptoms

Sl.No.	Type of Cancer	Signs and Symptoms
1.	Adult acute Lymphoblastic leukemia	Weakness, fever and night sweats, bleeding, shortness of breath, weight loss and loss of appetite.
2.	Bile duct cancer	Jaundice, pain in abdomen, fever and itchy skin
3.	Bladder cancer	Blood in urine and frequent urination, pain during urination, lower back pain
4.	Brain tumors	Morning headache, loss of balance, weakness
5.	Breast cancer	A lump or thickening in or near the breast, change in size and shape of the breast, a dimple or puckering in the skin of the breast, fluid other than breast milk, scaly, red and swollen skin on breast or nipple, a nipple tuned inward into the breast.
6.	Cervical cancer	Vaginal bleeding, unusual vaginal discharge, pelvic pain, pain during sexual intercourse
7.	Ewing sarcoma	Pain and swelling in arms, legs, chest, back or pelvis, a lump in arms, legs and chest, fever for no reason, a bone breaks for no reason
8.	Hypo pharyngeal cancer	A sore throat, ear pain, pain and difficulty in swallowing, change in voice
9.	Lip and oral cavity cancer	A sore on a lip or mouth, a lump or thickening on the lips, gums or in mouth, a white or red patch on lips, tongue, tonsil, bleeding, pain or numbness in the lip or mouth, change of voice, loose teeth, swelling of jaw, trouble in chewing, sore throat.
10.	Lung cancer	Chest discomfort or pain, a cough that doesn't go away, trouble in breathing, blood in sputum, loss of appetite, weight loss, trouble in swallowing, swelling in face
11.	Pancreatic cancer	Jaundice, pain in upper or middle abdomen, weight loss, loss of appetite, fatigue

system and second leading cause of death in both men and women worldwide (Mukherjee *et al.*, 2001; Eisenberg *et al.*, 1998; Russo *et al.*, 2001). Cancer is responsible for 12 per cent of the world's mortality and the second-leading cause of death in the Western world (Newman and Cragg, 2007). The disease affects men and women alike. It is the second major cause of death after cardiovascular diseases (Hartwell, 1971). Between 2000 and 2020, the total number of cases of cancer is predicted to increase by 73 per cent in the developing world and by 29 per cent in the developed world (Parkin, 2001). Malignant neoplasm was the leading cause of death in Hongkong during 1996 to 2001 (Stanley, 2001). WHO (2002) reported that malignant neoplasm is the third (12.4 per cent) leading cause of death worldwide, the first (30 per cent) being cardiovascular disease, and the second (18.8 per cent) being infectious diseases, which include HIV/AIDS (Mathers *et al.*, 2001).

According to the studies, worldwide about 6 million new incidences are reported every year (Reddy *et al.*, 2003). Every year, 10 million people are diagnosed with cancer, and of these, 6 million dies of this disease (Joseph, 2004). Lung, colon, prostate and breast cancer account for more than half of the cancer deaths (Srivastava *et al.*,

2005). It was estimated that there were 10.9 million new cases, 6.7 million deaths and 24.6 million persons living with cancer around the world in 2002 (Parkin *et al.*, 2005; Shoeb, 2006). In the US, cancer is the second leading cause of death (Jemal *et al.*, 2005), where one in four deaths is due to cancer (Shoeb, 2006). Cancer kills about 3500 million people annually all over the world. Several chemopreventive agents are used to treat cancer, but they cause toxicity that prevents their usage (Kathiresan *et al.*, 2006). Breast cancer is the most common form of cancer in women worldwide (Sharma and Pandey, 2009; Koduru *et al.*, 2007). Current estimates from the American Cancer Society and from the International Union against cancer indicate that 12 million cases of cancer were diagnosed in 1997, with 7 million deaths worldwide; these numbers are expected to double by 2030 (27 million cases with 17 million deaths) (Kutluk and Kars, 1998).

Because of high death rate associated with cancer and because of the serious side effects of chemotherapy and radiation therapy, many cancer patients seek alternative and/or complementary methods of treatment. The important preventive methods for most of the cancers include dietary changes, stopping the use of tobacco products, treating inflammatory diseases effectively and taking nutritional supplements that aid immune functions. Recent researches revolve round the urgency to evolve suitable chemotherapy consistent with new discoveries in cell biology for treatment of cancer with no toxic effect. Chemotherapy, being a major treatment modality used for the control of advanced stages of malignancies and as a prophylactic against possible metastasis, exhibits severe toxicity on normal tissues (Somkumar *et al.*, 2003; Pandey and Sharma, 2006). Thus, research and development on anticancer agents has become a worldwide scientific effort in both private and public institutions.

Cancer chemotherapy now plays a significant role in the treatment of many malignancies, either curative (by itself or as an adjuvant to surgery and/or radiation) or palliative care, depending upon the specific tumor situation (Carter and Livingston, 1982). The objective of cancer chemotherapy is to kill cancer cells with as little damage as possible to normal cells (Halliwell and Gutteridge, 1988).

Conventional cancer treatment can include surgery, radiation, chemotherapy, hormone therapy and biological therapy. But there are some side effects of conventional therapies like chemotherapy and radiation therapy. Chemotherapy drugs in addition to cancerous cells also kill some regular healthy cells, causing side effects such as the fatigue, nausea and hair loss. Like chemotherapy, radiation therapy is not perfectly precise in its targeting of cancer cells and some normal, healthy cells can also be damaged (Kumar *et al.*, 2013). Limited chances for cure by chemotherapy are a major contributing factor to this situation. Despite much progress in recent years, a key problem in tumor therapy with established cytostatic compounds is the development of drug resistance and threatening side effects. Most established drugs suffer from insufficient specificity toward tumor cells. Hence, the identification of improved antitumor drugs is urgently needed. Several approaches have been delineated to search for novel antitumor compounds. Combinatorial chemistry, a technology conceived about 20 years ago, was envisaged as a promising strategy to this demand. The expected surge in productivity, however, has hardly materialized (Newman and Cragg, 2007).

Therefore, any discovery of anticancer agents must be related to novel molecular targets; *i.e.* they should be effective against specific types of cancer cells but less toxic to normal cells, or have a unique mechanism of action for specific types of cancer (Pezzuto, 1997). Better antitumor drugs with minimal disadvantages and maximum therapeutic benefits in cancer cure and prevention are still being researched for (Peuzzuto, 1997) and drugs resourced from plants have been successfully used in cancer therapy (Pal *et al.*, 2003). Cancer chemoprevention involves pharmacologic intervention with synthetic or naturally occurring chemicals to prevent, inhibit or reverse carcinogenesis or prevent the development of invasive cancer. Out of an estimated 250,000 higher plants, less than 1 per cent has been screened pharmacologically (El-Shemy *et al.*, 2007). In recent years, focus on plant research has increased all over the world.

The Mechanism of Cancer Therapy

1. Inhibiting cancer cell proliferation directly by stimulating macrophage phagocytosis, enhancing natural killer cell activity.
2. Promoting apoptosis of cancer cells by increasing production of interferon, interleukin-2 immunoglobulin and complement in blood serum.
3. Enforcing the necrosis of tumor and inhibiting its translocation and spread by blocking the blood source of tumor tissue.
4. Enhancing the number of leukocytes and platelets by stimulating the hemopoietic function.
5. Promoting the reverse transformation from tumor cells into normal cells.
6. Promoting metabolism and preventing carcinogenesis of normal cells.
7. Stimulating appetite, improving quality of sleep, relieving pain, thus benefiting patients health (Sakarkar and Deshmukh, 2011).

Ayurveda, a traditional Indian medical practice using plant drugs has been successful from very early times in using these natural drugs and preventing or suppressing various tumors with different lines of treatment (Balachandran and Govindrajan, 2005). In India, people of different ethnic groups inhabiting various terrains, possess their own distinct cultures, religious rites, food habit and a rich knowledge of traditional medicine (Parinitha *et al.*, 2005). They practice herbal medicine to cure a variety of diseases. Natural products, especially plants have been used in the treatment of various diseases for thousands of years. Terrestrial plants have been used as medicines in Egypt, China, India and Greece from ancient times and an impressive number of modern drugs have been developed from them. The first written records on the medicinal uses of plants appeared about 2600 BC from the Sumerians and Akkaidians (Samuelsson, 1999).

Traditional medicine (TM) refers to the application, approach, knowledge, and belief in incorporating plant or animal based properties in remedies, singularly or in combination, for the purpose of treating or preventing disease as well as to maintain the well-being of an individual. Population rise, inadequate supply of drugs, prohibitive cost of treatments, side effects of several allopathic drugs and development of resistance to currently used drugs for infectious diseases have led to increased emphasis on the use of plant materials as a source of medicines for a wide variety of human ailments (Joy *et al.*, 2001). As such herbal remedies have been used to cure a variety of disorders or conditions such diabetes, cardiovascular problems, weight control, dermal infirmities, sexual malfunction and of course cancer. According to the World Health Organization, more than 70 per cent of the world's population uses TM in order to fulfill their health necessities (Hernandez, 2002).

Over the past decade, herbal medicines have been accepted universally and they have an impact on both world health and international trade. Hence, medicinal plants continue to play an important role in the healthcare system of a large number of the world's population (Akerele, 1988). The herbal products have been classified under 'dietary supplements' and are included with vitamins, minerals, amino acids and 'other products intended to supplement the diet' (Rao *et al.*, 2004). In fact there are several medicinal plants all over the world, including India, which are being used traditionally for the prevention and treatment of cancer. However, only few medicinal plants have attracted the interest of scientists to investigate the remedy for neoplasm (tumor or cancer). Hence an attempt has been made to review some medicinal plants used for the prevention and treatment of cancer in foreign countries (Sharma and Pandey, 2009).

The principles underlying herbal medicines are relatively simple, although they are quite distinct from conventional medicine and herbal medicine (Anonymous, 2005). India is a rich source of medicinal plants and a number of plant extracts are used against diseases in various systems of medicine such as Ayurveda, Unani and Siddha. Only a few of them have been scientifically explored. Plant derived natural products such as flavonoids, terpenes and alkaloids (Osawa *et al.*, 1990; Di Carlo *et al.*, 1999; Keith *et al.*, 1990) and soon has received considerable attention in recent years, due to their diverse pharmacological properties including cytotoxic and cancer chemo preventive effects (Roja and Heble, 1994).

The National Cancer Institute, U. S. collected about 35,000 plant samples from 20 countries and has screened around 114,000 extracts for anticancer activity (Mohammad, 2006). Over 3000 species of plants with antitumor properties have been reported (Hartwell, 1982). Cancer is one of the most prominent diseases in humans and currently there is considerable scientific and commercial interest in the continuing discovery of new anticancer agents from natural product sources (Kinghorn *et al.*, 2003).

Nature has long been an important source of medicinal agents. An impressive number of modern drugs have been isolated or derived from natural sources, based on their use in traditional medicine (Cragg and Newman, 2001). Plants have formed a basis for traditional medicine systems that have been used for thousand of years in countries with ancient civilizations such as China (Chang and But, 1986), India (Kapoor, 1990) and Thailand (Subchareon, 1998a). The use of plants in traditional medicine systems of many other cultures has been extensively documented (Schultes and Raffauf, 1990; Arvigo and Balick, 1993; Gupta, 1995; Ayensu, 1981; Iwu, 1993; Jain, 1991).

Plant-based systems continue to play an essential role in healthcare and it has been estimated by the WHO that approximately 80 per cent of the world's inhabitants rely mainly on traditional medicine for their primary healthcare (Farnsworth *et al.*, 1985). Plant products also play an important role in the healthcare systems of the remaining 20 per cent of the population who reside mainly in developed countries. Analysis of data on prescriptions dispensed from community pharmacies in the United States from 1959 to 1980 indicates that about 25 per cent contained plant extracts or active principles derived from higher plants. Furthermore, at least 119 chemical substances derived from 90 plant species can be considered as important drugs currently in use in one or more countries (Farnsworth *et al.*, 1985). About 74 per cent of these 119 drugs were discovered as a result of chemical studies directed at isolation of the active substances from plants used in traditional medicine (Cragg *et al.*, 1997). Ethnopharmacological or traditional use of plants often results in the discovery of new biologically active molecules (Houghton, 1995). However it is important that the investigators understand the principles of folk medicine or mode of action of folk herbs (Nakanishi, 1999).

Medicinal plants possess immunomodulatory and antioxidant properties, leading to anticancer activities. They are known to have versatile immunomodulatory activity by stimulating both non-specific and specific immunity (Pandey and Sharma, 2006; Agrawala *et al.*, 2001). Plants contain several phytochemicals, which possess strong antioxidant activities. The antioxidants may prevent and cure cancer and other diseases by protecting the cells from damage caused by 'free radicals' – the highly reactive oxygen compounds. Thus consuming a diet rich in antioxidant plant foods (*e.g.* fruits and vegetables) will provide a milieu of phytochemicals, non-nutritive substances in plants that possess health-protective effects. Many naturally occurring substances present in the human diet have been identified as potential chemopreventive agents; and consuming relatively large amounts of vegetables and fruits can prevent the development of cancer (Pandey and Sharma, 2006; Vecchia and Tavani, 1998). Compared with meat eaters, most, but not all, studies have found that vegetarians are likely to be diagnosed with cancer. Vegetarians have also been shown to have stronger immune function, possibly explaining why they may be partially protected against cancer (Sharma and Pandey, 2008; Armstrong *et al.*, 1981). Many plant-derived products have been reported to exhibit potent antitumor activity against several rodent and human cancer cell lines (Lin *et al.*, 1996).

Phytochemicals such as vitamins (A, C, E, K), carotenoids, terpenoids, flavonoids, polyphenols, alkaloids, tannins, saponins, pigments, enzymes and minerals have been found to elicit antioxidant activities (Kathiresan *et al.*, 2006; Heber, 2004; Kaur and Kapoor, 2002). Ellagic acid and a whole range of flavonoids, carotenoids and terpenoids present in *Fragaria vesca* (raspberries) have been reported to be responsible for antioxidant activity. These chemicals block various hormone actions and metabolic pathways that are associated with the development of cancer (Caragay, 1992; Steinmetz and Potter, 1991). *Rosmarinus officinalis* (rosemary) contains substantial amounts of carnosol and ursolic acid, the potent antioxidants that possess antitumor activity (Ho *et al.*, 1994).

Medicinal plants maintain the health and vitality of individuals, and also cure various diseases, including cancer without causing toxicity. In this review, some anticancer medicinal plants have been listed. These medicinal plants possess good immunomodulatory and antioxidant properties, leading to anticancer activities. The antioxidant phytochemicals protect the cells from oxidative damage. Thus, consuming a diet rich in antioxidant plant foods (*e.g.*, fruits and vegetables) will provide health-protective effects. The medicinal plants contain many antioxidants such as vitamins (A, C, E, K), carotenoids, flavonoids (flavones, isoflavones, flavonones, anthocyanins, catenchins, isocatechins), polyphenols (Ellagic acid, gallic acid, tannins), saponins, enzymes and minerals (selenium, copper, manganese, zinc, chromium, iodine, etc) (Gupta and Sharma, 2006). Plants continue to be used against various types of tumors such as sarcoma, lymphoma, carcinoma and leukemia. Many of these medicinal plants have been found to be very effective in experimental as well as clinical cases of tumors/cancers (Sharma and Pandey, 2009).

Natural dietary agents including fruits, vegetables, and spices have drawn a great deal of attention from both the specific community and the general public owing to their demonstrated ability to suppress cancers. Recent studies by Block *et al.* (1992) suggested that the consumption of food rich in fruits, vegetables and spices have a lower incidence of cancers (stomach, esophagus, lung, oral cavity and pharynx, endometrium, pancreas and colon). The medicinal plants and their products, particularly vegetables have antioxidant activity leading to anticancer effect. Many doctors recommend that people wish to reduce the risk of cancer must eat vegetables everyday in their diet. Oncologists are trying to identify antioxidants present in consumable fruits and vegetables rich in vitamins, amino acids and carotenes which can be utilized in the prevention and treatment of cancer. Nutritional experts are searching for suitable naturally occurring dietary factors which are or may be anti-carcinogenic (Kaor, 1990).

Currently, over 50 per cent of drugs used in clinical trials for anticancer activity were isolated from natural sources or are related to them (Cragg and Newman, 2000). Hence, the search for natural products to be used in cancer therapy represents an area of great interest in which the plant kingdom has been the most important source, providing many anti-tumor agents with novel structures and unique mechanism of action (Ramos *et al.*, 2003). Over the past 10 years, research for new drugs to be used in oncology has refocused on natural products, which led to the finding of some new compounds such as taxanes and camptothecins (Yuan *et al.*, 2007). Many substances derived from dietary or medicinal plant known to be effective and versatile chemo preventive and antitumor agents in a number of experimental models of carcinogensis (Russo *et al.*, 2001). The cytotoxicity of plant material is considered to be due to the presence of antitumor compounds (Kawsar *et al.*, 2008). Even for populations which use herbs traditionally, encouraging the use of species with chemoprevention could be helpful as part of life expectancy improvement strategies: herbs have usually little or no toxicity during long-term oral administration and are relatively available at large scale and cost effective (Geetha *et al.*, 2002).

The practice of herbal medicine dates back to the very early periods of known human history. There is evidence of herbs having been used in the treatment of diseases and for revitalizing body systems in almost all ancient civilizations such as the Indian, the Egyptian, the Chinese, the Greek and the Roman civilizations. Plants were the mainstay of medicine and credited with mystical and almost supernatural powers of healing. Plants have a vast potential for their use as curative medicine. In the recent times the trend in the research in the field of cancer is once again shifting towards identifying new medicines for the treatment of cancer from natural sources. Wide varieties of compounds are in use in current cancer therapeutic practices. Chemical adjuvants of bacterial origin such as Bacillus Calmette Guerin (BCG) have been shown to exert therapeutic effects in the treatment of cancer. But, the effect is limited due to number of undesirable side effects (Ribi *et al.*, 1981.). Agents such as levamisole and interferons were widely used to treat cancers in the mid 1970s to early 1980s (Gomi *et al.*, 1983).

Science has long acknowledged the value of healing substances found in nature, such as digitalis, aspirin, penicillin, insulin, steroids, etc. There has been a resurgence of interest, both specifically and popularly, in the utilization of natural approaches. Experiments on cell lines and in animals demonstrated that herbal drugs anticancer role by inducing apoptosis and differentiation, enhancing the immune system, inhibiting angiogenesis and reversing multidrug resistance (Romero-Jimenez *et al.*, 2005). However, the mechanism of the anticancer role has not yet been fully elucidated. Further research is needed to explore the molecular mechanism of herbal drugs. Although the clinical trials showed that herbs were helpful against cancer, these outcomes require further confirmation with rigorously controlled trials, many clinical trials focusing on the anticancer effects of herbal formulae have been conducted. Though many of them demonstrated that herbs are helpful against cancer, especially useful in improving survival and quality of life in patients suffering from advanced cancer, the lack of controls and reporting bias have been severe flaws (Das, 2002). In future research is required to determine which ingredients are effective which will provide valuable clues for researching and developing anticancer drugs in the future.

Anticancer properties of many natural compounds isolated from different Indian plant extracts have been reported. Research is being carried out throughout the world to find a lead compound which can block the development of cancer in humans. Nature has always been a great contributor towards this goal. Plant-derived natural products such as flavonoids, Terpenoids and steroids have received considerable attention due to their diverse pharmacological properties, which include cytotoxic and chemopreventive effects (Abdullaev, 2001). The isolation of Vinca alkaloids, Vinblastine and Vincristine from the Madagascar, periwinkle, *Catharanthus roseus* introduced a new era in the use of plant material as anticancer agents. They were the first agents to advance into clinical use for the treatment of cancer (Cragg and Newman, 2005). These facts lead us to pursue the search for new bioactive lead structures with antitumor activity by a strategy of bioactivity-guided isolation from plants used in traditional folk medicines (Heinrich and Bremner, 2006).

Screening Methods of Plant Extracts for Anticancer Activity

The search for natural products as potent anticancer agents dates back at least to the Ebers papyrus in 1550 B. C. However, the scientific period of this search is much more recent, beginning with the investigation by Hartwell and his co-workers on the application of podophyllotoxin and its derivatives as anticancer agents (Kingston *et al.*, 1990). Plants offer scientists searching for novel bioactive compounds the added advantage of Ethnobotanical observations, since many species are used in traditional medicine, principally in developing countries.

The study of bioactive compounds from plants has required the development of bioassay techniques, especially *in vitro* methods which allow a large number of plant extracts to be screened for activity, especially cytotoxicity, against many types of cancer cell lines. *In vitro* assays are particularly useful for bioassay-guided fractionation of plant extracts, since it is not always possible to test against cancer in animal models. *In vitro* assays are more sensitive to most anti-tumor agents than *in vivo* assays and usually cost less and require less test material and time.

The US National Cancer Institute (NCI) had an established program for the development of methods for initial screening of anticancer compounds since 1955. The initial screening program or primary screening used the *in vivo* L-1210 and P388 mouse leukemia model for the selection of anticancer compounds. The NCI developed an *in vitro* assay using KB cells, which derived from a human carcinoma of nasopharynx, as an anti-tumor assay for the screening of plant extracts since 1960 (Purdue, 1982). Plant extracts in the pre-screening assay are considered to have cytotoxic activity against KB cells when they show an IC_{50} of <30 µg/ml. Thus, it might be appropriate to screen the materials first with this *in vitro* assay and choose only *in vitro*- active compounds or natural products for further *in vivo* tests. It took approximately five years to develop the *in vitro* cell line screening process (1985-1990). The process was implemented and became fully operational in 1990. It is capable of screening 20,000 compounds per year. The screening process utilizes 60 different human tumor cell lines, representing leukemia, melanoma and cancers of lung, colon, brain, ovary, breast, prostate and kidney. Selective growth inhibition or cell killing of particular tumor cell lines indicates a positive result. The evaluation uses a pattern recognition algorithm to assign a putative mechanism of action for the compounds. In addition to characteristics associated with various cellular targets in the 60 cell lines, it may be possible to select compounds most likely to interact with a specific target (Boyd, 1997).

The *in vitro* screening has contributed to discoveries and developments of new clinically useful anticancer drugs. Tens of thousands of pure compounds from plant, marine, and microbial agents were tested initially in the *in vitro* primary screening; subsets were selected for *in vivo* preclinical follow up from 1990 to 1995 (Boyd, 1997). A bioassay-guided fractionation procedure, was, thus, designed for the isolation of active compounds (Pezzuto, 1997).

The terms 'cytotoxic', 'anti-tumor' and 'anticancer' were defined by the NCI program. A cytotoxic agent is toxic to tumor cells *in vitro* and if this toxicity transfers to tumor cells *in vivo*, the agent is said to have anti-tumor activity. The term anticancer is reserved for materials that are toxic to tumor cells in clinical trial on humans.

In vitro Cytotoxic Assays

The *in vitro* assay can be divided into two main groups, a cellular assay and a molecular assay (Suffness and Pezzuto, 1991). The cellular assay (cell-based assay or cytotoxicity-based bioassay) uses intact cells while the molecular assay (based on mechanism) aims for specific inhibition of the expression of an oncogene or oncoproducts or inhibition of a specific biochemical target at the subcellular level, such as enzymes and receptors.

In vitro Methods

1. **Trypan blue dye exclusion assay** (Unnikrishnan and Ramadasan, 1998)
2. **Lactic dehydrogenase (LDH) Assay** (Russo *et al.*, 2006)
3. **MTT assay** (Mossman, 1983)
4. **XTT assay** (Economou *et al.*, 2008)
5. **Sulforhodamine B assay** (Skehan *et al.*, 1990)

In vivo Assay

The *in vivo* assay is the secondary stage for screening; it is usually carried out in rats, mice or hamsters, which have been implanted subcutaneously. Induced tumor cells are applied depending on each type of tumor model. For example, L-1210 and P-388 were implanted intraperitoneally (*i. p*), Lewis lung carcinoma was induced intravenously (*i. v*) and colon 38 tumor cells were implanted subcutaneously (*s. c.*). The number of days for the treatment schedule depends on each tumor cell model. For example, the administration of test drug for P-388 begins at one day after implantation and continues for 5 days via the *i. p.* route. Anti-tumor activity has been defined in terms of a therapeutic index or the ratio of the 50 per cent lethal dose to the ED_{90} (the dose required to reduce tumor mass by 90 per cent) or the growth rate of the tumor cell. The therapeutic index is the packed cell volume or weight of the tumor cells of the test group/control group (Suffness, 1989).

In vivo Model

1. Induction of Ehrlich ascites carcinoma (Devi *et al.*, 1998)

Some Success Stories of Plants and Plant Phytoconstituents Used as Anticancer Agents

Plants have a long history of use in the treatment of cancer (Hartwell, 1982). However, many of the claims for the efficacy of such treatments should be viewed with some skepticism because cancer, as a specifc disease entity, is likely to be poorly defined in terms of folklore and traditional medicine (Cragg *et al.*, 1994). Among all the plant-derived anticancer drugs in clinical use, the best known is the so-called Vinca alklaoids, which include vinblastine and vincristine. These alkaloids are isolated from the Madagascar periwinkle, *Catharenthus roseus* (Linn.) G. Don, Apocynaceae, known in Thailand as Phaeng phuai farang. Vinblastine and vincristine were first discovered during an investigation of the plant for oral hypoglycemic agents. Therefore, their discovery as anticancer agents may be indirectly attributed to the observation of an unrelated medicinal use of the source plant.

The two clinically-active agents, Etoposide and teniposide, which are semi-synthetic derivatives of the natural product epipodophyllotoxin, may be considered to be more closely linked to a plant originally used for the treatment of cancer. Epipodophyllotoxin is an isomer of podophyllotoxin, which was isolated as the active anti-tumor agent from the roots of various species of the genus *Podophyllum* (Berberidaceae). These plants possess a long history of medicinal use by early American and Asian cultures, including the treatment of skin cancers and warts (Cragg *et al.*, 1994). From the time of Galen (about AD180) the juice expressed from woody nightshade (*Solanum dulcamara* L. Family Solanaceae) has been used to treat cancers, tumors and warts. The active tumor-inhibitory principle has been identified as the steroidal alkaloid glycoside β-solamarine.

Various lichens (*e.g.*, species of *Cladonia*, *Cetraria* and *Usnea*) also have a history of use in folk medicine against cancer since about AD 970. These are all rich sources of usnic acid, a compound recognized for many years as an antibacterial and antifungal agent, but only more recently as an anti-tumor compound. Similarly, many centuries ago, the Druids claimed that mistletoe (*Viscum album*) could be used to cure cancer. Protein fractions with marked anti-tumor activity has been isolated from mistletoe extract. The benzophenanthridine derivatives are present in *Chelidonium majus* (Papavaraceae), a plant with substantial folklore history of use in the treatment of cancers (Dewick, 2002).

Most recent additions to the armamentarium of the naturally derived chemotherapeutic agents are the taxanes and camptothecins. Paclitaxel (Taxol) was initially isolated from the bark of the Pacific or American yew tree, *Taxus brevifolia* Nutt. (Taxaceae), collected in Washington State as part of a random collection program by the U.S. Department of Agriculture for the National Cancer Institute (NCI)(Cragg *et al.*, 1993). The use of various parts of *T. brevifolia* Nutt. and other Taxus species by several native American tribes for the treatment of some non-cancerous conditions has been reported (Cragg *et al.*, 1994). The leaves of *T. baccata* are used in the traditional Asiatic Indian (Ayurvedic) medicine systems (Kapoor, 1990), with one reported use in the treatment of cancer (Hartwell, 1982).

Paclitaxel, along with several key precursors (the baccatins), occurs in the leaves of various *Taxus* species, and the ready semi-synthetic conversion of the relatively abundant baccatins to Paclitaxel, as well as active Paclitaxel analogs, such as docetaxel (Cortes and Pazdur, 1995), has provided a major renewable natural source of this important class of drugs. Likewise, the clinically active agents, Topotecan (hycamptamine), Irinotecan (CPT-11), 9-amino and 9-nitrocamptothecin, are semi-synthetically derived from camptothecin, isolated from the Chinese ornamental tree, *Camptotheca acuminate* Decne (Family Cornaceae) (Potmeisel and Pinedo 1995). Camptothecin (as its sodium salt) was advanced to clinical trials by the NCI in the 1970s, but was dropped because of severe bladder toxicity (Cragg, 2001).

Phytoconstituents derived from the herbs *Vinca rosea*, *Taxus species*, *Achyranthes bidentata*, *Allium sativum*, *Aloe vera*, *Angelica sinensis*, *Astragals membranaceus*, *Glycine max*, *Glycyrrhiza glabra*, *Hordeum vulgare*, *Hydrocotyle asiatica*, *Medicago sativa*, *Morinda citrifolia*, *Panax pseudoginseng*, *Saussurea lappa*, *Taxus wallichiana*, *Tinospora cordifolia*,

Viscum album, Withania somnifera, Zingiber officinale etc. have been used in various formulations to enhance activity of immune cells of the body that promotes production of cytokines including interleukin, interferon, tumor necrosis factor and colony stimulating factor. These formulations help the body to fight cancer more effectively and reduce toxic side effects of chemotherapy and radiotherapy stages of cancer (Suran *et al.*, 2013).

Some medicinal plants have been studied in various *in vivo* and *in vitro* experimental models of cancer and have shown significant inhibition of cancer cell proliferation.

Table 21.2: Plants Used against Cancer

Sl.No.	*Name of Plant*	*Type of Cancer*	*References*
1.	*Abrus precatorius*	Yoshida's sarcoma, carcinoma and Dalton's lymphoma ascites cancer	Sivakumar and Alagesaboopathi, 2008; Suba and Sirsi, 1969.
2.	*Alstonia scholaris*	Ehrlich ascites carcinoma	Jagetia and Baliga, 2006; Kulkarni and Juvekar, 2008.
3.	*Cymbopogon flexuosus*	Ehrlich ascites carcinoma, leukemia and sarcoma 180	Sharma *et al.*, 2009
4.	*Ocimum gratissimum*	Breast cancer	Makker *et al.*, 2007
5.	*Phellinus rimosus*	Lymphoma and Carcinoma	Ajith and Janardhanan, 2002; Ajith and Janardhanan, 2003
6.	*Punica gratum*	Prostate cancer	Malik *et al.*, 2005
7.	*Zingiber officinale*	Carcinoma	Shukla *et al.*, 2007 and Stoilova *et al.*, 2007
8.	*Moringa oleifera*	Skin cancer and Human multiple myeloma cancer	Guevara *et al.*, 1999 and Verma *et al.*, 2009
9.	*Allium sativum*	Sarcoma 180	Ejaz *et al.*, 2003 and Balasenthila, 2001
10.	*Asparagus racemosus*	Liver cancer	Agrawal *et al.*, 2008 and Kamata *et al.*, 2000
11.	*Catharanthus roseus*	P-1534 leukemia	Sayed and Cordell, 1981; Johnson *et al.*, 1960; Jaleel *et al.*, 2008
12.	*Indigofera aspalathoides*	Ehrlich's ascites carcinoma	Rajkapoor *et al.*, 2004 and Bakasso *et al.*, 2008
13.	*Mangifera indica*	Lung cancer	Rajendran *et al.*, 2008
14.	*Nigella sativa*	Colon cancer	Johar *et al.*, 2008 and Swamy and Tan, 2000
15.	*Tephrosia purpurea*	Oral carcinoma	Kavitha and Manoharan, 2006
16.	*Tinospora cordifolia*	Ehrlich's ascites carcinoma	Rao *et al.*, 2008, Prince and Menon, 1999
17.	*Withania somnifera*	Skin carcinoma	Padmavathi *et al.*, 2005 and Visavadiya and Narasimhacharya, 2007

Contd...

Table 21.2–*Contd...*

Sl.No.	*Name of Plant*	*Type of Cancer*	*References*
18.	*Woodfordia fruticosa*	Sarcoma 180	Yoshida *et al.*, 1990; Kumaraswamy and Satish, 2008
19.	*Azadirachta indica*	Prostate cancer	Gangar *et al.*, 2008 and Kumar *et al.*, 2006
20.	*Beta vulgaris*	Skin and Lung cancer	Kapadia *et al.*, 1996 and Jiratanan *et al.*, 2004
21.	*Emblica officinalis*	Liver cancer	Sultana *et al.*, 2008; Anila and Vijayalakshmi, 2003
22.	*Ephedra sinica*	Murine melanoma	Nam *et al.*, 2003
23.	*Ocimum sanctum*	Skin cancer	Rastogi *et al.*, 2007
24.	*Viscum album*	Ehrlich's carcinoma	Cebovic *et al.*, 2008 and Ucar *et al.*, 2006
25.	*Jatropha curcas*	Skin cancer	Hirota *et al.*, 1988 and Yan *et al.*, 2008
26.	*Andrographis paniculata*	Lymphoma and Carcinoma	Geethangili *et al.*, 2008
27.	*Annona reticulate*	Kidney and Colorectal carcinoma cancer	Mondal *et al.*, 2007 and Baskar *et al.*, 2007
28.	*Bacopa monniera*	Sarcoma	Rohini and Shyamala, 2008
29.	*Berberis vulgaris*	Breast cancer	Tomosaka *et al.*, 2008
30.	*Bidens pilosa*	Cervix cancer	Sundararajan *et al.*, 2006 and Abajo *et al.*, 2004
31.	*Citrullus colocynthis*	Breast cancer	Tannin-Spitz *et al.*, 2007 and Spitz *et al.*, 2007
32.	*Crocus sativus*	Cervical epithelioid carcinoma cancer	Abdullaev *et al.*, 2002 and Escribano *et al.*, 1996
33.	*Curculigo orchioides*	Breast cancer	Singh and Gupta, 2008; Venukumar and Latha, 2002
34.	*Ipomoea aquatica*	Larynx epithelial carcinoma and small lung carcinoma cancer	Prasad *et al.*, 2005
35.	*Lantana camara*	Lung carcinoma	Raghu *et al.*, 2004
36.	*Pinus resinosa*	Colorectal adenocarcinoma cell, Lung carcinoma cell and Normal skin Fibroblast	Simard *et al.*, 2008; Pietarinen *et al.*, 2006
37.	*Rubia cordifolia*	Carcinoma	Kaur *et al.*, 2008; Son *et al.*, 2008
38.	*Tiliacora racemosa*	Leukaemia and Carcinoma	Chakraborty *et al.*, 2004
39.	*Calycopteris floribunda*	Colon cancer	Ali *et al.*, 2008
40.	*Cedrus deodara*	Acute lymphoblastic leukemia, Prostate and Lung cancer	Sharma *et al.*, 2008; Tiwari *et al.*, 2001
41.	*Curcuma longa*	Colon cancer	Lee *et al.*, 2009; Hsu *et al.*, 2007
42.	*Ipomoea squamosa*	Ovarian cancer	Cao *et al.*, 2007

Contd...

Table 21.2–*Contd...*

Sl.No.	*Name of Plant*	*Type of Cancer*	*References*
43.	*Melia azedarach*	Lung cancer and Glioma cancer	Wu *et al.*, 2009; Szewczuk *et al.*, 2006
44.	*Morinda citrifolia*	Colon cancer	Kamiya *et al.*, 2009; Anekpankul *et al.*, 2007
45.	*Polyalthia longifolia*	Colon and Leukemia HL-60 cancer	Verma *et al.*, 2008
46.	*Psidium gujava*	Prostate carcinoma cancer	Chen *et al.*, 2007
47.	*Tragia involucrata*	Carcinoma cancer	Joshi *et al.*, 2011
48.	*Semecarpus anacardium*	Acute myeloblastic leukaemia, Chronic myelogenic leukaemia, Breast adenocarcinoma, Cervical epithelial carcinoma and Colon carcinoma cancer	Reddy *et al.*, 2009
49.	*Terminalia chebula*	Colon cancer	Reddy *et al.*, 2009

Table 21.3: List of Plants having Anticancer Activity (Kirtikar and Basu, 1984)

Sl.No.	*Name of the Plant*	*Family*	*Part Used*
1.	*Annona squamosa*	Annonaceae	Ripe fruit
2.	*Brassica nigra*	Cruciferae	Leaves
3.	*Raphanus sativus*	Cruciferae	Radish
4.	*Cleome viscosa*	Capparidaceae	Plant
5.	*Gynandropsis gynandra*	Capparidaceae	Root
6.	*Capparis sepiaria*	Capparidaceae	Plant
7.	*Garcinia indica*	Guttiferae	Raw fruit
8.	*Mesua ferrea*	Guttiferae	
9.	*Sida rhombifolia*	Malvaceae	Leaves
10.	*Ceiba pentandra*	Bombaceae	Gum
11.	*Pterspermum acerifolium*	Sterculiaceae	Flowers
12.	*Triumfetta bartramia*	Tiliaceae	Root
13.	*Corchorus olitorius*	Tiliaceae	Leaves
14.	*Corchorus fascicularis*	Tiliaceae	Plant
15.	*Corchorus depressus*	Tiliaceae	Plant
16.	*Zanthoxylum alatum*	Rutaceae	Fruit
17.	*Commiphora mukul*	Burseraceae	Gum
18.	*Commiphora agallocha*	Burseraceae	Gum
19.	*Azadirachta indica*	Meliaceae	Young branches, unripe fruit
20.	*Melia azedarach*	Meliaceae	Root
21.	*Vitis quadrangularis*	Vitaceae	Stem

Contd...

Table 21.3–*Contd...*

Sl.No.	*Name of the Plant*	*Family*	*Part Used*
22.	*Anacardium occidentale*	Anacardiaceae	Fruit
23.	*Semecarpus anacardium*	Anacardiaceae	Fruit
24.	*Moringo oleifera*	Moringaceae	Root-bark, flowers, fruit
25.	*Indigofera aspalathoides*	Papilionaceae	Whole plant with butter
26.	*Indigofera tinctoria*	Papilionaceae	Root, stem
27.	*Tephrosia purpurea*	Papilonaceae	Root
28.	*Butea monosperma*	Burseraceae	Bark, fruit, seed
29.	*Cajanus indicus*	Caesalpinaceae	Seed
30.	*Pongamia glabra*	Polypodiaceae	Root, bark
31.	*Caesalpinia pulcherrima*	Cactaceae	Plant
32.	*Cassia obtusifolia*	Caryophyliaceae	Fruit, seeds
33.	*Cassia angustifolia*	Caryophyliaceae	Plant
34.	*Saraca indica*	Sapotaceae	Bark
35.	*Bauhinia tomentosa*	Caesalpinaceae	Bark
36.	*Bauhinia racemosa*	Caesalpinaceae	Bark, leaves
37.	*Terminalia chebula*	Combretaceae	Fruit
38.	*Terminalia citrina*	Combretaceae	Fruit
39.	*Terminalia arjuna*	Combretaceae	Bark
40.	*Careya arborea*	Myrtaceae	Bark
41.	*Momordica dioica*	Cucurbitaceae	Fruit
42.	*Citrullus colocynthis*	Cucurbitaceae	Fruit
43.	*Randia dumetorum*	Rubiaceae	Fruit
44.	*Xanthium strumarium*	Compositae	Root
45.	*Calotropis gigantea*	Asclepediaceae	Plant, flower, milk
46.	*Adhatoda vasica*	Acanthaceae	Plant
47.	*Clerodendron serratum*	Verbenaceae	Root
48.	*Clerodendron infortunatum*	Verbenaceae	Leaves, roots
49.	*Boerhavia diffusa*	Nyctaginaceae	Leaves
50.	*Mallotus philippinensis*	Euphorbiaceae	Fruit
51.	*Dioscorea ulbifera*	Dioscoriaceae	Tuber
52.	*Asparagus racemosus*	Liliaceae	Roots

Plants have been used for treating various diseases of human beings and animals since time immemorial. They maintain the health and vitality of individuals, and also cure diseases, including cancer without causing toxicity. More than 50 per cent of all modern drugs in clinical use are of natural products, many of which have the ability to control cancer cells (Rosangkima and Prasad, 2004). A recent survey shows that more than 60 per cent of cancer patients use vitamins or herbs as therapy (Sharma and Pandey, 2008; Sivalokanathan *et al.*, 2005).

This review provides information on a number of plants which show promising anticancer activity. It lists various methods for evaluating anticancer activity so it will be easy for the experimenter. It emphasizes that *in vitro* anticancer assays have been carried out for most of the plants, but *in vivo* remains to be done in majority of them.

Conclusion

Cancer is one of the most widespread diseases in humans and there is considerable scientific and commercial interest in the continuing discovery of new anticancer agents from natural product sources. Currently, over 50 per cent of drugs used in clinical trials for anticancer activity were isolated from natural sources or are related to them. A number of active compounds have been shown to possess anticancer activity; these include flavonoids, diterpenoids, triterpenoids and alkaloids. Several mechanisms have been proposed to explain the cancer-preventive effects of plants. These include inhibition of mutagenesis by inhibiting the metabolism, inhibition of DNA adduct formation, free-radical scavenging and effects on cell proliferation and tumor growth.

In this review, some anticancer medicinal plants of Indian origin have been presented. These medicinal plants possess good antioxidant properties, leading to anticancer activities. The aim of this study was to give an overview on the progress of anticancer medicinal plant research around the continental India, focusing on the most important findings of scientists in this field. We have tried to explore the discovered plants components with proved anticancer activity both *in vitro* and *in vivo.* India is one of the most promising regions for discovering novel biologically-active substances from its flora. More efforts are needed to explore potent anticancer plants from the mother earth and save humans around the world from cancer.

References

Abajao, C., Boffill, M. A., Campo, J., Alexandra Mendez M., Gonzalez, Y., Mitjans, M., and Pilar Vinardell, M. (2004). *In vitro* study of the antioxidant and immunomodulatory activity of aqueous infusion of *Bidens pilosa. J Ethnopharmacol.*, **93**: 319-323.

Abdullaev, F. I. (2001). Plant derived agents against cancer. In: Gupta, S. K., editor. Pharmacology and therapeutics in the new millennium. Narosa Publishing House: New Delhi, India, p. 345-354.

Abdullaev, F. I. (2002). Cancer chemopreventive and tumoricidal properties of *Crocus sativus* L. *Exp Biol Med.*, **227**: 20-25.

Acharaya, P. K. (1979). Encyclopedia of Hindu architecture. New Delhi: oriental Book reprints Co.

Agrawal, A., Sharma, M., Rai, S. K., Singh, B., Tiwari, M., and Chandra, R.(2008). The effect of the aqueous extract of the roots of *Asparagus racemosus* on hepatocarcinogenesis initiated by diethyl nitrosamine. *Phytother Res.*, **22**: 1175-1182.

Agrawala, S. K., Chatterjee, S., and Misra, S. K. (2001). Immunepotentiation activity of a polyherbal formulation 'Immu-21' (research name). *Phytomedica.*, **2**: 1-22.

Ajith, T. A., and Janardhanan, K. K. (2002). Antioxidant and hepatotoxic activities of *Phellinus rimosus* (Berk) Pilat. *J Ethnopharmacol.*, **81**: 387-391.

Ajith, T. A., and Janardhanan, K. K. (2003). Cytotoxic and antitumor activities of a polypore macrofungus, phellinus rimosus Pilat. J *Ethnopharmacol.*, **84**: 157-162.

Akerele, O. (1988). Medicinal plants and primary health care: an agenda for action. *Fitoterapia*, **59**: 355-363.

Ali, H. A., Chowdhury, A. K., Rahman, A. K., Borkowski, T., Nahar, L., and Sarker, S. D. (2008). Pachypodol a flavonol from the leaves of *Calycopteris floribunda*, inhibits the growth of CaCo-2 colon cancer cell line *in vitro*. *Phytother Res.*, **22**: 1684-1687.

Ames, B. N., Gold, L. S., and Willet, W. C. (1995). The causes and prevention of cancer. *Proc. Natt. Acad. Sci. USA.*, **92**: 5258-5265.

Anekpankul, T., Goto, M., Sasaki, M., Pavasant, P., and Shotipruk, A. (2007). Extraction of anticancer damnacanthal from roots of *Morinda citrifolia* by subcritical water. *Sep Purif Technol.*, **55**: 343-349.

Anila, L., and Vijayalakshmi, N. R. (2003). Antioxidant action of flavonoids from *Mangifera indica* and *Emblica officinalis* in hypercholesterolemic rats. *Food Chem.*, **83**: 569-574.

Anonymous (2005). An introductory overview seminars in oncology nursing, **21(3)**: 102-105.

Armstrong, B. K., Brown, J. B., and Clarke, H. T. (1981). Diet and reproductive hormones: a study of vegetarian and nonvegetarian postmenopausal women. *J. Natl. Cancer Inst.*, **67**: 761-767.

Arvigo, R., and Balick, M. (1993). Rainforest Remedies, Lotus Press, Twin Lakes, Wisconsin.

Ayensu, E. S. (1981). Medicinal plants of the West Indies, Reference Publications, Algonac, Michigan.

Badmaev, V., and Majeed, M. (1995). Effects of Ayurvedic herbs. *Health supplement Retailer Magazine*, 22-25.

Bakasso, S., Meda, L. A., Lamien, C. E., Kiendrebeogo, M., Millogo, J. Ovedraogo, A. G., and Nacoulma, O. G. (2008). Polyphenol contents and anioxidant activities of five Indigofera species (Fabaceae) from Burkina Faso. *Pakistan J Biol Sci.*, **11**: 1429-1435.

Balachandran, P., and Govindarajan, R. (2005). Cancer – an Ayurvedic perspective. *Pharmacol Res.*, **51**: 19-30.

Balasenthila, S., Ramachandra, C. R., and Naginia, S. (2001). Prevention of 4-nitroquinoline 1-oxide-induced rat tongue carcinogenesis by garlic. *Fitoterapia,* **72**: 524-531.

Baskar, R., Rajeshwari, V., and Kumar, T. S. (2007). *In vitro* antioxidant studies in leaves of Annona species. *India J Exp Biol.,* **45**: 480-485.

Bhishagratna, K. L. (1991). Sushruta Samhita, English translation, Nidana-sthana, Sarira-sthana, chikitsa-sthana and Kalpa-sthana. Vol. 2. Varanasi: Chowkambha Sanskrit Series office; 571.

Block, G., Patterson, B., and Subar, A. (1992). Fruit, vegetables and cancer prevention: A review of the epidemiological evidence. *Nutr Cancer,* **18(1)**: 1-29.

Boyd, M. R. (1997). The NCI *in vitro* anticancer drug discovery screen. In Teicher, B. (Ed.). Anticancer drug development guide; preclinical screening, clinical trials and approval, Human Press, Totowa, p. 30.

Cao, S., Norris, A., Wisse, J. H., Miller, J. S., Evans, R., and Kingston, D. G. (2007). Ipomoeassin F, a new cytotoxic macrocyclic glycoresin from the leaves of *Ipomoea squamosa* from the Suriname rain forest. *Nat Prod Res.,* **21**: 872-876.

Caragay, A. B. (1992). Cancer-preventive foods and ingredients. *Food Technol.,* **46**: 65-68.

Carter, S., and Livingston, R. (1982). Principle of cancer chemotherapy, in Carter, S., Glatstein and E., Livingston, R (eds.). Principles of Cancer Treatment. New York, McGraw-Hill. Pp. 95-110.

Cebovic, T., Spasic, S., and Popovic, M. (2008). Cytotoxic effects of the *Viscum album* L. extract on Ehrlich tumor cells *in vivo. Phytother Re.,* **22**: 1097-1103.

Chakraborty, S., Roy, M., Taraphdar, A. K., and Bhattacharya, R. K. (2004). Cytotoxic effect of root extract of *Tiliacora racemosa* and oil of *Semecarpus anacardium* nut in human tumor cells. *Phytother Res.,* **18**: 595-600.

Chang, H. M., and Butt, P. P. H. (1986). Pharmacology and Applications of Chinese Materia Medica, Vols. 1 and 2, World Scientific Publishing, Singapore.

Chen, K. C., Hsieh, C. L., Peng, C. C., Hsieh-Li HM, Chiang, H. S., Huang, K. D., and Peng, R. Y. (2007). Brain derived metastatic prostate cancer DU-145 cells are effectively inhibited *in vitro* by guava (*Psidium gujava* L.) leaf extracts. *Nutr Cancer,* **58**: 93-106.

Cortes, J. E., and Pazdur, R. (1995). Docetaxel. *J. Clin. Oncol.,* **13**: 2643-2655.

Cragg, G. M., and Newman, D. J. (2000). Antineoplastic agents from natural sources: achievements and future directions. *Expert Opin Investig Drugs,* **9**: 1-15.

Cragg, G. M., and Newman, D. J. (2001). National product drugs discovery in next millennium, National Cancer Institute, Frederick, USA.

Cragg, G. M., and Newman, D. J. (2005). Plants as source of anticancer agents. *J Ethnopharmacol.,* **100**: 72-79.

Cragg, G. M., Boyd. M. R., Cardellina, J. H., Newman, D. J., Snader, K. M., and McCloud, T. G. (1994). Ethnobotany and the search for new drugs in Ciba foundation symposium, vol. 185, Chadwick, D. J. and Marsh, J. (eds.), pp.178-196, Wiley and Sons, Chichester, U. K.

Cragg, G. M., Newman, D. J., and Snader, K. M. (1997). Natural products in drug discovery and development. *J. Nat. Prod.*, **60**: 52-60.

Cragg, G. M., Schepartz, S. A., Suffness, M., and Grever, M. R. (1993). The Taxol supply crisis. New NCI policies for handling the large scale production of novel natural product anticancer anti anti-HIV agents. *J. Nat. Prod.*, **56**: 1657-1668.

Das, U. N. (2002). A radical approach to cancer. *Med. Sci. Monit.*, **8**: 79-92.

Devi, P. U., Rao, B. S. S., and Solomon, F. E. (1998). Effect of Plumbagin on the radiation induced cytogenetic and cell cycle changes in mouse Ehrlich ascites carcinoma *in vivo*. *Indian J Exp Biol.*, **36**: 891-895.

Dewick, P. M. (2002). Tumor inhibitors from plants. Pp. 394-407. In Evans, W. C. (ed.) Trease and Evans Pharmacognosy, London, W. B. Saunders.

Di Carlo, G., Mascolo, N., Izzo, A. A., and Capassao, F. (1999). Flavonoids: Old and new aspects of a class of natural therapeutic drugs. *Life Sci.*, **65**: 337-353.

Economou, M. A, Andersson, S., Vasilcanu, D.; Ericsson, C. A., Menu, E., Girnita, A., Girnita, L., Axelson, M., Seregard, S., and Larsson, O. (2008). Oral picropodophyllin (PPP) is well tolerated *in vivo* and inhibits IGF-1R expression and growth of uveal melanoma. *Acta Ophthalmologica*, **86**: 35-41.

Eisenberg, D. M., Davis, R. B., Ettner, S. L., Wilkey, S., Van Rompay, V., and Kessler, R. C. (1998). Trends in alternative medicine use in the united States, 1990-1997: Results of a follow-up national survey. *J Am Med Assoc.*, **280**: 1569-1575.

Ejaz, S., Woong, L. C., and Ejaz, A. (2003). Extract of garlic (Allium sativum) in cancer chemoprevention. *Exp Oncol.*, **25**: 93-97.

El-Shemy, H. A.; Aboul-Enein, A. M.; Aboul-Enien, K. M., and Fujita, K. (2007). Willow leaves extracts contain anti-tumor agents effective against three cell types. *Plos one.*, **2(1)**: 178.

Escribano, J., Alonso, G., Coca-Prados, M., and Fernandez, J. A. (1996). Crocin, Safranaland picrocrocin from *Crocus sativus* L. inhibit the growth of human cancer cells *in vivo*. *Cancer Let.t*, **100**: 23-30.

Farnsworth, N. R., Akerele, O., Bingel, A. S., Soejarto, D. D., and Guo, Z. (1985). Medicinal plants in therapy. Bull. *WHO.*, **63**: 968-981.

Gangar, S. C., and Koul, A. (2008). *Azadirachta indica* modulates carcinogen biotransformation and reduced glutathione at peri-initiation phase of benzo(a)pyrene induced murine forestomach tumorigenesis. *Phytother Res.*, **22**: 1229-1238.

Geetha, S., Sairam, M., Sing, V., Ilavazhagan, G., and Sawhney, R. C. (2002). Effect of seabuckthorn on sodium nitroprusside-induced cytotoxicity in murine macrophages. *J Ethnopharmacol.*, **79**: 373-378.

Geethangili, M., Rao, Y. K., Fang, S., and Tzeng, Y. (2008). Cytotoxic constituents from *Andrographis paniculata* induce cell cycle arrest in jurkat cells. *Phytother Res.*, **22**: 1336-1341.

Gomi, K., Morinto, M., and Nomoto, K. (1983). Influence of surgical removal and effect of levamisole on cytotoxic T-cell mediated anti-tumor immunity in mice. *Cancer Res.*, **43**: 5120.

Guevara, A. P., Vargas, C., Sakurai, H., Fujiwara, Y., Hashimoto, K., Maoka, T., Kozuka, M., Ito, Y., Tokuda, H., and Nishino H. (1999). An antitumor promoter from *Moringa oleifera* Lam. *Mutation Res.*, **440**: 181-188.

Gupta, M. P. (1995). 270 Plantas Medicinales Iberoamericans, Tallares de Editorial Presencia Ltda., Bogota, Colombia.

Gupta, V. K., and Sharma, S. K. (2006). Plants as natural antioxidants. *Nat Prod Rad.*, **17**: 326-334.

Halliwell, B., and Gutteridge, J. M. C. (1988). Free radicals in biology and medicine 2 edn. Pp. 481, Oxford, Charendon Press.

Hartwell, J. L. (1982). Plants used against cancer, Quarterman, Lawrence, Massachusetts.

Hartwell, L. (1971). Plants used against cancer. A survey. *Lloyida*, **32(1)**: 78-107.

Heber, D. (2004). Vegetables, fruits and phytoestrogens in the prevention of diseases. *J. Postgrad. Med.*, **50**: 145-149.

Heinrich, M., and Bremner, P. (2006). Ethnobotany and Ethnopharmacy - Their role for anti-cancer drug development. *Curr drug targets*, **7**: 239-45.

Hernandez, E. G., Contreras, A. A., Santamaria, A., Ramos, R. R., Miranda, A. A. C., Vega, L. M. G., Saenz, J. L. F., and Aguilar, F. J. A. (2002). Studies on Hypoglycemic activity of Mexican Medicinal Plants. Proc. *West Pharmacol. Soc.*, **45**: 118-124.

Hirota, M., Suttajit, M., Suguri, H., Endo, Y., Shudo, K., Wongchai, V., Hecker, E., and Fujiki, H. (1988). A new tumor promoter from the seed oil of *Jatropha curcas* L.; an intramolecular diester of 12-Deoxy-16-hydroxyphorbol. *Cancer Res.*, **48**: 5800-5804.

Ho, C.T., Ferraro, T., Chen, Q., and Rosen, R. T. (1994). Phytochemical in teas and rosemary and their cancer-preventive properties. In: Ho, C.T., Osawa, T., Huang, M.T., Rosen, R.T. (Eds.), Food Phytochemicals for Cancer Prevention. II. Tea, Spices and Herbs. ACS Symposium Series 547, American Chemical Society, Washington, DC, pp. 2–9.

Houghton, P. (1995). The role of plants in traditional medicine and current therapy. *J. Alt. and Comple. Med.*, **1(3)**: 131-143.

Hsu, Y., Weng, H., Lin, S., and Chien, Y. W. (2007). Curcuminoids-Cellular uptake by human primary colon cancer cells as quantified by a sensitive HPLC assay and its relation with the inhibition of proliferation and apoptosis. *J Agric Food Chem.*, **55**: 8213-8222.

Iwu, M. M. (1993). Handbook of African Medicinal Plants, CRC Press, Boca raton, Florida.

Jagetia, G. C., and Baliga, M. S. (2006). Evaluation of anticancer activity of the alkaloid fraction of *Alstonia scholaris in vitro* and *in vivo. Phytother Res.*, **20**: 103-109.

Jain, S. K. (1991). Medicinal plants of India, vols. 1 and 2, Reference Publications, Algonac, Michigan.

Jaleel, C. A., Manivanan, P., Murali, P. V., Gomathinayagam, M., and Panneerselvam, R. (2008). Antioxidant potential and indole alkaloid profile variations with water deficits along different parts of two varities of *Catharanthus roseus. Colloids Surf B Biointerfaces*, **62**: 312-318.

Jiratanan, T., and Liu, R. H. (2004). Antioxidant activity of processed table beets (*Beta vulgaris*) and green beans (*Phaseolus vulgaris*). *J Agric Food Chem.*, **52**: 2659-2670.

Johar, D. A., Shinwari, N., Arif, J., Sanea, N., Jabbar, A. A., Sayed, R., Mashhour, A., Billedo, G., Doush, I., and Saleh, I. (2008). Role of *Nigella sativa* and a number of its antioxidant constituents towards Azoxymethane-induced genotoxic effects and colon cancer in rats. *Phytother Res.*, **22**: 1311-1323.

Johnson, I. S., Wright, H. F., Svoboda, G. H., and Vlantis, J. (1960). Antitumor principles derived from *Vinca rosea* L. *Cancer Res.*, **20**: 1016-1022.

Joseph, P. (2004). Stem cell Research. Facts on file Inc, New York, 42-54.

Joshi, C. G., Gopal, M., and Kumari, N. S. (2011). Antitumor activity of hexane and ethyl acetate extracts of *Tragia involucrata. International Journal of Cancer Research*, **7**: 267-277.

Joy, P. P., Thomas, J., Mathew, S., Jose, G., and Joseph, J. (2001). Medicinal plants. In: Bose, T. K., Kabir, J., Das, P. And Joy, P. P. Editors. Tropical horticulture Vol. 2. Calcutta: Naya Prokash, p. 449-632.

Kamata, J. P., Boloora, K. K., Devasagayam, T. P., and Venkatachalam, S. R. (2000). Antioxidant properties of *Asparagus racemosus* against damage induced by γ-radiation in rat liver mitochondria. *J Ethnopharmacol.*, **71**: 425-435.

Kamiya, K., Hamabe, W., Tokuyama, S., Hirano, K., Satake, T., Kumamoto-Yonezawa, Y., Yoshida, H., and Mizushina, Y. (2009). Inhibitory effect of Anthraquinones isolated from the *Morinda citrifolia* root on animal A, B and Y families of DNA polymerases and human cancer cell proliferation. *Food chem.*, **118**: 725-730.

Kaor, L. D. (1990). CRC Handbook of Ayurvedic Medicinal Plants, Boca Raton, Florida, CRC Press; 416-417.

Kapadia, G. J., Tokuda, H., Konoshima, T., and Nishino, H. (1996). Chemoprevention on lung and skin cancer by beta vulgaris root extract. *Cancer Lett.*, **100**: 211-214.

Kapoor, L. D. (1990). Handbook of Ayurveda Medicinal Plants, CRC Pres, Boca Raton, Florida.

Kathiresan, K., Boopathy, N. S., and Kavitha, S. (2006). Coastal vegetation – An underexplored source of anticancer drugs. *Nat. Prod. Rad.*, **5**: 115-119.

Kaur, C., and Kapoor, H. C. (2002). Antioxidants activity and total phenolic content of some Asian vegetables. *Int. J. Food Sci. Technol.*, **37**: 153-161.

Kaur, P., Singh, B., Kumar, S., and Kaur, S. (2008). *In vitro* evaluation of free radical scavenging activity of *Rubia cordifolia* L. *J Chinese Clin Med.*, **3**: 278-284.

Kavitha, K., and Manoharan, S. (2006). Anticarcinogenic and antilipidperoxidative effects of *Tephrosia purpurea* L. in 7, 12 – dimethylbenz(a)anthracene (DMBA) induced hamster buccal pouch carcinoma. *Indian J Pharmacol.*, **38**: 185-189.

Kawsar, S. M. A., Huq, E., and Nahar, N. (2008). Cytotoxicity assessment of the aerial parts of *Macrotyloma uniflorum* Linn. *Intl J Pharmacol.*, **4(4)**: 297-300.

Keith, M. W., Sally, A. L., Michael, W. S., Thomas, J. G., and Garry, M. M. (1990). Needles contain amounts of tax oil comparable to the stem bark of *Taxus brevifolia:* analysis and isolation. *Nat prod.*, **53**: 1249-1255.

Kinghorn, A. D., Farnsworth, N. R., Soejarto, D. D., Cordell, G. A., Swanson, S. M., Pezzuto, J. M., Wani, M. C., Wall, M. E., Oberlies, N. H., Kroll, D. J., Kramer, R. A., Rose, W. C., Vite, G. D., Fairchild, C. R., Peterson, R. W., and Wild, R. (2003). Novel strategies for the discovery of plant-derived anticancer agents. *Pharmaceutic Biol.*, **41**: 53-67.

Kingston, D. G. I., Samarayanake, G., and Ivey, C. A. (1990). The chemistry of Taxol, a clinically useful anticancer agent. *J. Nat. Prod.*, **53(1)**: 1-12.

Kirtikar, K. R., and Basu, B. D. (1984). Indian Medicinal Plants. 2nd ed. Allahabad, India: Lalit Mohan Basu

Koduru, S., Grierson, D. S., and Afolayan, A. J. (2007). Ethnobotanical information of medicinal plants used for treatment of cancer in the Eastern Cape Province, South *Africa. Curr. Sci.*, **92**: 906-908.

Kulkarni, M. P., and Juvekar, A. R. (2008). Effect of *Alstonia scholaris* Linn. on stress and cognition in mice. *Indian J Exp Biol.*, **47**: 47-52.

Kumar, S., Singh, B. B., Kaur, B., Singh, K., and Nandan, D. (2013). Herbal plants as potential anticancer agents: A review. *Research journal of Pharmaceutical, Biological and Chemical Sciences*, **4(3)**: 233-251.

Kumar, S., Suresh, P. K., Vijayababu, M. R., Arunkumar, A., and Arunakaran, J. (2006). Anticancer effects of ethanolic neem leaf extract on prostate cancer cell line. *J Ethnopharmacol.*, **105**: 246-250.

Kumaraswamy, M. V., and Satish, S. (2008). Free radical scavenging activity and lipoxygenase inhibition of *Woodfordia fructicosa* Kurz and *Betula utilis* Wall. *Afr J Biotechnol.*, **7**: 2013-2016.

Kutluk, T., and Kars, A. (1998). General knowledge about cancer, Ankara. *Turkey cancer investigation and fight society publications*, 7-15.

Lee, Y. K., Lee, W. S., Hwang, J. T., Kwon, D. Y., Surh, Y. J., and Park, O. J. (2009). Curcumin exerts anti-differentiation effect through AMPKα-PPAR-γ IN 3T3-L1 adipocytes and antiproliferatory effect through AMPKα-COX-2 in cancer cells. *J Agric Food Chem.*, **57**: 305-310.

Lin, Y. L., Juan, I. M., Chen, Y. L., Liang, Y. C., and Lin, J. K. (1996). Composition of polyphenols in fresh tea leaves and associations of their oxygen-radial absorbing capacity with antiproliferative actions in fibroblast cells. *J. Agric. Food. Chem.*, **44**: 1387-1394.

Makker, P. N., Tait, L., Shekhar, M. P. V., Palomino, E., Hogan, V., Piechocki, M. P., Funasaka, T., and Raz, A. (2007). Inhibition of breast tumor growth and angiogenesis by a medicinal herb *Ocimum gratissimum*. *Int J Cancer*, **121**: 884-894.

Malik, A., Afaq, F., Sarfaraz, S., Adhami, V. M., Syed, D. N., and Mukhtar, H. (2005). Pomegranate fruit juice for chemoprevention and chemotherapy of prostate cancer. *Proc Natl Acad Sci.*, **102**: 14813-14818.

Mathers, C. D., Boschi-Pinto, C., Lopez, A. D., and Murray, C. J. L. (2001). Cancer incidence, mortality and survival by site for 14 regions of the world. World Health Organization.

McNutt, K. (1995). Medicinals in foods. *Nutr Today*, **30**: 218-22.

Mohammad, S. (2006). Anticancer agents from medicinal plants. *Bangladesh J Pharmacol.*, **1**: 35-41.

Mondal, S., Mondal, N. B., and Mazumder, U. K. (2007). *In vitro* cytotoxic and human recombinant caspase inhibitory effect of *Annona reticulate* leaves. *Indian J Pharmacol.*, **39**: 253-254.

Mossman, T. (1983). Rapid colorimetric assay for cellular growth and survival: application to proliferation and cytotoxicity assays. *J Immunol methods*, **65**: 55-63.

Mukherjee, A. K., Basu, S., Sarkar, N., and Ghosh, A. C. (2001). Advances in Cancer Therapy with Plant Based Natural Products. *Curr Med Chem.*, **8**: 1467-1486.

Nakanishi, K. (1999). An historical perspective of natural products chemistry. In: Sankawa U. (ed.). Comprehensive natural products chemistry. Vol. I. Polyketides and other secondary metabolites including fatty acids and their derivatives. Pp. 23-30, Amsterdam, Elsevier.

Nam, N. H., Lee, C. W., Hong, D. H., Kim, H. M., Bae, K. H., and Ahn, B. Z. (2003). Antiinvasive, antiangiogenic and antitumor activity of *Ephedra sinica* extract. *Phytother Res.*, **17**: 70-76.

Newman, D. J., and Cragg, G. M. (2007). Natural products as sources of new drugs over the last 25 years. *J Nat Prod.*, **70**: 461-477.

Osawa, T., Kawakishi, S., and Namiki, M. (1990). In: Kuroda Y, Shankel, DM, Waters MD, Antimutagenesis and anticarcinogenesis mechanism II. NewYork: plenum;.p. 139-153.

Padmavathi, B., Rath, P. C., Rao, A. R., and Singh, R. P. (2005). Roots of *Withania somnifera* inhibit forestomach and skin carcinogenesis in mice. *Adv Access Publi.*, **2**: 99-105.

Pal, S. K., Pandey, G. S., Kesari, A., Choudhuri, G., and Meltal, B. (2003). Fighting cancer in the information age: The role of Internet. *Ind. J. Exp. Biol.*, **41**: 189-200.

Pandey, G., and Sharma, M. (2006). Medicinal plants: better remedy for neoplasm. *Indian Drugs*, **43**: 869-874.

Parinitha, M., Srinivasa, B. H., and Shivanna, M. B. (2005). Medicinal plant wealth of local communities in some villages in Shimoga distinct of Karnataka. *India J Ethnopharmaco.*, **98**: 307-312.

Parkin, D. M. (2001). Global cancer statistics in the year 2000. *Lancet Oncol.*, **2**: 533-543.

Parkin, D. M., Bray, F., Ferlay, J., and Pisani, P. (2005). Global cancer statistics, 2002. CA: *Cancer J Clin.*, **55**: 74-108.

Pezzuto, J. M. (1997). Plant-derived anticancer agents. *Biochem. Pharmacol.*, **53**: 121-133.

Pietarinen, S. P., Willfor, S. M., Ahotupa, M. O., Hemming, J. E., and Holmbon, B. R. (2006). Knotwood and bark extracts: strong antioxidants from waste materials. *J Wood Sci.*, **52**: 436-444.

Potmeisel, M., and H. Pinedo. 1995. Camptothecins. New anticancer agents. CRC Press, Boca Raton, FL.

Prasad, K. N, Ashok, G., Raghu, C., Shivamurthy, G. R., Vijayan, P., and Aradhya, S. M. (2005). *In vitro* cytotoxic properties of *Ipomoea aquatica* leaf. *Indian J Pharmacol.*, **37**: 397-398.

Prince, P. S. M., and Menon, V. P. (1999). Antioxidant activity of *Tinospora cordifolia* roots in experimental diabetes. *J. Ethnopharmacol.*, **65**: 277-281.

Purdue, R. E. (1982). Kb cell culture. A role in discovery of antitumor agents from higher plants. *J. Nat. Prod.*, **45**: 418-426.

Raghu, C., Ashok, G., Dhanaraj, S. A., Suresh, B., and Vijayan, P. (2004). *In vitro* cytotoxic activity of *Lantana camara* Linn. *Indian J Pharmacol.*, **36**: 93-95.

Rajendran, P., Ekambaram, G., and Sakthisekaran, D. (2008). Cytoprotective effect of mangiferin on benzo(a)pyrene-induced lung carcinogenesis in Swiss albino mice. *Basic Clin Pharmacol.*, **103(2)**: 137-142.

Rajkapoor, B., Jayakar, B., and Murugesh, N. (2004). Antitumor activity of *Indigofera aspalathoides* on Ehrlic ascites carcinoma in mice. *Indian J Pharmacol.*, **36**: 38-40.

Ramos, A., Visozo, A., Piloto, J., Garcia, A., Rodriguez, C. A., and Rivero, R. (2003). Screening of antimutagenicity via antioxidant activity in Cuban medicinal plants. *J Ethnopharmacol.*, **87**: 241–246.

Rao, K. V. K., Schwartz, S. A., Nair, H. K., Aalinkeel, R., Mahajan, S., Chawda, R., and Nair, M. P. N. (2004). Plant derived products as a source of cellular growth inhibitory phytochemicals on PC-3M, DU-145 and LNCap prostate cancer cell lines. *Curr. Sci.*, **87**: 1585-1588.

Rao, S. K., Rao, P. S., and Rao, B. N. (2008). Preliminary investigation of the radiosensitizing activity of guduchi *(Tinospora cordifolia)* in tumor bearing mice. *Phytother Res.*, **22**: 1482-1489.

Rastogi, S., Shukla, Y., Paul, B. N., Chowdhuri, D. K., Khanna, S. K., and Das, M. (2007). Protective effect of *Ocimum sanctum* on 3-methylcholanthrene, 7, 12 – dimethylbenz(a)anthracene and aflatoxin B1 induced skin tumorigenesis in mice. *Toxicol Appl Pharmacol.*, **224**: 228-240.

Reddy, D. B., Reddy, T. C. M., Jyotsna, G., Sharan, S., Priya, N., Lakshmipathi, V., and Reddanna, P. *et al.* (2009). Chebulagic acid, a COX-LOX dual inhibitor isolated from the fruits of *Terminalia chebula* Retz., induces apoptosis in COLO-205 cell line. *J Ethnopharmacol.*, **124**: 506-512.

Reddy, L., Odhav, B., and Bhoola, K. D. (2003). Natural products for cancer prevention: A global perspective. *Pharmacol Ther.*, **99(1)**: 1-13.

Ribi, E., Canterall, J., Schwartzmans, S., and Parker, R. (1981). BCG cell wall skeleton P_3 MDP and other microbial components.structure activity studies in animal studies In: Hersh E. M.; Chingos M. A.; Materangelo, M. A. (Eds) Augmenting agents in cancer therapy, Raven Press, New York, 15.

Rohini, G., and Shyamala, D. C. S. (2008). *Bacopa monniera* extract induces apoptosis in murine sarcoma cells. *Phytother Res.*, **22**: 1595-1598.

Roja, G., and Heble, M. R. (1994). The quinoline alkaloid Camptothecin and 9-methoxy camptothecin from tissue culture and mature trees of *Nathapodytes foetida Phytochemistry*, **36**: 65-66.

Romero-Jimenez, M., Campos-Sanchez, J., Analla, M., Munoz-Serrano, A., and Alonso-Moraga, A. (2005). Genotoxicity and anti-genotoxicity of some traditional medicinal herbs. *Mutat. Res.*, **585**: 147-55.

Rosangkima, G., and Prasad, S. B. (2004). Antitumor activity of some plants from Meghalaya and Mizoram against Murine ascites dalton's lymphoma. *Indian J Exp. Biol.*, **42**: 981-988.

Russo, A. V., Cardile, L., Vanella, A., and Garbarino, J. A. (2001). Neoplastic properties of cell. *J Ethnopharmacol.*, **100**: 323–332.

Russo, A., Piovano, M., Lombardo, L., Vanella, L., Cardile, V., and Garbarino, J. (2006). Pannarin inhibits cell growth and induces cell death in human prostate carcinoma DU-145 cells. *Anti-Cancer Drugs*, **17**: 1163-1169.

Sakarkar, D. M., and Deshmukh, V. N. (2011). Ethnopharmacological review of traditional medicinal plants for anticancer activity. *International Journal of PharmTech Research*, **3(1)**: 298-308.

Samuelsson, G. (1999). Drugs of natural origin. A textbook of Pharmacognosy. 4th ed., Stockholm, Swedish Pharmaceutical Press.

Sayed, E. A., and Cordell, G. A. (1981). Catharanthus alkaloids atharanthamine, a new antitumor bisindole alkaloid from *Catharanthus roseus*. *J Nat Prod.*, **44**: 289-293.

Schultes, R. E., and Raffauf, R. F. (1990). The Healing Forest, Dioscorides Press, Portland, Oregon.

Sharma, M., and Pandey, G. (2008). Some dietary agricultural plants with anticancer properties. *Plant Arch.*, **8**: 13-16.

Sharma, M., and Pandey, G. (2009). Some anticancer medicinal plants of foreign origin. *Current Science*, **96(6)**: 779-783.

Sharma, P. R., Mondhe, D. M., Muthiah, S., Pal, H. C., Shahi, A. K., Saxena, A. K., and Qazi, G. N. (2009). Anticancer activity of an essential oil from *Cymbopogon flexuosus. Chemico-Biol Interact.*, **179**: 160-168.

Sharma, P. R., Shanmugavel, M., Saxena, A. K., and Qazi, G. N. (2008). Induction of apoptosis by a synergistic lignin composition from *Cedrus deodara* in human cancer cells. *Phyto Res.*, **22**: 1587-1594.

Shoeb, M. (2006). Anticancer agents from medicinal plants. *Bangladesh J Pharmacol.*, **1**: 35-41.

Shukla, Y., Prasad, S., Tripathi, C., Singh, M., George, J., and Kalra, N. (2007). *In vitro* and *in vivo* modulation of testosterone mediated alterations in apoptosis related proteins by [6] – gingerol. *Mol Nutr Food Res.*, **51**: 1492-1402.

Simard, F., Legault, J., Lavoie, S., Mshvildadze, V., and Pichette, A. (2008). Isolation and identification of cytotoxic compounds from the wood of *Pinus resinosa. Phytother Res.*, **22**: 919-922.

Singh, R., and Gupta, A. K. (2008). Antimicrobial and antitumor activity of the fractionated extracts of kalimusli (*Curculigo orchioides*). *Int J Green Pharm.*, **2**: 34-36.

Sivakumar, R., and Alagesaboopathi, C. (2008). Studies on cytotoxicity and antitumor screening of red and white forms of *Abrus precatorius* L. *Afr J Biotechnol.*, **7**: 3984-3988.

Sivalokanathan, S., Ilayaraja, M., and Balasubramanium, M. P. (2005). Efficacy of *Terminalia arjuna* (Roxb.) on N-nitrosodiethylamine induced hepatocellular carcinoma in rats. *Indian J Exp. Biol.*, **43**: 264-267.

Skehan, P., Storeng, R., Scudiero, D., Monks, A., McMahon, J., Vistica, D., Warren, J. T., Bokesch, H., Kenney, S., and Boyd, M. R. (1990). New colorimetric cytotoxicity assay for anticancer-drug screening. *J. Natl. Cancer Inst.*, **82**: 1107-1112.

Somkumar, A. P. (2003). Studies on anticancer effects of *Ocimum sanctum* and *Withania somnifera* o experimentally induced cancer in mice. Ph D thesis, J. N. K. V. V., Jabalpur.

Son, J. K., Jung, S. J., Jung, J. H., Fang, Z., Lee, C. S., Seo, C. S., Moon, D. C., Min, B. S., and Woo, M. H. (2008). Anticancer constituents from the roots of *Rubia cordifolia* L. *Chem Pharm Bull.*, **56**: 213-216.

Spitz, T. T., Bergman, M., and Grossman S. (2007). Cucurbitacin glucosides: Antioxidant and free-radical scavenging activities. *Biochem Biophy Res Commun.*, **364**: 181-186.

Srivastava, V., Negi, A. S., Kumar, J. K., Gupta, M. M., and Khanuja, S. P. (2005). Plant-based anticancer molecules: A chemical and biological profile of some important leads. *Bioorg Med Chem.*, **13(21)**: 5892-5908.

Stanley, H. U. I. (2001). Health and Physical Activity in Hong Kong: A Review. Pp. 4, The Chinese University of Hong Kong.

Steinmetz, K. A., and Potter, J. D. (1991). Vegetables, fruits and cancer. *I. Epidemiology. Cancer Causes Control (suppl.)*, **2**: 325-357.

Stoilova, I., Krastanov, A., Stoyanova, A., Denev, P., and Gargova, S. (2007). Antioxidant activity of a ginger extract (*Zingiber officinale*). *Food Chem.*, **102**: 764-770.

Suba, R. V. V., and Sirsi, M. (1969). Effect of *Abrus precatorius* L. on experimental tumors. *Cancer Res.*, **29**: 1447-1451.

Subchareon, P. (1998a). Handbook of anticancer: Thai traditional medicine: new concept for treated cancer. Pp 3. Thai Traditional medicine Institute, Ministry of Public Health.

Suffness, M. (1989). Development of antitumor natural products at the National Cancer Institute in Takeichi, T. Nitta, K. and Tanak, N. (Eds.). *Antitumor natural products*, 21-44, London, taylor and Francis.

Suffness, M., and Pezzuto, J. M. (1991). Assays related to cancer drug discovery. In: K. Hostettmann (ed.), Methods in Plant Biochemistry. Vol. 6. Assays for Bioactivity, Academic Press. Pp. 71-133.

Sultana, S., Ahmed, S., and Jahangir, T. (2008). *Emblica officinalis* and hepatocarcinogenesis: A chemopreventive study in Wistar rats. *J. Ethnopharmacol.*, **118**: 1-6.

Sundararajan, P., Dey, A., Smith, A., Doss, A. G., Rajappan, M., and Natarajan, S. (2006). Studies of anticancer and antipyretic activity of *Bidens pilosa* whole plant. *Afr Health Sci.*, **6**: 27-30.

Suran, P., Eapen, S. G., Kutty, S. V., Haribabu, Y., and Oommen, M. K. (2013). A Review on anticancer activity of traditional medicinal plants. *World Journal of Pharmacy and Pharmaceutical sciences*, **2(3)**: 1056-1076.

Swamy, S. M. K., and Tan, B. H. K. (2000). Cytotoxic and immunopotentiating effects of ethanolic extract of *Nigella sativa* L. seeds. *J Ethnopharmacol.*, **70**: 1-7.

Szewczuk, V. D., Mongelli, E. R., and Pomilia, A. B. (2006). *In vitro* antihelminthic activity of *Melia azedarch* naturalized in Argentina. *Phytother Res.*, **20**: 993-996.

Tannin-Spitz, T., Grossman, S., Dovrat, S., Gottlieb, H. E., and Bergman, M. (2007). Growth inhibitory activity of cucurbitacin glucosides isolated from *Citrullus colocynthis* on human breast cancer cells. *Biochem Pharmacol.*, **73**: 56-67.

Tiwari, A. K., Srinivas, P. V., Kumar, S. P., and Rao, J. M. (2001). Free radical scavenging active components from *Cedrus deodara. J Agric Food Chem.*, **49**: 4642-4645.

Tomosaka, H., Chin, Y. W., Salim, A. A., Keller, W. J., Chai, H., and Kinghorn, A. D. (2008). Antioxidant and cytoprotective compounds from *Berberis vulgaris. Phytother Res.*, **22**: 979-981.

Tyler, V. (1994). Herbs of choice. The therapeutic use of phytomedicinals. New York: Haworth Press, 24-26.

Ucar, E. O., Karagoz, A., and Arda, N. (2006). Antioxidant activity of *Viscum album* ssp. Album. *Fitoterapia,* **77**: 556-560.

Unnikrishnan, M. C., and Ramadasan, K. (1998). Cytotoxicity of extracts of spices to cultured cells. *Nutr Cancer,* **11**: 251-257.

Vecchia, C. L., and Tavani, A. (1998). Fruits, vegetables and human cancer. *Eur. J. Cancer,* **7**: 3-8.

Venukumar, M. R., and Latha, M. S. (2002). Antioxidant activity of *Curculigo orchioides* in carbon tetrachloride induced hepatopathy in arts. *Indian J Clin Biochem.,* **17**: 80-87.

Verma, A. R., Vijayakumar, M., Mathela, C. S., and Rao, C. V. (2009). *In vitro* and *in vivo* antioxidant properties of different fractions of *Moringa oleifera* leaves. *Food Chem Toxicol.,* **47**: 2196-2201.

Verma, M., Singh, S. K., Bhushan, S., Sharma, V. K., Datt, P., Kapahi, B. K., and Saxena, A. K. (2008). *In vitro* cytotoxic potential of *Polyalthia longifolia* on human cancer cell lins and induction of apoptosis through mitochondrial dependent pathway in HL-60 cells. *Chemico-Biol Interact.,* **171**: 45-56.

Visavadiya, N. P., and Narasimhacharya, A. V. R. L. (2007). Hypocholesteremic and antioxidant effects of *Withania somnifera* (Dunal) in hypocholesteremic rats. *Phytomedicine,* **14**: 136-142.

Wu, S. B., Ji, Y. P., Zhu, J. J., Zhao, Y., Xia, G., Hu, Y. H., and Hu, J. F. (2009). Steroids from the leaves of Chinese *Melia azedarch* and their cytotoxic effects of human cancer cell lines. *Steroids,* **74**: 761-765.

Yan, R., Gao, S., Yang, W., Cao, M., Wang, S., and Chen, F. (2008). Nickel toxicity induced antioxidant enzyme and phenylalanine ammonia-lyase activities in *Jatropha curcas* L. cotyledons. *Plant Soil Environ.,* **54**: 294-300.

Yoshida, T., Chou, T., Nitta, A., Miyamoto, K., Koshiura, R., and Okuda, T (1990). Woodfordin C, a micro-ring hydrolysable tannin dimer with antitumor activity and accompanying dimmers from *Woodfordia fruticosa* flowers. *Chem Pharm Bull.,* **38**: 1211-1217.

Yuan, L. L., Guo, P. G., Hui, Z. Z., He, Z. W., Chang, L. L., Yong, P. H., Yan, W. L., and Jian, W. L. (2007). A flavonoid glycoside isolated from *Smilax china* L. rhizome *in vitro* anticancer effects on human cancer cell lines. *J Ethnopharmacol.,* **113**: 115-124.

Previous Volume Contents

Bioactive Phytochemicals: Perspectives for Modern Medicine Vol 1/*Gupta, V K et al. eds*

2012, xi+516p., col. plts., figs., tabls., ind., 25 cm

ISBN 978-81-7035-779-7 Rs. 2800/US$ 122

Bioactive Phytochemicals: Perspectives for Modern Medicine Vol 2/*Gupta, V K et al eds*

2014, xiii+575p., col. plts., figs., tabls., ind., 25 cm

ISBN 978-81-7035-911-1 Rs. 3500/US$ 130

Index

A

N

O

Q

R

S

X

Y

Z